# Diseases of the Bladder and Prostate Gland

# Diseases of the Bladder and Prostate Gland

Editor: Smith Chaney

AMERICAN
MEDICAL PUBLISHERS
www.americanmedicalpublishers.com

AMERICAN
MEDICAL PUBLISHERS
www.americanmedicalpublishers.com

**Cataloging-in-Publication Data**

Diseases of the bladder and prostate gland / edited by Smith Chaney.
p. cm.
Includes bibliographical references and index.
ISBN 979-8-88740-065-5
1. Bladder--Diseases. 2. Prostate--Diseases. 3. Bladder--Diseases--Diagnosis.
4. Prostate--Diseases--Diagnosis. 5. Bladder--Diseases--Treatment.
6. Prostate--Diseases--Treatment. I. Chaney, Smith.
RC919 .D57 2023
616.62--dc23



American Medical Publishers,
41 Flatbush Avenue,
1st Floor, New York,
NY 11217, USA

ISBN 979-8-88740-065-5 (Hardback)

# Contents

# Preface

Bladder diseases are a group of diseases that affect the function of the bladder in the body. Different types of bladder diseases include bladder cancer, interstitial cystitis, overactive bladder, and urinary incontinence. These diseases can be diagnosed by performing tests, such as urine tests, bladder examination and X-rays. The prostate gland is a male reproductive organ that produces semen, which is the thick fluid that nourishes and protects sperms. The diseases that affect the prostate gland are referred to as prostate diseases. Some common prostate gland diseases are prostatitis, benign prostatic hyperplasia (BPH) and prostate cancer. The most common symptoms of these diseases include difficulty while urinating, painful urination, urine retention, and frequent urination. The clinical management of prostate diseases includes medications, therapies and surgeries. This book is compiled in such a manner, that it will provide in-depth knowledge about the clinical assessment and management of bladder and prostate gland diseases. It presents researches and studies performed by experts across the globe. Researchers and students in the field of urology will be assisted by this book.

The researches compiled throughout the book are authentic and of high quality, combining several disciplines and from very diverse regions from around the world. Drawing on the contributions of many researchers from diverse countries, the book's objective is to provide the readers with the latest achievements in the area of research. This book will surely be a source of knowledge to all interested and researching the field.

In the end, I would like to express my deep sense of gratitude to all the authors for meeting the set deadlines in completing and submitting their research chapters. I would also like to thank the publisher for the support offered to us throughout the course of the book. Finally, I extend my sincere thanks to my family for being a constant source of inspiration and encouragement.

**Editor**

# 1

# Preoperative pelvic floor muscle exercise for early continence after holmium laser enucleation of the prostate

Go Anan*, Yasuhiro Kaiho, Hiromichi Iwamura, Jun Ito, Yuki Kohada, Jotaro Mikami and Makoto Sato

**Abstract**

**Background:** Transient postoperative urinary incontinence is a bothersome complication of holmium laser enucleation of the prostate (HoLEP). The effects of preoperative pelvic floor muscle exercise (PFME) for early recovery of continence after HoLEP have never been elucidated. The aim of this study was to determine the benefit of preoperatively started PFME for early recovery of continence after HoLEP.

**Methods:** We randomly assigned patients to start PFME preoperatively and continue postoperatively (group A) or start PFME no earlier than the postoperative period (group B). The primary outcome was time to complete urinary control, defined as no pad usage. The secondary outcome was measured using the International Consultation on Incontinence Questionnaire-Short Form (ICIQ-SF) score. Univariate and multivariate analyses were performed to identify parameters associated with recovery of continence after HoLEP.

**Results:** Seventy patients were randomized across groups A ($n = 35$) and B ($n = 35$). Patients' characteristics were not different between groups A and B. The postoperative urinary incontinence rate significantly decreased in group A compared with that in group B at 3 months postoperatively [3% vs. 26% ($P = 0.01$)]. However, there were no significant differences between groups A and B at 3 days [40% vs. 54% ($P = 0.34$)], 1 month [37% vs. 51% ($P = 0.34$)], and 6 months [0% vs. 3% ($P = 1.00$)] postoperatively, respectively. The postoperative ICIQ-SF score was not significantly different between groups A and B at any time point postoperatively. In univariate analysis, patients who performed preoperative PFME had a 0.56-fold lower risk of urinary incontinence 1 month after HoLEP and a 0.08-fold lower risk of urinary incontinence 3 months after HoLEP.

**Conclusions:** Preoperatively started PFME appears to facilitate improvement of early urinary continence after HoLEP.
**Keywords:** Benign prostatic hyperplasia, Incontinence, HoLEP, Pelvic floor muscle exercise

* Correspondence: goanan@tohoku-mpu.ac.jp
Department of Urology, Tohoku Medical and Pharmaceutical University, Sendai, Japan, 1-15-1 Fukumuro, Miyagino-ku, Sendai, Miyagi 983-8536, Japan

## Background

Benign Prostatic Hyperplasia (BPH) is a common condition in elderly males and affects over half of all men aged > 60 years [1]. Holmium laser enucleation of the prostate (HoLEP) is widely used as a minimally invasive surgical procedure because it can be performed in patients with large-sized prostatic hyperplasia and is associated with lower volumetric blood loss and shorter periods of indwelling catheterization and hospitalization than transurethral resection of the prostate (TURP) [2]. However, postoperative transient urinary incontinence has been reported as a bothersome complication of HoLEP in 16–44% patients within 3 months [3–5]. Postoperative urinary incontinence remains a representative complication of HoLEP and can have a negative influence on the patient's quality of life (QOL) [5].

Pelvic floor muscle exercise (PFME) is one of the physiotherapies used for recovery of continence after prostate surgery. Although the efficacy of PFME for urinary incontinence after prostate surgery remains controversial [6–11], some recent studies demonstrated that PFME started preoperatively and continued postoperatively was associated with better outcomes than PFME started only postoperatively [6–8]. We herein present the first randomized clinical trial to compare the effects of preoperatively started PFME with postoperatively started PFME for early recovery of continence after HoLEP.

## Methods

### Study design

This randomized, prospective study enrolled patients with BPH who underwent HoLEP at a single institution (Tohoku Medical and Pharmaceutical University Hospital) between September 2017 and March 2019. Patients were randomly assigned in a ratio of 1:1 to one of the two groups using a simple randomization procedure (computerized random numbers generated using Microsoft Excel for Windows). Group A included patients who started PFME preoperatively 28 days before HoLEP and continued postoperatively. Group B included patients who started PFME postoperatively only.

The inclusion criteria were males between 50 and 90 years of age with symptoms of dysuria for ≥3 months before study entry. Patients with prostate volumes of ≥30 ml were eligible. Patients who could continue PFME on their own were eligible. We excluded patients who could not continue PFME on their own and those who had severe incontinence before HoLEP due to severe cerebrovascular disorder or spinal cord injuries.

The primary outcome measure was self-reported continence postoperatively. The condition of no incontinence was evaluated by defining complete urinary control as no pad usage. The secondary outcome measure gauged QOL as determined by International Consultation on Incontinence Questionnaire-Short Form (ICIQ-SF) score [12].

Urinary incontinence was evaluated on the day before surgery; 3 days after HoLEP, which was one day after catheter removal; and 1, 3, and 6 months after HoLEP. ICIQ-SF score was evaluated on the day before surgery and at 1, 3, and 6 months after HoLEP. Patients in group A received sufficient instructions for PFME by urological nurses to start the same 28 days before HoLEP and continue thereafter. Then, on the second day after HoLEP, which was the day of catheter removal, all patients in both groups A and B were instructed regarding PFME by the nurses sufficiently. For all patients, the instructions for PFME included illustrations; all patients were instructed to perform a set of 3 min at least three times a day and record it in a PFME performance table. The table was described by all patients, and the PFME implementation status was confirmed for each outpatient.

The ethical committee of Tohoku Medical and Pharmaceutical University Hospital School of Medicine, Sendai, Japan approved the study protocol. Written informed consent was obtained from all patients prior to participation in this study. This study was registered with the Tohoku Medical and Pharmaceutical University Hospital Medical Research Registry in Japan (Protocol 2017–2-056) on August 22, 2017 and was registered with the University Hospital Medical Information Network Clinical Trials Registry in Japan (UMIN000034713) on October 31, 2018.

### Surgical technique

The enucleation procedure was performed following the anteroposterior dissection HoLEP method (antegrade separation method), as reported by Endo et al. [13]. The three lobes technique was used in all cases. In this study, all surgeons used the same surgical techniques. We removed the urinary catheter on the second day after HoLEP and confirmed self-urination and degree of urinary incontinence.

### Predictive factors for postoperative urinary incontinence

Uni- and multivariate analyses were performed to investigate the predictive factors for postoperative urinary incontinence at 3 days and 1, 3, and 6 months after HoLEP, including potential factors. These factors included age, body mass index (BMI), preoperative international prostate symptom score (IPSS) and overactive bladder symptom score (OABSS), ICIQ-SF score, prostate volume, operation time, enucleate prostate weight, presence or absence of diabetes mellitus, and G8 score [14]. Urodynamic examination, including free uroflowmetry, filling cystometry, and pressure flow studies, was performed before HoLEP. We investigated the maximum detrusor pressure, detrusor overactivity, volume at the first desire to void, maximum cystometric capacity, and residual volume.

### Statistical analysis

Prior to this study, there were about 40% postoperative urinary incontinence 1–3 months after HoLEP at our institute. Therefore, between the study groups, we set a significant difference in the urinary incontinence rate of 16–20% as the threshold for clinical importance. This threshold was derived following discussions between clinicians and the project management group as well as inspection of the urinary incontinence rate reported in previous studies that reviewed the number of men who showed urinary incontinence at 1–3 months after HoLEP [3–5]. Using the two-sided test to differentiate between proportions, this study had an ability of 80% to detect a difference of 20% in the proportion of patients remaining incontinent at 1 and 3 months after HoLEP, assuming a total sample size of 70 patients and a type 1 error rate of 0.05.

Patient characteristics are described in terms of mean and standard deviation (SD) or range for continuous variables. We used the JMP version 9.0 (SAS Institute Inc., Cary, NC. USA) for statistical analyses. Intergroup differences were analyzed using Mann–Whitney U test for continuous variables and Fisher exact tests for categorical variables. Multivariate analysis was analyzed using logistic regression analysis. $P$ value of $< 0.05$ was considered statistically significant.

## Results

A total of 70 patients were randomized into groups A (PFME started preoperatively and continued thereafter, $n = 35$) and B (PFME postoperatively only, $n = 35$) for final analysis (Fig. 1). Among the patient and perioperative background characteristics, there were no differences in age, BMI, IPSS, OABSS, ICIQ-SF score, prostate volume, operation time, enucleate prostate weight, diabetes mellitus status, and G8 score between the two groups (Table 1). The postoperative urinary incontinence rate was significantly lower in group A than in group B at 3 months postoperatively (3% vs. 26%; $P = 0.01$); however, there were no significant differences in the urinary incontinence rate between groups A and B at 3 days (40% vs. 54%; $P = 0.34$), 1 month (37% vs. 51%; $P = 0.34$), and 6 months (0% vs. 3%; $P = 1.00$) postoperatively (Fig. 2). Furthermore, the postoperative ICIQ-SF score was not significantly different between groups A and B at 1 month (5.4 ± 4.9 vs. 5.6 ± 4.9; $P = 0.89$), 3 months (2.9 ± 3.4 vs. 3.8 ± 4.6; $P = 0.80$), and 6 months (1.5 ± 2.0 vs. 1.5 ± 2.4; $P = 0.83$) postoperatively.

We investigated the predictive factors for urinary incontinence at 3 days and 1, 3, and 6 months after HoLEP. As shown in Table 2, by univariate and

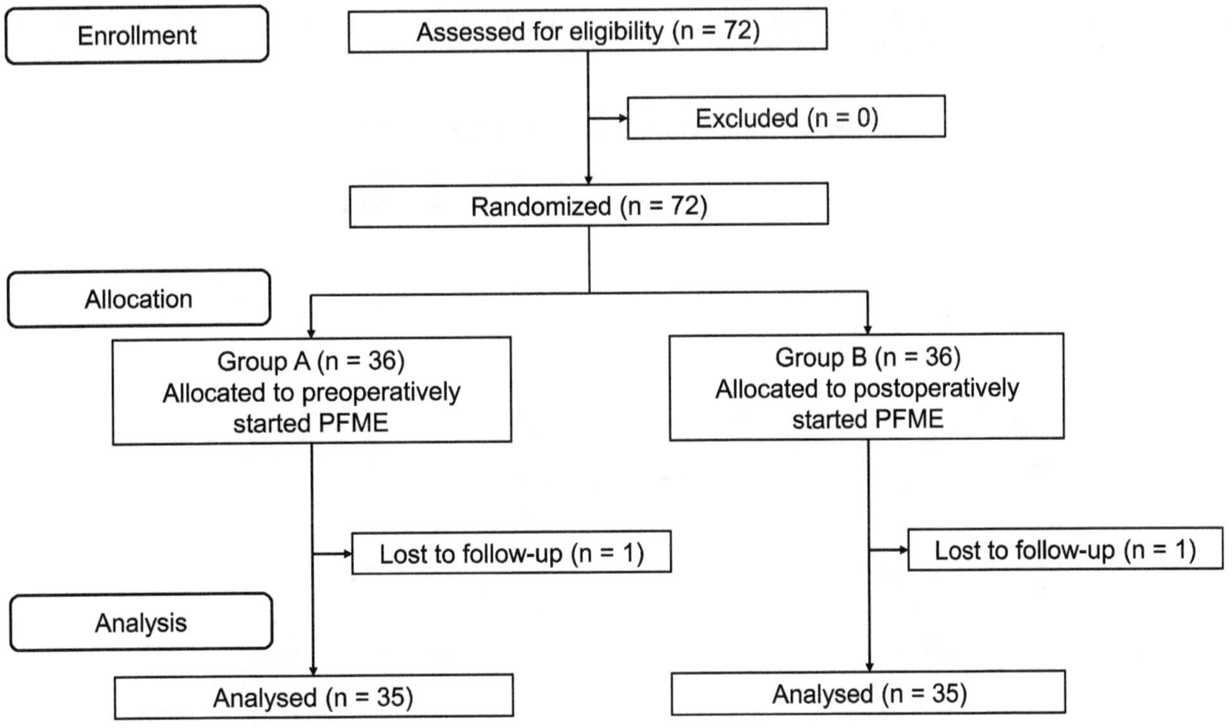


**Fig. 1** The study flow diagram. PFME: pelvic floor muscle exercise

**Table 1** Patients background (median, range)

| | Group A | Group B | *P*-value |
|---|---|---|---|
| Number of cases | 35 | 35 | |
| Age (years) | 72 (62–83) | 73 (57–86) | 0.55 |
| BMI (kg/m$^2$) | 24 (17–31) | 24 (19–32) | 0.37 |
| G8 | 15 (12–16) | 14 (12–17) | 0.60 |
| IPSS | 17 (5–34) | 19 (5–35) | 0.32 |
| OABSS | 6 (2–13) | 6 (2–15) | 0.94 |
| ICIQ-SF score | 0 (0–13) | 0 (0–13) | 0.83 |
| Diabetes mellitus (n, %) | 12 (34%) | 10 (29%) | 0.80 |
| Prostate volume (mL) | 56 (35–208) | 60 (35–114) | 0.89 |
| Operation time (min) | 89 (50–202) | 88 (34–160) | 0.88 |
| Enucleate prostate weight (g) | 31 (7–168) | 34 (5–94) | 0.81 |

*BMI* Body mass index, *ICIQ-SF* International consultation on incontinence questionnaire-short form, *IPSS* International prostate symptom score, *OABSS* Overactive bladder symptom score

multivariate analyses, preoperative PFME was a significant predictive factor for urinary incontinence at 3 months after HoLEP [odds ratio (OR), 0.08; $P = 0.01$ (univariate), OR, 0.10; $P = 0.01$(multivariate)]. At 3 days and 1 month after HoLEP, there were no significant predictive factors for urinary incontinence. At 6 months postoperatively, predictive factors could not be evaluated and were thus not included in Table 2 because there remained only one case with urinary incontinence in 70 cases. In univariate analysis, patients who performed preoperative PFME had a 0.56-fold lower risk of being incontinent 1 month after HoLEP and a 0.08-fold lower risk of being incontinent 3 months after HoLEP (Table 2).

Regarding the urodynamic examination results, there were no differences between groups A and B in terms of the maximum detrusor pressure (76 ± 33 $cmH_2O$ vs. 73 ± 29 $cmH_2O$; $P = 0.85$), detrusor overactivity (18% vs. 12%; $P = 0.73$), volume at the first desire to void (274 ± 118 ml vs. 288 ± 145 ml; $P = 0.79$), maximum cystometric capacity (422 ± 171 ml vs. 366 ± 180 ml; $P = 0.12$), and residual volume (127 ± 145 ml vs. 135 ± 178 ml; $P = 0.91$). We also investigated the predictive factors for postoperative urinary incontinence among the factors obtained on urodynamic examination, and no significant predictive factors were found at 3 days, 1 month, 3 months, and 6 months after HoLEP.

## Discussion

Urinary incontinence is one of the common complications after prostate surgeries such as radical prostatectomy (RP) for prostate cancer and TURP as well as HoLEP for BPH. Urinary incontinence after surgery is a challenging complication that may discourage patients from seeking surgery and reduces patient QOL [5]. PFME, which was shown to be effective primarily in females with stress urinary incontinence [15], is one of the physiotherapy approaches used for recovery of continence after prostate surgery. However, to the best of our knowledge, no study has examined the effects of PFME on urinary continence after HoLEP. Although the period is relatively short in most patients, postoperative urinary incontinence seriously decreases the

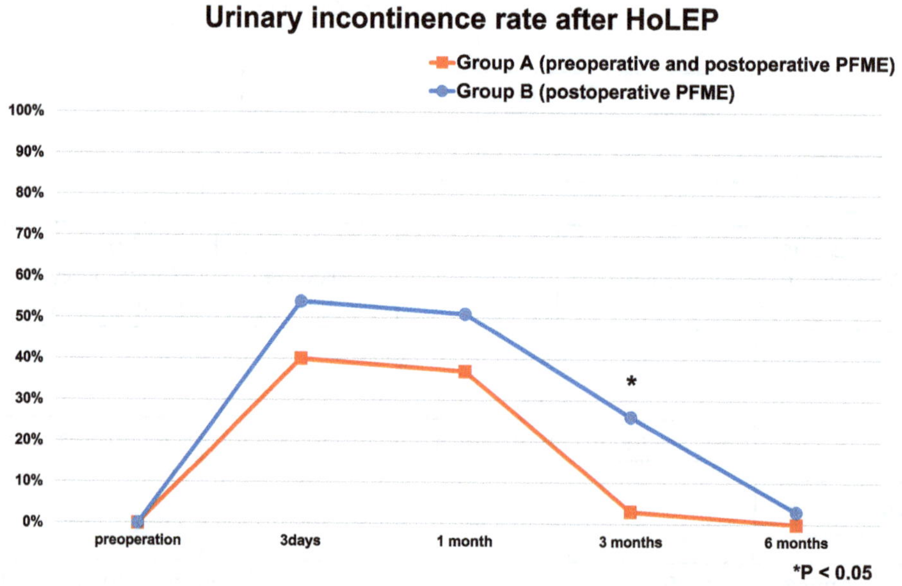


**Fig. 2** Comparison of postoperative urinary incontinence rate after HoLEP between group A (preoperative and postoperative PFME) and group B (postoperative PFME alone). PFME: pelvic floor muscle exercise

**Table 2** Predictive factors for urinary incontinence at 3 days, 1 month, and 3 months after HoLEP

| Variable | | Univariate | | | Multivariate | | |
|---|---|---|---|---|---|---|---|
| | | Odds ratio | 95%CI | *P*-value | Odds ratio | 95%CI | *P*-value |
| Age (years) (≧75 vs <75) | 3 days | 0.82 | 0.31-2.20 | 0.80 | 0.83 | 0.30-2.28 | 0.72 |
| | 1 month | 1.26 | 0.47-3.37 | 0.80 | 1.34 | 0.48-3.76 | 0.57 |
| | 3months | 2.00 | 0.52-7.72 | 0.48 | 1.42 | 0.29-6.56 | 0.65 |
| BMI (kg/m$^2$) (≧24 vs <24) | 3 days | 1.24 | 0.48-3.17 | 0.81 | | | |
| | 1 month | 0.76 | 0.29-1.97 | 0.63 | | | |
| | 3months | 1.96 | 0.50-7.68 | 0.50 | | | |
| Diabetes mellitus (yes vs no) | 3 days | 0.53 | 0.19-1.48 | 0.30 | | | |
| | 1 month | 1.07 | 0.39-2.96 | 1.00 | | | |
| | 3months | 1.56 | 0.39-6.19 | 0.71 | | | |
| Prostate volume (mL) (≧60 vs <60) | 3 days | 0.83 | 0.32-2.15 | 0.81 | 0.80 | 0.30-2.10 | 0.65 |
| | 1 month | 1.67 | 0.64-4.35 | 0.34 | 1.66 | 0.63-4.46 | 0.30 |
| | 3months | 2.44 | 0.56-10.7 | 0.29 | 2.43 | 0.54-13.2 | 0.25 |
| Operation time (min) (≧90 vs <90) | 3 days | 0.78 | 0.30-2.00 | 0.64 | | | |
| | 1 month | 1.21 | 0.47-3.13 | 0.81 | | | |
| | 3months | 3.27 | 0.77-13.9 | 0.17 | | | |
| Enucleate prostate weight (g) (≧50 vs <50) | 3 days | 1.01 | 0.35-2.91 | 1.00 | | | |
| | 1 month | 2.13 | 0.73-6.21 | 0.19 | | | |
| | 3months | 3.29 | 0.83-13.0 | 0.12 | | | |
| Pelvic floor muscle exercise (preoperative vs postoperative) | 3 days | 0.56 | 0.22-1.45 | 0.34 | 0.51 | 0.19-1.33 | 0.17 |
| | 1 month | 0.56 | 0.22-1.45 | 0.34 | 0.54 | 0.20-1.42 | 0.21 |
| | 3months | 0.08 | 0.01-0.71 | 0.01 | 0.10 | 0.005-0.60 | 0.01 |

*BMI* Body mass index, *HoLEP* Holmium laser enucleation of the prostate

postoperative QOL not only after HoLEP but also other prostate surgeries.

The current study demonstrated that preoperatively started PFME promoted early recovery of continence after HoLEP. We started PFME preoperatively to promote early recovery of continence after HoLEP based on several recent studies demonstrating that preoperatively started PFME was associated with improved outcomes compared with postoperatively started PFME in patients undergoing RP [6–8]. A recent meta-analysis showed that preoperatively started PFME significantly reduced the risk of postoperative urinary incontinence by 36% at 3 months after RP [8]. Conversely, the same meta-analysis also showed that there were no differences in long-term outcomes beyond the first 6 months postoperatively, suggesting that preoperatively started PFME might aid in early recovery of short-term continence and not long-term continence [8]. These results regarding preoperatively started PFME in RP are consistent with our findings which show that preoperatively started PFME promoted early recovery of continence at 3 months after HoLEP but did not have an effect on long-term continence.

The mechanism underlying the effect of preoperatively started PFME on urinary incontinence after HoLEP is unclear. One potential explanation is that PFME requires a certain time period to exhibit the beneficial effect. One study previously reported that a minimum of 1 month was required for the increase in the contraction strength of the pelvic floor muscle after PFME [9]. We considered that PFME affected postoperative urinary incontinence after at least 1 month from the start of PFME. Therefore, in the group that underwent preoperative PFME from 1 month before HoLEP, a significant effect on postoperative urinary incontinence was observed 1–3 months after HoLEP. In this study, only at 3 months after HoLEP, there was a significant difference in the urinary incontinence rate between the two groups. The same rationale might also underlie the disappearance of the beneficial effect of PFME by 6 months postoperatively. However, the study sample size was small; therefore, further randomized studies involving larger groups of patients are necessary. Another possibility underlying the benefit of preoperatively started PFME for postoperative urinary incontinence is the additional instruction timing provided to the patients by the nurses, which might have allowed for improved acquisition of appropriate PFME techniques. Therefore, it is critical for the patients to learn to perform PFME appropriately [16], as noted by several reports emphasizing the importance of repeated education [16, 17].

Several studies examined the effect of PFME on postoperative urinary incontinence in TURP, a standard surgery for BPH, as well as HoLEP. The efficacy of PFME for urinary incontinence after TURP continues to be a topic of debate [9–11]. Chang et al. reported that patients performed postoperative PFME showed improvement in urinary continence at 3 and 4 weeks after TURP compared with patients who did not receive the intervention [9]. Conversely, Glazener et al. reported that PFME started 6 weeks after TURP did not lead to an improvement in urinary continence at 3, 6, 9, or 12 months after TURP [10]. One study investigating preoperatively started PFME found that preoperatively started PFME was not associated with an improvement in urinary continence after TURP compared with the control group [11], which is not consistent with the finding of the current study. Although the initiation time and duration of preoperative PFME were not described in that report, one potential reason for the discrepant finding is short or insufficient exercise duration for the emergence of the beneficial effect of preoperatively started PFME. Another possibility is that patients might have recovered from postoperative urinary incontinence after TURP relatively early; the number of patients with postoperative urinary incontinence in that case would be too low to detect any significant differences regardless of preoperative PFME.

There are several limitations to this study. First, the number of cases was small. Second, we did not investigate the severity, type, or continuation of incontinence using objective tests, such as the pad test. However, we believe that preoperative PFME contributed to the improvement of early urinary continence after HoLEP because the current study was conducted as a prospective randomized trial including two groups with no differences in patient background characteristics. Additionally, the multivariate analysis showed that preoperative PFME was the only significant predictive factor for early recovery of continence at 3 months after HoLEP (Table 2). Nonetheless, larger randomized prospective studies that investigate the efficacy of preoperatively started PFME will be beneficial to further elucidate definitive treatment strategies of PFME for recovery of continence after HoLEP.

## Conclusions

Preoperatively started PFME may promote early recovery of continence at 3 months after HoLEP. Preoperative PFME is a costless and minimally invasive treatment that can be adapted to individuals attempting to recover urinary continence. However, the study sample size was small; therefore, further randomized studies involving larger groups of patients are necessary.

### Abbreviations

BMI: Body mass index; BPH: Benign prostatic hyperplasia; HoLEP: Holmium laser enucleation of the prostate; ICIQ-SF: International Consultation on Incontinence Questionnaire-Short Form; IPSS: International prostate symptom score; OABSS: Overactive bladder symptom score; PFME: Pelvic floor muscle exercise; QOL: Quality of life; RP: Radical prostatectomy; TURP: Transurethral resection of the prostate

### Acknowledgements

We would like to acknowledge the support and assistance provided by all the staff of the Department of Urology, Tohoku Medical and Pharmaceutical University School of Medicine.

### Declarations

The paper adhered to the CONSORT guidelines.

### Authors' contributions

GA and YK1 made study conception and design. GA, YK1, HI, JI, YK2, JM and MS participated in the patient's medical treatment. GA, HI, JI, YK2, and JM collected data and GA performed statistical analysis. GA drafted the first version of the manuscript and YK1 and MS helped to draft the revised manuscript. All authors have read and approved of this submission.

### References

1. Roehrborn CG. Benign prostatic hyperplasia: an overview. Rev Urol. 2005; 7(Suppl 9):3–14.
2. Cornu JN, Ahyai S, Bachmann A, de la Rosette J, Gilling P, Gratzke C, et al. A systematic review and meta-analysis of functional outcomes and complications following transurethral procedures for lower urinary tract symptoms resulting from benign prostatic obstruction: an update. Eur Urol. 2015;67(6):1066–96.
3. Montorsi F, Naspro R, Salonia A, Suardi N, Briganti A, Zanoni M, et al. Holmium laser enucleation versus transurethral resection of the prostate: results from a 2-center, prospective, randomized trial in patients with obstructive benign prostatic hyperplasia. J Urol. 2008;179(Suppl 5):87–90.
4. Nam JK, Kim HW, Lee DH, Han JY, Lee JZ, Park SW. Risk factors for transient urinary incontinence after holmium laser enucleation of the prostate. World J Mens Health. 2015;33(2):88–94.
5. Cho MC, Park JH, Jeong MS, Yi JS, Ku JH, Oh SJ, et al. Predictor of de novo urinary incontinence following holmium laser enucleation of the prostate. Neurourol Urodyn. 2011;30(7):1343–9.
6. Centemero A, Rigatti L, Giraudo D, Lazzeri M, Lughezzani G, Zugna D, et al. Preoperative pelvic floor muscle exercise for early continence after radical prostatectomy: a randomised controlled study. Eur Urol. 2010;57(6):1039–43.
7. Patel MI, Yao J, Hirschhorn AD, Mungovan SF. Preoperative pelvic floor physiotherapy improves continence after radical retropubic prostatectomy. Int J Urol. 2013;20(10):986–92.
8. Chang JI, Lam V, Patel MI. Preoperative pelvic floor muscle exercise and Postprostatectomy incontinence: a systematic review and meta-analysis. Eur Urol. 2016;69(3):460–7.
9. Chang PL, Tsai LH, Huang ST, Wang TM, Hsieh ML, Tsui KH. The early effect of pelvic floor muscle exercise after transurethral prostatectomy. J Urol. 1998;160(2):402–5.
10. Glazener C, Boachie C, Buckley B, Cochran C, Dorey G, Grant A, et al. Urinary incontinence in men after formal one-to-one pelvic-floor muscle training following radical prostatectomy or transurethral resection of the prostate (MAPS): two parallel randomised controlled trials. Lancet. 2011;378(9788): 328–37.
11. Tibaek S, Klarskov P, Lund Hansen B, Thomsen H, Andresen H, Schmidt Jensen C, et al. Pelvic floor muscle training before transurethral resection of the prostate: a randomized, controlled, blinded study. Scand J Urol Nephrol. 2007;41(4):329–34.
12. Gotoh M, Homma Y, Funahashi Y, Matsukawa Y, Kato M. Psychometric validation of the Japanese version of the international consultation on incontinence questionnaire-short form. Int J Urol. 2009;16(3):303–6.

13. Endo F, Shiga Y, Minagawa S, Iwabuchi T, Fujisaki A, Yashi M, et al. Anteroposterior dissection HoLEP: a modification to prevent transient stress urinary incontinence. Urology. 2010;76(6):1451–5.
14. Bellera CA, Rainfray M, Mathoulin-Pélissier S, Mertens C, Delva F, Fonck M, et al. Screening older cancer patients: first evaluation of the G-8 geriatric screening tool. Ann Oncol. 2012;23(8):2166–72.
15. Dumoulin C, Cacciari LP, Hay-Smith EJC. Pelvic floor muscle training versus no treatment, or inactive control treatments, for urinary incontinence in women. Cochrane Database Syst Rev. 2018;10:CD005654.
16. Marchiori D, Bertaccini A, Manferrari F, Ferri C, Martorana G. Pelvic floor rehabilitation for continence recovery after radical prostatectomy: role of a personal training re-educational program. Anticancer Res. 2010;30(2):553–6.
17. Porru D, Campus G, Caria A, Madeddu G, Cucchi A, Rovereto B, et al. Impact of early pelvic floor rehabilitation after transurethral resection of the prostate. Neurourol Urodyn. 2001;20(1):53–9.

2

# Rectal perforation following endorectal prostate MRI: An unexpected complication

I Hsu[1*], Chia-Chen Lee[2] and Ming-Jenn Chen[3,4]

**Abstract**

**Background:** Prostate cancer is a common cancer among men in developed countries. Prostate magnetic resonance imaging (MRI) has been widely employed for early diagnosis of prostate cancer and recommending a treatment plan. The incidence of rectal perforation during endorectal prostate MRI is rare and has never been reported before. Herein, we present a case of rectal perforation after a prostate MRI examination that was subjected to emergency surgical intervention because of the acute presentation of generalized peritonitis. Patients with systemic comorbidities are reportedly at greater risks of encountering colonoscopic perforation. Endorectal prostate MRI is a safe diagnostic modality, but inadequate lubrication of the endorectal coil or over-insufflation of the balloon during the procedure may also lead to serious complications such as hollow organ perforation. Early surgery will be necessary should peritoneal symptoms persist.

**Case presentation:** In 2015, a 56-year-old man came to our ER due to acute abdominal pain after he finished his MRI exam. The exam indicated diffuse tenderness over his abdomen and at the ER, his abdominal CT (computerized tomography) was checked. The images revealed extraluminal air in the perirectal fat and the pneumoperitoneum. In response, exploratory laparotomy, simple closure of rectal perforation, and loop-S colostomy were performed and the patient was discharged 1 month after operation.

**Conclusions:** Prostate MRI is a secure procedure with few complications. Clinicians must keep in mind the possibility of perforation when using ultrasound probe. Hollow organ perforation can result in serious morbidity or death. As a result, patients need to be informed of the complications of prostate MRI. When performing the procedure, clinicians must be cautioned about the potential problems for patients with high-anesthetic risk.

**Keywords:** Rectal perforation, Endorectal prostate MRI, Prostate cancer, Complication

## Background

Endorectal prostate MRI has shown to be a safe and useful modality that provides better image resolution in assessing prostate tumor localization, volume estimation, and staging. It not only improves the early diagnosis of prostate cancer by transrectal–ultrasound guided biopsy and serum PSA blood test, but also facilitates subsequent therapeutic planning. In general, prostate MRI rarely poses risks to average patients. The risks of prostate MRI include excessive sedation, allergic reactions to contrast materials, and contrast-induced nephrogenic systemic fibrosis. While an endorectal coil is applied, a gentle and meticulous operative technique is always required to minimize the chance of iatrogenic complications. The incidence of rectal perforation has not been reported elsewhere. The etiologic factors may link to the systemic comorbidities of the individuals, whereas endorectal coil insertion and latex balloon insufflation during the procedure may also impose direct trauma to the rectum.

* Correspondence: Polarbear558@hotmail.com; Polarbear558@yahoo.com.tw
[1]Division of plastic surgery, Department of Surgery, Chi-Mei Medical Center, Tainan, Taiwan
Full list of author information is available at the end of the article

## Case presentation

A 56-year-old man who had diabetes mellitus and a recent diagnosis of prostate cancer presented with acute abdomen to the emergency room about two hours after having received endorectal prostate MRI examination. Prior to the event, he had been initially referred to our hospital because of one-month history of gross hematuria. Serum prostate-specific antigen (PSA) was 3.99 ng per milliliter. Examination of transrectal ultrasound-guided (TRUS) biopsy specimen of the prostate revealed prostate adenocarcinoma in the right anterior and posterior aspect with Gleason score of 9 (4 + 5). A whole-body bone scan reported bone metastasis to the thoracic spine (T11). Therefore, endorectal prostate MRI was arranged to evaluate the extent of cancer for the best treatment path. Patient had a light diet 1 day before and undergone cleansing enema early morning at the hospital prior to the procedure, while metal and electronic objects were removed. A 1.5 T endorectal MRI/MRSI was used (Fig. 1). The endorectal coil was covered with latex condom to prevent contamination. During endorectal prostate MRI examination, patient maintained a left lateral decubitus position. The probe was lubricated with xylocaine jelly adequately and inserted through the anus to the rectum with mild force in cephalad fashion. Slight painful sensation of the lower abdomen was experienced momentarily but soon dissipated. The intrarectal balloon was inflated with 70 to 80 ml of carbon dioxide (Fig. 2) to reach maximal image resolution. Patient tolerated the procedure well without immediate complications and was sent home afterwards. The MRI result revealed advanced prostate cancer with transcapsular invasion to periprostatic tissue, right seminal vesicle and urinary bladder, metastatic regional lymphadenopathies and multiple bony metastases.

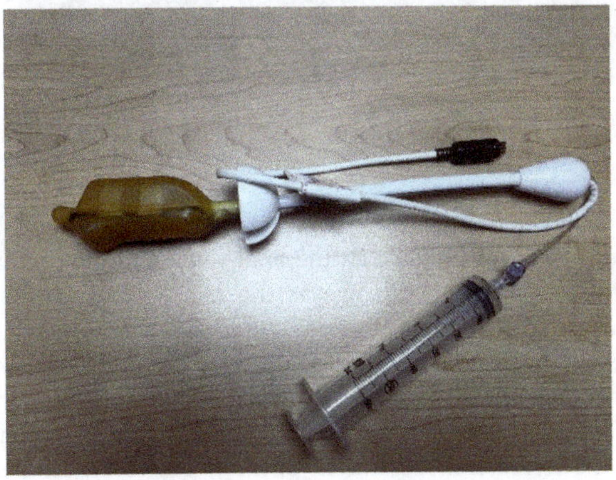

**Fig. 1** Medrad® Prostate eCoil MR Endorectal Coil. The probe improve your ability to visualize the internal architecture of the prostate and periprostatic structures, including prostate capsule and neurovascular bundles

Approximately two hours following the examination, patient was seen in the emergency room because of a sudden onset of severe lower abdominal pain. A supine abdominal computed tomography (CT) showed diffuse pneumoperitoneum and perirectal extraluminal air with fat stranding (Fig. 3), prompting an emergency exploratory laparotomy. Intra-operatively, a rectal perforation about 2 cm in diameter at the anterior wall of the upper rectum was identified, suggesting an iatrogenic relation during endorectal prostate MRI examination (Fig. 4). A primary closure of the rectal perforation with sigmoid loop colostomy was performed. Nasogastric decompression was applied until the third day post-operatively. The intraoperative ascites culture result revealed ESBL-producing *Escherichia coli* infection. A concomitant urinary tract infection with *Pseudomonas aeruginosa* was reported. A colonoscopy was performed to evaluate the perforation site 10 days later. An approximately 8-mm residual perforation still presented in the anterior wall of the rectum, which was repaired by intraluminal endoclipping for perforation closure. The follow-up computed tomoraphy scan 20 days later showed absence of intra-abdominal free air. A good healing process of the perforation was seen during the colonoscopic examination.

## Discussion and conclusion

This is the first reported case of iatrogenic rectal perforation following endorectal prostate MRI. Endorectal prostate MRI is a safe modality that provides better image resolution for prostate cancer staging. Compared with other endoscopic procedures, the incidence of iatrogenic rectal perforation resulted from colonoscopic retroflexion was as low as 0.01% [1, 2], and such complication during endorectal prostate MRI examination is even rare. Despite the uncommonness, colonic or rectal perforations usually bring about serious mortality and morbidity. The most common site of colonic perforation is the rectosigmoid colon [2, 3]. In a 15-year study of Lüning et al. [ 4], most endoscopic perforations were diagnosed shortly after the procedure due to the presentation of acute abdomen as all perforations were subjected to surgery the same day. Patient with comorbidities of diabetes mellitus, chronic pulmonary disease, cardiovascular disease, cerebrovascular disease, liver or kidney diseases are at greater risks of encountering iatrogenic bowel perforations [2]. Gaetano et al. [5]reported a case of rectal perforation during defecography, causing extraluminal barium impaction, which successfully removed by TEM (Transanal Endoscopic Microsurgery). With the risk factors in mind, recognizing early signs of perforation, and directing early, and optimal treatment may reduce the chance of complications and death from iatrogenic colon or rectal perforations.

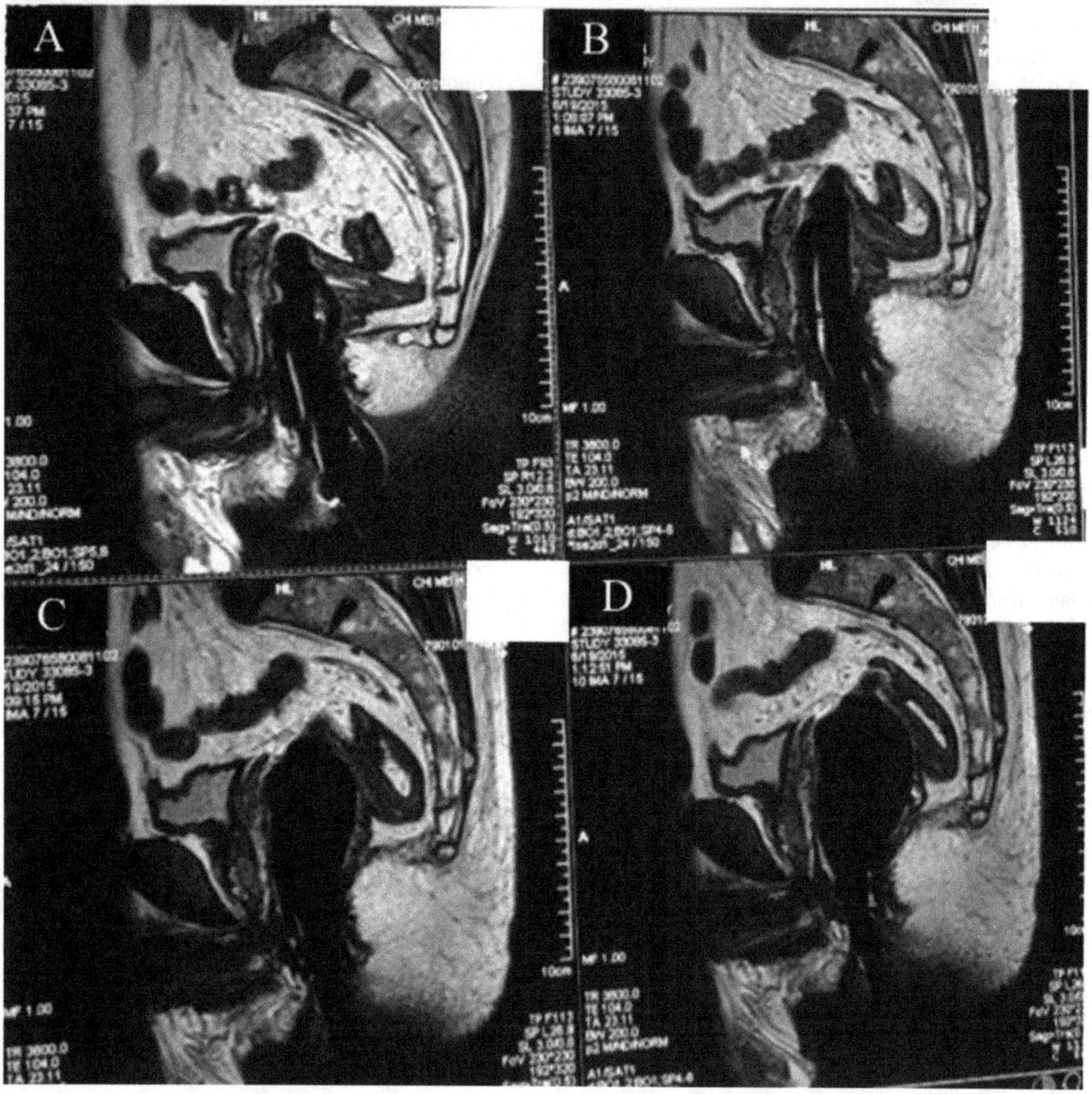

**Fig. 2** Balloon inflation with 30 ml (left) and 70–80 ml (right) of carbon dioxide, respectively

Endorectal prostate MRI is an excellent diagnostic tool for prostate cancer assessment. The mechanism of iatrogenic perforations during the procedure includes mechanical trauma from insufficient lubrication of the endorectal coil and barotrauma due to over-insufflation of the balloon. Meanwhile, we have to take into account the pre-existing morbidity of the patient. In our case, an experienced radiologist was in charge of performing endorectal insufflation technique during the examination, whilst there was no procedural abnormality encountered. However, the perforation injury might be related to the method of coil insertion and the distance of catheter insertion. Kayo Haruta et al. [6] pointed out that the distance between the anal verge and the rectum tends to increase with age as the maximum and minimum values for this distance differ for each age group. Rectal injury may occur at catheter insertion beyond 5.4 cm (sum of the anatomical length of the anal canal by 2.5 cm and the minimum measured distance by 2.9 cm) in the left lateral recumbent position. However, the best management of scope induced perforation remains controversial as the clinical condition and comorbidity of each patient should be considered. Patient of the case had metastatic prostate cancer, but the bowel was free

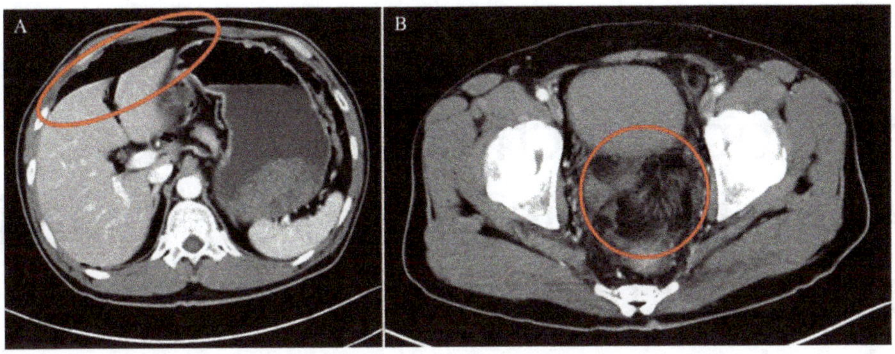


**Fig. 3** A supine abdominal CT showed diffuse pneumoperitoneum with mainly collected free-air around hepatic flexure (**a**) and perirectal extraluminal air with fat stranding (**b**)

from the involvement of prostate malignancy. Hence, tumor-related intestinal rupture was less likely. In addition, adequate bowel preparation during rectal probing of endorectal prostate MRI examination, good general health of patient, no underlying colonic pathology, absent or localized peritoneal sign, conservative management may be primarily considered before resorting to surgery [7]. If the vital signs are unstable or signs, surgical intervention will be necessary.

With an experienced operator, endorectal prostate MRI is a safe procedure with few complications. However, previous studies showed that high-anesthetic risk patients having a colonic perforation have relatively poor recovery and prognosis. Clinicians must be cautious about the possibility of iatrogenic perforation when introducing the endorectal coil and balloon inflation. Early diagnosis with appropriate management is the best strategy for patients with hollow organ perforation, which may progress to peritonitis or sepsis, resulting in serious morbidity or death. Hence, patients need to be informed of the complications of endorectal prostate MRI, and clinicians must be aware of the potential problems for patients with higher risk factors when performing the examination.

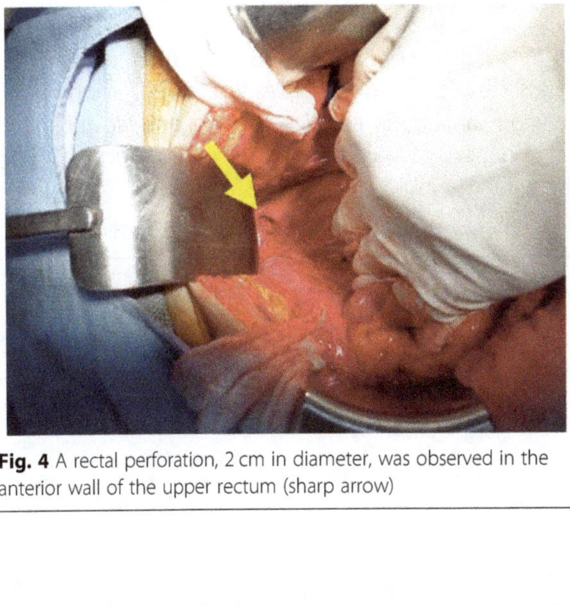

**Fig. 4** A rectal perforation, 2 cm in diameter, was observed in the anterior wall of the upper rectum (sharp arrow)

### Abbreviations

CT: Computerized tomography; MRI: Magnetic resonance imaging; PSA: Prostate-specific antigen; TEM: Transanal Endoscopic Microsurgery; TRUS: Transrectal ultrasound-guide

### Acknowledgements

The authors thank the patient for allowing us to publish this case report.

### Authors' contributions

I, CC, MJ provided clinical care; All authors contributed to the final manuscript and approved it.

### Author details

[1]Division of plastic surgery, Department of Surgery, Chi-Mei Medical Center, Tainan, Taiwan. [2]Department of surgery, Kaohsiung Medical University Hospital, Kaohsiung, Taiwan. [3]Department of Surgery, Chi-Mei Medical Center, No.901, Zhonghua Rd., Yongkang Dist., Tainan City 710, Taiwan, Republic of China. [4]Department of Sports Management, College of Leisure and Recreation Management, Chia Nan University of Pharmacy and Science, Tainan, Taiwan, Republic of China.

### References

1. Quallick MR, Brown WR. Rectal perforation during colonoscopic retroflexion: a large, prospective experience in an academic center. Gastrointest Endosc. 2009;69:960–3.
2. Lohsiriwat V. Colonoscopic perforation: incidence, risk factors, management and outcome. World J Gastroenterol. 2010;16(4):425–30.
3. Panteris V, Haringsma J, Kuipers E. Colonoscopy perforation rate, mechanisms and outcome: from diagnostic to therapeutic colonoscopy. Endoscopy. 2009;41(11):941.
4. Lüning TH, Keemers-Gels ME, Barendregt WB, Tan ACITL, Rosman C. Colonoscopic perforations: a review of 30,366 patients. Surg Endosc. 2007; 21:994–7.
5. Gallo G, Clerico G, Tutino R, De Luca E, Luc AR, Trompetto M. Rectal perforation during defecography: extraluminal barium impaction removed by TEM (Transanal endoscopic microsurgery). Ann Ital Chir. 2016;28:87.
6. Haruta KYA, Shinoda K, Ito M, Kasugai K, Suzumura H. Safe length for enema catheter insertion: estimation based on lower gastrointestinal series imaging findings in adults (in Japanese). Kango Kenkyu. 2011;34:71–5.
7. Ker TS, Wasserberg N, Beart RW Jr. Colonoscopic perforation and bleeding of the colon can be treated safely without surgery. Am Surg. 2004;70(10): 922.

# 3

# Prostate biopsy techniques and pre-biopsy prophylactic measures: Variation in current practice patterns in the Netherlands

Sofie C. M. Tops[1*], Evert L. Koldewijn[2], Diederik M. Somford[3], Anita M. P. Huis[4], Eva Kolwijck[1], Heiman F. L. Wertheim[1], Marlies E. J. L. Hulscher[4] and J. P. Michiel Sedelaar[5]

**Abstract**

**Background:** The clinical landscape of prostate biopsy (PB) is evolving with changes in procedures and techniques. Moreover, antibiotic resistance is increasing and influences the efficacy of pre-biopsy prophylactic regimens. Therefore, increasing antibiotic resistance may impact on clinical care, which probably results in differences between hospitals. The objective of our study is to determine the (variability in) current practices of PB in the Netherlands and to gain insight into Dutch urologists' perceptions of fluoroquinolone resistance and biopsy related infections.

**Methods:** An online questionnaire was prepared using SurveyMonkey® platform and distributed to all 420 members of the Dutch Association of Urology, who work in 81 Dutch hospitals. Information about PB techniques and periprocedural antimicrobial prophylaxis was collected. Urologists' perceptions regarding pre-biopsy antibiotic prophylaxis in an era of antibiotic resistance was assessed. Descriptive statistical analysis was performed.

**Results:** One hundred sixty-one responses (38.3%) were analyzed representing 65 (80.3%) of all Dutch hospitals performing PB. Transrectal ultrasound guided prostate biopsy (TRUSPB) was performed in 64 (98.5%) hospitals. 43.1% of the hospitals (also) used other image-guided biopsy techniques. Twenty-three different empirical prophylactic regimens were reported among the hospitals. Ciprofloxacin was most commonly prescribed (84.4%). The duration ranged from one pre-biopsy dose (59.4%) to 5 days extended prophylaxis. 25.2% of the urologists experienced ciprofloxacin resistance as a current problem in the prevention of biopsy related infections and 73.6% as a future problem.

**Conclusions:** There is a wide variation in practice patterns among Dutch urologists. TRUSPB is the most commonly used biopsy technique, but other image-guided biopsy techniques are increasingly used. Antimicrobial prophylaxis is not standardized and prolonged prophylaxis is common. The wide variation in practice patterns and lack of standardization underlines the need for evidence-based recommendations to guide urologists in choosing appropriate antimicrobial prophylaxis for PB in the context of increasing antibiotic resistance.

**Keywords:** Antibiotic prophylaxis, Antibiotic resistance, Healthcare research, Prostate biopsy, Transrectal biopsy

* Correspondence: sofie.tops@radboudumc.nl

[1]Department of Medical Microbiology, Radboud Center Infectious Diseases, Radboudumc, huispost 777, Geert Grooteplein Zuid 10, 6525, GA, Nijmegen, the Netherlands

Full list of author information is available at the end of the article

## Background

In the Netherlands, prostate biopsy (PB) is performed in approximately 40,000 patients every year [1]. Biopsies are performed to diagnose prostate cancer and form the basis for further staging patients with prostate cancer in either low, intermediate or high risk prostate cancer groups. Random systematic transrectal ultrasound guided prostate biopsy (TRUSPB) has been the preferred method for years. The field of PB, however, is undergoing rapid, significant change. Very recently, the European Association of Urology (EAU) guideline on prostate cancer has been updated [2]. An important modification in this guideline is the recommendation to also perform multiparametric magnetic resonance imaging (mpMRI) before PB in biopsy-naïve patients and, when mpMRI is positive (i.e. PI-RADS ≥3), to combine targeted and systematic biopsies. In addition, several more or less equivalent techniques are introduced to improve targeted biopsies [3]. These developments may have significant impact on the urological care provided in daily clinical practice, whereby it seems plausible that diagnostic differences exist between hospitals.

Moreover, (inter) national urological guidelines are unclear and lack standardization with regard to the recommended periprocedural prophylactic measures in PB [2, 4–7]. In Table 1 an overview of these guidelines is given [2, 4–7]. Guidelines strongly recommend the use of antimicrobial prophylaxis, generally with fluoroquinolones (FQ). The EAU guidelines on urological infections, however, states that the choice of regimen remains debatable [5]. An important reason for this is the increase in FQ resistant faecal flora, ranging from 10.6 to 92% between different countries, and 22% in the Netherlands, which is a potential threat for patients undergoing transrectal PB [8, 9].

In the guidelines, there is no cut-off point in the level of resistance at which FQ would be deemed ineffective and no recommendations about what equally effective other prophylactic regimens could be used [2, 4–7]. Therefore, urologists must assess the risk of carrying FQ resistant faecal flora and consider alternatives for each patient individually, which affects daily care and leads to variation in prostatic biopsy practices.

There are already signs that differences in PB care exist between health care providers. Studies from various countries (Sweden, Germany, Australia and New Zealand, Ireland and the United States) showed a lack of uniformity in PB techniques and pre-biopsy prophylaxis [10–15].

The objective of our study is to gain insight into current Dutch prostatic biopsy practices and to determine the variation in practice patterns among Dutch urologists in the context of the risk of post-biopsy infections. In addition urologists' perceptions of FQ resistance and biopsy related infections is assessed. It should be noted that at the time of our survey, the EAU guideline update was not published yet [2]. At that moment, guidelines stated to only perform mpMRI before repeat biopsy to allow targeted biopsies of suspicious lesions in addition to standard biopsies [4, 16].

**Table 1** Overview of guidelines on the prevention of infectious complications after transrectal prostate biopsy

| ***Recommendations*** | EAU guidelines on prostate cancer [2] | EAU guidelines on urological infections [5] | AUA guidelines [4] | Dutch guidelines [6, 7] |
|---|---|---|---|---|
| *First choice antimicrobial prophylaxis* | Fluoroquinolones with ciprofloxacin being superior to ofloxacin | Debatable, most commonly FQ are applied | Fluoroquinolones *or* 1st/2nd/3rd gen. Cephalosporin | Fluoroquinolones |
| *Alternative antimicrobial prophylaxis* | Not mentioned | Fosfomycin trometamol[a] | Co-trimoxazole *or* Aminoglycoside (Aztreonam) | If recent culture shows FQ resistance: antibiotics based on the resistance pattern, preferably co-trimoxazole |
| *Duration of prophylaxis* | Not mentioned | Debatable, meta-analysis by the guideline panel ongoing | ≤ 24 h | Single dose |
| *Timing of prophylaxis* | Not mentioned | Not mentioned | ≥ 1 h before prostate biopsy | Not mentioned |
| *Culture-guided prophylaxis* | Regional and local resistance patterns should be taken into account when deciding on the choice of antibiotics | Mentioned[a] | Not mentioned | There is no indication to routinely perform a urine or rectum culture |
| *Topical preparation* | Rectal disinfection with povidone-iodine may be considered. | Use rectal cleansing with povidone-iodine | No standard for topical preparation has been established | Not mentioned |

[a]No strong recommendations are made

## Methods

### Design and study population

In this observational study, a 5 min online questionnaire was prepared using SurveyMonkey® platform. Pilot testing was performed by members of the research team. Thereafter, the online questionnaire was distributed by the Dutch Association of Urology (DUA) to all its members. From the 81 Dutch hospitals, a total of 420 urologists and residents were approached to gain insight into the practices in their hospital. In April 2018, all DUA-members received an e-mail containing a unique link to complete the questionnaire. A reminder was sent after 2 weeks. Respondents were excluded from analysis if they only answered demographic questions or if the hospital of employment was unknown. Urologists from the Netherlands Antilles were also excluded from analysis.

All participants were informed about the voluntary nature of their participation and that their responses were kept confidential. They were able to access the questionnaire multiple times to allow for possible changes and completion at later times. No financial compensation was given in exchange for participation.

### Survey

The survey consisted of three parts (25 items), and mainly multiple-choice questions were used. In the first part (five items) general information was collected regarding gender, position, number of years working in the current position, hospital name and location.

The second part consisted of 12 questions about biopsy technique and pre-prostate biopsy patient preparation. More specifically, urologists were asked about the route of PB, type(s) of procedural imaging guidance, number of biopsy cores, whether prophylactic antibiotics were used, the name(s), route(s) of administration, dosage(s), timing and duration of antibiotics, prophylactic strategy (empirical or culture-guided) and whether other prophylactic measures were applied.

In the third part (eight items), respondents' perceptions of FQ resistance and infectious complications in PB was assessed. Unfortunately, the answers to two questions were not interpretable due to methodological shortcomings. The full questionnaire is available in Supplementary Appendix I.

### Statistical analysis

Descriptive statistical analysis was performed using SPSS version 25.0 (IBM Corp., Armonk, NY, USA). Both completed and partially completed questionnaires were analyzed using the number of completed responses per item as the denominator.

To describe Dutch PB practice, answers to questions on biopsy technique and pre-biopsy patient preparation (part 2) were analyzed on hospital level, i.e. answers of different professionals from the same hospitals were counted once. In case of discrepancies in the answers of urologists from the same hospital, the urology department of the concerning hospital was contacted to reach consensus.

All answers to questions on characteristics of the study population and professionals perceptions on biopsy related infections (part 1 and 3) were analyzed on individual level, i.e. answers of different professionals from the same hospitals were counted separately.

## Results

Demographic characteristics are shown in Table 2. A total of 176 responses were received. Twelve respondents that only answered the demographic questions and three respondents from the Netherlands Antilles were excluded from the analysis. Questionnaires of 161 professionals (38.3%) were included in the final analyses, providing data on 65 (80.3%) Dutch hospitals [17]. Three of the professionals only partially answered the other questions. There were 41 (50.6%) hospitals where more than one urologist completed the questionnaire.

### PB techniques

There was a wide variation in combinations of applied PB techniques between Dutch hospitals: in total ten different combinations were used (Fig. 1). Schematic TRUSPB was performed in 64 (98.5%) hospitals. TRUSPB was the only method to obtain prostate tissue in 37 (56.9%) hospitals and was the most common procedure in 21 of the 27 hospitals with additional PB techniques. In four (6.2%) hospitals, transrectal MRI/TRUS fusion-guided PB was the most used method. Perineal MRI/TRUS fusion-guided PB and transrectal MRI guided PB was most frequently applied in

**Table 2** Demographic characteristics

| *Parameter* | *n (%)* |
|---|---|
| **Function** | |
| Urologist | 141 (87.6) |
| Residents | 20 (12.4) |
| **Sex** | |
| Male | 106 (65.8) |
| Female | 55 (34.2) |
| **Number of years working in the current position** | |
| 0–5 years | 37 (23.0) |
| 5–10 years | 52 (32.3) |
| ≥ 10 years | 72 (44.7) |
| **Working at** | |
| Academic hospital | 24 (14.9) |
| Peripheral hospital or other institution | 136 (84.5) |
| Unknown | 1 (0.6) |

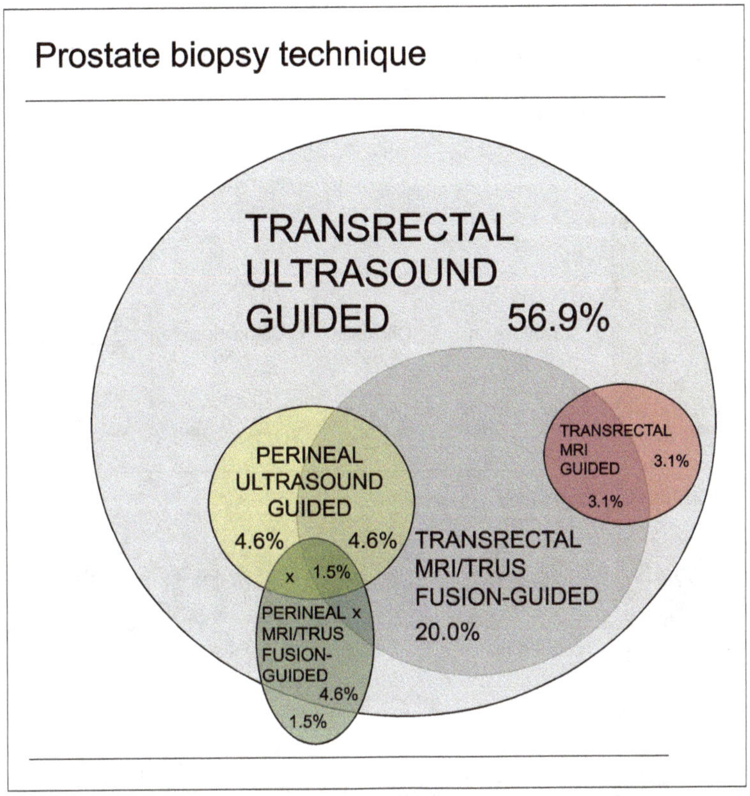


**Fig. 1** Variation in combinations of prostate biopsy techniques in the different hospitals. *Certain combinations do not exist, these are indicated with X*

respectively two (3.1%) and one (1.5%) hospital(s). Digitally directed PB was occasionally used in 12 (18.5%) hospitals.

In 57 of the 58 hospitals (98.5%) where TRUSPB was the most common procedure, urologists routinely obtained 8–12 cores per biopsy session. In one (1.5%) hospital, the number of biopsy cores during TRUSPB amounted to 12–16. In case MRI/TRUS fusion-guided or MRI guided PB was the most common method, there was a wide variation in the number of biopsy cores between hospitals. In four (57.1%) hospitals, targeted biopsies of mpMRI suspicious lesions were taken in addition to systematic biopsies (12–14 cores per biopsy session) and in three (42.9%) hospitals targeted biopsies were taken alone (2–6 cores per biopsy session).

We received one or more responses from all eight academic hospitals in the Netherlands. With regard to PB techniques, almost all academic hospitals also used methods other than TRUSB (87.5%). In two academic hospitals MRI/TRUS fusion-guided PB and in one academic hospital MRI guided PB was the most used method.

#### Perioperative antimicrobial prophylaxis

Oral antimicrobial prophylaxis for transrectal PB was prescribed in all hospitals. There was a wide inter-hospital variation in antibiotic choice, duration and timing combinations: 23 different antibiotic regimens with five different antibiotics were reported. The antibiotics most frequently used were FQ, either alone (98.5%) or combined with another antibiotic (1.6%) (Fig. 2). In case (a combination with) ciprofloxacin was used (84.4%), a single dose consisted of 500 mg (90.7%), 750 mg (3.7%) or 1000 mg (5.6%). The duration of the prophylaxis ranged from one pre-biopsy dose to 5 days extended prophylaxis with most hospitals (59.4%) giving a single dose of antibiotics 1 hour prior to PB (Fig. 2).

In all hospitals, antimicrobial prophylaxis was given empirically according to a standardized protocol. Urologists from four hospitals (6.3%) reported to use rectal swab cultures prior to PB in patients at risk for FQ resistance. Other measures reported to prevent infectious complications after PB were screening for urinary tract infection by urine sediment and/or urine culture (3.1%), washing the biopsy needle with povidone-iodine solution (1.6%) and the use of laxative suppositories (3.1%). A rectal enema was included in the preparation in one hospital (1.6%).

With regard to antimicrobial prophylaxis, no differences between academic and peripheral hospitals were detected nor were there any differences according to regions. The antimicrobial prophylaxis regimens as specified by the

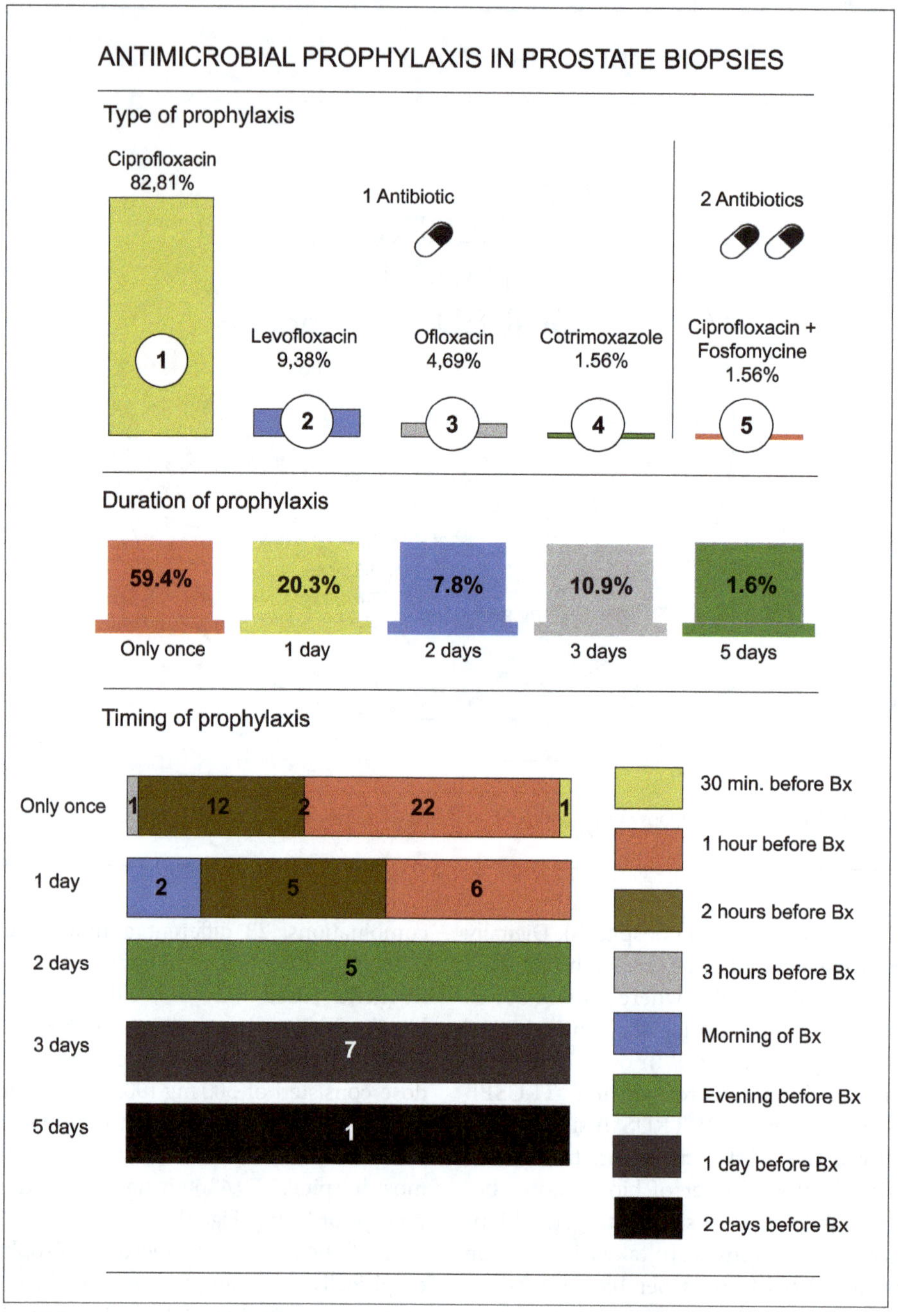


**Fig. 2** Variation in antimicrobial prophylaxis in prostate biopsies

respondents on hospital and individual level are described in Supplementary Appendix II.

#### Urologists' perception regarding antimicrobial prophylaxis in PB

According to 89 respondents (57.4%) the degree of infectious complications after PB in their hospital was stable, while 17 respondents (11.0%) indicated that they (subjectively) observed a decreasing number and 28 respondents (18.1%) an increasing number of infectious complications after PB. The other 21 respondents (13.5%) indicated that they did not know the trend of infectious complications after PB in their hospital.

After stating in our questionnaire that in urological patients the percentage of FQ resistant Gram-negative bacteria has increased from 7% in 2000 to 19% in 2017, we asked professionals if they were aware of this increasing level of FQ resistance [8]. Except for one respondent, all respondents (99.4%) indicated to be aware of the increasing FQ resistance. However, the degree of FQ resistance was assumed to be lower by 52 respondents (33.6%) and to be higher by four respondents (2.6%).

A total of 39 respondents (25.2%) (strongly) agreed with the statement that FQ resistance currently poses a problem in the empirical use of ciprofloxacin alone as prophylaxis around PB. One hundred fourteen respondents (73.6%) anticipate future problems in this area (Fig. 3). The preferred solutions of urologists to the increasing resistance for FQ can be found in Fig. 3. Besides the solutions provided in the questionnaire, urologists also suggested several solutions in the category *Other*. The most often mentioned 'other' solutions were: 'if necessary, adapt antimicrobial prophylaxis based on local resistance data in consultation with the medical microbiologist or based on evidence-based guidelines' (3.9%) and 'perform more transperineal biopsies' (3.2%).

## Discussion

This online survey among Dutch urologists showed a wide variation between hospitals both in PB techniques and in antimicrobial prophylaxis regimens.

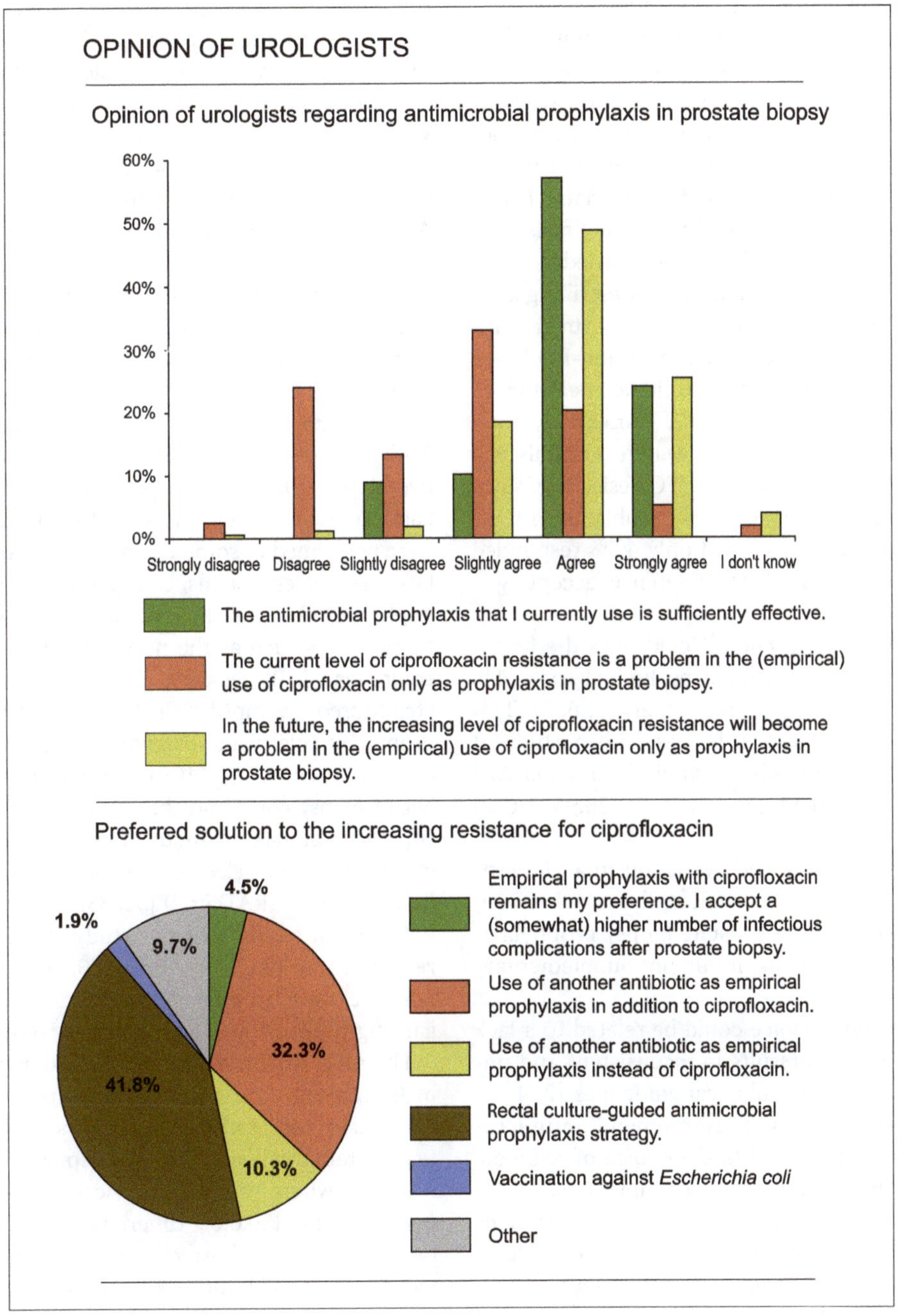


**Fig. 3** Urologists' perception of antimicrobial prophylaxis in prostate biopsy

Our survey showed that systematic TRUSPB with 8–12 cores per biopsy session was most frequently used (89.3%), which was in line with the guidelines at that moment [18]. Although our survey was performed before the recently published update of the EAU guidelines, urologists from 41.5% of the hospitals reported that they already perform MRI guided or MRI/TRUS fusion guided PB [2]. It suggests that (some) urologists, prior to guideline updates, already adjusted their practice patterns based on recent literature [19], which contributes to variation in daily care. In the Netherlands, saturation biopsies are not commonly performed.

Antimicrobial prophylaxis for PB is still dominated by ciprofloxacin monotherapy (84.4%), reflecting the recommendations in urological guidelines. However, given the rising prevalence of FQ resistance among relevant pathogens, antimicrobial prophylaxis with ciprofloxacin monotherapy is an increasingly doubtful policy. Many Dutch urologists are aware of the increased risk of FQ resistance and about a quarter of all urologists acknowledge rising FQ resistance as a current problem when prescribing antimicrobial prophylaxis. At this moment, only a small number of the Dutch hospitals are opting for a non-FQ based antibiotic regimen or have taken additional measures to address the problem of FQ resistance. We expect, however, that in the (near) future more Dutch hospitals will take measures trying to address rising FQ resistance, since 73.6% of all urologists anticipate future problems with regard to ciprofloxacin resistance and only 4.5% responded that ciprofloxacin remains their preference accepting a higher risk of urosepsis.

Furthermore, according to current guidelines the length of antimicrobial prophylaxis should be limited to < 24 h, which is not followed by 20% of the centers [4, 6, 7]. This deviation from the guidelines is in line with a study of Branch-Elliman et al. in which surgical antimicrobial prophylaxis was continued for > 24 h in 26.9% of all patients [20].

It is known that there is a wide variation in antimicrobial prophylaxis regimens internationally and between centers. Prior surveys on pre-prostate biopsy prophylaxis published since 2010 can be found in Supplementary Appendix III [10–15].

Variation in antibiotic choice could be related to a lack of strong evidence, which results in inconsistent and unclear recommendations in urological guidelines [2, 4–7]. While these guidelines generally recommend antimicrobial prophylaxis in transrectal PB, the choice of regimen, duration and the starting moment are ambiguous.

Moreover, the EAU guidelines leave individual clinicians to determine which patients may benefit from culture-guided prophylaxis [5]. It should be noted that although a recent meta-analysis [21] provided evidence for the use of culture-guided antimicrobial prophylaxis in reducing infectious complications after transrectal PB, a large prospective multicenter trial evaluating the effectiveness of rectal swab culture-guided antimicrobial prophylaxis, cost-effectiveness and optimal implementation is missing, but is currently being performed (NCT03228108).

Finally, the EAU guidelines recommend to use rectal cleansing with povidone-iodine prior to transrectal PB [5]. This is based on a meta-analysis of six trials including 1373 men that showed that the use of pre-biopsy rectal povidone-iodine preparation in addition to antimicrobial prophylaxis resulted in lower rates of infectious complications [0.58 (0.43 to 0.76); RR (95% CI)] [22–27]. However, not a single Dutch urologist reported to use rectal povidone-iodine cleansing prior to PB.

There is no cut-and-dried solution to the increasing resistance against FQ in the context of the risk of post-biopsy infection, which is supported by our finding that Dutch urologists have various preferred solutions to this problem. Although, in our survey, we asked urologists mainly for solutions with in the field of antimicrobial prophylaxis, it is important to note that the solution does not have to be (solely) based on the use of adapted or rectal culture-guided antimicrobial prophylaxis. Various studies found favourable infection rates for transperineal PB compared to TRUSB with similar rates of prostate cancer detection [2, 28–31]. Therefore, transperineal PB is an obvious alternative biopsy approach to avoid infections from FQ resistant bacteria. Our survey showed that transperineal biopsies were performed to some extent in 16.9% of all Dutch hospitals. In the Netherlands, transperineal biopsy is slow to be implemented in the clinic because of the consequent logistic problems such as the necessity for specialized staff and equipment, MRI capacity, greater labor time, higher costs etc. Moreover, mpMRI is likely to play an increasingly prominent role in the diagnostic pathway of prostate cancer. In the future, mpMRI could possibly reduce the number of biopsy cores and thereby possibly lower (infectious) complication rates without compromising detection rates or avoid PB in selected patients with negative mpMRI (index lesion PI-RADS ≤2) [32, 33].

The main strength of our study is that due to the high response rate (38.3% covering 80.2% of all Dutch hospitals) we were able to get a nationwide impression regarding the current Dutch prostatic biopsy practices.

The most important limitation of our study is that most of the results were analyzed at hospital level in order to obtain a representative picture of the variation in PB practice patterns between Dutch hospitals. Unfortunately, in hospitals where more than one urologist completed the questionnaire (50.6%), differences were also found between these intra-hospital urologists with regard to PB technique (41.5%) and antimicrobial prophylaxis (48.8%). However, in all cases the local protocol could be clarified. These intra-hospital differences again emphasize the lack of standardization in PB techniques and antimicrobial prophylaxis regimens in the Netherlands even among urologists who work in the same center. On individual level, 41 different antimicrobial prophylaxis regimens were reported instead of the 23 regimens we identified at hospital level (Supplementary Appendix II). In daily clinical practice, the variation is therefore probably even wider than the variation described in this article. Another limitation is that between the performance of our survey and publication of the results, the EAU guideline on prostate cancer [2] has been updated. Therefore, this survey does no longer depict the current international guidelines regarding prostate biopsy technique. This is, however, illustrative for the rapid evolutions in this area. Moreover, two questions were difficult to analyze due to methodological shortcomings and were left out. However, these questions were not critical for our analysis.

## Conclusions

The diversity of the reported prophylactic regimens is likely due to a lack of good evidence. Therefore, there is need for well designed, adequately powered trials of good quality in the field of urological pre-biopsy prophylactic measures. High quality research will result in evidence-based, clear-cut recommendations and offers urologists more guidance regarding antimicrobial prophylaxis around PB in the context of increasing antibiotic resistance. Professionals in daily practice have a need for dynamic, regularly updated guidelines that address changes in procedures, antimicrobial resistance patterns or new scientific insights. This study shows that the lack of standardized, clear guidelines lead to (undesirable) practice variation between health care professionals, which implies that patients in one hospital may receive better care than in another hospital. Moreover, this study shows that in an evolving clinical landscape of PB with changes in procedures, techniques and antimicrobial resistance, current urological guidelines lead to urologists making their own policies, resulting in an over-prescription of prophylactic antibiotics. This is ironically exactly what these guidelines aim to prevent.

## Supplementary information

**Additional file 1 Supplementary appendix I** Full questionaire. *The full online questionnaire that was distributed by the Dutch Association of Urology (DUA) to all its members.*

**Additional file 2 Supplementary file II** Antimicrobial prophylaxis regimens on hospital level and as specified by the (individual) respondents. *The antimicrobial prophylaxis regimens as specified by the respondents on hospital and individual level are described.*

**Additional file 3 Supplementary file III** Prior surveys on pre-prostate biopsy prophylaxis published since 2010. *Schematic overview of surveys conducted by others since 2010 about prophylactic measures around transrectal prostate biopsy.*

### Abbreviations

DUA: Dutch Association of Urology; EAU: European Association of Urology; FQ: Fluoroquinolones; mpMRI: Multiparametric magnetic resonance imaging; PB: Prostate biopsy; TRUSPB: Transrectal ultrasound guided prostate biopsy; ZonMw: The Netherlands Organisation for Health Research and Development

### Acknowledgements

We thank ZonMw for their financial support.

### Authors' contributions

Study design: ST, EKD, RS, AH, EKW, HW, MH, MS. Data collection: ST, MS. Data analysis: ST. Writing the manuscript: ST, MH. Critical review of the manuscript: EKD, RS, AH, EKW, HW, MS. All authors have read and approved the manuscript.

### Author details

[1]Department of Medical Microbiology, Radboud Center Infectious Diseases, Radboudumc, huispost 777, Geert Grooteplein Zuid 10, 6525, GA, Nijmegen, the Netherlands. [2]Department of Urology, Catharina Hospital, Eindhoven, the Netherlands. [3]Department of Urology, Canisius-Wilhelmina Hospital, Nijmegen, the Netherlands. [4]Scientific Center for Quality of Healthcare, Radboud Institute for Health Sciences, Radboudumc, Nijmegen, the Netherlands. [5]Department of Urology, Radboudumc, Nijmegen, the Netherlands.

### References

1. Volksgezondheidenzorg.info [Updated 12th July 2017. RIVM Bilthoven: [Available from: https://www.volksgezondheidenzorg.info/onderwerp/prostaatkanker/cijfers-context/huidige-situatie#!node-prevalentie-prostaatkanker.
2. Mottet N, van den Bergh R, Briers E, Cornford P, De Santis M, Fanti S, et al. Guidelines on prostate cancer. Eur Assoc Urol. 2019;65(1):124.
3. Wegelin O, Exterkate L, van der Leest M, Kummer JA, Vreuls W, de Bruin PC, et al. The FUTURE trial: a multicenter randomised controlled trial on target biopsy techniques based on magnetic resonance imaging in the diagnosis of prostate Cancer in patients with prior negative biopsies. Eur Urol. 2019; 75(4):582–90.
4. Wolf JS Jr, Bennett CJ, Dmochowski RR, Hollenbeck BK, Pearle MS, Schaeffer AJ, et al. Best practice policy statement on urologic surgery antimicrobial prophylaxis. J Urol. 2008;179(4):1379–90.
5. Bonkat G, Bartoletti RR, Bruyère F, Cai T, Geerlings SE, Köves B, et al. EAU Guidelines on Urological Infections 2019. Uroweb. Available from: http://uroweb.org/guideline/urological-infections/.
6. van Haarst EP, Bootsma AMJ, Elzevier HW, Froeling FMJA, Geerlings SE, Jansen FH, et al. NVU richtlijn: Bacteriële urineweginfecties bij adolescenten en volwassenen. 2009. Available from: https://www.nvu.nl/Portals/_default/Skins/NVU/DocumentHandlerPublic.ashx?id=817db8b4-e657-40d0-bc20-52ebc1d286ff&filename=bijlage%20C58%20urineweginfectie%202009.pdf.
7. Antibioticabeleid SW. SWAB Richtlijn Peri-operatieve profylaxe. 2018.
8. De Greef SC, Mouton JW, Schoffelen AF, Verduin CM. NethMap 2019: consumption of antimicrobial agents and antimicrobial resistance among medically important bacteria in the Netherlands in 2018. RIVM Bilthoven; 2019. Available from: https://www.rivm.nl/sites/default/files/2019-09/Nethmap%20Maran%202019%20beveiligd.pdf.
9. Van Besien J, Uvin P, Van den Abeele AM, Merckx L. Prevalence, risk factors, and clinical relevance of Fluoroquinolone-resistant organisms in rectal cultures: should we target antibiotic prophylaxis prior to prostate biopsy? Ther Adv Urol. 2016;2016:5392107.
10. Boehm K, Siegel FP, Schneidewind L, Kranz J, Spachmann P, Frank T, et al. Antibiotic prophylaxis in prostate biopsies: contemporary practice patterns in Germany. Front Surg. 2018;5:2.
11. Carlsson S, Bratt O, Stattin P, Egevad L. Current routines for transrectal ultrasound-guided prostate biopsy: a web-based survey by the Swedish urology network. Scand J Urol Nephrol. 2012;46(6):405–10.
12. Davis P, Paul E, Grummet J. Current practice of prostate biopsy in Australia and New Zealand: a survey. Urol Ann. 2015;7(3):315–9.

13. Hillelsohn JH, Duty B, Blute ML Jr, Okhunov Z, Kashan M, Moldwin R, et al. Variability of transrectal ultrasound-guided prostate biopsy prophylactic measures. Can J Urol. 2012;19(6):6573–7.
14. Smyth LG, Mulvin DW. Antibiotic prophylaxis for transrectal ultrasound biopsy of the prostate in Ireland. Ir J Med Sci. 2012;181(1):33–5.
15. Johnson JR, Polgreen PM, Beekmann SE. Transrectal prostate biopsy-associated prophylaxis and infectious complications: report of a query to the emerging infections network of the infectious diseases society of america. Open Forum Infect Dis. 2015;2(1):ofv002.
16. Grabe M, Bartoletti R, Bjerklund-Johansen TE, Çek HM, Pickard RS, Tenke P, et al. EAU Guidelines on Urological Infections 2015. Uroweb. Available from: https://uroweb.org/wp-content/uploads/19-Urological-infections_LR2.pdf.
17. ZorgkaartNederland. Patiëntenfederatie Nederland. [Available from: https://www.zorgkaartnederland.nl/uroloog.
18. Mottet N, Bellmunt J, Briers E, van den RCN B, Bolla M, van NJ C, et al. Guidelines on prostate cancer. Eur Assoc Urol. 2015;65(1):124.
19. Rouviere O, Puech P, Renard-Penna R, Claudon M, Roy C, Mege-Lechevallier F, et al. Use of prostate systematic and targeted biopsy on the basis of multiparametric MRI in biopsy-naive patients (MRI-FIRST): a prospective, multicentre, paired diagnostic study. Lancet Oncol. 2019;20(1):100–9.
20. Branch-Elliman W, O'Brien W, Strymish J, Itani K, Wyatt C, Gupta K. Association of Duration and Type of Surgical Prophylaxis With Antimicrobial-Associated Adverse Events. JAMA Surg. 2019;154(7):590.
21. Scott S, Harris PN, Williamson DA, Liss MA, Doi SAR, Roberts MJ. The effectiveness of targeted relative to empiric prophylaxis on infectious complications after transrectal ultrasound-guided prostate biopsy: a meta-analysis. World J Urol. 2018;36(7):1007–17.
22. Kanjanawongdeengam P, Viseshsindh W, Santanirand P, Prathombutr P, Nilkulwattana S. Reduction in bacteremia rates after rectum sterilization before transrectal, ultrasound-guided prostate biopsy: a randomized controlled trial. J Med Assoc Thail. 2009;92(12):1621–6.
23. Brown RW, Warner JJ, Turner BI, Harris LF, Alford RH. Bacteremia and bacteriuria after transrectal prostatic biopsy. Urology. 1981;18(2):145–8.
24. Melekos MD. Efficacy of prophylactic antimicrobial regimens in preventing infectious complications after transrectal biopsy of the prostate. Int Urol Nephrol. 1990;22(3):257–62.
25. Sharpe JR, Sadlowski RW, Finney RP, Branch WT, Hanna JE. Urinary tract infection after transrectal needle biopsy of the prostate. J Urol. 1982;127(2):255–6.
26. Abughosh Z, Margolick J, Goldenberg SL, Taylor SA, Afshar K, Bell R, et al. A prospective randomized trial of povidone-iodine prophylactic cleansing of the rectum before transrectal ultrasound guided prostate biopsy. J Urol. 2013;189(4):1326–31.
27. Ghafoori M, Shakiba M, Seifmanesh H, Hoseini K. Decrease in infection rate following use of povidone-iodine during transrectal ultrasound guided biopsy of the prostate: a double blind randomized clinical trial. Iran J Radiol. 2012;9(2):67–70.
28. Lo KL, Chui KL, Leung CH, Ma SF, Lim K, Ng T, et al. Outcomes of transperineal and transrectal ultrasound-guided prostate biopsy. Hong Kong Med J. 2019;25(3):209–15.
29. Xue J, Qin Z, Cai H, Zhang C, Li X, Xu W, et al. Comparison between transrectal and transperineal prostate biopsy for detection of prostate cancer: a meta-analysis and trial sequential analysis. Oncotarget. 2017;8(14):23322–36.
30. Huang GL, Kang CH, Lee WC, Chiang PH. Comparisons of cancer detection rate and complications between transrectal and transperineal prostate biopsy approaches - a single center preliminary study. BMC Urol. 2019;19(1):101.
31. Grummet J. How to biopsy: Transperineal versus Transrectal, saturation versus targeted, What's the evidence? Urol Clin North Am. 2017;44(4):525–34.
32. Venderink W, van Luijtelaar A, van der Leest M, Barentsz JO, Jenniskens SFM, Sedelaar MJP, et al. Multiparametric magnetic resonance imaging and follow-up to avoid prostate biopsy in 4259 men. BJU Int. 2019;124(5):775–84.
33. Kasivisvanathan V, Rannikko AS, Borghi M, Panebianco V, Mynderse LA, Vaarala MH, et al. MRI-targeted or standard biopsy for prostate-Cancer diagnosis. N Engl J Med. 2018;378(19):1767–77.

# 4

# Survival and mortality of elderly men with localized prostate cancer managed with primary androgen deprivation therapy or by primary observation

Heikki Seikkula[1*], Peter J. Boström[2,3], Karri Seppä[4], Janne Pitkäniemi[4,5,6], Nea Malila[4,7] and Antti Kaipia[8]

**Abstract**

**Background:** Androgen deprivation therapy (ADT) remains a primary treatment for localized prostate cancer (PCa) even though there is no evidence that its use is beneficial in the absence of curative treatment.

**Methods:** Men aged ≥70 years ($n = 16,534$) diagnosed with localized PCa from 1985 to 2014 and managed either with primary observation or ADT in the absence of curative treatment were included. The cases were identified from the population-based Finnish Cancer Registry. We estimated the standardized mortality ratios (SMR) for overall mortality by treatment group. We determined the relative risk (RR) of PCa-specific mortality (PCSM) and other-cause mortality between the two treatment groups. Survival was determined using the life table method. Two age groups (70–79 years and ≥ 80 years) and three calendar time cohorts (1985–1994, 1995–2004, and 2005–2014) were compared following adjustment of propensity score matching between the treatment groups with four covariates (age, year of diagnosis, educational level, and hospital district). Follow-up continued until death or until December 31, 2015.

**Results:** Patients in the observation group had lower overall SMRs than those in the ADT group in both age cohorts over the entire study period. PCSM was higher in men aged 70–79 years undergoing primary ADT compared to those managed by observation only (RR: 1.70, 95% confidence interval [CI]: 1.29–2.23 [1985–1994]; RR 1.55, 95% CI: 1.35–1.84 [1995–2004]; and RR 2.71, 95% CI: 2.08–3.53 [2005–2014]); $p = 0.005$ for periodic trend. A similar trend over time was also observed in men aged > 80 years; ($p$ for age–period interaction = 0.237). Overall survival was also higher among men in their 70's managed by observation compared to those undergoing ADT.

**Conclusions:** Primary ADT within four months period from diagnosis is not associated with improved long-term overall survival or decreased PCSM compared to primary conservative management for men with localized PCa. However, this observational study's conclusions should be weighted with confounding factors related to cancer aggressiveness and comorbidities.

**Keywords:** Prostate cancer survival, Prostate cancer–specific mortality, Localized prostate cancer, Androgen deprivation therapy

* Correspondence: heikki.seikkula@ksshp.fi
[1]Department of Surgery, Central Hospital of Central Finland, Jyväskylä, Finland
Full list of author information is available at the end of the article

## Background

Androgen deprivation therapy (ADT) has been the cornerstone of treatment for locally advanced and metastatic (M+) prostate cancer (PCa) since the 1940s [1]. Immediate ADT or ADT combined with docetaxel or abiraterone acetate is the current treatment of choice for M+ PCa [2]. However, the use of ADT increased sharply between 1989 and 2001 in the USA despite the fact that ≤5% of patients with newly diagnosed PCa have distant metastases at first presentation compared with 20–25% ≥20 years ago [3, 4]. While the increased use of ADT is partly accounted for by the uptake of neoadjuvant and adjuvant treatment along with radiation therapy, it is primarily elucidated by ADT for localized disease, especially for elderly patients [5]. Thus, ADT is commonly used to treat localized PCa although it has not been shown to improve survival [6].

The risk of metastases or death from conservatively managed clinical stage T1/T2 cancers was estimated in a meta-analysis of six studies from the era prior to prostate-specific antigen (PSA) [7]. The risk of metastasis at 10 years was found to be 19, 42, and 74% for well-differentiated, moderately differentiated, and poorly differentiated tumors, respectively [7]. Similarly, the long-term clinical outcomes of localized PCa without initial treatment with curative intent during the PSA era were assessed [8]. Thirty per cent of the patients died of PCa and 30% of other causes within a 12-year period [8]. A landmark Swedish study demonstrated a benign course of well- or intermediately differentiated PCa in the absence of initial treatment with curative intent [9]. Thus, the clinical course of localized high-risk PCa can be progressive, but the majority of cancers are indolent and slow to progress [2]. According to current guidelines, observation with the option of later treatment in the case of disease progression (i.e., watchful waiting) is recommended for localized and locally advanced PCa in elderly patients with competing comorbidities.

The objective of this observational study was to investigate mortality in elderly PCa patients primarily managed with ADT or observation only during long follow-ups in Finland.

## Methods

### Study population

The Finnish Cancer Registry is a nationwide population-based register of all incident cancer cases diagnosed in Finland since 1953. The health care personnel in hospitals, outpatient clinics, and healthcare facilities are obligated to notify of new cases. Additionally, pathology notifications are received from all histopathological laboratories in Finland. The registry coverage is estimated at 99% for male genital cancers [10]. The spreading into localized, locally advanced, or metastatic are classified by tumor size, regional node involvement, and presence of metastasis for cases covered by the Finnish Cancer Registry.

The Finnish Cancer Registry data can be linked with the population register center database for dates of death or emigration and causes of death and education levels from Statistics Finland.

We identified all PCa patients aged 70 years or older at diagnosis with localized cancer (clinical stage T1/T2) from 1985 to 2014 and managed by primary ADT or observation in the absence of radical treatment with curative intent (Table 1). Of the total patients identified ($n$ = 16,534), 11,572 were aged 70–79 years and 4962 were ≥ 80. Within four months of diagnosis, the primary treatment was ADT (ADT group $n = 9704$), while 6830 received no treatment (observation group) (Table 1). The regional data included 22 hospital districts taking care of specialized care. The survival rates of the patients were compared by age and treatment group over three periods (1985–1994, 1995–2004, and 2005–2014).

### Statistical analysis

Overall survival was evaluated using the life table method [11]. The Poisson regression model was used to quantify differences in patient mortality between the defined groups. The results were reported as relative risk (RR) of PCa-specific mortality (PCSM) and mortality due to causes other than PCa. We also estimated the standardized mortality ratio (SMR) for overall mortality among the patients. The SMR is estimated as the ratio of observed and expected numbers of deaths. The latter was derived from the mortality rates of the male population in Finland stratified by age (1-year intervals), calendar year and education. We used a nearest neighbor matching with a logistic regression–based propensity score [12] to identify a cohort of 5715 paired patients. In the logistic regression, the probability of a given treatment was modeled as a function of age and calendar period (in 5-year groups), education, and hospital district. Interactions between calendar period and each of the covariates were also included in the model. Statistical analysis was performed with R (version 3.2.3) using the packages popEpi [13] and MatchIt [14].

The study protocol was approved by the institutional review board of the Hospital District of Southwest Finland. The National Institute for Health and Welfare (Finland) approved access to the registry data (study number 182/5.05.00/2015). Statistics Finland approved access to the data on the cause of death (study number TK-53-86-17).

## Results

The stage distribution of all prostate cancer patients from 1985 to 2014 ($n = 95{,}959$) in Finland is shown in

**Table 1** Study population of prostate cancer patients

| | All patients | | | |
|---|---|---|---|---|
| | ADT | | Observation | |
| Variable | N | % | N | % |
| **Age at diagnosis** | | | | |
| 70–74 | 3096 | 31.9 | 2850 | 41.7 |
| 75–79 | 3411 | 35.2 | 2215 | 32.4 |
| 80–84 | 2170 | 22.4 | 1227 | 18.0 |
| 85–89 | 832 | 8.6 | 438 | 6.4 |
| > 90 | 195 | 2.0 | 100 | 1.5 |
| Total | 9704 | 100 | 6830 | 100 |
| **Year of diagnosis** | | | | |
| 1985–1989 | 785 | 8.1 | 208 | 3.0 |
| 1990–1994 | 1197 | 12.3 | 337 | 4.9 |
| 1995–1999 | 1724 | 17.8 | 797 | 11.7 |
| 2000–2004 | 2159 | 22.2 | 1313 | 19.2 |
| 2005–2009 | 2280 | 23.5 | 2194 | 32.1 |
| 2010–2014 | 1559 | 16.1 | 1981 | 29.0 |
| Total | 9704 | 100 | 6830 | 100 |
| **Education level** | | | | |
| Basic | 6920 | 71.3 | 4421 | 64.7 |
| Secondary | 1325 | 13.7 | 1074 | 15.7 |
| High | 1459 | 15.0 | 1335 | 19.5 |
| Total | 9704 | 100 | 6830 | 100 |
| **Hospital district** | | | | |
| Uusimaa | 932 | 9.6 | 786 | 11.5 |
| Helsinki | 812 | 8.4 | 698 | 10.2 |
| Varsinais-Suomi | 835 | 8.6 | 628 | 9.2 |
| Satakunta | 500 | 5.2 | 281 | 4.1 |
| Kanta-Hame | 471 | 4.9 | 322 | 4.7 |
| Pirkanmaa | 1187 | 12.2 | 614 | 9.0 |
| Paijat-Hame | 668 | 6.9 | 304 | 4.5 |
| Kymenlaakso | 433 | 4.5 | 182 | 2.7 |
| Etela-Karjala | 321 | 3.3 | 179 | 2.6 |
| Etela-Savo | 158 | 1.6 | 102 | 1.5 |
| Ita-Savo | 76 | 0.8 | 64 | 0.9 |
| Pohjois-Karjala | 149 | 1.5 | 178 | 2.6 |
| Pohjois-Savo | 466 | 4.8 | 403 | 5.9 |
| Keski-Suomi | 374 | 3.9 | 557 | 8.2 |
| Etela-Pohjanmaa | 522 | 5.4 | 386 | 5.7 |
| Vaasa | 285 | 2.9 | 182 | 2.7 |
| Keski-Pohjanmaa | 136 | 1.4 | 128 | 1.9 |
| Pohjois-Pohjanmaa | 610 | 6.3 | 372 | 5.4 |
| Kainuu | 265 | 2.7 | 99 | 1.4 |
| Lansi-Pohja | 280 | 2.9 | 132 | 1.9 |
| Lappi | 190 | 2.0 | 177 | 2.6 |
| Åland | 34 | 0.4 | 56 | 0.8 |
| Total | 9704 | 100 | 6830 | 100 |

*ADT* androgen deprivation therapy, *N* number

Supplementary Table 1. Approximately half of the patients were classified as having localized PCa. The proportion of metastatic disease decreased from 28 to 17% between the periods 1985–1994 and 2005–2014. However, the PCa stage was missing in nearly one-third of the patients over the study period (Supplementary Table 1). In this study, we included only PCa patients aged 70 years or older at diagnosis who received primary treatment with ADT or no treatment within four months of diagnosis (Table 1).

SMR analysis showed that overall mortality was lower in the observation group than in the ADT group in all three time periods. However, a declining trend in SMR over time was seen in both groups. Furthermore, over the most recent period (2005–2014), patients in both age cohorts had lower overall mortality than the general male population in Finland (SMR: 0.93, 95% CI: 0.88–0.98) (Table 2). Propensity score matching did not change any of these results.

In both age cohorts, we observed higher PCSM in patients undergoing primary ADT compared to those managed by observation only (Table 3). The relative risk of prostate cancer mortality increased significantly over time in the ADT group compared to the observation group ($p$ for trend = 0.05). On the other hand, the risk of death from causes other than PCa decreased over time in patients aged 70–79 years undergoing primary ADT compared to those managed by observation only, but the same was not true in patients aged 80 years or older (Table 3).

Overall survival of PCa patients aged 70–79 years was higher in the observation group than in the ADT group throughout the study period. However, a rising trend was observed in both treatment groups. Among patients over 80 years of age, overall survival improved over time in both treatment groups with no significant differences between them until the most recent period (from 2005 to 2014), when overall survival in the observation group was higher than in the ADT group (Fig. 1). The results remained similar after propensity score matching.

## Discussion

In this population-based study, we investigated whether the survival and mortality outcomes in elderly male

**Table 2** Overall mortality of the study patients compared to that of the male population of Finland

| All patients | Period | | | | | |
|---|---|---|---|---|---|---|
| | 1985–1994 | | 1995–2004 | | 2005–2014 | |
| | ADT | Observation | ADT | Observation | ADT | Observation |
| Age | SMR (95% confidence interval) | | | | | |
| All (> 70) | 1.48 (1.41–1.54) | 1.20 (1.10–1.30) | 1.19 (1.15–1.23) | 1.03 (0.98–1.08) | 1.08 (1.03–1.13) | 0.93 (0.88–0.98) |
| 70–79 | 1.57 (1.48–1.65) | 1.17 (1.05–1.30) | 1.24 (1.19–1.29) | 1.05 (0.99–1.11) | 1.11 (1.04–1.19) | 0.95 (0.88–1.01) |
| ≥80 | 1.39 (1.22–1.42) | 1.25 (1.08–1.43) | 1.10 (1.04–1.17) | 1.00 (0.92–1.09) | 1.04 (0.97–1.11) | 0.89 (0.82–0.97) |
| Matched pairs | | | | | | |
| All (> 70) | 1.50 (1.38–1.63) | 1.19 (1.09–1.30) | 1.19 (1.13–1.25) | 1.03 (0.98–1.08) | 1.09 (1.03–1.15) | 0.93 (0.87–0.98) |
| 70–79 | 1.57 (1.41–1.74) | 1.16 (1.04–1.29) | 1.23 (1.16–1.30) | 1.05 (0.99–1.11) | 1.12 (1.05–1.20) | 0.94 (0.87–1.01) |
| ≥ 80 | 1.39 (1.21–1.60) | 1.25 (1.08–1.44) | 1.12 (1.02–1.21) | 1.00 (0.91–1.08) | 1.03 (0.94–1.12) | 0.91 (0.82–0.99) |

Population mortality stratified by age and calendar year and education level
*ADT* androgen deprivation therapy, *SMR* standardized mortality ratio

patients (aged ≥70 years) with localized PCa is different between those managed by primary observation and those undergoing primary ADT over a long period of time. We showed that the overall SMR of patients in the observation cohort was lower than those in the ADT cohort in both age groups over the entire study period. PCSM and mortality due to causes other than PCa were lower in patients monitored with primary observation compared to those managed with primary ADT. This difference was particularly evident in patients aged 70–79 years at the time of diagnosis. Overall survival was also higher in subjects in this age group managed by primary observation. By contrast, a smaller difference in PSCM was observed between patients undergoing ADT and those managed by primary observation, while a clear difference in mortality due to other causes was not seen in patients aged 80 or older. This implies a better general health condition and a healthier lifestyle among patients in the observation cohort.

An increased risk of PCSM was observed in patients undergoing primary ADT compared to those managed by primary observation, while a lower risk of other-cause mortality was seen in the younger patient group managed by primary observation. This suggests that in recent times, primary ADT without curative treatment was generally selected for patients with aggressive disease. A 10-year threefold risk of PCSM was associated with poorly differentiated PCa among patients with conservatively managed localized PCa in the Surveillance, Epidemiology, and End Results (SEER) Program [15]. Most male patients with conservatively managed localized PCa aged > 66 years with competing comorbidities died from causes other than PCa in a period of 10 years, irrespective of age and tumor aggressiveness [16]. The use of primary ADT was beneficial for patients with aggressive disease and few comorbidities [16]. However, overall mortality was lower in subjects managed by observation than with ADT. We assumed that a shift from ADT to a more radical treatment may have occurred in patients with a good general health status. Since an increasing number of PCa cases has been diagnosed in recent years, and observation is widely utilized in Finland, it is likely that observation was selected for patients with less aggressive histology and without advanced disease. Consequently, fewer male patients died of cancer owing to the slow, natural course of disease.

Overall survival was reduced in patients aged 70–79 years initially treated with. It is still difficult to draw a

**Table 3** Risk of PCa and other-cause mortality among men on primary ADT compared to observation only

| Time period (age) | Relative risk of PCa mortality (95% CI) | | Relative risk of mortality due to causes other than PCa (95% CI) | |
|---|---|---|---|---|
| | ADT | Observation | ADT | Observation |
| 1985–1994 **(70–79y)** | 1.70 (1.29–2.23) | 1.00 (ref) | 1.22 (1.00–1.49) | 1.00 (ref) |
| 1995–2004 | 1.55 (1.31–1.84) | 1.00 (ref) | 1.07 (0.97–1.18) | 1.00 (ref) |
| 2005–2014 | 2.71 (2.08–3.53) | 1.00 (ref) | 1.03 (0.92–1.16) | 1.00 (ref) |
| 1985–1994 **(>80y)** | 1.30 (0.89–1.88) | 1.00 (ref) | 1.09 (0.85–1.39) | 1.00 (ref) |
| 1995–2004 | 1.49 (1.13–1.97) | 1.00 (ref) | 1.05 (0.92–1.20) | 1.00 (ref) |
| 2005–2014 | 1.65 (1.19–2.29) | 1.00 (ref) | 1.06 (0.91–1.23) | 1.00 (ref) |

*p*-value for age–period interaction = 0.237; *p* for age effect = 0.052; *p* for period effect = 0.005. Analysis is based on propensity matched pairs
*PCa* prostate cancer, *CI* confidence interval, *ADT* androgen deprivation therapy, *ref.* reference

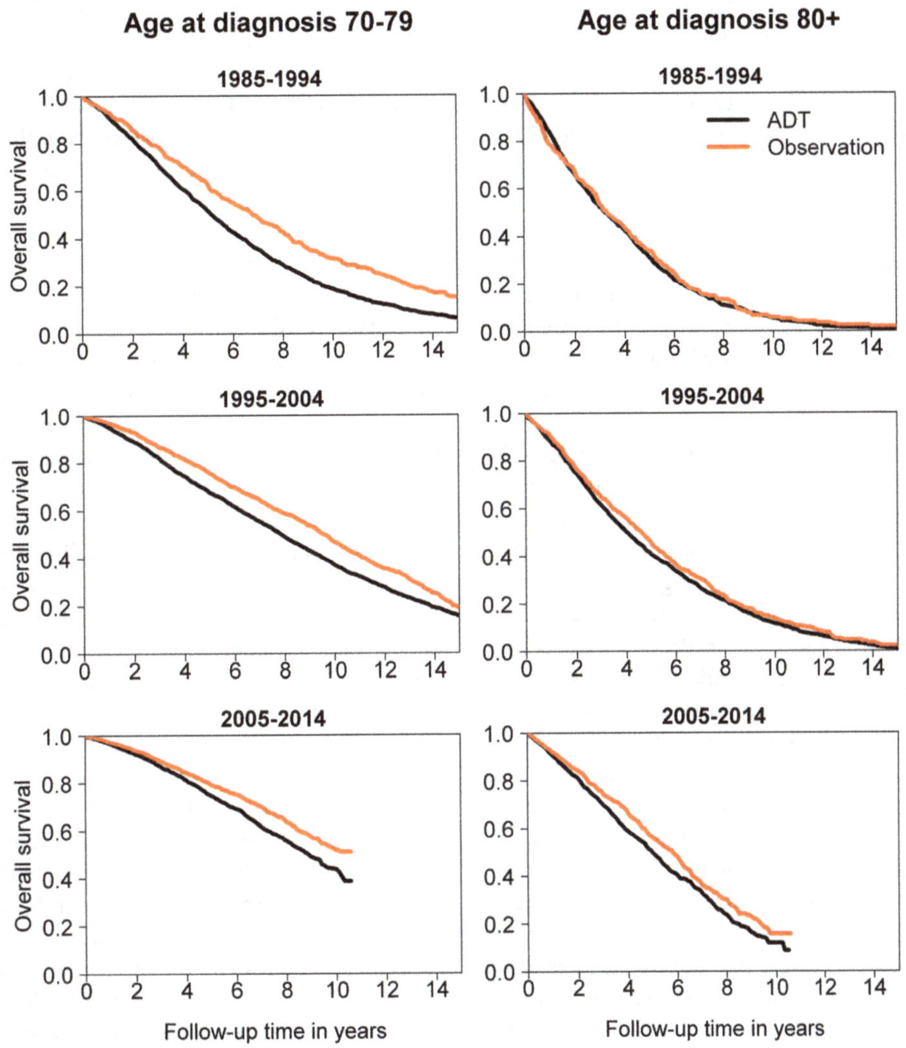


**Fig. 1** Overall survival among men aged 70–79 years and among men aged 80 or older

conclusion from this finding owing to the absence of data on patient comorbidities. However, increased morbidity and mortality from ADT-related side effects is possible. Thus, the survival benefits of ADT are partly offset by its high toxicity. These findings can also be explained by a better general health condition among patients in the observation group. In our cohort, patients in the observation group had a clearly lower risk of overall mortality compared to patients undergoing primary ADT. Since in epidemiological studies the only endpoint that is free from bias is mortality, we can assume that patients in observation cohort were healthier than those in the ADT cohort.

Many population-based analyses suggest that gonadotropin-releasing hormone (GnRH) agonist use is associated with a greater risk of coronary artery disease, myocardial infarction, and diabetes mellitus (DM) [17–19]. Subsequent reports have suggested that male patients with comorbidities or prior cardiovascular disease treated with GnRH agonists might be at increased risk of cardiovascular mortality [20, 21]. Based on these observations, a science advisory consensus statement on GnRH agonist therapy and cardiovascular risk was issued, together with a U.S. Food and Drug Administration safety warning to address concerns of increased risk of myocardial infarction, stroke, sudden cardiac death, and DM [22]. However, conflicting results have been reported. In a recent meta-analysis, ADT use was not associated with an increased risk of cardiovascular death, but with a lower risk of PCSM and all-cause mortality [23]. Studer et al. also reported that ADT for localized PCa may even reduce cardiovascular mortality if started immediately after diagnosis [24].

The current study findings did not support the life-prolonging effects of primary ADT for localized PCa. Several reports have shown similar results: In a prior population-based cohort study on 66,717 Medicare patients diagnosed between 1992 and 2009, and who received no definitive local therapy within 180 days of prostate cancer diagnosis, primary ADT was not associated with improved overall long-term CSS or the CSS of patients with localized PCa [25]. Instead, there is evidence that primary ADT led to inferior outcomes [24]. Low overall survival rates were reported for male patients with localized disease treated with primary ADT rather than observation in a previous population-based study [26]. In addition, Potosky et al. reported that primary ADT was neither associated with an enhanced risk of all-cause mortality (hazard ratio [HR] of 1.04, 95% CI: 0.97–1.11) nor PCa-specific mortality (HR of 1.03; 95% CI: 0.89–1.19) after adjusting for the sociodemographic and clinical characteristics of patients with localized PCa. However, primary ADT was associated with a decreased risk of all-cause mortality, but not PCSM, among patients at high risk of PCa progression [27].

PSA screening practices have increased exponentially over a 30-year period, and regular PSA testing is used frequently among all socioeconomic groups in Scandinavia and Finland [28, 29]. In the early years of the present study, a diagnosis of localized PCa was generally performed via a digital rectal examination or using pathological specimens obtained following a transurethral resection of the prostate. In recent years, most localized PCa cases have been diagnosed by prostate biopsies prompted by elevated PSA values. Moreover, although a proven benefit of the PSA screening of older males has not been shown, PSA testing is frequently performed for elderly patients [30]. The wide-stage migration of PCa from advanced to indolent disease has been reported over ≥20 years [31]. Thus, a commonly employed but poorly organized screening policy explains the increased rate of PCa in past decades in Finland. Consequently, the number of elderly male patients with PCa has also increased. This implies that the more favorable outcomes associated with the use of primary observation compared to ADT in patients with PCa, especially those in their 70s, can be attributed to PSA-related "lead time" rather than life extension.

Over the study period, staging of metastatic disease in Finland was performed by bone scan examination according to national guidelines until the mid-2000s, after which low-risk PCa patients typically underwent no imaging. The proportion of de novo metastatic PCa in Finland was nearly one-third from 1985 to 1994. This implies that staging procedures of PCa by bone scans were widely performed even in the earlier years of the study period, suggesting a good quality of the TNM classification data of PCa in the Finnish Cancer Registry database. In the Finnish Cancer Registry reports, the proportion of de novo metastatic PCa has recently been around 17%, higher than in Sweden [32], where the incidence of PCa is high and PSA screening is widely performed. This might also indicate a more aggressive PCa histology in cases that are classified as localized by the TNM system, and thus more commonly treated with immediate ADT than cases with less aggressive histology.

A few points are worthy of further consideration. As information on patient comorbidities and detailed PCa characteristics (i.e., Gleason scores and PSA values) was not collected, it was not possible to adjust for differences in morbidity and mortality with a potential link to ADT. Thus, a comparison of study outcomes in terms of PCSM and overall survival between the different groups was not possible. Also, due to the absence of data on patient comorbidities and PCa characteristics, it was not possible to determine who would benefit from primary ADT in localized PCa. However, propensity score matching, particularly when applied to socioeconomic status/education level, may have mitigated some of the comorbidity-related limitations. Detailed information on cancer treatment was also incomplete for both treatment groups. Although men in the observation group did not receive ADT or radical treatment in the four months following diagnosis, it is conceivable that some of them may have received treatment later. This limitation may have had a substantial effect on the study outcomes. Furthermore, although the study population included patients with localized PCa, the reliability of the staging procedures over time is debatable. TNM staging was based on mandatory reports obtained from hospitals and pathological laboratories. In other words, clinical practices in Finland were governed by national and/or European prostate cancer guidelines of the time. Consequently, the risk of metastases was evaluated according to these guidelines.

Notwithstanding these limitations, the study had several strengths. It was an observational population-based study estimating trends in cancer survival and mortality over time. While we did not directly compare different types of cancer treatments, population-based cohorts yield important information about PCa treatment in real-life situations, as the populations in randomized controlled trials are selected using stringent criteria by excluding out substantial proportion of real-life patients. However, in population-based studies patients are also allocated to different treatments, and results based on those can be subject to errors when comorbidities are involved. From an epidemiological perspective, these data determine the Finnish results obtained for patients managed with primary ADT or by observation. This study was based on nationwide data for PCa and included nearly 100% of patients in Finland over a nearly 30-year period. No previous population-based results from Finland on this subject have been published. Similar complete population-based coverage is not available in many European countries.

## Conclusion

Primary ADT within four months period from diagnosis is not associated with improved long-term overall survival or decreased PCSM than primary conservative management for men with localized PCa. However, the study's results may have been affected by patient selection or treatment intention as a consequence of general health and healthcare service–related factors.

## Supplementary information

**Additional file 1: Table S1.** Stage distribution of prostate cancer patients by TNM-classification in Finland from 1985 to 2014.

### Abbreviations

ADT: androgen deprivation therapy; PCa: prostate cancer; PCSM: prostate cancer–specific mortality; RR: relative risk; SMR: standardized mortality ratio

### Acknowledgements

Not applicable.

### Authors' contributions

AK, PB, NM, and JP designed the study. HS and KS performed the data acquisition. KS, HS, and JP analyzed and interpreted the data regarding prostate cancer and androgen deprivation therapy. HS, AK, and NM wrote the manuscript draft. AK, NM, JP, and PB revised the text for important intellectual content. AK, PB, and NM supervised the work. All authors read and approved the final manuscript.

### Author details

[1]Department of Surgery, Central Hospital of Central Finland, Jyväskylä, Finland. [2]Department of Urology, Turku University Hospital, Turku, Finland. [3]Department of Urology, University of Turku, Turku, Finland. [4]Finnish Cancer Registry, Helsinki, Finland. [5]Faculty of Social Sciences (Health Sciences), Tampere, Finland. [6]Department of Public Health, University of Helsinki, Helsinki, Finland. [7]School of Health Sciences, University of Tampere, Tampere, Finland. [8]Department of Urology, Tampere University Hospital, Tampere, Finland.

### References

1. Huggins C, Stevens R, Hodges C. Studies on prostatic cancer: II. The effects of castration on advanced carcinoma of the prostate gland. Arch Surg. 1941;43(2):209–23.
2. European Association of Urology Guidelines. 2018 Edition. ESTRO – ESUR – SIOG Prostate Cancer Guidelines Panel. EAU – ESTRO – ESUR – SIOG Guidelines on Prostate Cancer. Available from: [https://uroweb.org/guideline/prostate-cancer/]. Accessed 3 June 2019.
3. Ryan CJ, Small EJ. Early versus delayed androgen deprivation for prostate cancer: new fuel for an old debate. J Clin Oncol. 2005;23(32):8225–1.
4. Cooperberg MR, Grossfeld GD, Lubeck DP, Carroll PR. National practice patterns and time trends in androgen ablation for localized prostate cancer. J Natl Cancer Inst. 2003;95(13):981–9.
5. Basaria S, Bhasin S. Targeting the skeletal muscle–metabolism axis in prostate-cancer therapy. N Engl J Med. 2012;367(10):965–7.
6. Lu-Yao GL, Albertsen PC, Moore DF, Shih W, Lin Y, DiPaola RS, et al. Survival following primary androgen deprivation therapy among men with localized prostate cancer. JAMA. 2008;300(2):173–81.
7. Chodak GW, Thisted RA, Gerber GS, Johansson JE, Adolfsson J, Jones GW, et al. Results of conservative management of clinically localized prostate cancer. N Engl J Med. 1994;330(4):242–8.
8. Kattan MW, Cuzick J, Fisher G, Berney DM, Oliver T, Foster CS, et al. Nomogram incorporating PSA level to predict cancer-specific survival for men with clinically localized prostate cancer managed without curative intent. Cancer. 2008;112(1):69–74.
9. Johansson JE, Andren O, Andersson SO, Dickman PW, Holmberg L, Magnuson A, et al. Natural history of early, localized prostate cancer. JAMA. 2004;291(22):2713–9.
10. Leinonen MK, Miettinen J, Heikkinen S, Pitkaniemi J, Malila N. Quality measures of the population-based Finnish Cancer registry indicate sound data quality for solid malignant tumours. Eur J Cancer. 2017;77:31–9.
11. Cutler SJ, Ederer F. Maximum utilization of the life table method in analyzing survival. J Chronic Dis. 1958;8(6):699–712.
12. Ho D, Imai K, King G, Stuart E. Matching as nonparametric processing for reducing model dependence in parametric causal inference. Polit Anal. 2007;15(3):199–236.
13. popEpi: Functions for epidemiological analysis using population data. R package version 0.2.1. http://cran.r-project.org/package=popEpi. Accessed 2 Apr 2019.
14. Ho D, Imai K, King G, Stuart E. MatchIt: nonparametric preprocessing for parametric causal inference. J Stat Softw. 2011;42(8):1–28.
15. Lu-Yao GL, Albertsen PC, Moore DF, Shih W, Lin Y, DiPaola RS, et al. Outcomes of localized prostate cancer following conservative management. JAMA. 2009;302(11):1202–9.
16. Albertsen PC, Moore DF, Shih W, Lin Y, Li H, Lu-Yao GL. Impact of comorbidity on survival among men with localized prostate cancer. J Clin Oncol. 2011;29(10):1335–41.
17. Keating NL, O'Malley AJ, Smith MR. Diabetes and cardiovascular disease during androgen deprivation therapy for prostate cancer. J Clin Oncol. 2006; 24(27):4448–56.
18. Keating NL, O'Malley AJ, Freedland SJ, Smith MR. Diabetes and cardiovascular disease during androgen deprivation therapy: observational study of veterans with prostate cancer. J Natl Cancer Inst. 2010;102(1):39–46.
19. D'Amico AV, Denham JW, Crook J, Chen MH, Goldhaber SZ, Lamb DS, et al. Influence of androgen suppression therapy for prostate cancer on the frequency and timing of fatal myocardial infarctions. J Clin Oncol. 2007; 25(17):2420–5.
20. Saigal CS, Gore JL, Krupski TL, Hanley J, Schonlau M, Litwin MS. Androgen deprivation therapy increases cardiovascular morbidity in men with prostate cancer. Cancer. 2007;110(7):1493–500.
21. Nanda A, Chen MH, Braccioforte MH, Moran BJ, D'Amico AV. Hormonal therapy use for prostate cancer and mortality in men with coronary artery disease-induced congestive heart failure or myocardial infarction. JAMA. 2009;302(8):866–73.
22. Levine GN, D'Amico AV, Berger P, Clark PE, Eckel RH, Keating NL, et al. Androgen-deprivation therapy in prostate cancer and cardiovascular risk: a science advisory from the American Heart Association, American Cancer Society, and American urological association: endorsed by the American Society for Radiation Oncology. CA Cancer J Clin. 2010;60(3):194–201.
23. Nguyen PL, Je Y, Schutz FA, Hoffman KE, Hu JC, Parekh A, Beckman JA, Choueiri TK. Association of androgen deprivation therapy with cardiovascular death in patients with prostate cancer: a meta-analysis of randomized trials. JAMA. 2011;306(21):2359–66.
24. Studer UE, Whelan P, Albrecht W, Casselman J, de Reijke T, Hauri D, et al. Immediate or deferred androgen deprivation for patients with prostate cancer not suitable for local treatment with curative intent: European Organisation for Research and Treatment of Cancer (EORTC) trial 30891. J Clin Oncol. 2006;24(12):1868–76.
25. Lu-Yao GL, Albertsen PC, Moore DF, Shih W, Lin Y, DiPaola RS, et al. Fifteen-year survival outcomes following primary androgen-deprivation therapy for localized prostate cancer. JAMA Intern Med. 2014;174(9):1460–7.
26. Wong YN, Freedland SJ, Egleston B, Vapiwala N, Uzzo R, Armstrong K. The role of primary androgen deprivation therapy in localized prostate cancer. Eur Urol. 2009;56(4):609–16.
27. Potosky AL, Haque R, Cassidy-Bushrow AE, Ulcickas Yood M, Jiang M, Tsai HT, et al. Effectiveness of primary androgen-deprivation therapy for clinically localized prostate cancer. J Clin Oncol. 2014;32(13):1324–30.
28. Nordstrom T, Bratt O, Ortegren J, Aly M, Adolfsson J, Gronberg H. A population-based study on the association between educational length, prostate-specific antigen testing and use of prostate biopsies. Scand J Urol. 2016;50(2):104–9.
29. Kilpelainen TP, Pogodin-Hannolainen D, Kemppainen K, Talala K, Raitanen J, Taari K, et al. Estimate of opportunistic prostate specific antigen testing in the Finnish randomized study of screening for prostate Cancer. J Urol. 2017; 198(1):50–7.

30. Vickers AJ, Sjoberg DD, Ulmert D, Vertosick E, Roobol MJ, Thompson I, et al. Empirical estimates of prostate cancer overdiagnosis by age and prostate-specific antigen. BMC Med. 2014;12:26.
31. Stamey TA, Caldwell M, McNeal JE, Nolley R, Hemenez M, Downs J. The prostate specific antigen era in the United States is over for prostate cancer: what happened in the last 20 years? J Urol. 2004;172(4 Pt 1):1297–301.
32. Westerberg M, Franck Lissbrant I, Damber JE, Robinson D, Garmo H, Stattin P. Temporal changes in survival in men with de novo metastatic prostate cancer: nationwide population-based study. Acta Oncologica. 2020;59(1): 106–11.

# 5

# Burkitt's lymphoma of the prostate presenting as acute urinary retention

Marcus Derigs[1*], Anika Pehl[2], Jorge Riera-Knorrenschild[3], Rainer Hofmann[1] and Axel Hegele[1]

**Abstract**

**Background:** Non-Hodgkin lymphomas, which include Burkitt's lymphoma, affect the prostate in only 0.1% of cases. They most commonly present as painless lymphadenopathy elsewhere in the body and can cause abdominal or thoracic pain and systemic symptoms such as fever, weight loss and night sweats. Here we report a rare case of sporadic Burkitt's lymphoma of the prostate whose initial clinical presentation was acute urinary retention.

**Case presentation:** A 28-year-old Caucasian male presented repeatedly with urinary retention. First, he was misdiagnosed with alcohol-induced urinary retention and later with benign prostatic hyperplasia. After the appearance of new symptoms, including hematuria and hydronephrosis, endoscopic and radiographic evaluation was performed. Transurethral biopsy of the prostate secured the diagnosis of Burkitt's lymphoma. The symptoms receded under chemotherapy and complete remission of the disease was established.

**Conclusion:** This case report brings lymphomas into focus as a differential diagnosis for urinary retention in young males. Early use of extensive diagnostic measures is advised in patients with urinary retention for uncertain reasons to make prompt diagnosis and start appropriate treatment early.

**Keywords:** Urinary retention, Burkitt's lymphoma of the prostate, Non-Hodgkin lymphoma of the prostate

## Background

Burkitt's lymphoma is a specific non-Hodgkin B-cell lymphoma which first was described by Denis Burkitt in 1958 [1]. It makes up less than 1% of all non-Hodgkin lymphomas but is the most common non-Hodgkin lymphoma in childhood [2].

It can be divided into three subtypes: endemic, sporadic and immunodeficiency-associated. The endemic type is associated almost always with Epstein-Barr virus (EBV) infection and occurs frequently in African children. In western countries the sporadic form is more common. The immunodeficiency-associated type is seen in patients with HIV infection [3].

Sporadic Burkitt's lymphoma most commonly presents as abdominal lymphadenopathy with abdominal pain and other gastrointestinal symptoms [4]. It less commonly affects the head and neck region and only seldom occurs extranodally [5]. Non-Hodgkin's lymphomas affect the prostate in only 0.1% of cases [6]. A couple of case reports exists of prostatic Burkitt's lymphoma in childhood [7, 8]. In adults only four cases have been described [6, 9–11].

We report another case of prostatic Burkitt's lymphoma in a young male whose initial clinical sign was urinary retention. This case report and review of the literature are indented to reintroduce Burkitt's lymphoma and lymphomas as a whole to the list of differential diagnoses for acute urinary retention. Thereby it is supposed to sharpen diagnostic and clinical skills of urologists, oncologists and pathologists with special regard to treating young adult patients.

* Correspondence: derigs@med.uni-marburg.de
[1]Department of Urology and Pediatric Urology, University Hospital, Philipps-University Marburg, Baldingerstr. 1, 35043 Marburg, Germany
Full list of author information is available at the end of the article

## Case presentation

A 28-year-old Caucasian male (80 kg, 178 cm) was admitted to the emergency room with acute urinary retention and lower abdominal pain. The patient had consumed 1 l of wine and several beers within the last few hours. Otherwise, he was in a good general condition and had not complained about any urinary symptoms beforehand. The patient did not have any pre-existing conditions and his family history was negative for genitourinary disease including renal calculi. He admitted to smoking cigarettes and drinking alcohol regularly for more than 10 years. He did not take any illicit drugs or prescription medication. He had no known allergies. Physical examination revealed a distended lower abdomen. Digital rectal examination and all other physical findings did not show any abnormalities. Neurological examination was non-contributory. Ultrasound showed normal kidneys and a full bladder without any wall irregularities. The prostate was unremarkable and its size was not documented. Hence, the first working diagnosis was alcohol-induced urinary retention. Consequently, a Foley catheter was placed without any problems. It drained 1 l of clear urine. The complaints of the patient diminished gradually. Urinalysis showed normal values. A therapy trial with the nonsteroidal anti-inflammatory drug diclofenac (75 mg, twice daily) was initiated. The patient came back 2 days later for a trial without catheter (TWOC). Hereafter, he was able to urinate sufficiently. A month later, the patient suffered acute urinary retention again, this time without being under the influence of alcohol or other drugs. Physical examination and abdominal ultrasound now both revealed an enlarged prostate measuring approximately 50 ml. Laboratory tests did not show any abnormal values, including those of prostate-specific antigen (PSA) and lactate dehydrogenase (LDH). The working diagnosis was changed to urinary retention caused by benign prostatic hyperplasia. Alpha-blocker therapy with tamsulosin (0.4 mg, once daily) was started. Three days later another TWOC failed and a new Foley catheter was inserted. During the following weeks intermittent vesical tenesmus developed. Symptomatic treatment with the muscarinic antagonist trospium chloride (15 mg, twice daily) was started. Cystoscopy revealed diffusely erythematous and villous epithelium of the prostatic urethra up to the bladder neck and large obstructive lobes. An appointment was arranged for a transurethral resection of the prostate and bladder in a month's time. In the meantime, the patient developed persistent right-sided flank pain. Urinalysis showed leukocyturia and right-sided pyelonephritis was diagnosed. Antibiotic treatment with ciprofloxacin (500 mg, twice daily) was started by his general practitioner. Two days later the patient presented with hematuria and right-sided 2$^{nd}$ degree

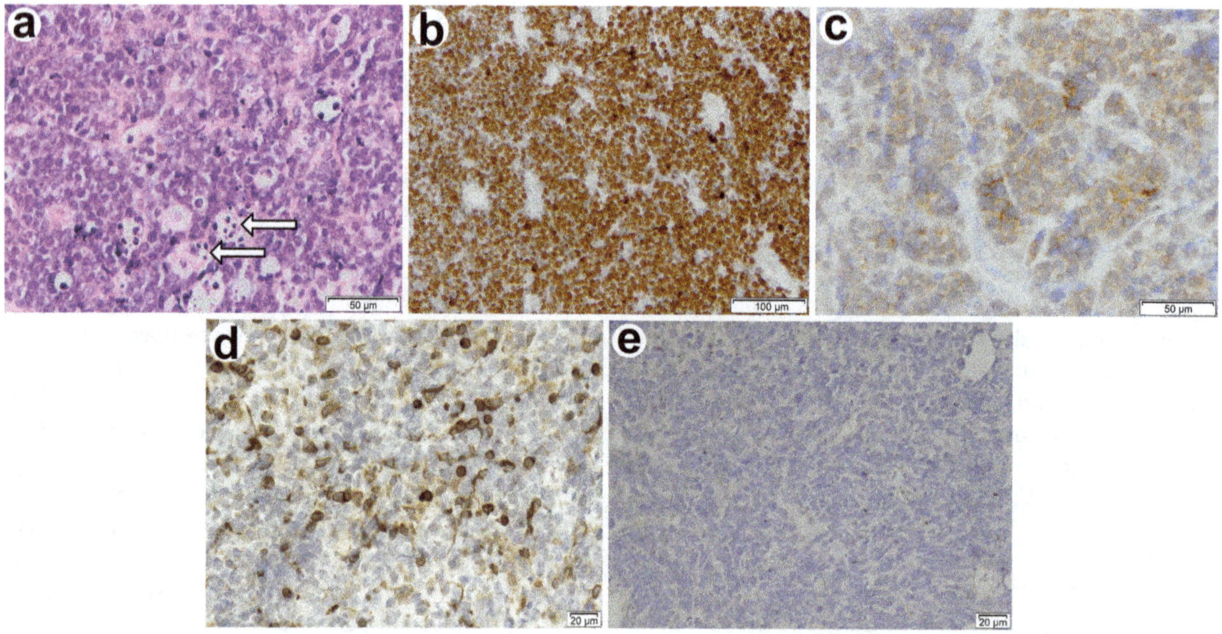


**Fig. 1** Histological and immunophenotypic features of prostatic Burkitt's lymphoma. Microscopic observation of transurethral biopsy of the prostate and bladder neck. Homogeneously basophilic, poorly differentiated B-cells and scattered tingible body macrophages with pale cytoplasm creating the characteristic starry sky appearance **a**. Lymphoma cells are almost 100% Ki-67 positive **b**, show moderate CD10 expression **c**, atypical Bcl-2 positivity **d** and negative results for EBER **e**. **a** Haematoxylin and eosin stain (200x magnification) revealing tingible body macrophages (arrows). **b** Ki-67 reactivity (100x magnification). **c** CD10 reactivity (200x magnification). **d** Bcl-2 reactivity (400x magnification). **e** EBER in situ hybridization (400x magnification)

hydronephrosis in the emergency room. Right-sided renal colic and hemorrhagic cystitis was suspected and the patient referred to the Department of Urology. Spasmoanalgesic therapy with metamizole (1 g, four times daily) was initiated and antibiotic treatment continued. A low-dose CT scan did not show urolithiasis but a tumor of the prostate. Cystoscopy revealed obstructive lobes of the prostate and an erythematous epithelium of the prostatic urethra and bladder neck again. The new working diagnosis was an unnoticed passing of the ureteral calculus alongside cystitis and benign prostatic hyperplasia, albeit persisting right-sided hydronephrosis. Flank pain and hematuria receded under analgesic therapy and Foley catheter placement. Transurethral biopsy of the prostate was scheduled. Until then left-sided flank pain and concomitant 2$^{nd}$ degree hydronephrosis developed while 2$^{nd}$ degree hydronephrosis on the right side persisted. Creatinine levels were elevated slightly and LDH levels were still within normal range. Cystoscopy now revealed a partly villous and solid tumor formation of the prostatic urethra which was infiltrating the trigone of the bladder including the ureteric orifices. Biopsies were taken endoscopically and ureteral stents were inserted bilaterally.

The histologic specimen provided evidence for a highly malignant Burkitt's lymphoma and proved the diagnosis of benign prostatic hyperplasia wrong (Fig. 1). It showed diffuse infiltration of the prostatic parenchyma by sheets of monomorphic medium-sized lymphoid cells with basophilic nucleoli. They were highly proliferative, indicated by many mitotic figures and also had a high number of apoptotic cells. Scattered among them were numerous tingible body macrophages. Due to their pale cytoplasm with incorporated apoptotic bodies they created a so called starry sky appearance, which is characteristic for Burkitt's lymphoma. Immunohistochemistry confirmed this diagnosis and showed the typical reactivity for CD20, a co-expression for CD10 and a strong expression for Ki-67 of nearly all tumor cells. Untypical for Burkitt's lymphoma was the relatively strong Bcl-2 expression of B-cells, which is only expressed by about 10% of Burkitt's lymphomas [12]. The Ebstein-Barr virus-encoded small RNAs (EBER) in situ hybridization stain was negative.

Diagnosis was further confirmed by fluorescence in situ hybridization that gave normal results for the *BCL6* probe, but showed the typical translocation t(8;14) with probes for *MYC* and t (8;14) (Fig. 2). This translocation induces the fusion of *MYC* and *IGH* gene loci and thereby leads to the dysregulation of the protooncogene *MYC* [13].

The patient was referred to the Department of Oncology and was scheduled for staging CT scan in preparation for chemotherapy 1 week later. His general condition was progressively declining as he experienced night sweats, melena and constipation. Laboratory results showed anemia (8.2 g/dl), increased C-reactive protein (CRP) levels and normal LDH levels. Contrast-enhanced staging CT of thorax and abdomen revealed an 85 × 65 × 44 mm tumor of the prostate with seminal vesicle and bladder invasion. Also, retroperitoneal and iliac chain lymphadenopathy (up to 17 × 13 mm in size) and gastric wall thickening were present (Fig. 3).

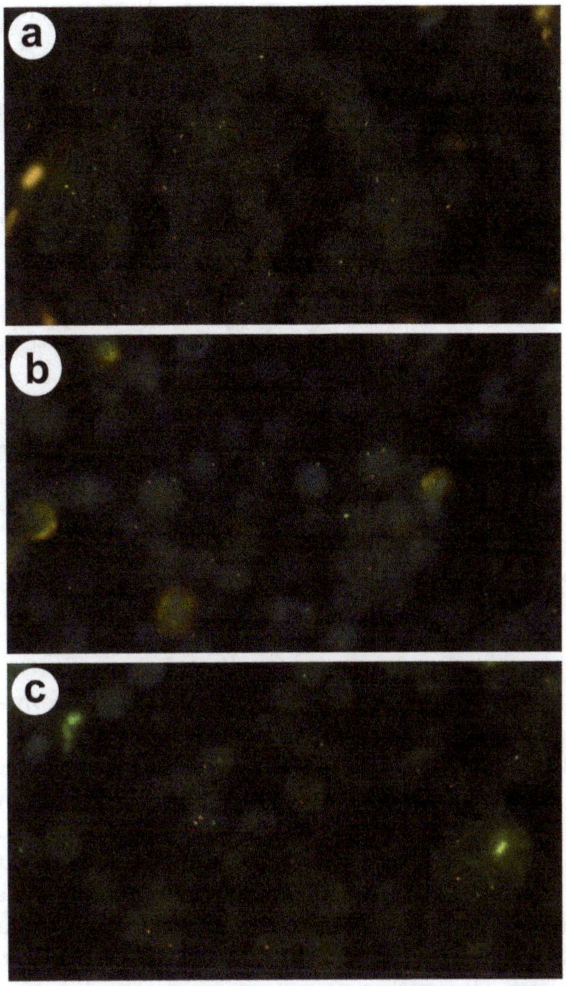


**Fig. 2** FISH analyses of prostatic Burkitt's lymphoma. Microscopic observation of transurethral biopsy of the prostate and bladder neck. **a** FISH for *MYC*. Break apart assay to detect breakpoints in the *MYC* gene, showing separation of the probes (red and green) on one allele (1000x magnification). **b** FISH for *BCL6*. The break apart assay shows no evidence of breakpoints in the *BCL6* gene (1000x magnification). **c** FISH for t(8;14). Fusion assay confirming the typical translocation t(8;14) (1000x magnification)

Gastroscopy ruled out upper gastrointestinal bleeding and confirmed diagnosis of gastric involvement of Burkitt's lymphoma via biopsy. Bone marrow biopsy and lumbar puncture excluded involvement of bone marrow and liquor concluding a stage IV Burkitt's lymphoma according to the Lugano staging system [14]. Before

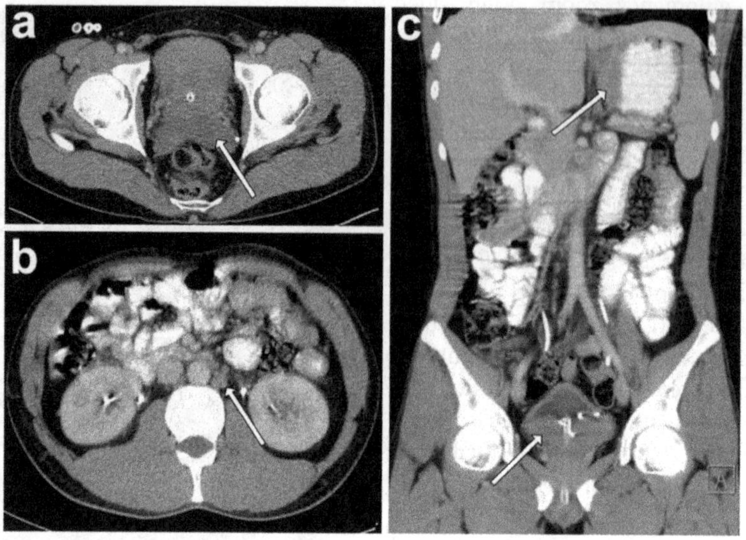


**Fig. 3** Radiographic extent of Burkitt's lymphoma. Contrast enhanced staging CT scan after diagnosis of prostatic Burkitt's lymphoma. **a** Axial view showing prostatic involvement and infiltration of the seminal vesicles (arrow). **b** Axial view showing involvement of paraaortic lymph nodes (arrow). **c** Coronal view showing bladder infiltration and gastric involvement (arrows). Ureteral stents and Foley catheter are visible

chemotherapy was initiated, the patient performed sperm cryopreservation.

Ultimately, the diagnosis of Burkitt's lymphoma was made 4 months after initial presentation and only 6 days later systemic chemotherapy according to the GMALL (German Multicenter Study Group for Adult Acute Lymphoblastic Leukemia) B-ALL/NHL 2002 protocol was started. It consisted of a total of 6 cycles of 3 different drug regimen including dexamethasone, cyclophosphamide, rituximab, dexamethasone, vincristine, ifosfamide, etoposide, cytarabine and high-dose methotrexate. Concurrent medication was composed of acyclovir, trimethoprim/sulfamethoxazole, ciprofloxacin, pantoprazole, G-CSF, amphotericin B mouth rinse and Glandomed® mouthrinse. The first cycle was given as a milder regimen with dexamethasone and cyclophosphamide together with hydration, allopurinol and urinary alkalization in order to prevent tumor lysis syndrome. Nonetheless, the patient developed neutropenic fever and grade 4 mucositis and required extensive analgesic and antibiotic treatment. Due to increasing abdominal pain a CT scan was done which excluded a tumor lysis with gastric perforation. It rather showed a response to treatment according to Lugano treatment response criteria (Fig. 4) [14].

During the following cycles there was one more episode of neutropenic fever. Mucositis persisted only on a lower level. The Foley catheter was removed 2 months after initiation of chemotherapy. Hereafter satisfactory voiding with insignificant post-void residual volume was established. After finishing chemotherapy, a CT scan showed complete response. Following this, both ureteral stents were removed. Subsequent sonography of the

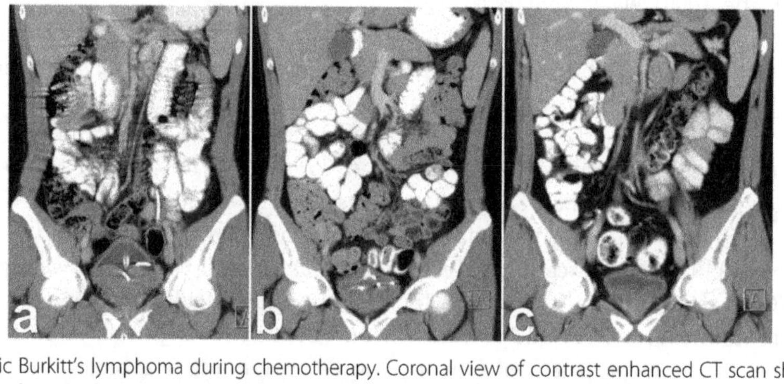


**Fig. 4** Regression of prostatic Burkitt's lymphoma during chemotherapy. Coronal view of contrast enhanced CT scan showing prostatic Burkitt's lymphoma before (**a**), during (**b**) and after (**c**) chemotherapy. Burkitt's lymphoma caused urinary retention and bilateral hydronephrosis. **a** Foley catheter and ureteral stents were inserted and chemotherapy started. **b** After one of 6 cycles significant downsizing of the lymphoma was seen. **c** Foley catheter and ureteral stents could be removed after 6 cycles of chemotherapy

kidneys could exclude persisting hydronephrosis. Another CT scan 3 months later confirmed complete remission of Burkitt's lymphoma (Fig. 4c). The patient recovered completely and is now participating in follow-up care.

## Discussion and conclusion

Acute urinary retention (AUR) is one of the most common urologic emergencies and will be encountered by physicians of every specialty. It is described as the sudden inability to urinate and is usually managed by transurethral catheterization [15]. The incidence of AUR is reported in 2.2 events per 1000 man-years in men over 45 years old [16]. Almost all patients with AUR are men at the age of over 60 with an identifiable predisposing risk factor. In general, there are three reasons for AUR. Firstly, any event that increases the resistance to subvesical urinary flow. This is mainly achieved by mechanical obstruction by a variety of reasons (Table 1). The most common cause is forward displacement of the internal urethral orifice by benign prostatic hyperplasia (BPH) in men above the age of 50.

However, AUR is a rare event in young adults. In this age group the most common cause for AUR are urethral calculi, urethral strictures or urinary tract infections such as cystitis, urethritis or prostatitis [17, 18]. Hence, younger patients have to be carefully evaluated. Only very rarely BPH leads to acute urinary retention in young adult males below the age of 40. A few case reports exist of such patients as well as for children [19–21]. Other reasons causing obstruction are pelvic and prostatic tumors of any kind. Also, a dynamic obstruction due to an increase in the smooth and/or striated muscle tone has to be considered. Secondly, interrupted sensory innervation of the bladder wall or motor supply of the detrusor muscle is a reason for AUR. This might be caused by demyelination or spinal cord compression [22]. The depression of the cortical areas for voluntary micturition or of the detrusor nuclei in the brainstem and interference of neurotransmission at the bladder or urethra by a number of drugs can also cause AUR [23]. Frequent triggers are central nervous depressants such as alcohol and medication like anticholinergics, sympathomimetics and antineoplastic agents [24].

Thirdly, AUR is precipitated by any situation that leads to an overdistension of the bladder (post-surgery, drugs) [25].

The reason for obstructive urinary retention in the presented case turned out to be prostatic Burkitt's Lymphoma, a subtype of non-Hodgkin lymphoma. Less than 0.1% of all non-Hodgkin lymphomas affect the prostate of which diffuse large B-cell lymphoma is the most common entity [6]. In younger aged patients malignant rhabdomyosarcomas are the most common prostatic malignancy [26]. Only a couple of case reports exists of prostatic Burkitt's lymphoma in childhood [7, 8]. To date in adults only four cases have been described [6, 9–11]. Lymphoma of the prostate is very rare and is usually not considered in patients with urinary retention. On the other hand, adenocarcinoma of the prostate or BPH are equally rare entities in young males and should not be assumed without further investigation either. In this case a young male was treated for urinary retention and was misdiagnosed twice. Initially, the consumption of alcohol by the patient and a lack of other findings led to the working-diagnosis of alcohol-induced urinary retention. Even though the pathophysiologic reasoning for alcohol-induced urinary retention are CNS-depression and bladder overdistention, an anti-inflammatory therapy with diclofenac was started. In the beginning, the diagnosis was affirmed by a successful TWOC, so no other diagnostic tests were performed.

**Table 1** Reasons for urinary retention. Modified after [18, 25]

| Reasons for urinary retention |
|---|
| **Reasons for mechanical obstruction** |
| Adenocarcinoma or sarcomatoid carcinoma of the prostate |
| Benign prostatic hyperplasia |
| Prostatic, appendiceal abscess |
| Prostatitis, cystitis, urethritis |
| Chronic lymphocytic leukemia |
| Sarcoma, lymphoma of the prostate |
| Urolithiasis |
| Ectopic Ureterocele |
| Constipation |
| Urethral valves, strictures |
| Uterine fibroids or other tumors |
| Impacted retroverted uterus |
| Gastrointestinal tumors |
| Haematocolpos |
| Cystocele or rectocele |
| Foreign bodies (external or internal) |
| Trauma |
| Phimosis, paraphimosis |
| Blood clots from bleeding in the bladder or upper urinary tract |
| **Reasons for increased sphincter tone** |
| Neurofibromatosis in the prostate |
| Anorectal surgery |
| Fowler's syndrome |
| **Reasons for interference with sensory or motor innervation to the bladder** |
| Diabetic cystopathy |
| Herpes zoster in the sacral dermatomes (S2-S4) |
| Drug-induced |
| Cauda equina syndrome/Elsberg syndrome/Guillan-Barré syndrome |
| Psychogenic |
| Transverse myelitis in Lyme disease |

More common causes for AUR in this age group were not suspected due to absent flank pain, normal urinalysis and unremarkable micturition in the past. After urinary retention recurred, clinical and sonographic examination revealed an enlarged prostate. Notwithstanding the rarity in this age group, BPH was diagnosed without further workup. Prompt performance of cystoscopy or other imaging techniques would have led to the correct diagnosis earlier. Instead, progression of the lymphoma caused both-sided hydronephrosis, hematuria and systemic symptoms.

In conclusion, this case shows that the unlikely event of urinary retention in a young adult male has to be of great concern. After all, it can be the first manifestation of a serious prostatic malignancy. Thorough interviewing of previous and current symptoms and physical examination have to be performed to narrow down differential diagnoses. If benign reasons are ruled out or if initial treatment fails, more extensive diagnostic tests including cystoscopy and imaging techniques like CT or MRI scan are mandatory. Subsequent biopsy of the prostate should be performed urgently to secure the diagnosis. In our case systemic chemotherapy led to complete remission and possibly cure of the Burkitt's lymphoma.

### Abbreviations

AUR: Acute urinary retention; Bcl-2: B-cell Lymphoma 2; BPH: Benign prostatic hyperplasia; CRP: C-reactive protein; CT: Computed tomography; G-CSF: Granulocyte-colony stimulating factor; GMALL : German Multicenter Study Group for Adult Acute Lymphoblastic Leukemia; LDH: Lactate dehydrogenase; HIV: Human immunodeficiency virus; FISH: Fluorescence in situ hybridization; MRI: Magnetic resonance imaging; PSA: Prostate-specific antigen; TWOC: Trial without catheter

### Acknowledgements

Not applicable.

### Authors' information (optional)

MD is a 3rd year resident in the Department of Urology of the University Hospital Marburg.

### Authors contributions

MD and AH were the main treating physicians. MD wrote the manuscript and conducted the literature review. AH revised the manuscript. AP performed the histopathological analysis. JRK carried out chemotherapy and revised the part describing the treatment of the disease. RH made supervision and reviewed the manuscript. All authors read and approved the final manuscript.

### Author details

[1]Department of Urology and Pediatric Urology, University Hospital, Philipps-University Marburg, Baldingerstr. 1, 35043 Marburg, Germany. [2]Department of Pathology, University Hospital, Philipps-University Marburg, Baldingerstr 1, 35043 Marburg, Germany. [3]Department of Hematology and Oncology, University Hospital, Philipps-University Marburg, Baldingerstr. 1, 35043 Marburg, Germany.

### References

1. Burkitt D. A sarcoma involving the jaws in African children. Br J Surg. 1958;46:218–23.
2. Linch DC. Burkitt lymphoma in adults. Br J Haematol. 2012;156(6):693–703.
3. Ferry JA. Burkitt's lymphoma Clinicopathologic features and differential diagnosis. Oncologist. 2006;11:375–83.
4. Mbulaiteye SM, Biggar RJ, Bhatia K, Linet MS, Devesa SS. Sporadic childhood Burkitt lymphoma incidence in the United States during 1992-2005. Pediatr Blood Cancer. 2009;53(3):366–70.
5. Molyneux EM, Rochford R, Griffin B, Newton R, Jackson G, Menon G, et al. Burkitt's lymphoma. Lancet. 2012;379(9822):1234–44.
6. Pereira Aras JG. Primary prostatic infiltration by Burkitt's lymphoma. Arch Esp Urol. 1997;50(8):906–8.
7. Sinclair N, Babyn P, Kinloch M, Sinha R. A rare and unusual case of Burkitt's lymphoma presenting with a prostate mass in a 12-year-old boy. Case Rep Radiol. 2014;2014:106176.
8. Bostwick DG. Malignant lymphoma involving the prostate: report of 62 cases. Cancer. 1998;83(4):732–8.
9. Gardella S. Prostatic tumor as the presenting form of a Burkitt-type undifferentiated lymphoma. Med Clin (Barc). 1986;86(11):466–8.
10. Boe S. Burkitt's lymphoma mimicking prostatitis. J Urol. 1981;125(6):891–2.
11. Lewis RH. Burkitt's lymphoma presenting as urinary outflow obstruction. J Urol. 1983;130(1):120–4.
12. Pervez S, Raza MQ, Mirza A, Pal A. Strong BCL2 expression in Burkitt lymphoma is not uncommon in adults. Indian J Pathol Microbiol. 2011;54(2):290–3.
13. Maifrede S, Skorski T. IGH/MYC translocation in Burkitt lymphoma is associated with BRCA2 deficiency and synthetic lethality by PARP1 inhibitors. Blood. 2016;128(22):4111.
14. Cheson BD, Fisher RI, Barrington SF, Cavalli F, Schwartz LH, Zucca E, et al. Recommendations for initial evaluation, staging, and response assessment of Hodgkin and non-Hodgkin lymphoma: the Lugano classification. J Clin Oncol. 2014;32(27):3059–68.
15. Dawson CWH. Urological Emergencies in general practice. BMJ. 1996;(312):838–40.
16. Verhamme KM, Dieleman JP, van Wijk MA, Bosch JL, Stricker BH, Sturkenboom MC. Low incidence of acute urinary retention in the general male population: the triumph project. Eur Urol. 2005;47(4):494–8.
17. Singh V, Sinha RJ. Acute urinary retention in young adult and middle-aged males due to calculi in the urethra: a single Centre experience from North India. Actas Urologicas Espanolas. 2011;36:75–8.
18. Selius BA, Subedi R. Urinary retention in adults- diagnosis and initial management. Am Fam Physician. 2008;77(5):643–50.
19. Georgiades F, Demosthenous S, Antoniades G, Kouriefs C. Giant benign prostatic hyperplasia in a young adult male. Urology. 2014;84(2):e4–5.
20. Sumiya H. Benign prostatic hypertrophy in a young male. Eur Urol. 1987;13(5):355–7.
21. Harada M. A case of prostatic hyperplasia in a young male. Hinyokika Kiyo. 1991;37:768–73.
22. Tintinalli JE. Acute urinary retention as a presenting sign of spinal cord compression. Ann Emerg Med. 1986;15(10):147–9.
23. Gillenwater JY. The pathophysiology of urinary obstruction. Campbell's Urology. 1986:542–72.
24. McGuire J. Neuromuscular dysfucntion of the lower urinary tract. Campbell's Urology. 1986:616–30.
25. Emberton MAK. Acute urinary retention in men- an age old problem. BMJ. 1999;318:921–5.
26. Humphrey PA, Moch H, Cubilla AL, Ulbright TM, Reuter VE. The 2016 WHO classification of Tumours of the urinary system and male genital organs-part B: prostate and bladder Tumours. Eur Urol. 2016;70(1):106–19.

# 6

# miR-185 inhibits prostate cancer angiogenesis induced by the nodal/ALK4 pathway

Youkong Li[1*†], Wen Zhong[2†], Min Zhu[1], Mengbo Li[1] and Zhenwei Yang[1]

**Abstract**

**Background:** Inhibition of angiogenesis in prostatic cancer could be a brand-new method to suppress tumour progression. Nodal/ALK4 has been associated with vascularization in many cancers. However, the relationship between and role of Nodal/ALK4 and miR-185 in human prostatic cancer is still unknown.

**Methods:** Prostatic cancer DU145 cells and LNCaP cells were used to investigate the angiogenic effect induced by Nodal and the anti-angiogenic roles of miR-185. Colony formation assay, MTT assay, transwell assay and tube formation assay were used to explore cell proliferation, migration and tube-forming ability, respectively. A luciferase reporter assay confirmed the binding relationship between miR-185 and ALK4. The expression levels of miR-185, ALK4 and VEGF were detected by qRT-PCR and Western blotting. The effects of miR-185 and Nodal in prostate cancer were also investigated in animal experiments.

**Results:** VEGF expression was increased in DU145 cells and LNCaP cells after Nodal incubation, and Nodal activated the proliferation ability of prostatic cancer cells and the migration and tube-forming ability of human umbilical vein endothelial cells (HUVECs), which were all inhibited by treatment with the Nodal inhibitor SB431524. Bioinformatics analysis and luciferase assay were used to verify miR-185 as a target of ALK4. Prostatic cancer cell proliferation was inhibited by overexpression of miR-185, which was shown to regulate the migration and angiogenesis of HUVECs by targeting ALK4 for suppression. miR-185 also showed a significant inverse correlation with Nodal treatment and reversed the angiogenic effects induced by Nodal. More importantly, for the first time, xenograft experiments indicated that overexpression of miR-185 suppressed tumour development.

**Conclusion:** The Nodal/ALK4 pathway is important in the angiogenesis of prostate cancer and can be inhibited by targeting miR-185 to downregulate ALK4. These findings provide a new perspective on the mechanism of prostate cancer formation.

**Keywords:** Nodal, miR-185, ALK4, Angiogenesis, Prostate cancer

## Background

Prostate cancer is the most common malignant tumour among men and has the second highest mortality rate among cancers in developed countries and regions such as Europe and the United States [1]. The incidence of prostate cancer in Asia is lower than that in Europe, but it has shown a rapid upward trend in recent years [2]. The blood supply of malignant tumours is a key factor in tumour growth. It is known that some tumour cells play a role in the angiogenesis pathway to provide sufficient oxygen and nutrients for tumour growth, invasion

* Correspondence: liyoukong@126.com
†Youkong Li and Wen Zhong are co-first authors
[1]Department of Urology, Jingzhou Central Hospital and The Second Clinical Medical College, Yangtze University, No.60 Jingzhong Road, Jingzhou District, Jingzhou 434020, Hubei Province, People's Republic of China
Full list of author information is available at the end of the article

and metastasis and have different characteristics than conventional vascular endothelial cells [3]. Inhibition of tumour vascularization has been found to increase the necrosis of tumour cells. Thus, in-depth exploration of the molecular mechanism of angiogenesis in prostate cancer is of great significance for its treatment.

Nodal, a member of the transforming growth factor beta (TGFβ) superfamily, has properties that promote tumour cell plasticity and tumourigenicity [4, 5]. It was reported in the literature that Nodal was highly expressed in prostate cancer cells such as WPE, DU145, and LNCaP and could regulate prostate cancer proliferation by activating smad 2/3 phosphorylation by activin receptor-like kinase 4 (ALK4) [6]. Another report indicated that Nodal could promote the formation of tumour angiogenesis mimicry in malignant tumours such as breast cancer [7]. However, whether the Nodal/ALK4 pathway is related to the regulation of prostate cancer angiogenesis has not been reported in the literature.

In recent years, miRNAs have been shown to have an important effect on the progression of tumours, especially by acting as oncogenes or tumour suppressor genes in tumourigenesis and the regulation of tumour molecular mutations. Each miRNA has many potential target genes, and finding a true target gene that acts on tumour cell behaviour is crucial. miR-185 was shown to be expressed at low levels in prostate cancer cell lines and tissues and to inhibit prostate cancer progression by inducing apoptosis [8]. A previous study demonstrated that in human microvascular endothelial cells, miR-185 could inhibit angiogenesis by targeting STIM1 [9], but the function of miR-185 in prostate cancer angiogenesis has not been reported. We found that there was a binding site for miR-185 on ALK4 through bioinformatics analysis. Therefore, we wanted to test whether miR-185 inhibited the Nodal/ALK4 pathway, thereby inhibiting prostate cancer angiogenesis.

In this study, the relationship between the Nodal/ALK4 pathway and angiogenesis was first evaluated in prostate cancer cells. Then, whether miR-185 could regulate the Nodal/ALK4 pathway was investigated. The anti-angiogenic effects of miR-185 in prostate cancer cells were explored via an in vitro cell model and with animal experiments. Therefore, our results could determine whether miR-185 inhibited the Nodal/ALK4 pathway and angiogenesis in prostate cancer.

## Methods

### Cell culture and treatment

Human umbilical vein endothelial cells (HUVECs) and the human prostate cancer DU145 cells and LNCaP cells were purchased from American Type Culture Collection (ATCC, Manassas, VA, USA). RPMI 1460 medium (Gibco, Waltham, MA, USA) supplemented with 10% foetal bovine serum (HyClone, Logan, UT) and 1% penicillin–streptomycin (Gibco, Waltham, MA, USA) was used for cell culture at 37 °C in 7% $CO_2$ for 3–4 days. To study the relationship between the Nodal/ALK4 pathway and angiogenesis, both cell lines were treated with Nodal (Sigma, St Louis, MO, USA) for 8 h at a concentration of 5 μM. To explore the effect of prostate cancer on angiogenesis, HUVECs were co-cultured with DU145 cells and LNCaP cells.

### Quantitative reverse-transcription polymerase chain reaction (qRT-PCR)

miR-185 was verified using a TaqMan primer and probe set from Applied Biosystems. Total RNA was isolated from human DU145 cells and LNCaP cells using TRIzol reagent (TransGen Biotechnology Co., Ltd., Beijing, China). A cDNA Reverse Transcription kit (TransGen Biotechnology Co., Ltd., Beijing, China) was used to obtain cDNA following the manufacturer's instructions. Single-stranded cDNA was generated by TaqMan PCR Master Mix (TransGen Biotechnology Co., Ltd., Beijing, China), and U6 and GAPDH acted as internal controls. The primers used for the analysis were as follows: miR-185 forward: 5′-CGCTGGAGAGAAAGGCAGT-3′, reverse: 5′-GTCGTATCCAGTGCAGGGTCCGAGGT ATTCGCACTGGATACGACTCAGGA-3′; ALK4 forward: 5′-CTGCAACAGGATCGACTTGA-3′, reverse: 5′-GGAGCGTCTTGTCTTTGGAG-3′; VEGF forward: 5′-GGGCAGAATCATCACGAAGT-3′, reverse: 5′- TG GTGATGTTGGACTCCTCA-3′; U6 forward: 5′-CT CGCTTCGGCAGCACA-3′, reverse: 5′-AACGCTTC ACGAATTTGCGT-3′; GAPDH forward: 5′-TGTGGG CATCAATGGATTTGG-3′, reverse: 5′-ACACCATG TATTCCGGGTCAAT-3′. PCRs were run three times, and the experiment was conducted in triplicate. According to the formula $2^{-\Delta\Delta Ct}$, the relative fold changes in mRNA expression were verified [10].

### Western blot analysis

Total proteins were extracted from tissues and cells by RIPA buffer, and the concentration was determined by a BCA protein assay kit. Protein (30 μg) was separated by 10% sodium dodecyl sulfate (SDS) polyacrylamide gel electrophoresis (PAGE) and transferred onto polyvinylidene fluoride (PVDF) membranes (Santa Cruz Biotech, USA). After blocking with 15% blocking solution, the membranes were incubated with a primary rabbit polyclonal antibody against VEGF (1:800, Abcam, Cambridge, MA, USA) and primary mouse monoclonal antibody against ALK4 (1:500, Santa Cruz Biotechnology, Inc., Dallas, TX, USA) overnight at 4 °C. A primary rabbit polyclonal antibody against β-actin (1:2000, Abcam, Cambridge, MA, USA) was then applied as an internal reference. Following three washes with TBST, a horseradish peroxidase-conjugated antibody against the corresponding species (1:2000, Santa Cruz Biotech, USA) was added for a 1 h incubation at room temperature, and then an ECL detection kit (Jiancheng Bioengineering Institute, Nanjing, China) was used for band detection. All bands were visualized and quantified by ImageJ software (NIH, Bethesda, Maryland, USA). The experiment was conducted in triplicate. The result was expressed as the band intensity ratio of the target protein to the internal reference protein.

#### Colony formation assay

After 14 days of culture, the corresponding treated DU145 cells and LNCaP cells were fixed with methanol. Crystal violet dye solution was used to stain colonies, and then the colony-forming units were counted under an optical microscope (Leica, Wetzlar, Germany) with a 20-fold objective.

#### MTT assay

Cell viability was assessed by the MTT assay. Human prostate cancer DU145 cells and LNCaP cells were co-cultured with HUVECs and then subjected to specific treatment, which included Nodal or Nodal+SB431524 incubation for 8 h, or miR-185 mimics or miR-NC transfection. After treatment, MTT (0.5 mg/ml in pH 7.4 PBS, Sigma, USA) was added to each well for 4 h at 37 °C. The supernatant was removed. After washing with phosphate-buffered saline (PBS) three times, 150 µl dimethyl sulfoxide (DMSO, Sigma, USA) was added, and the plate was agitated to dissolve the precipitates. The absorbance was measured by a multiwell spectrophotometer (Biotek Instruments Inc., Burlington, Vermont) at 490 nm. The experiment was conducted in triplicate.

#### Transwell assay

In 8-mm pore 24-well transwell chambers, HUVECs were first cultured for 8 h before invasion towards the conditioned medium. The upper chamber was filled with 200 µl serum-free medium, while the lower chamber contained 10% FBS medium. After 48 h of incubation, cells in the upper chamber were collected with a cotton swab. Then, cells were fixed with 5% glutaraldehyde in PBS for 15 min, and 0.1% crystal violet was applied to the lower chamber for microscopic inspection (Leica, Wetzlar, Germany). At least five different fields were randomly selected for each sample. The cell migration capacity was verified by calculating the number of cells passing through the membrane.

#### Tube formation assay

Basement membrane matrix (BMM) was added to each well and then allowed to harden at 37 °C for 30 min. HUVECs were cultured on top of the BMM-coated wells for 48 h at 37 °C. The morphology of HUVECs was observed under an optical microscope (Leica, Wetzlar, Germany) with a 20-fold objective. Images were obtained using an Olympus IX70 microscope (Tokyo, Japan).

#### Cell transfection

Human miR-185 mimics and their relative control mimics (mimics NC) and human miR-185 inhibitor and its relative control inhibitor (inhibitor NC) were purchased from GenePharma (Shanghai, China). Full-length human ALK4 cDNA was amplified and cloned into the pcDNA3.1 vector (OE-ALK4). DU145 cells or LNCaP cells were cultured, and Lipofectamine 2000 (Invitrogen, California, USA) containing nucleotide fragments was added to Opti-MEM at room temperature for a 0.5-h incubation and then added to cells for a 6-h incubation. After removing the above culture medium, cells were cultured under normal conditions for detection after 48 h.

#### Luciferase activity assay

To obtain the reporter vector ALK4-wild-type, the fragment from the 3′-untranslated region (3'UTR) of ALK4 containing the predicted miR-185 binding site was synthesized and cloned into the pmirGLO vector (Promega, Madison, WI, USA). Sites were mutated to generate ALK4-mutated to disrupt the predicted miR-185 binding site. miR-185 mimics or miR-185 inhibitor and vectors (WT-ALK4–3'UTR or MUT-ALK4–3'UTR) were cotransfected into cells. After 48 h, cells were analysed by the dual-luciferase kit (Promega, California, USA) for luciferase activity. Each experiment was performed in triplicate. The results are presented as relative luciferase activity (firefly LUC/Renilla LUC).

#### Xenograft experiments in nude mice

All animal experiments were performed in accordance with protocols approved by the Animal Research Committee of the Second Clinical Medical College of Yangtze University. Male BALB/c nude mice (approximately 20 g) at 6 weeks of age were purchased from SJA Laboratory Animal Co., Ltd. (Hunan, China). DU145 cells ($2 \times 10^6$) and LNCaP cells ($2 \times 10^6$) were subcutaneously injected into the right side of the armpits of BALB/c nude mice. To assess the antitumour activity in a xenograft model in vivo, the mice were randomly divided into four groups: control, Nodal, mimics NC, and miR-185 mimics ($n = 6$ per group). After palpable tumours developed a volume of approximately 50 mm$^3$, the mice were injected with a PBS solution as a control, Nodal, mimics NC, or miR-185 mimics through intratumor injection, and tumour growth was examined during the course of 28 days. The tumour width and length were measured by a micrometre. The tumour volumes were calculated as (length × width$^2$)/2. Tumour growth was observed for 28 days, at which time the mice were euthanized. The largest diameters of the formed tumours were measured macroscopically, and the tumours were weighed with an electronic balance at the end of the experiment.

### Immunohistochemical staining

Tumour tissues were obtained from euthanized mice after the indicated treatments and fixed with paraformaldehyde (Sigma-Aldrich, St Louis, MO, USA) diluted to 10% in PBS for 24 h. For immunohistochemical staining, the sections were cut serially (5 μm) and boiled at 121 °C for 20 min in 10 mM citrate buffer solution (pH 6.0) for antigen retrieval. After endogenous peroxidase activity was blocked with 0.3% hydrogen peroxide, the sections were incubated with a primary rabbit polyclonal antibody against CD31 (1:800, Abcam, Cambridge, MA, USA) overnight at 4 °C. After adding a goat anti-rabbit secondary antibody (1:1200, Abcam, Cambridge, MA, USA) for 30 min incubation at room temperature, the sections were incubated with a DAB detection kit (Jiancheng Bioengineering Institute, Nanjing, China). Following dehydration and clearing, the sections were analysed by general microscopy (Leica, Wetzlar, Germany).

### Statistical analysis

Statistical analysis of the data was performed in SPSS 16.0. All values are shown as the average ± SD. Student's t-test and one-way analysis of variance (ANOVA) were used to perform comparisons between two groups and multiple groups, respectively. Statistically significant differences were considered at $P < 0.05$.

## Results

### Nodal promoted prostate cancer cell-induced angiogenesis

To determine whether Nodal treatment affected prostate cancer cell angiogenesis, DU145 cells and LNCaP cells were divided into three groups: control, Nodal, and Nodal+SB431524, where SB431524 is an inhibitor of Nodal. Western blot analysis of VEGF in DU145 cells and LNCaP cells was first performed. The results are shown in Fig. 1a. This finding suggested that Nodal induced VEGF expression in both DU145 cells and LNCaP cells, which was inhibited by SB431524. Then, a colony formation assay was used to detect the proliferation of prostate cancer cells. The results in the two cell types consistently demonstrated that the proliferative capacity of the Nodal group was stronger than that of the control group, while there was no significant difference between the control group and the Nodal+SB431524 group (Fig. 1b). The results of cell viability at 8 h after incubation with Nodal or Nodal+SB431524 in HUVECs co-cultured with DU145 cells or LNCaP cells were consistent with the colony formation assay results detected by MTT (Fig. 1c). Additionally, the migration ability of HUVECs co-cultured with DU145 cells or LNCaP cells was detected by transwell assay. Nodal induced HUVEC migration in co-culture with DU145 cells or LNCaP cells. Compared to DU145 cells or LNCaP cells treated with Nodal alone, HUVECs co-cultured with DU145 cells or LNCaP cells decreased the number of migrated HUVECs after treatment with Nodal+SB431524 (Fig. 1d). Angiogenesis mimicry in co-culture of HUVECs with DU145 cells or LNCaP cells in three-dimensional culture was observed. Slight angiogenesis mimicry was observed in the control group at 48 h in the three-dimensional culture, but obvious angiogenesis mimicry was observed in the Nodal group (Fig. 1e). By adding SB431524, the observed angiogenesis mimicry induced by Nodal was relieved (Fig. 1e). These results indicated that Nodal promoted prostate cancer cell-induced angiogenesis.

### miR-185 inhibited ALK4 expression by binding to the 3'-UTR of ALK4

By using StarBase, we predicted the miRNAs that may interact with ALK4 to investigate interactions between ALK4 and miRNAs. The bioinformatics prediction results shown in Fig. 2a indicate the presence of a binding site of miR-185 on ALK4. We also performed a luciferase reporter assay to further verify whether ALK4 was a functional target of miR-185. The results demonstrated that miR-185 mimics decreased the luciferase activity of ALK4-WT, whereas it had no influence on the luciferase activity of ALK4-MUT (Fig. 2b). qRT-PCR (Fig. 2c&d) and Western blotting (Fig. 2e) were performed to verify the expression levels of miR-185 and ALK4. In DU145 cells and LNCaP cells, miR-185 inhibitor decreased the gene expression level of miR-185 and consequently increased the gene and protein expression of ALK4, while miR-185 mimics increased the gene expression level of miR-185 and thus decreased the gene and protein expression of ALK4. The Western blot and qRT-PCR results were consistent and suggested a potential role of miR-185 in regulating ALK4 expression.

### miR-185 targets ALK4 to regulate angiogenesis induced by prostate cancer cells

We have demonstrated the relationship between miR-185 and ALK4. To further prove whether miR-185 could regulate angiogenesis through ALK4, DU145 cells or LNCaP cells were divided into four groups: control, mimics NC, miR-185 mimics, and miR-185 mimics+OE-ALK4. Western blot analysis of VEGF in DU145 cells and LNCaP cells was first performed (Fig. 3a). miR-185

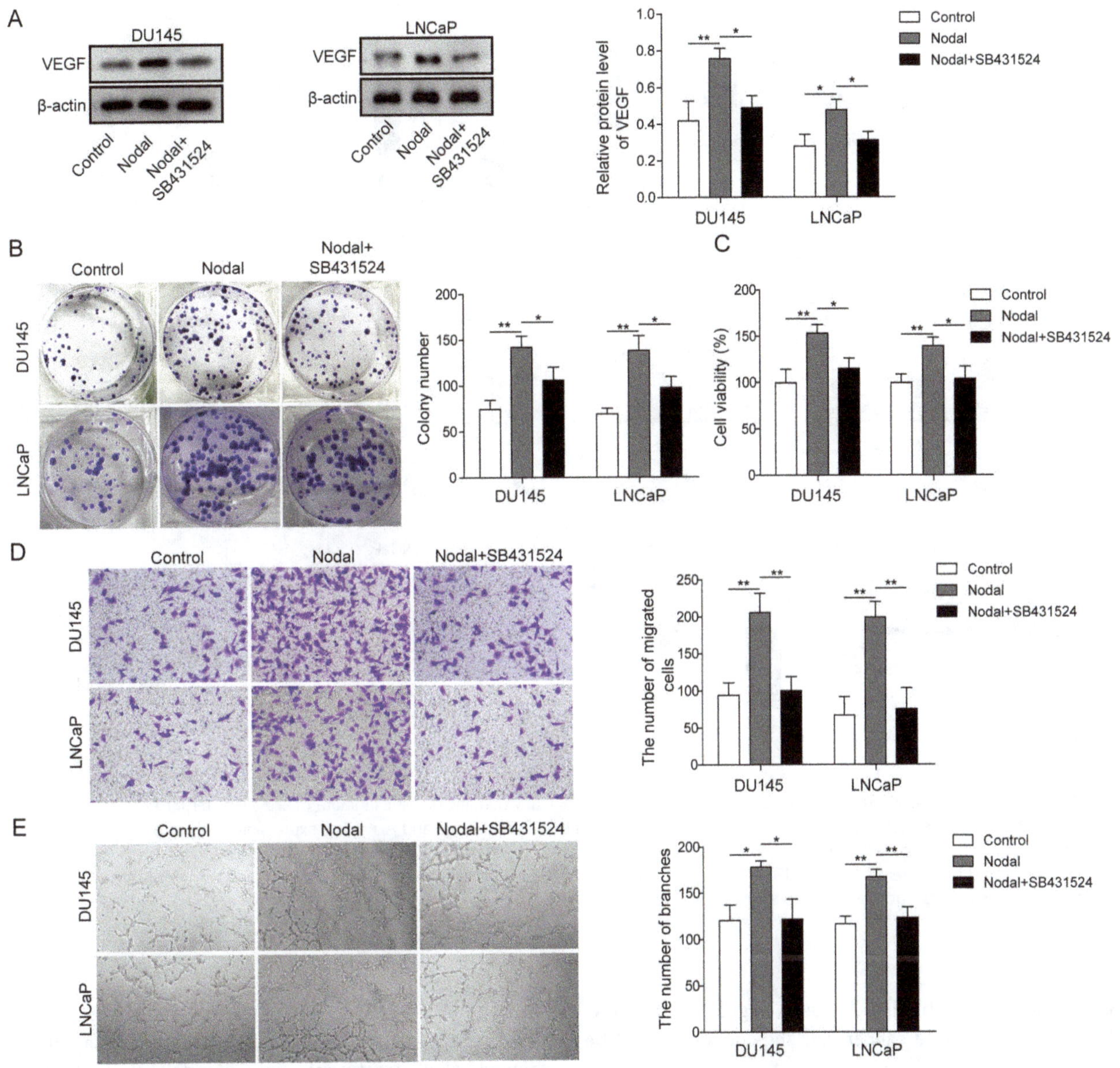


**Fig. 1** Nodal promoted prostate cancer cell-induced angiogenesis. **a** Protein levels of VEGF were assessed by Western blot in DU145 cells and LNCaP cells treated with Nodal or SB431524. **b** Representative photomicrographs of the colony formation assay and quantification of colony numbers in DU145 cells and LNCaP cells treated with Nodal or SB431524. **c** Cell viability of co-cultured HUVECs was evaluated by MTT assay and was determined as the percentage of the value relative to that of the control group. **d** The migration ability of co-cultured HUVECs was detected by transwell assay. **e** Tube forming ability of HUVECs was observed after the indicated treatment. The data represent one of three independent experiments. Error bars denote the mean ± SD. $^{*}P < 0.05$, $^{**}P < 0.01$

mimics significantly inhibited VEGF expression compared with that in the control group and mimics NC group, while overexpression of ALK4 reversed the above effect of miR-185 mimics (Fig. 3a). The colony formation assay shown in Fig. 3b clearly demonstrated that miR-185 mimics inhibited prostate cancer cell proliferation, which was blocked by ALK4 overexpression. The viability of HUVECs co-cultured with DU145 cells or LNCaP cells displayed the same trends (Fig. 3c). With miR-185 mimic treatment, HUVEC viability was reduced, and simultaneous overexpression of miR-185 and ALK4 could restore viability to the level of the control group (Fig. 3c). Cell migration was inhibited in HUVECs co-cultured with DU145 cells or LNCaP cells treated with miR-185 mimics, while miR-185 mimics plus OE-ALK4 increased the number of migrated HUVECs (Fig. 3d). Additionally, Fig. 3e verified that miR-185 mimics + OE-ALK4 reversed HUVEC angiogenesis inhibited by miR-

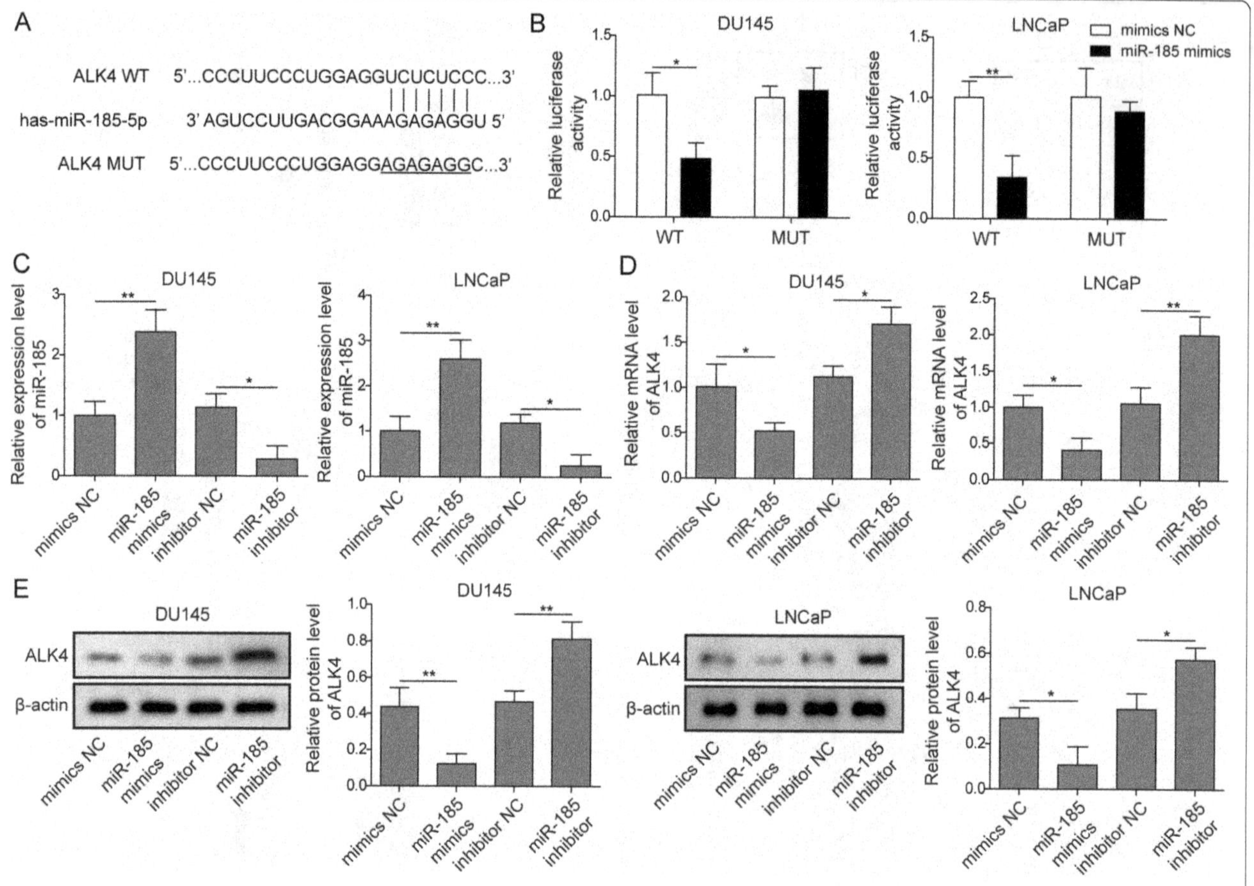

**Fig. 2** miR-185 inhibited ALK4 expression by binding to the 3'-UTR of ALK4. **a** Schematic of the candidate miRNAs that target ALK4 predicted by StarBase. **b** Dual-luciferase assay was performed to study the interaction between miR-185 and ALK4. The expression levels of miR-185 **c** and ALK4 **d** were quantified by qRT-PCR in DU145 cells and LNCaP cells transfected with miR-185 mimics or miR-185 inhibitor. **e** Protein levels of ALK4 were assessed by Western blotting in DU145 cells or LNCaP cells with the indicated treatments. The data represent one of three independent experiments. Error bars denote the mean ± SD. *$P < 0.05$, **$P < 0.01$

185 mimics. Undoubtedly, ALK4 is regulated by miR-185, and thus prostate cancer cell angiogenesis could be affected.

### miR-185 inhibited angiogenesis through the nodal/ALK4 pathway

To explore the role of miR-185 in Nodal/ALK4 pathway-induced angiogenesis, DU145 cells or LNCaP cells were divided into four groups: control, Nodal, Nodal+mimics NC, and Nodal+miR-185 mimics. qRT-PCR (Fig. 4a) and Western blotting (Fig. 4b) of ALK4 and VEGF in DU145 cells and LNCaP cells were first conducted. The results of qRT-PCR and Western blot consistently suggested the potential role of miR-185 mimics in regulating the Nodal/ALK4 signalling pathway. Nodal treatment induced ALK4 expression, thereby increasing VEGF levels (Fig. 4a&b). However, with miR-185 mimic treatment, the expression of ALK4 was significantly decreased compared with that in the Nodal+mimics NC group, thus reversing the level of VEGF (Fig. 4a&b). The colony formation assay results showed that treatment with Nodal alone induced prostate cancer cell proliferation, and miR-185 mimics inhibited the above effect of Nodal (Fig. 4c). In HUVECs co-cultured with DU145 cells or LNCaP cells, Nodal induced HUVEC proliferation, and the viability of HUVECs was higher than that of the control group, which was restored by miR-185 mimics (Fig. 4d). The migration ability results in HUVECs was confirmed with the cell viability results in HUVECs (Fig. 4e), displaying the opposite effect between Nodal and miR-185 mimics. In the angiogenesis test of HUVECs co-cultured with DU145 cells or LNCaP cells, Nodal induced HUVEC angiogenesis, and miR-185 mimics inhibited the angiogenic effect of Nodal (Fig. 4f). Therefore, miR-185 showed a significant inverse correlation with Nodal treatment, reversing the angiogenesis effects induced by Nodal.

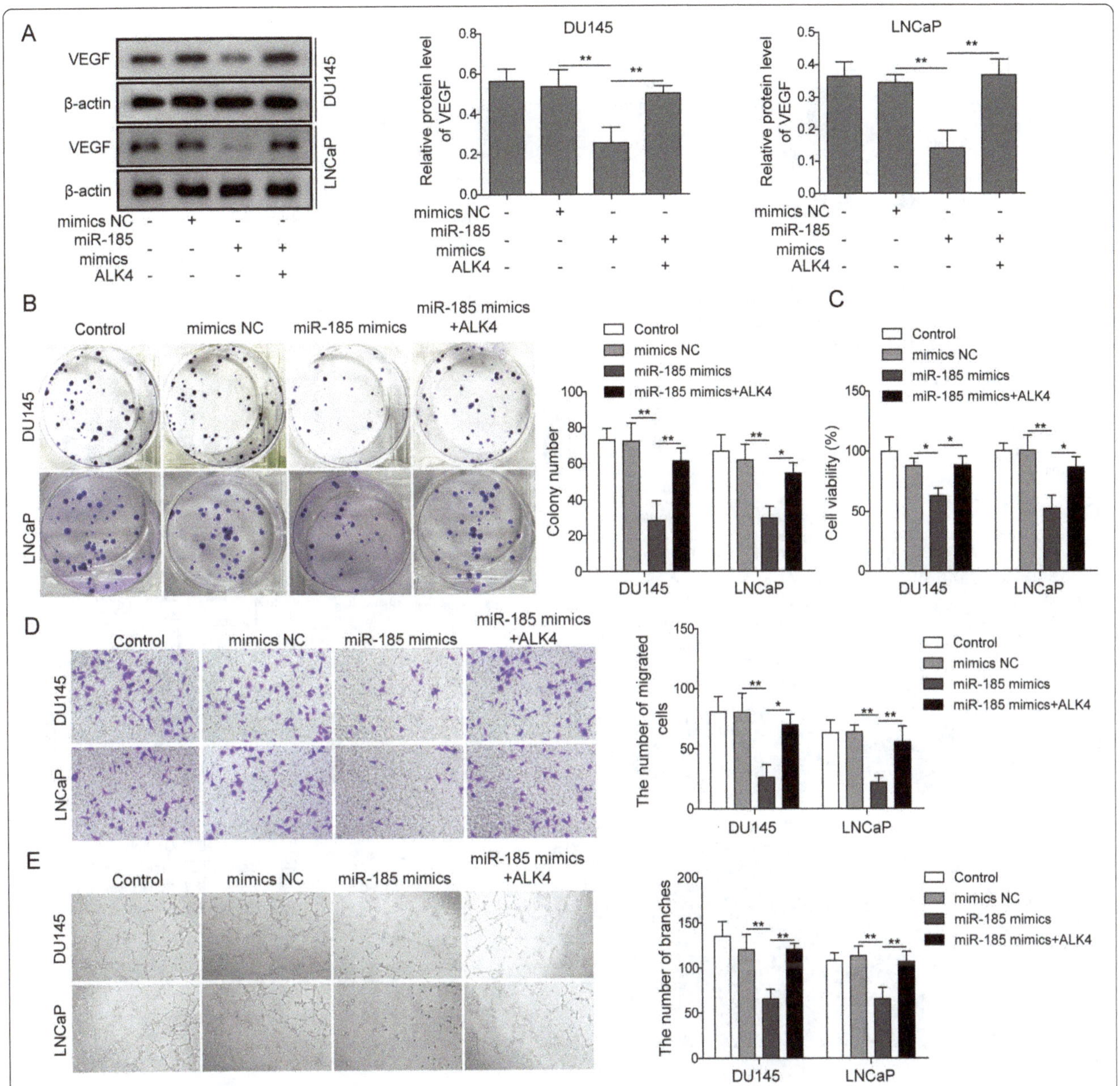


**Fig. 3** MiR-185 targeted ALK4 to regulate angiogenesis induced by prostate cancer cells. **a** Protein levels of VEGF were assessed by Western blot in DU145 cells and LNCaP cells transfected with miR-185 mimics or pcDNA3.1-ALK4. **b** Representative photomicrographs of the colony formation assay and quantification of colony numbers in DU145 cells and LNCaP cells transfected with miR-185 mimics or pcDNA3.1-ALK4. **c** Cell viability of co-cultured HUVECs was evaluated by MTT assay and was determined as the percentage of the value relative to that of the control group. **d** The migration ability of co-cultured HUVECs was detected by transwell assay. **e** Tube forming ability of HUVECs was observed after the indicated treatment. The data represent one of three independent experiments. Error bars denote the mean ± SD. $^*P < 0.05$, $^{**}P < 0.01$

### Overexpression of miR-185 exerted antitumor activity against tumor growth in nude mice

To determine the in vivo effects of miR-185 and Nodal on tumor growth in a xenograft model, DU145 cells or LNCaP cells were injected subcutaneously into 6-week-old male athymic nude mice (BALB/c-nu/nu). The mice were randomly divided into control, Nodal, mimics NC and miR-185 mimics group. The macroscopic appearance of the dissected tumor tissues after 28 days from specific treatments was shown in Fig. 5a. Obviously, the tumors in the Nodal-treated group were significantly larger than those in the control group, and after overexpressing miR-185, the tumors were the smallest. The statistical results of tumor size (Fig. 5b) and tumor weight (Fig. 5c) were consistent with the above trends. The results of Western blotting in Fig. 5c verified that Nodal treatment accelerated the expression of VEGF while overexpression of miR-185 inhibited this abnormal

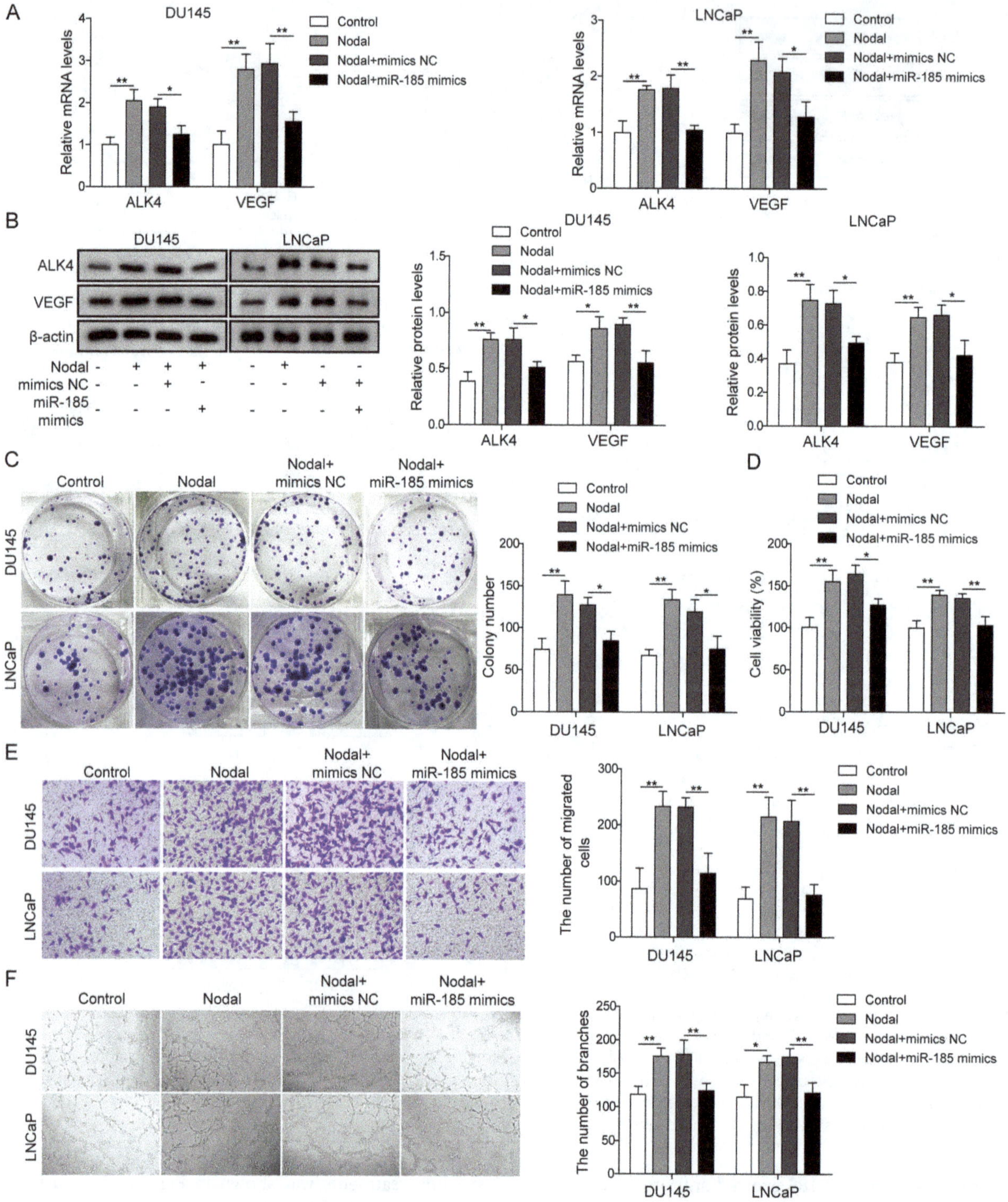


**Fig. 4** miR-185 inhibited angiogenesis through the Nodal/ALK4 pathway. **a** The mRNA levels of ALK4 and VEGF were quantified by qRT-PCR in DU145 cells and LNCaP cells treated with Nodal or transfected with miR-185 mimics. **b** Protein levels of ALK4 and VEGF were assessed by Western blot in DU145 cells and LNCaP cells with the indicated treatments. **c** Representative photomicrographs of the colony formation assay and quantification of colony numbers in DU145 cells and LNCaP cells treated with Nodal or transfected with miR-185 mimics. **d** Cell viability of co-cultured HUVECs was evaluated by MTT assay and was determined as the percentage of the value relative to that of the control group. **e** The migration ability of co-cultured HUVECs was detected by transwell assay. **f** The tube forming ability of HUVECs was observed after the indicated treatment. The data represent one of three independent experiments. Error bars denote the mean ± SD. *$P < 0.05$, **$P < 0.01$

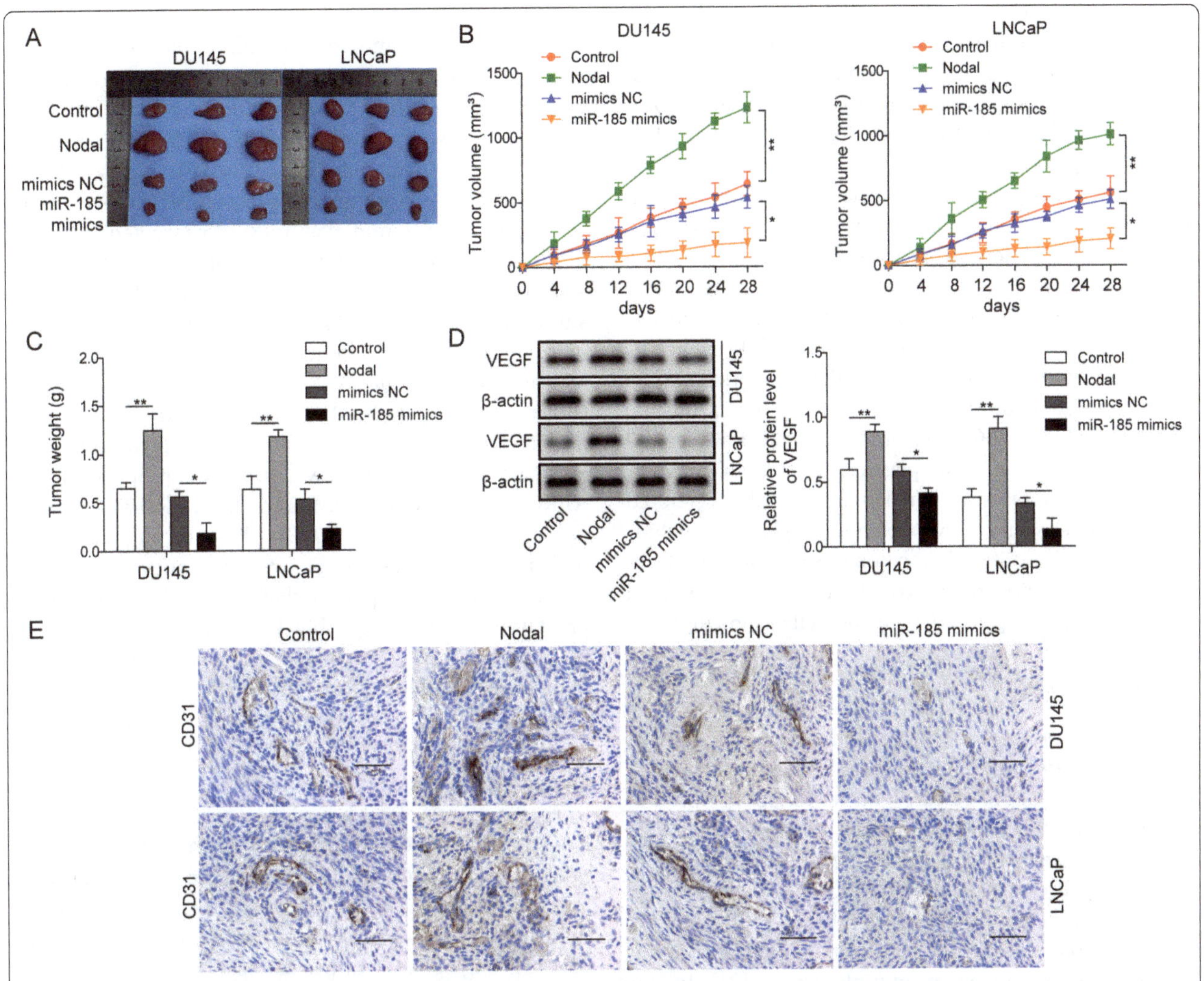


**Fig. 5** Overexpression of miR-185 exerted antitumour activity against tumour growth in nude mice. **a** The macroscopic appearance of the dissected tumour tissues 30 days after the treatments. **b** The tumour size was calculated in nude mice subjected to specific treatments. **c** The tumour weight was calculated in nude mice subjected to specific treatments. **d** Protein levels of VEGF were assessed by Western blot in nude mice treated with specific treatments. **e** The distribution of CD31 was detected by immunohistochemistry. Scale bar: 50 μM. The data represent one of three independent experiments. Error bars denote the mean ± SD. *$P < 0.05$, **$P < 0.01$

expression. Based on basic level of VEGF in control group, miR-185 overexpressed attenuated the tumor progression. As shown in Fig. 5e, there was significantly abundant expression of angiogenesis biomarker CD31 observed in Nodal group, while miR-185 mimics could reduce the expression of CD31. Analysis of the data of xenograft experiments revealed that overexpression of miR-185 suppressed tumor growth in an in vivo xenograft model.

## Discussion

In this study, we provided evidence of the association between Nodal and prostatic cancer. The results suggest that Nodal/ALK4 is involved in the regulation of angiogenesis in pancreatic cancer. miR-185 could decrease prostatic cancer cell proliferation and HUVEC migration and angiogenesis, while overexpression of ALK4 in DU145 cells or LNCaP cells could suppress the effect of miR-185, indicating that miR-185 targeted ALK4 to regulate angiogenesis in prostate cancer. The animal experiments clearly showed that overexpression of miR-185 suppressed prostate carcinoma development in vivo. All the results implied that miR-185 may act as a tumour suppressor in the angiogenesis of prostate cancer by inhibiting the Nodal/ALK4 pathway.

Angiogenesis is the basis of reproduction, growth and repair and is also a necessary condition for tumour growth and metastasis. Studies have shown that high protein expression in prostate cancer tissue can promote blood vessel growth [11]. In our study, we found that Nodal incubation could increase the expression of VEGF, resulting in HUVEC proliferation and migration, which is characteristic of vascularization. Nodal is a member of the transforming growth factor beta superfamily. It has been found that Nodal expression is limited to human embryonic stem cells and embryonic tissues [12]. However, the Nodal protein was found to be highly expressed in some tumour tissue cells, suggesting that Nodal expression is associated with tumourigenesis, development, invasion and metastasis. Taylor et al. found that the protein expression of Nodal was lower in benign prostatic disease tissues than in prostate cancer tissues [13]. Stable expression of the Nodal gene enhanced LNCaP cell growth on Matrigel [14], which is consistent with our findings in the migration assay. Nodal promoted tumour angiogenesis by increasing the expression of the VEGF receptor [15], and downregulation of Nodal inhibited the plasticity of tumour cells [4]. In the study by Dueng-Yuan Hueng, Nodal accelerated the angiogenesis and growth of human gliomas, including glioma cell proliferation, colony formation, VEGF secretion, and angiogenesis [16]. Our research obtained similar results in prostatic cancer cells, showing that Nodal dramatically increased HUVEC viability and tube-forming ability.

miR-185 is located on chromosome 22q11.21, and its precursor consists of 82 nucleotides [17]. Although there has been no in-depth research on its function, miR-185 is considered to be a tumour suppressor gene in a variety of tumours and inhibits the proliferation of lung cancer [18], breast cancer [19], and colon cancer [20], which may indicate diverse effects of miR-185 in inhibiting cell proliferation. In lung cancer cells, miR-185 inhibited the expression of multiple cyclins [21]. In our study, Nodal increased the expression of VEGF, while overexpressing miR-185 inhibited the concentration of VEGF. miR-185 inhibited VEGF expression and HUVEC viability, migration and tube-forming ability, thus resulting in a reduced trend of angiogenesis. To further explore the inhibition mechanism of miR-185 on the angiogenesis of prostate cancer cells, we found through bioinformatics analysis that ALK4 had a miR-185 binding site. Overexpression of ALK4 in the Nodal pathway could significantly reverse the effects of miR-185 overexpression on VEGF levels, cell proliferation, migration and angiogenesis, but it could not be reversed to the same level as the control group, indicating that miR-185 exerted its antitumour effect through the Nodal/ALK4 pathway. In addition to Nodal/ALK4, miR-185 might exert its antitumour effect through other signalling pathways. It was demonstrated that miR-185 could suppress Wnt/β-catenin signalling and modulate the transcription and translation levels of downstream molecules of this pathway, including MYC and CCND1, in human colorectal cancer, thus exerting tumour suppressor effects [22]. Pan et al. found that lncAGER had an inhibitory effect on cell proliferation through upregulation of advanced glycosylation end-product specific receptor (AGER) by competitively binding to miR-185 in lung cancer [23]. It is possible that miR-185 inhibits cell proliferation by different mechanisms in different tumour cells. Zhu et al. found that miR-185 targeted Six2 and inhibited cell proliferation and epithelial-mesenchymal transition in hepatocellular carcinoma [24]. Another study showed that miR-185 inhibited angiogenesis in human microvascular endothelial cells by targeting stromal interaction molecule 1 [25]. Moreover, our results showed that miR-185 not only inhibited the proliferation of prostate cancer cells but also inhibited the migration and tube formation of HUVECs by inhibiting the Nodal/ALK4 pathway. Qu et al. found that miR-185 regulated cell cycle arrest at the G0/G1 phase through CDC6 to prevent the progression of prostate cancer [26]. Additionally, Li et al. reported that miR-185 is involved in prostate cancer through blockade of the SREBP metabolic pathway [27]. Therefore, we suspect that miR-185 may have multiple effects in prostate cancer, but in-depth studies are still needed to verify this assumption.

## Conclusions

In recent years, research on Nodal protein has become a new trend. At present, there are no reports on the expression and target significance of Nodal/ALK4 in prostate cancer cells. The results of this experiment showed that miR-185 could regulate Nodal/ALK4 pathway to inhibit the angiogenesis of prostate cancer, which provided a new perspective on the mechanism of prostate cancer formation.

**Abbreviations**

ALK4: Activin receptor-like kinase 4; GADPH : Glyceraldehyde-3-phosphate dehydrogenase; HUVEC: Human umbilical vein endothelial cells; qRT-PCR : Quantitative real-time polymerase chain reaction; STIM1: Stromal interaction molecule 1; TGFβ: Transforming growth factor β; VEGF: Vascular endothelial growth factor

**Acknowledgements**

Not applicable.

,

**Authors contributions**

YL, WZ: protocol/project development; YL, WZ, MZ, ML: data collection or management; MZ, ZY: data analysis; YL, WZ: manuscript writing; YL, WZ: critical revision of the manuscript. All authors read and approved the final manuscript.

**Author details**

[1]Department of Urology, Jingzhou Central Hospital and The Second Clinical Medical College, Yangtze University, No.60 Jingzhong Road, Jingzhou District, Jingzhou 434020, Hubei Province, People's Republic of China. [2]Department of Endocrine, Jingzhou Central Hospital and The Second Clinical Medical College, Yangtze University, Jingzhou 434020, Hubei Province, People's Republic of China.

**References**

1. Torre LA, Bray F, Siegel RL, Ferlay J, Lortet-Tieulent J, Jemal A. Global cancer statistics, 2012. CA Cancer J Clin. 2015;65(2):87–108.
2. Chen R, Ren S, Yiu MK, Fai NC, Cheng WS, Ian LH, et al. Prostate cancer in Asia: a collaborative report. Asian J Urol. 2014;1(1):15–29.
3. Byrne AM, Bouchier-Hayes DJ, Harmey JH. Angiogenic and cell survival functions of vascular endothelial growth factor (VEGF). J Cell Mol Med. 2005; 9(4):777–94.
4. Bodenstine TM, Chandler GS, Seftor REB, Seftor EA, Hendrix MJC. Plasticity underlies tumor progression: role of nodal signaling. Cancer Metastasis Rev. 2016;35(1):21–39.
5. Gong W, Sun B, Sun H, Zhao X, Zhang D, Liu T, et al. Nodal signaling activates the Smad2/3 pathway to regulate stem cell-like properties in breast cancer cells. Am J Cancer Res. 2017;7(3):503.
6. Vo BT, Khan SA. Expression of nodal and nodal receptors in prostate stem cells and prostate cancer cells: autocrine effects on cell proliferation and migration. Prostate. 2011;71(10):1084–96.
7. Liu TJ, Sun BC, Zhao XL, Zhao XM, Sun T, Gu Q, et al. CD133+ cells with cancer stem cell characteristics associates with vasculogenic mimicry in triple-negative breast cancer. Oncogene. 2013;32(5):544.
8. Gordanpour A, Nam RK, Sugar L, Seth A. MicroRNAs in prostate cancer: from biomarkers to molecularly-based therapeutics. Prostate Cancer Prostatic Dis. 2012;15(4):314.
9. Hou J, Liu L, Zhu Q, Wu Y, Tian B, Cui L, et al. MicroRNA-185 inhibits angiogenesis in human microvascular endothelial cells through targeting stromal interaction molecule 1. Cell Biol Int. 2016;40(3):318–28.
10. Livak KJ, Schmittgen TD. Analysis of relative gene expression data using real-time quantitative PCR and the 2– ΔΔCT method. Methods. 2001;25(4): 402–8.
11. Quail DF, Walsh LA, Zhang G, Findlay SD, Moreno J, Fung L, et al. Embryonic protein nodal promotes breast cancer vascularization. Cancer Res. 2012; 72(15):3851–63.
12. Strizzi L, Hardy KM, Kirsammer GT, Gerami P, Hendrix MJC. Embryonic signaling in melanoma: potential for diagnosis and therapy. Lab Investig. 2011;91(6):819.
13. Taylor RA, Fraser M, Livingstone J, Espiritu SMG, Thorne H, Huang V, et al. Germline BRCA2 mutations drive prostate cancers with distinct evolutionary trajectories. Nat Commun. 2017;8:13671.
14. Lawrence MG, Margaryan NV, Loessner D, Collins A, Kerr KM, Turner M, et al. Reactivation of embryonic nodal signaling is associated with tumor progression and promotes the growth of prostate cancer cells. Prostate. 2011;71(11):1198–209.
15. van Iterson V, Leidenius M, von Smitten K, Bono P, Heikkilä P. VEGF-D in association with VEGFR-3 promotes nodal metastasis in human invasive lobular breast cancer. Am J Clin Pathol. 2007;128(5):759–66.
16. Hueng D-Y, Hsieh C-H, Cheng Y-C, Tsai W-C, Chen Y. Cordycepin inhibits migration of human glioblastoma cells by affecting lysosomal degradation and protein phosphatase activation. J Nutr Biochem. 2017;41:109–16.
17. Fang M, Li Y, Wu Y, Ning Z, Wang X, Li X. MiR-185 silencing promotes the progression of atherosclerosis via targeting stromal interaction molecule 1. Cell Cycle. 2019 (just-accepted).
18. Takahashi Y, Forrest ARR, Maeno E, Hashimoto T, Daub CO, Yasuda J. MiR-107 and MiR-185 can induce cell cycle arrest in human non small cell lung cancer cell lines. PLoS One. 2009;4(8):e6677.
19. Tang H, Liu P, Yang L, Xie X, Ye F, Wu M, et al. miR-185 suppresses tumor proliferation by directly targeting E2F6 and DNMT1 and indirectly upregulating BRCA1 in triple-negative breast cancer. Mol Cancer Ther. 2014; 13(12):3185–97.
20. Liu M, Lang N, Chen X, Tang Q, Liu S, Huang J, et al. miR-185 targets RhoA and Cdc42 expression and inhibits the proliferation potential of human colorectal cells. Cancer Lett. 2011;301(2):151–60.
21. Sun C-C, Zhang L, Li G, Li S-J, Chen Z-L, Fu Y-F, et al. The lncRNA PDIA3P interacts with miR-185-5p to modulate oral squamous cell carcinoma progression by targeting cyclin D2. Mol Ther Nucleic Acids. 2017;9:100–10.
22. Dong-Xu W, Jia L, Su-Juan Z. MicroRNA-185 is a novel tumor suppressor by negatively modulating the Wnt/β-catenin pathway in human colorectal cancer. Indian J Cancer. 2015;52(7):182.
23. Pan Z, Liu L, Nie W, Miggin S, Qiu F, Cao Y, et al. Long non-coding rna ager-1 functionally upregulates the innate immunity gene ager and approximates its anti-tumor effect in lung cancer. Mol Carcinog. 2018;57(3): 305–18.
24. Zhu SM, Chen CM, Jiang ZY, Yuan B, Ji M, Wu FH, et al. MicroRNA-185 inhibits cell proliferation and epithelial-mesenchymal transition in hepatocellular carcinoma by targeting Six2. Eur Rev Med Pharmacol Sci. 2016;20(9):1712–9.
25. Zeng Q, Tao X, Huang F, Wu T, Wang J, Jiang X, et al. Overexpression of miR-155 promotes the proliferation and invasion of oral squamous carcinoma cells by regulating BCL6/cyclin D2. Int J Mol Med. 2016;37(5): 1274–80.
26. Qu F, Cui X, Hong Y, Wang J, Li Y, Chen L, et al. MicroRNA-185 suppresses proliferation, invasion, migration, and tumorigenicity of human prostate cancer cells through targeting androgen receptor. Mol Cell Biochem. 2013; 377(1–2):121–30.
27. Li X, Chen Y-T, Josson S, Mukhopadhyay NK, Kim J, Freeman MR, et al. MicroRNA-185 and 342 inhibit tumorigenicity and induce apoptosis through blockade of the SREBP metabolic pathway in prostate cancer cells. PloS one. 2013;8(8).

7

# Serum omentin-1 level in patients with benign prostatic hyperplasia

Haiqing He[1,2], Shuiqing Wu[1], Jun Hao[2], Long Wang[3], Kai Ai[1], Xuan Zhu[1], Ran Xu[1*], Xiaokun Zhao[1], Yinhuai Wang[1] and Zhaohui Zhong[1]

**Abstract**

**Backgroud:** To evaluate the relationship between omentin-1 and benign prostatic hyperplasia (BPH). BPH is the most common urological disease in elderly men worldwide. Lower serum omentin-1 levels were reported to be negatively associated with the incidence of inflammation, diabetes, obesity and metabolic syndrome, which all play a role in the development of BPH. To the best of our knowledge, the relationship between omentin-1 and BPH has not been investigated previously.

**Methods:** A total of 70 males participated in this study, including forty patients diagnosed with BPH and thirty healthy males. The anthropometric measurements and the biochemical parameters were measured in this study. We evaluated serum omentin-1 levels and the correlation with those data. We also test the gene expression of IL-8, IL-18 in BPH group using the TURP tissues.

**Results:** The serum omentin-1 levels were lower in the BPH patients than in the control group ($27.95 \pm 4.18$ versus $32.03 \pm 5.46$, $p < 0.001$). The general characteristics and biochemical parameters were investigated, and a negative correlation was found between serum omentin-1 levels and BMI in the BPH group ($r = -0.391$, $p = 0.013$) as well as the whole group ($r = -0.457$, $p < 0.001$). Multiple-factor binary regression analysis revealed that serum omentin-1was a protective factor of BPH development. Furthermore, lower serum omentin-1 levels were associated with higher mRNA expression of IL-8 or IL-18 in the BPH group.

**Conclusion:** Omentin-1 may suppress the development of BPH and Lower serum omentin-1 levels in BPH patients might associated with higher prostate volume and higher IL-8 and IL-18 expression levels in their prostatic cells.

**Keywords:** Benign prostatic hyperplasia (BPH), Omentin/Omentin-1, Adipokine, Prostate volume, Interleukin-8, Interleukin-18

## Backgroud

Benign prostatic hyperplasia (BPH) is the most common urological disease in elderly men worldwide. BPH causes prostate enlargement and is associated with bladder outlet obstruction and various lower urinary tract symptoms (LUTS) [1]. BPH can also cause the deterioration of urinary function and quality of life and increase the risk of both urinary tract infection (UTI) and acute urinary retention, which requires surgical attention. Moreover, the medical costs for managing BPH are high, despite the fact that many men with BPH remained underdiagnosed and undertreated.

Although the mechanisms are not fully clear, metabolic status, inflammation, and hormonal status may contribute to the pathogenesis of BPH. Previous studies demonstrated evidence of strong correlations between metabolic syndrome and chronic inflammation in BPH pathogenesis and progression [2].

* Correspondence: xuran@csu.edu.cn
[1]Department of Urology, The Second Xiangya Hospital, Central South University, Changsha 410011, Hunan, China
Full list of author information is available at the end of the article

Omentin was primarily identified from cDNA library of human omental adipose tissue [3]. Omentin-1 (Gene name ITLN1), which is an isoform of omentin, shows its abundance in human plasma. Decreased serum omentin-1 levels are detected in patients with endocrine diseases such as type2 diabetes and obesity [4]. Meanwhile, it was proved that reduced omentin-1 level plays pivotal role in the causation of inflammatory diseases [5].

Previous studies on the association of BPH and adipokines (e.g., C-peptide, leptin and adiponectin) have reported conflicting results [6–8]. To the best of our knowledge, there are no reports of a relationship between omentin and BPH. Therefore, this matched case-control study investigated the serum omentin concentrations in patients with BPH.

## Methods

### Subjects

This study was approved by the Ethics Committee of the Second Xiangya Hospital of Central South University. A total of 70 males seen from January 2017 to January 2018 gave informed consent before participating in this study. Forty patients diagnosed with BPH who needed transurethral resection of the prostate (TURP) and thirty healthy males matched by age were assigned into two groups: the BPH group and the control group (CG). BPH was diagnosed based on clinical findings, rectal examination, ultrasound and confirmed by histopathological results. The healthy males were defined by ultrasound and International Prostate Symptom Score (IPSS). The prostate size of CG measured by ultrasound is less than 4 cm × 3 cm × 2 cm and IPSS is less than 7. The PSA values of all these men were less than 4 ng/mL.

### Methods

The anthropometric measurements obtained in this study included height, weight, systolic blood pressure (SBP), diastolic blood pressure (DBP), and waist circumference (WC). Body mass index (BMI) was calculated as the body weight divided by the height squared (kg/m2). We measured the WC at the umbilicus level. Biochemical parameters were measured in venous blood samples taken after at least a 10-h fast. Fasting blood samples were obtained to analyze blood urea nitrogen (BUN), triglyceride (TG), total cholesterol (TC), high-density lipoprotein (HDL), creatinine, prostate-specific antigen (PSA) and glucose levels using standard methods. The estimated glomerular filtration rates (eGFRs) were assessed using the following equation: eGFR = α × (SC÷0.9)-β × 0.993age [Note: SC is the serum creatinine level in mg/ml. α is 128, and β is 0.015 for SC ≤ 0.9 mg/dl or 79.56 μmol/l; otherwise, α is 119, and β is 0.688]. Prostate size was measured by ultrasound and the prostate volume (PV) was calculated from transverse images by using the prolate-ellipsoid formula: 0.524 × height×width×length [9].

### Omentin-1 measurement

Venous blood was collected after fasting followed with centrifugation of 4000 rpm at room temperature. Afterward, enzyme-linked immunosorbent assay (ELISA) was performed to determine concentration of omentin-1 in human serum (Apotech, Inc.).

Quantification of gene expression in BPH tissues by quantitative real-time PCR.

Total RNA was extracted using an RNAsimple Total RNA Kit (TIANGEN Biotech) and miRcute miRNA Isolation Kit (TIANGEN Biotech) and reverse transcribed using a RevertAid First Strand cDNA Synthesis Kit (Thermo Fisher). Quantitative RT-PCR was performed using SuperReal PreMix Plus (TIANGEN Biotech) and the following primers:

IL-8:
Fwd: CCAGGAAGAAACCACCGGA
Rev: GAAATCAGGAAGGCTGCCAAG
IL-18:
Fwd: AAAACCTGGAATCAGATTACTTTGG
Rev: TCCGGGGTGCATTATCTCTA
β-actin:
Fwd: TTCCTTCCTGGGCATGGAGTC
Rev: TCTTCATTGTGCTGGGTGCC

Specific gene expression was quantified using the 2-ΔΔCT method. Gene expression normalization was performed using β-actin as a reference gene.

### Statistical analysis

SPSS 22.0 software was used for the statistical analyses. The results are presented as the mean ± standard deviation (SD). Student's t-test was used to determine the significance between two groups. Spearman's rank correlation coefficient analyses (r) and the coefficient of determination ($r^2$) were conducted to test for associations between omentin-1 levels and general clinical characteristics, biochemical parameters and relative gene expression. The influential factors for omentin-1 levels were identified using multiple-factor binary logistic regression analysis for meaningful clinical characteristics and biochemical parameters. Finally, the influential factors for BPH development were identified using multiple-factor binary logistic regression analysis for meaningful clinical characteristics and biochemical parameters. $P < 0.05$ was considered statistically significant, * indicates $p < 0.05$, ** indicates $p < 0.01$, *** indicates $p < 0.001$.

## Results

The general characteristics and biochemical parameters of the two groups are listed in Table 1. There were no statistically significant differences in age, WC, fasting

**Table 1** Comparison of the general characteristics and biochemical parameters

| | BPH ($n = 40$) | CG ($n = 30$) | p |
|---|---|---|---|
| Age (years) | 59.15 ± 7.382 | 59.07 ± 7.593 | 0.963 |
| BMI (kg/m$^2$) | 26.20 ± 3.48 | 22.56 ± 3.01 | **< 0.001** |
| SBP (mmHg) | 126.6 ± 10.8 | 124.5 ± 11.8 | 0.706 |
| DBP (mmHg) | 76.1 ± 8.3 | 72 ± 9.2 | 0.059 |
| Waist circumference (cm) | 90.33 ± 14.06 | 88.93 ± 12.89 | 0.671 |
| TG (mmol/L) | 1.81 ± 0.26 | 1.71 ± 0.18 | 0.091 |
| TC (mmol/L) | 4.56 ± 0.86 | 4.14 ± 1.01 | 0.073 |
| HDL (mmol/L) | 1.22 ± 0.31 | 1.18 ± 0.24 | 0.561 |
| Fasting glucose (mmol/L) | 4.76 ± 0.96 | 4.34 ± 0.94 | 0.076 |
| BUN (mmol/L) | 5.40 ± 1.57 | 4.80 ± 1.12 | 0.084 |
| eGFR (mL/min/1.73 m$^2$) | 76.18 ± 8.37 | 79.97 ± 7.64 | 0.055 |
| Creatinine (μmol/L) | 81.46 ± 17.26 | 72.92 ± 17.63 | **0.047** |
| PSA (ng/mL) | 2.29 ± 0.89 | 1.72 ± 0.73 | **0.005** |
| Omentin-1 (ng/mL) | 27.31 ± 4.56 | 33.47 ± 4.92 | **< 0.001** |
| Prostate volume (mL) | 62.00 ± 30.26 | 10.64 ± 1.29 | **< 0.001** |

glucose, SBP, DBP, TG, TC, HDL, fasting glucose, BUN and eGFR between the two groups. BMI, BUN, creatinine, PSA levels were significantly higher in the BPH group than in the CG. The omentin-1 levels were lower in the BPH group than in the CG (Fig. 1a).

Multiple-factor binary regression analysis was performed to reveal the risk factors for BPH development from various meaningful clinical characteristics and biochemical parameters, including BMI, creatinine, PSA and omentin-1 (Table 2). Among these data, BMI and omentin-1 level were significantly associated with the BPH development.

Correlations between the serum omentin-1 level and the biochemical properties in the BPH, CG and whole group were determined with Spearman's rank correlation coefficient analysis. It was suggestive that serum omentin-1 levels have little correlation with age, SBP, DBP, WC, TG,TC,HDL, fasting glucose, BUN, eGFR or creatinine while negative correlations were found between serum omentin-1 levels and BMI in the BPH group ($r = -0.391$, $p = 0.013$) as well as the whole group ($r = -0.457$, $p < 0.001$) (Supplementary Table 1).

The BPH patients have been divided in two group according to the IPSS level, IPSS 8–19 and IPSS 20–35. The serum omentin-1 level in these two group showed no significantly difference (Fig. 1b). And also, there was no significant correlation between serum omentin-1 and IPSS in either BPH group or CG (Fig. 2a, b). Alternative, serum omentin-1 level showed significant negative correlations with prostate volume in BPH group (Supplementary Table 2, Fig. 2c, d).

Interleukin-8 (IL-8) and interleukin-18 (IL-18) are two cytokines secreted mainly by prostatic cells and functionally related to Omentin-1 (Supplementary Figure 1) [10–13]. It has been shown that the mRNA expression of these two cytokines was significantly higher in BPH patients with LUTS [11–13]. Thus, in this study, we also checked the expression levels of IL-8 and IL-18 in our BPH patient samples. We found that the mRNA expression levels of IL-8 and IL-18 were significantly higher in the low serum omentin-1 group (levels lower than the median) (Fig. 3a, b). Moreover, there were significant negative correlations between serum omentin-1 levels

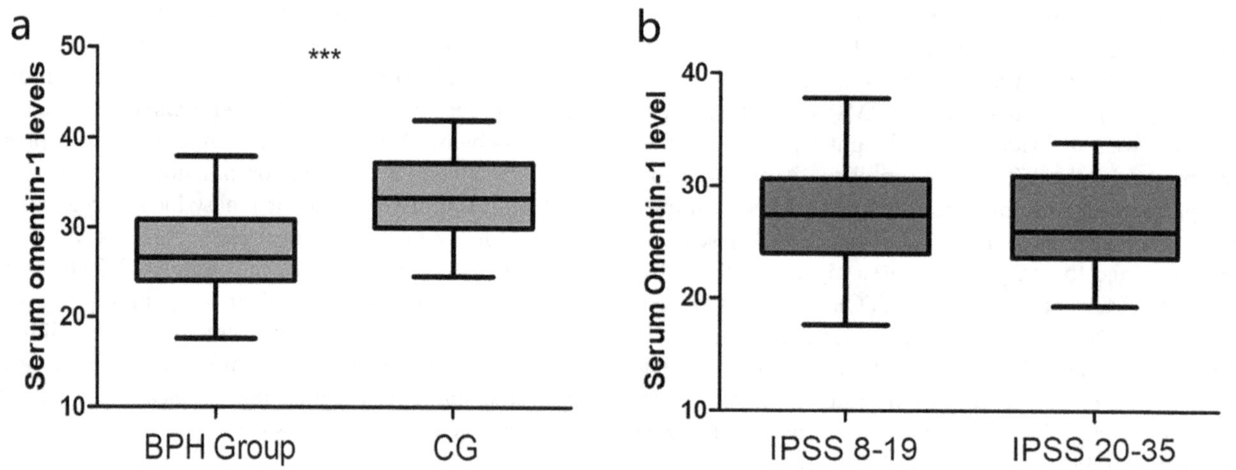


**Fig. 1** Serum omentin-1 levels. **a**. Serum omentin-1 levels in the BPH groups and CG. The concentrations of omentin-1 in human serum were determined using an enzyme-linked immunosorbent assay (ELISA) kit. **b**. The serum omentin-1 level in different IPSS level in BPH group. The BPH patients have been divided in two group according to the IPSS level. IPSS 8–19 indicates Level 2. IPSS 20–35 indicates level 3. The Vertical histograms show means ± SD

**Table 2** Multiple-factor binary logistic regression analysis

| Variables | B value | SE value | OR value | 95%CI | *P* value |
|---|---|---|---|---|---|
| BMI (kg/m$^2$) | 0.242 | 0.120 | 1.274 | 1.008–1.611 | **0.043** |
| PSA (ng/mL) | 0.457 | 0.390 | 1.579 | 0.720–3.395 | 0.242 |
| Creatinine (μmol/L) | 0.036 | 0.019 | 1.036 | 0.998–1.077 | 0.065 |
| Omentin-1 (ng/mL) | −0.206 | 0.077 | 0.813 | 0.699–0.946 | **0.008** |

*SE* standard error, *OR* odds ratio, *CI* confidence interval

and IL-8 and IL-18 mRNA expression in the BPH group (Supplementary Table 2, Fig. 3c, d).

## Discussion

With the changing demographic profile and an increasingly aging population in almost all societies, it is inevitable that the prevalence of BPH will increase.

Obesity is often comorbid with BPH. Body weight, BMI, and WC have been reported to be positively associated with prostate volume. Moreover, obesity was also associated with an increased risk of symptomatic BPH in several different international studies [14, 15]. In the present study, WC was greater in patients in the BPH group than those in the CG, but the difference was not statistically significant. BMI was significantly greater for the patients in the BPH group than for those in the CG, which suggests that increased body weight could be a factor in the etiology of BPH.

Several studies were done to examine the influence of diabetes using more objective measures of BPH, specifically prostate gland size. Increased prostate size and BPH surgery have strong association with the diagnosis of diabetes and increased serum insulin fasting plasma glucose level [16, 17]. In our study, glucose levels were not statistically significantly higher in the BPH group.

It is likely that inflammation plays a role in the development and progression of BPH [1, 18] because inflammatory cytokines are overexpressed in BPH tissues [19]. It remains unclear how inflammation mediates BPH. Obesity is considered a hormone-regulated disease when the secretion of pro-inflammatory cytokines and chemokine can promote the enlargement of adipocytes and at the mean time, influence prostate health [20]. These active hormones are known as adipokines, such as adiponectin. High adiponectin concentrations were associated with a reduced risk of symptomatic BPH [6].

Omentin is an anti-inflammatory adipokine in human with a higher expression in visceral adipose tissue than those found subcutaneously [21]. Omentin-1 is the major circulating form of omentin. Omentin showed a strong negative correlation with the incidence of inflammation, diabetes, obesity and metabolic syndrome [4],

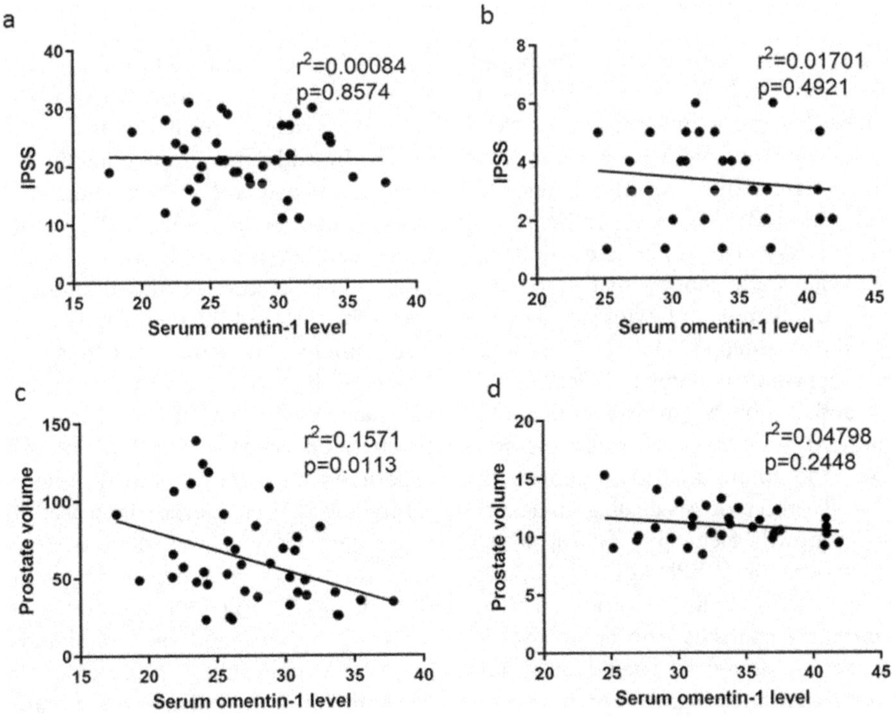


**Fig. 2** The correlation between serum omentin-1 and IPSS/Prostate volume. **a**. The coefficient of determination for IPSS and serum omentin-1 level in BPH group was established. **b**. The coefficient of determination for for IPSS and serum omentin-1 level in CG was established. **c**. The coefficient of determination for prostate volume and serum omentin-1 level in BPH group was established. **d**. The coefficient of determination for prostate volume and serum omentin-1 level in CG was established. The trend line is shown

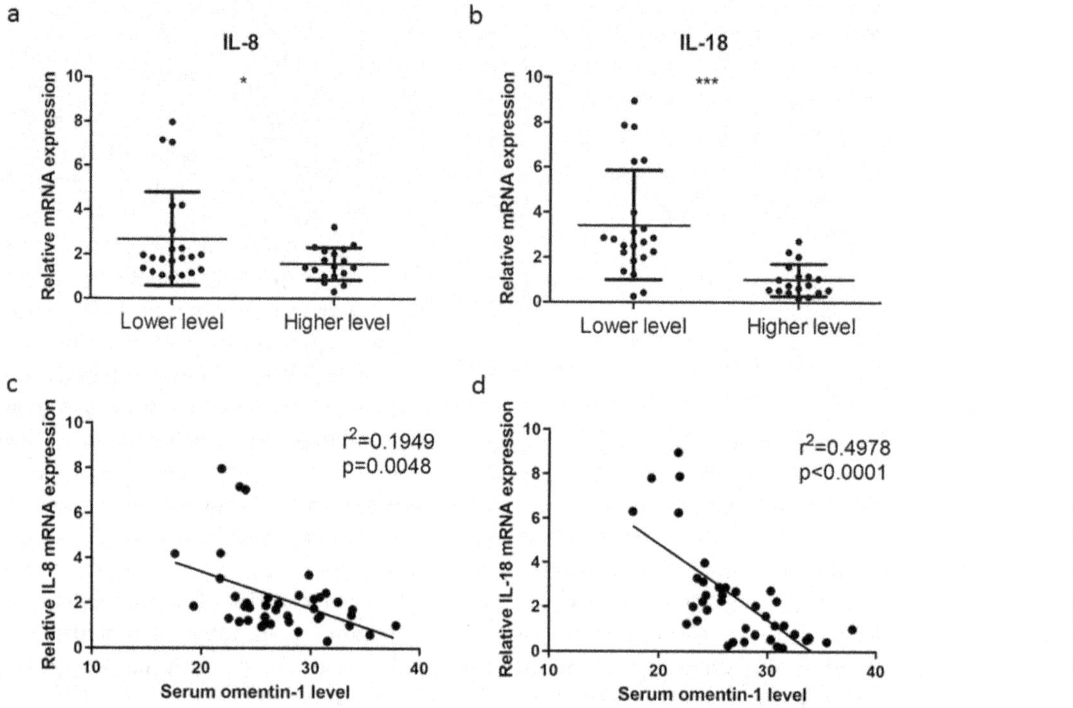


**Fig. 3** Relative gene mRNA expression according to omentin-1 Levels and their correlation. **a**, **b**. IL-8 and IL-18 mRNA expressions in clinical BPH specimen were determined by qRT-PCR. BPH patients were divided into two groups based on their serum omentin-1 levels. Results are presented as means ± SD. Specific gene expression was quantified using the 2-ΔΔCT method. Gene expression normalization was performed using β-actin as a reference gene. **c**. The coefficient of determination for IL-8 mRNA expression and serum omentin-1 level was established. **d**. The coefficient of determination for IL-18 mRNA expression and serum omentin-1 level was established. The trend line is shown

which all contribute to BPH progression. Decreased omentin-1 levels may play a role in the development of insulin resistance, type 2 diabetes mellitus and particularly obesity [22]. Through homeostasis model assessment, it was demonstrated that omentin-1 level is negatively correlated with BMI, WC and insulin resistance while it is positively associated HDL and adiponectin level [23]. A previous study showed that omentin-1 could downregulate pro-inflammatory cytokines to prevent inflammation-induced osteoporosis [5]. Di has reported that omentin suppresses pulmonary inflammation and promotes the endothelial barrier to prevent lipopolysaccharide (LPS)-induced acute respiratory distress syndrome (ARDS) [24]. Yao found that during prostatic hyperplasia, LPS/Toll-like receptor 4 signaling could upregulate transforming growth factor-β (TGF-β), which plays a role in the pathogenesis of BPH [25, 26]. Patients diagnosed with inflammatory bowel diseases such as Crohn's disease or ulcerative colitis have lower level of circulating omentin-1 [27]. Uyeturk reported that serum omentin-1 levels were significantly higher in prostate cancer (PCa) patients than in BPH patients [28]. However, serum omentin-1 levels have not been previously examined in BPH patients and healthy people. In our present study, omentin-1 levels were dysregulated in patients in the BPH group compared to those in the CG. PSA levels were significantly different between the two groups but were negatively correlated with omentin-1 in the whole group. In addition, serum omentin-1 levels were negatively correlated with BMI in the BPH group and in the whole group. Serum omentin-1 level also showed significant negative correlation with prostate volume in BPH group. Furthermore, we found that omentin-1 might be a protective factor of BPH development.

In patients with acute myocardial infarction, omentin-1 negatively correlated with IL-18, and IL-18 remained an independent determinant of omentin-1 levels [29]. In research on obese people who participated in training experiments, serum omentin-1 levels decreased significantly, and IL-18 levels increased significantly after detraining [30]. These studies showed that serum omentin-1 levels may negatively correlate with IL-18 in BPH tissues. IL-18 could be secreted by prostatic epithelial cells and respond to several inflammatory stimuli [31]. IL-18 itself directly influences prostatic stromal cell proliferation [12]. Similarly, our results suggested that in the BPH group, serum omentin-1 levels were significantly negatively correlated with IL-18 expression in prostatic cells. IL-8, produced by BPH prostate epithelial cells as a reliable biomarker of inflammation in BPH, can promote the proliferation of non-senescent epithelial and stromal cells and contributes to the increased tissue growth in BPH [11, 13]. IL-8 expression was also significantly negatively correlated with serum omentin-1 levels in our investigation, which supports the findings that omentin-1 could reduce IL-8 production in kidney tissue [32]. From all these data, what can be hypothesized is that men with higher BMI might show lower serum omentin-1 level, thereby contribute to the development of BPH via facilitating the activation of prostatic inflammation.

## Conclusion

In summary, we found that serum omentin-1 levels were decreased in patients with BPH. Omentin-1 may suppress the development of BPH and Lower serum omentin-1 levels in BPH patients might associated with higher prostate volume and higher IL-8 and IL-18 expression levels in their prostatic cells. Further studies establishing the mechanism underlying this phenomenon would allow better management of BPH development.

## Supplementary information

**Additional file 1: Figure S1**. Functional protein association networks of Omentin-1 (ITLN1). The functional protein association networks of Omentin-1 (Gene name: ITLN1) was shown. Cytokines such as Interleukin-18 (IL18) were reported to be closely linked to ITLN1.

**Additional file 2: Table S1**. Spearman's rank correlation coefficient analysis of serum omentin-1 levels with the general clinical characteristics and biochemical parameters.

**Additional file 3: Table S2**. Spearman's rank correlation coefficient analysis of serum omentin-1 levels with the general clinical characteristics and biochemical parameters.

### Abbreviations

BPH: benign prostatic hyperplasia; BMI: Body mass index; SBP: Systolic blood pressure; DBP: Diastolic blood pressure; WC: Waist circumference; BUN: Blood urea nitrogen; TG: Triglyceride; TC: Total cholesterol; HDL: High-density lipoprotein; PSA: Prostate-specific antigen; eGFRs: Estimated glomerular filtration rates; PV: Prostate volume; CG: Control group; IL-8: Interleukin-8; IL-18: Interleukin-18

### Acknowledgements

Not applicable.

### Authors' contributions

Conception and design: R.X. Acquisition of data: H. H, S.W, J.H, K.A, X.Z1, R.X. Analysis and interpretation of data: H.H, S.W, J.H, K.A. Drafting of the manuscript: H.H, J.H, R.X. Critical revision of the manuscript for important intellectual content: H.H, J.H, X.Z2, Y.W, Z.Z. Obtaining funding: Y.W, R.X, Z.Z, L.W. Supervision: R.X, X.Z2. The authors read and approved the final manuscript.

### Author details

[1]Department of Urology, The Second Xiangya Hospital, Central South University, Changsha 410011, Hunan, China. [2]Vancouver Prostate Centre, Department of Urologic Sciences, Faculty of Medicine, University of British Columbia, Vancouver, BC, Canada. [3]Department of Urology, Xiangya Hospital, Central South University, Changsha 410008, Hunan, China.

### References

1. Inamura S, et al. Prostatic stromal inflammation is associated with bladder outlet obstruction in patients with benign prostatic hyperplasia. Prostate. 2018;78(10):743-52.
2. De Nunzio C, Presicce F, Tubaro A. Inflammatory mediators in the development and progression of benign prostatic hyperplasia. Nat Rev Urol. 2016;13(10):613–26.
3. Yang RZ, et al. Identification of omentin as a novel depot-specific adipokine in human adipose tissue: possible role in modulating insulin action. Am J Physiol Endocrinol Metab. 2006;290(6):E1253–61.
4. Watanabe T, et al. Adipose tissue-derived Omentin-1 function and regulation. Compr Physiol. 2017;7(3):765–81.
5. Rao SS, et al. Omentin-1 prevents inflammation-induced osteoporosis by downregulating the pro-inflammatory cytokines. Bone Res. 2018;6:9.
6. Schenk JM, et al. Serum adiponectin, C-peptide and leptin and risk of symptomatic benign prostatic hyperplasia: results from the prostate Cancer prevention trial. Prostate. 2009;69(12):1303–11.
7. Grosman H, et al. Complex relationship between sex hormones, insulin resistance and leptin in men with and without prostatic disease. Aging Male. 2016;19(1):40–5.
8. Fu S, et al. Adiponectin deficiency contributes to the development and progression of benign prostatic hyperplasia in obesity. Sci Rep. 2017;7: 43771.
9. Eri LM, et al. Accuracy and repeatability of prostate volume measurements by transrectal ultrasound. Prostate Cancer Prostatic Dis. 2002;5(4):273–8.
10. Szklarczyk D, et al. The STRING database in 2017: quality-controlled protein-protein association networks, made broadly accessible. Nucleic Acids Res. 2017;45(D1):D362–8.
11. Castro P, et al. Interleukin-8 expression is increased in senescent prostatic epithelial cells and promotes the development of benign prostatic hyperplasia. Prostate. 2004;60(2):153–9.
12. Hamakawa T, et al. Interleukin-18 may lead to benign prostatic hyperplasia via thrombospondin-1 production in prostatic smooth muscle cells. Prostate. 2014;74(6):590–601.
13. Liu L, et al. Evaluation of interleukin-8 in expressed prostatic secretion as a reliable biomarker of inflammation in benign prostatic hyperplasia. Urology. 2009;74(2):340–4.
14. Dahle SE, et al. Body size and serum levels of insulin and leptin in relation to the risk of benign prostatic hyperplasia. J Urol. 2002;168(2):599–604.
15. Kristal AR, et al. Race/ethnicity, obesity, health related behaviors and the risk of symptomatic benign prostatic hyperplasia: results from the prostate cancer prevention trial. J Urol. 2007;177(4):1395–400 quiz 1591.
16. Sarma AV, et al. Diabetes and benign prostatic hyperplasia/lower urinary tract symptoms--what do we know? J Urol. 2009;182(6 Suppl):S32–7.
17. Kim WT, et al. Prostate size correlates with fasting blood glucose in non-diabetic benign prostatic hyperplasia patients with Normal testosterone levels. J Korean Med Sci. 2011;26(9):1214–8.
18. Zlotta AR, et al. Prevalence of inflammation and benign prostatic hyperplasia on autopsy in Asian and Caucasian men. Eur Urol. 2014;66(4): 619–22.
19. Schenk JM, et al. Biomarkers of systemic inflammation and risk of incident, symptomatic benign prostatic hyperplasia: results from the prostate cancer prevention trial. Am J Epidemiol. 2010;171(5):571–82.
20. Di Silverio F, et al. Distribution of inflammation, pre-malignant lesions, incidental carcinoma in histologically confirmed benign prostatic hyperplasia: a retrospective analysis. Eur Urol. 2003;43(2):164–75.
21. Martinez-Garcia MA, et al. Evidence for masculinization of adipokine gene expression in visceral and subcutaneous adipose tissue of obese women with polycystic ovary syndrome (PCOS). J Clin Endocrinol Metab. 2013;98(2): E388–96.
22. Zhang Q, et al. Changes of serum omentin-1 levels in normal subjects, type 2 diabetes and type 2 diabetes with overweight and obesity in Chinese adults. Ann Endocrinol (Paris). 2014;75(3):171–5.
23. de Souza Batista CM, et al. Omentin plasma levels and gene expression are decreased in obesity. Diabetes. 2007;56(6):1655–61.
24. Qi D, et al. Omentin protects against LPS-induced ARDS through suppressing pulmonary inflammation and promoting endothelial barrier via an Akt/eNOS-dependent mechanism. Cell Death Dis. 2016;7(9):e2360.
25. He Y, et al. LPS/TLR4 signaling enhances TGF-beta response through Downregulating BAMBI during prostatic hyperplasia. Sci Rep. 2016;6:27051.

26. Wang L, et al. Aberrant transforming growth factor-beta activation recruits Mesenchymal stem cells during prostatic hyperplasia. Stem Cells Transl Med. 2017;6(2):394–404.
27. Yin J, et al. Decreased levels of serum omentin-1 in patients with inflammatory bowel disease. Med Sci Monit. 2015;21:118–22.
28. Uyeturk U, et al. Serum omentin level in patients with prostate cancer. Med Oncol. 2014;31(4):923.
29. Kadoglou NP, et al. Serum levels of novel adipokines, omentin-1 and chemerin, in patients with acute myocardial infarction: KOZANI STUDY. J Cardiovasc Med (Hagerstown). 2015;16(5):341–6.
30. Nikseresht M, Hafezi Ahmadi MR, Hedayati M. Detraining-induced alterations in adipokines and cardiometabolic risk factors after nonlinear periodized resistance and aerobic interval training in obese men. Appl Physiol Nutr Metab. 2016;41(10):1018–25.
31. Wang X, et al. Increased infiltrated macrophages in benign prostatic hyperplasia (BPH): role of stromal androgen receptor in macrophage-induced prostate stromal cell proliferation. J Biol Chem. 2012;287(22):18376–85.
32. Song J, et al. Omentin-1 protects renal function of mice with type 2 diabetic nephropathy via regulating miR-27a-Nrf2/Keap1 axis. Biomed Pharmacother. 2018;107:440–6.

8

# Early upregulation of AR and steroidogenesis enzyme expression after 3 months of androgen-deprivation therapy

Agus Rizal A. H. Hamid[1*], Harun W. Kusuma Putra[1], Ningrum Paramita Sari[2], Putri Diana[1], Saras Serani Sesari[1], Eka Novita[3], Fajar Lamhot Gultom[3], Meilania Saraswati[3], Budiana Tanurahardja[3], Asmarinah[2], Rainy Umbas[1] and Chaidir A. Mochtar[1]

**Abstract**

**Background:** Androgen deprivation therapy (ADT) is a standard treatment for advanced prostate cancer (PCa). However, PCa recurrence and progression rates during ADT are high. Until now, there has been no evidence regarding when progression begins. This study evaluated the gene expression of intraprostatic androgen receptor (AR) and steroidogenic enzymes in the early stages of ADT.

**Methods:** Prostate tissue samples were taken from PCa patients with urinary retention who received ADT (ADT-PCa; $n = 10$) and were further subgrouped into ADT ≤12 months ($n = 4$) and ADT > 12 months ($n = 6$). The ADT-PCa tissues were then compared with BPH ($n = 12$) and primary (no treatment) PCa tissues ($n = 16$). mRNA for gene expression analysis of AR and steroidogenic enzymes was extracted from formalin-fixed paraffin embedded (FFPE) tissues and analyzed by real-time PCR. Protein expression was evaluated by immunohistochemistry with specific antibodies.

**Results:** AR gene expression was higher in the ADT-PCa group than in the BPH or primary PCa group. Both the ADT ≤12 and > 12 months subgroups had significantly higher relative gene expression levels of AR ($p < 0.01$ and 0.03, respectively) than the primary PCa group. In the ADT-PCa group, AR protein expression showed an increasing trend in the ADT ≤12 months subgroup and was significantly elevated in the ADT > 12 months subgroup compared with the PCa group (100%; $p < 0.01$). Half (50%) of the patients in the ADT ≤12 months subgroup were found to have upregulation of AR, and one showed upregulation beginning at 3 months of ADT. A trend toward elevated relative gene expression of SRD5A3 was also apparent in the ADT groups.

**Conclusion:** AR and steroidogenic enzymes are upregulated in ADT-PCa patients as early as 3 months, without PSA elevation. Steroidogenic enzymes, particularly SRD5A3, were also upregulated before PSA rose.

**Keywords:** Androgen receptor, Steroidogenic enzyme, AKR3C1 SRD5A1, SRD5A2, SRD5A3

* Correspondence: rizalhamid.urology@gmail.com
[1]Department of Urology, CiptoMangunkusumo Hospital - Faculty of Medicine Universitas Indonesia, Jl. Diponegoro No.71, RW.5, Kenari, Senen, RW.5, Kenari, Senen, Kota Jakarta Pusat, Daerah Khusus Ibukota Jakarta 10430, Indonesia
Full list of author information is available at the end of the article

## Background

Over the years, there have been notable improvements in the development of prostate cancer (PCa) treatment, resulting in better prognoses [1]. However, 40% of patients with early PCa are still at risk of disease progression to a more advanced stage [1] and thus need androgen deprivation therapy (ADT), the current standard palliative treatment [2]. Although ADT may prolong overall survival [3], prolong the occurence of metastasis [4], and decrease PSA levels [5], these effects are only temporary. The disease often progresses further after 2–3 years of treatment [6]. This form of late-stage PCa is called castration-resistant prostate cancer (CRPC), as PCa cells have evolved and become capable of both hormone-dependent and hormone-independent cell proliferation and survival [7].

The existence of CRPC has motivated an increased focus on the disease. The androgen receptor (AR) signaling pathway is an important mechanism of PCa and plays a key role in PCa progression [8–10]. The known mechanisms of resistance include AR overexpression, AR gene amplification, AR hypersensitivity, AR mutations, AR variants (ARVs), androgen-independent AR activation, and intratumoral and alternative androgen production [8–10]. Furthermore, data have suggested that the increased level of intraprostatic AR can lead to disease progression [10]. Other downstream steroidogenic enzymes within the AR signaling pathway, 5α-reductase and AKR1C3, have also become targets of interest [7–12]. These enzymes are responsible for the conversion of androgens into dihydrotestosterone (DHT), which is needed by PCa cells [11]. Currently, there are three identified isozymes of SRD5A encoded by 3 different genes: SRD5A1, SRD5A2, and SRD5A3 [11]. AKR1C3, SRD5A1 and SRDA2 have been extensively studied [7–12], and marked changes in their levels were reported to occur during the course of PCa development and progression [7–12]. SRD5A1 and SRD5A3 are associated with androgen response elements (AREs) that promote the transcription of target genes, leading to cell homeostasis, angiogenesis, differentiation, and apoptosis [13]. It is also believed that the two isozymes play important roles in androgen production in prostate cells [11]. On the other hand, the role of SRD5A3 is still obscure, although associations with DHT production and AR activation have been suggested [14]. Based on these findings, AR, AKR1C3, and 5α-reductase are indicative of PCa progression, as differences in their levels between malignant and nonmalignant cells have been documented. However, changes in the levels of these genes following ADT treatment have never been reported, although they have been associated with further disease progression and recurrence.

Currently, no study has reported the start of disease progression after ADT. This study hypothesized that progression of the disease would likely occur within a short time interval after commencement of ADT. Therefore, this study evaluated the early effects of ADT by investigating the levels of AR and steroidogenic enzymes as an indicator of disease progression. To this end, we compared the levels of these factors within the intraprostatic cells of benign prostatic hyperplasia (BPH) and primary PCa cases to those of PCa cases after ADT treatment.

## Methods

### Samples

Formalin-fixed paraffin embedded (FFPE) prostate tissue was obtained from the Department of Pathology Anatomy, Cipto Mangunkusumo General Hospital (RSCM). The study included three groups of patients: 1) the BPH group ($n = 12$), 2) the primary PCa group ($n = 16$, sampled from 2009 to 2015), and 3) the PCa after ADT (ADT-PCa) group ($n = 10$). The sample retrieval method for BPH and primary PCa are through biopsy, TUR-P, or Radical prostatectomy, while ADT-PCa tissues were taken primarily from TUR-P. The ADT-PCa group was categorized as the ADT ≤12 months and ADT > 12 months subgroups based on the duration of ADT. All use of specimens was in compliance with the guidelines of the local review board and Ethics Committee 520/UN2, F1/ETIK/2015, and prostatic tissues were obtained with patient consent at the time of the procedure.

### RNA extraction from FFPE tissue

Paraffinization was performed by prior isolation of the RNA using a High Pure RNA Paraffin Kit (Roche, Germany). The sample used was FFPE prostate tissues, which were cut to a thickness of 5–10 μM from each tissue sample from each group (BPH, primary PCa, and ADT-PCa). DNA extraction was performed from the FFPE samples. Total RNA was extracted in 50 μl and stored in a – 80 °C freezer.

### Quantitative real-time PCR

Quantification of gene expression (by qPCR) was performed for AR, AKR1C3, SRD5A1, SRD5A2, and SRD5A3 using a QuantiTect SYBR Green RT-PCR kit. The 18S gene was the housekeeping gene used as the internal control due to its constitutive expression across tissues and cells. qPCR mix (2x QuantiTect SYBR Green RT-PCR Mix, Forward Primer, Reverse Primer, free water nuclease) was used to set up the reactions, and 2 μL of the cDNA sample was used as the template. The specific primers used in this study are shown in Table 1. Measurements were performed using the Mx3000P (Agilent) tool with an amplification program. The cycle

**Table 1** Primers for rtPCR

| Gene | Forward | Reverse |
|---|---|---|
| AR | CAT TGA GCC AGG TGT AGT GT | CCA GTT CAT TGA GGC TAG AGA G |
| AKR1C3 | TGC AGG TTT TTG AGT TCC AGT | TGG CTA GCA AAA CTA TCA CGT T |
| SRD5A1 | ACG GGC ATC GGT GCT TAA T | CCA ACA GTG GCA TAG GCT TTC |
| SRD5A2 | GGAGTCCTTCAAGGCTACTATCT | CACCCAAGCTAAACCGTATGT |
| SRD5A3 | GTC ATC TGC CCA TCA GTA TAA | GAA TGA CCA CTC CTG CTT TAT |
| 18 S | AAA CGG CTA CCA CAT CCA AG | CCT CCA ATG GAT CCT CGT TA |

threshold (Ct) was obtained by using MxPro (Agilent) software. Relative gene expression was measured by using the Livak method, also known as the delta threshold cycle (ΔΔCt).

### Immunohistochemistry

Immunohistochemistry was performed by using the FFPE preparation. Each sample was cut into 4-μm sections, warmed at 58 °C, and deparaffinized using xylol I, II, and III. The specimens were rehydrated in a 100, 96, and 80% graded ethanol series and were then subjected to heat-induced epitope retrieval (HIER) at pH 6 in a pressure boiler at 125 °C and cooled at 90 °C. A dual endogenous enzyme block was performed using 0.3% $H_2O_2$ and 95% ethanol. Staining for analysis of the expression of AR, AKR1C3 and steroidogenic enzymes SRD5A1, SRD5A2, and SRD5A3 was performed using antibodies obtained from Sigma Aldrich (St Louis, Missouri) [15]: mouse monoclonal anti-AR (WH0000367M1) [15, 16], mouse monoclonal anti-AKR1C3 (A6229) [15, 17], rabbit polyclonal anti-SRD5A1 (HPA051402) [15], rabbit polyclonal anti-SRD5A2 (SAB2105567) [15], and rabbit polyclonal anti-SRD5A3 (HPA027006) [15, 18]. All of the antibodies were validated, referenced (Human Protein Atlas project) and peer-reviewed and are widely used in the immunohistochemistry research field, as referenced by Sigma Aldrich. Additional information is provided in Supplementary Table 1.

Tissues were incubated with an HRP-labeled polymer followed by chromogenization in DAB (substrate DAB: chromogen DAB was 1:20) using the DAKO autostainer Kit. The specimens were then counterstained using hematoxylin and dehydrated (100, 80, 96%), cleared (xylol I, II, III), and mounted onto slides with coverglass.

Slides were assessed visually by three examiners who were blinded to the patient groups, and the results were confirmed by an experienced pathologist. Microscopic semiquantitative examination was performed on 10 random fields per specimen containing a minimum of 500 cells using ImageJ (Research Service Branch, NIH.gov) at 400× magnification. Protein expression was considered positive if the cells staining was brownish in the cytoplasm or if the nuclei had a granular pattern.

### H-score calculation to measure protein expression

Positively stained epithelial cells were then quantified using a semiquantitative scoring method of 0, + 1, + 2, and + 3 with expression scores for each cell. A score of + 1 was defined as low positive, + 2 as moderate positive, and + 3 as high positive. Quantification of protein expression was performed by measuring the H-score. The H-score was measured using the following formula:

$$[(1\ x\% + 1\ \text{cells}) + (2\ x\% + 2\ \text{cells}) + (3\ x\% + 3\ \text{cells})]$$

The mean H-score of the BPH group was set as the cut-off to determine which samples showed upregulated or downregulated protein expressionand the results were further analyzed for statistical comparisons. The percentage of samples with upregulation is presented

### Statistical analysis

Statistical analysis was performed using GraphPad Prism 7 (La Jolla, CA). The Mann-Whitney U test was used to compare gene expression among the groups as follows: ADT versus BPH and ADT versus PCa. $P < 0.05$ was defined as statistically significant. Fisher's exact test was used for comparisons of protein expression between specified groups and the associations with clinicopathological parameters.

## Results

### Sample characteristics

From 2007 to 2015, we were able to evaluate 10 patients who still had urinary retention after ADT treatment (ADT-PCa group), and their mean age was 67.27 ± 9.69. The group was then subdivided into two groups: one received ADT for under 12 months (4 samples), with a median treatment time of 5 (3–9) months, and the other received ADT for more than 12 months (6 samples), with a median treatment time of 30 (15–70) months. The initial PSA levels were 93.3 (58.14–784.60) in the ADT ≤ 12 months group and 176.9 (104.23–200.40) in the ADT > 12 months group. The Gleason scores of most of the patients were high [8–10], and the T-stages and prostate volumes were comparable between the two groups. The ADT types used were similar and comparable between the two groups: in the ADT ≤ 12 months group, 50% of the patients underwent orchiectomy and 50% received LHRH agonist and antiandrogen, while in the ADT > 12 months group, these proportions were 67 and 33% respectively. We also compared these patients to the BPH group (12 samples) and primary PCa group (16 samples). The detailed characteristics of the patients are presented in Table 2. There was statistically significant difference of PSA level between the groups, with the highest PSA level found in the ADT > 12 months group.

### Relative gene expression

AR gene expression was higher in the ADT-PCa group than in the BPH (median difference of 1.1; *p*-value 0.05) and primary PCa (median difference of 1.83; $p < 0.01$) groups. Patients with ADT ≤12 months had the highest relative AR gene expression (median 5.14). AKR1C3 showed an increasing trend in the ADT-PCa subgroups compared with the BPH and primary PCa groups (Fig. 1).

There were no significant differences in the gene expression of SRD5A1 or SRD5A2 between the groups. However, a decreasing trend in SRD5A2 gene expression was noted (Fig. 1). In contrast, an overall increasing trend in SRD5A3 expression was observed between the BPH and ADT-PCa subgroups, with the ADT ≤12 months subgroup having the highest relative SRD5A3 expression (median difference of 9.39 in ADT ≤12 months vs the primary PCa group, $p = 0.13$; median difference of 11.3 in the ADT ≤12 months group vs the BPH group, $p = 0.02$) (Fig. 1).

### Protein expression by immunohistochemistry

AR and AKR1C3 expression was found in both the nucleus and cytoplasm, while the protein expression of SRD5A1, SRD5A2, and SRD5A3 was found predominantly in the cytoplasm (Fig. 2). Upregulation of protein

**Table 2** Basic characteristics of patients

| | BPH *n* = 12 | Prostate Cancer | | | *P*-Value[c] |
|---|---|---|---|---|---|
| | | Primary PCa *n* = 16 | ADT-PCa *n* = 10 | | |
| | | | Duration ≤ 12 Months *n* = 4 | Duration > 12 Months *n* = 6 | |
| **Age** | 64.2 ± 8.6 | 63.4 ± 7.0 | 58.75 ± 3.4 | 72 ± 9.3 | 0.05 |
| **Sample retrieval method** | | | | | |
| Biopsy | 5 (71%) | 5 (31%) | – | – | – |
| TUR-P | 2 (29%) | 5 (31%) | 4 (100%) | 6 (100%) | |
| Radical Prostatectomy | – | 6 (38%) | – | – | |
| **Gleason Score** | | | | | 0.76 |
| ≤ 7 | – | 4 (25%) | – | 1 (17%) | |
| 8–10 | – | 12 (75%) | 4 (100%) | 5 (83%) | |
| **T Staging**[a] | | | | | 0.91 |
| 1 | – | 6 (37%) | – | – | |
| 2 | – | 4 (25%) | 2 (50%) | 3 (50%) | |
| 3 | – | 3 (19%) | – | 1 (17%) | |
| 4 | – | 3 (19%) | 2 (50%) | 2 (33%) | |
| **Lymphatic Involvements** | – | 1 (7%) | NE | NE | – |
| **PSA**[a] | 9.5 (1.4–36.7) | 49.3 (4.6–600) | 24.13 (10.1–303.2) | 203.2 (10.2–689) | **0.01*** |
| **Prostate volume**[a] | 51.6 (28–73.6) | 43.6 (13.4–80.5) | 30.5 (28.6–36.68) | 39.7 (27.6–94.2) | 0.39 |
| **ADT Type** | | | | | 0.76 |
| Orchyde | – | – | 2 (50%) | 4 (67%) | |
| LHRH agonist ± antiandrogen | – | – | 2 (50%) | 2 (33%) | |
| **ADT Treatment Duration** | – | – | 5 (3–9) | 30 (15–70) | - |

*N.E* not evaluated
[a] PSA and prostate volume are presented in median (min-max)
[b] Sample retrieval method, T staging, and Lymphatic involvements are presented as percentages
[c] Statistical significance was measured by comparing Primary PCa, ADT-PCa ≤ 12 months and > 12 months using Pearson chi square for Gleason score, and ADT Type; ANOVA for age; Kurskall Wallis test for T-stage, PSA level, and Prostate Volume
[d] ADT treatment duration is presented in months
[*] *P*-value < 0.05 is significant

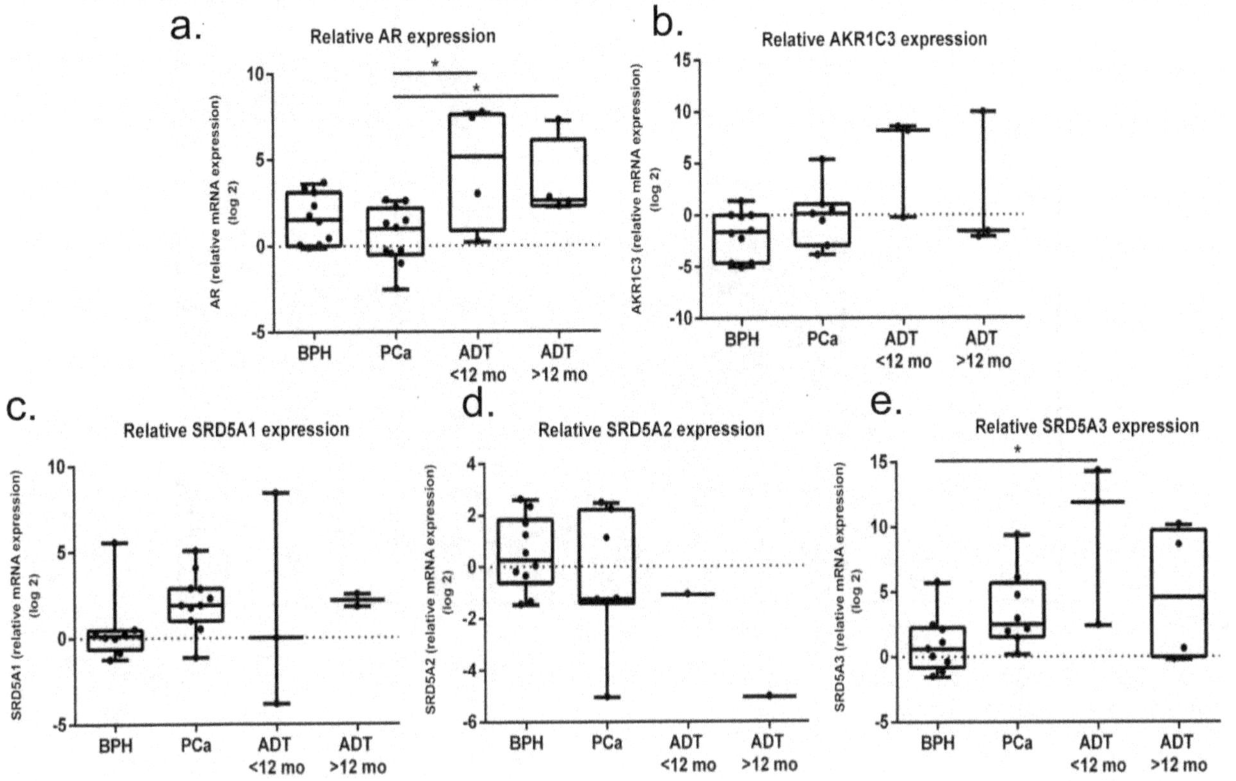


**Fig. 1** Gene expression analysis. Analysis of the relative expression of five different genes was performed by quantification of real-time one-step RT-PCR using the Mx3000P (Agilent) tool in tissue samples of the BPH group ($n = 12$), primary PCa group ($n = 13$), ADT ≤12 months group ($n = 4$) and ADT > 12 months group ($n = 6$). The included AR (**a**), AKR1C3 (**b**), SRD5A1 (**c**), SRD5A2 (**d**), and SRD5A3 (**e**). Statistical analysis was performed by using the Mann-Whitney test, comparing each group to another in a paired manner. * $p < 0.05$ and ** $p < 0.01$. Standard errors of the means are indicated by bars. **a-e** All experiments were performed at least two times

expression is described in Table 3. AR protein expression in the ADT-PCa group was increased by 80% compared with that in the primary PCa group ($p < 0.01$), showing an increasing trend in the ADT ≤12 months subgroup compared with the PCa group ($p = 0.2$), and AR protein expression was significantly higher in the ADT > 12 months subgroup (100; $p < 0.01$) (Table 3). No upregulation in AKR1C3 was found in either ADT-PCa subgroup.

### Associations between protein expression in the prostatic tissue of ADT-PCa patients and clinicopathological parameters

A further analysis of the ADT-PCa patients was performed by examining the association between increased protein expression and the clinical status of the patients (**data not shown**). This part of the study focused on the ADT-PCa subgroups. Specifically, we evaluated the ADT ≤12 months subgroup (Table 4) to determine whether the initial changes within the intraprostatic tissue were due to ADT. Half of the patients in the ADT ≤12 months group and all of the patients in the ADT > 12 months group had upregulated AR expression. Furthermore, one patient in the ADT ≤12 months subgroup had shown AR upregulation only 3 months after beginning ADT. However, there was no case of upregulation of AKR1C3 expression in the ADT ≤12 months subgroup. Additionally, there was no notable finding for SRD5A1, SRD5A2, and SRD5A3 protein expression. Moreover, there were no notable significant differences in the clinical or pathological parameters between the patients with upregulated and nonupregulated AR within the ADT ≤12 months subgroup.

Among the patients in the group given ADT for ≤12 months, one sample had increased protein expression of AR only, one sample had increased protein expression of SRDA1, 2, and 3 proteins, one sample increased protein expression of AR, SRDA1 and SRDA2, and one had no increase in protein expression. The specific H-scores for protein expression are available in Supplementary Table 2.

## Discussion

Although chemical castration by ADT has been the standard frontline therapy for advanced-stage PCa, disease progression is predicted to occur when cancer develops into CRPC. To better understand the changes

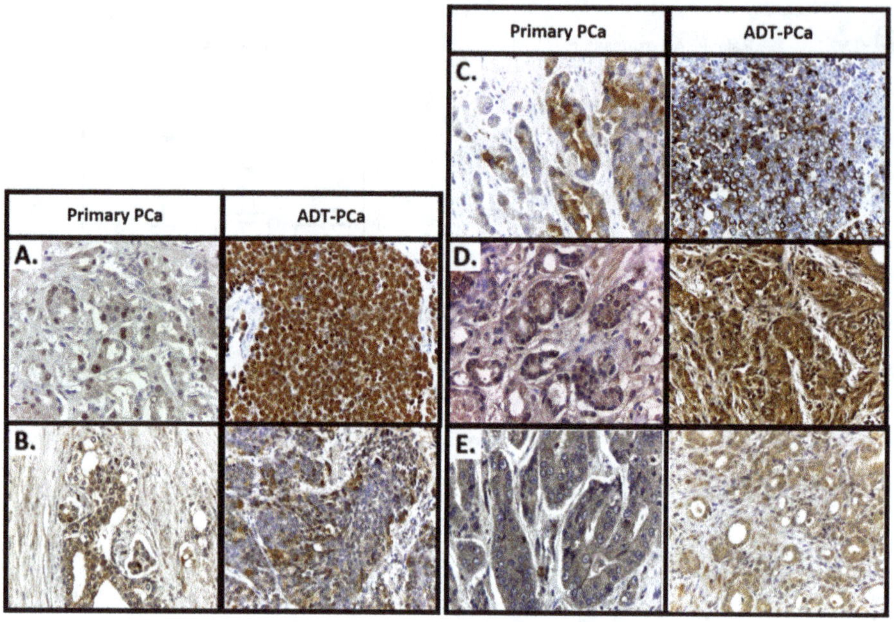


**Fig. 2** Immunohistochemistry of prostate cancer tissue stained for AR, AKR1C3, SRD5A1, SRD5A2, and SRD5A3. Comparison between the protein expression of AR and intraprostatic steroidogenic enzymes in the prostatic cells of the primary PCa and ADT-PCa groups: **a** AR, **b** AKR1C3, **c** SRD5A1, **d** SRD5A2, and **e** SRD5A3. Images were taken of sliced FFPE samples of patients obtained between 2009 and 2014 in RSCM. Images were captured at 400.000x magnification

involved in the transition to the progressive state, thorough study of the mechanisms of ADT resistance is important. The upregulation of components of the AR signaling pathway in intraprostatic tissue is one of the resistance mechanisms in CRPC. This study found upregulation of AR and steroidogenic enzymes in ADT-treated PCa patients. Furthermore, this study, in accordance with other studies, found that CRPC can develop in less than 12 months after the commencement of ADT [19] However, until now, no study has evaluated when the mechanism that triggers resistance to ADT becomes active in the prostate during ADT.

This study delves into the early response to ADT by evaluating intraprostatic AR and steroidogenic enzyme changes using prostate tissue from patients who still experienced urinary retention during ADT. It revealed a notably unique finding in the subgroup of patients who had ADT for only 12 months or less. Two patients had high intratumoral AR gene and protein expression after 3 months of ADT. It can be speculated that the resistance mechanism to ADT [10] through upregulation of AR might start as early as 3 months after the beginning of ADT. To the best of our knowledge, this is the first study to show early AR upregulation in human PCa

**Table 3** Expression of target proteins in the epithelial cells of the prostate tissue

| Expressions of proteins | H-score cut-off[a] | Upregulated cancer tissues | | | | | | | |
|---|---|---|---|---|---|---|---|---|---|
| | | Primary PCa (*n* = 7) | | ADT-PCa (*n* = 10) | | | | | |
| | | | | ≤ 12 months (*n* = 4) | | | > 12 months (*n* = 6) | | |
| | | n | % | n | % | Compared to primary PCa[b] | n | % | Compared to primary PCa[b] |
| AR | 57% | 1 | 14 | 2 | 50 | 0.2 | 6 | 100 | **< 0.01*** |
| AKR1C3 | 39% | 2 | 29 | **0** | **0** | 0.23 | 1 | 17 | 0.61 |
| SRD5A1 | 41% | 5 | 71 | 2 | 50 | 0.47 | 4 | 67 | 0.85 |
| SRD5A2 | 85% | 3 | 43 | 2 | 50 | 0.81 | 3 | 50 | 0.79 |
| SRD5A3 | 41% | 7 | 100 | 1 | 25 | **< 0.01*** | 3 | 50 | **0.03*** |

[a] H-Score cut-off was measured from mean H-score of BPH group (n = 6) as mentioned in the method, to determine upregulation of protein expressions in malignant tissues (Primary PCa and ADT ≤ 12 months and > 12 months)
[b] Statistical significance was measured for p-value by comparing the H score of ADT ≤ 12 months and > 12 months with Primary PCa using Pearson Chi Square
* *P*-value < 0.05 is significant

**Table 4** ADT-treated prostate cancer patients characteristics and clinical and pathological parameters

| Characteristics | AR | | | SRD5A1 | | | SRD5A2 | | | SRD5A3 | | |
|---|---|---|---|---|---|---|---|---|---|---|---|---|
| | ADT < 12 Months | | *P*-Value[b] | ADT < 12 Months | | *P*-Value[b] | ADT < 12 Months | | *P*-Value[b] | ADT < 12 Months | | *P*-Value[b] |
| | High (***n*** = 2) | No (***n*** = 2) | | High (***n*** = 2) | No (***n*** = 2) | | High (***n*** = 2) | No (***n*** = 2) | | High (***n*** = 1) | No (***n*** = 3) | |
| **Age** | 59.5 ± 0.7 | 58 ± 5.6 | 0.75 | 56.5 ± 3.5 | 61 ± 1.4 | 1 | 56.5 ± 3.5 | 61 ± 1.4 | 1 | 54 | 60.3 ± 1.5 | 0.07 |
| **T Stages** | | | 0.05 | | | 0.32 | | | 0.32 | | | 0.25 |
| 1 | – | – | | – | – | | – | – | | – | – | |
| 2 | 100% | – | | 50% | 50% | | 50% | 50%% | | – | 67% | |
| 3 | – | – | | – | – | | – | – | | – | – | |
| 4 | – | 100% | | 50% | 50% | | 50% | 50% | | 100% | 33% | |
| **Gleason score[a]** | | | 0.25 | | | 0.25 | | | 0.25 | | | 0.50 |
| ≤ 7 | 50% | – | | – | 50% | | – | 50% | | – | 33% | |
| 08–10 | 50% | 100% | | 100% | 50% | | 100% | 50% | | 100% | 67% | |
| **PSA level[a]** | 160.6 (17.9–303.3) | 20.2 (10.1–30.4) | 0.19 | 156.7 (10.1–303.3) | 22.3 (17.9–30.4) | 1 | 156.7 (10.1–303.3) | 22.3 (17.9–30.4) | 1 | 10.1 | 30.4 (17.9–303.3) | 0.5 |
| **ADT Type** | | | – | | | – | | | – | | | – |
| Orchyde | 2 | – | | 1 | 1 | | 1 | 1 | | – | 1 | |
| LHRH agonist ± antiandrogen | – | 2 | | 1 | 1 | | 1 | 1 | | 1 | 2 | |
| **ADT Treatment Duration** | 5 (3–7) | 6 (3–9) | – | 8 (7–9) | 3 | – | 8 (7–9) | 3 | – | 9 | 3 (3–7) | – |

+ is upregulated protein expression group; – is downregulated protein expression group

[a] Age is presented in mean ± SD; PSA level and prostate volume are presented in median (min-max)

[b] Statistical significance was measured by comparing the clinical parameters of upregulated and non-upregulated ADT-PCa samples using Independent T test for Age; Pearson chi square test for Gleason score; Mann-Whitney test for T-stages and PSA level

[*] *P*-value < 0.05 is significant

tissue during ADT. This early resistance mechanism should be a warning to clinicians that this process should be monitored when starting ADT [20].

Another interesting result is that AR was the only gene that was upregulated at the early stage (3 months). PCa cells might start to overcome low serum androgen levels due to ADT by increasing AR expression first [10–13]. This suggests that the early mechanism to overcome low serum androgen levels is increased AR expression [10–13]. Many in vitro studies have shown upregulation of AR expression, demonstrating the adaptations of prostatic cells that increase sensitivity to low androgen levels after treatment with ADT [21–23]. However, these phenomena can be seen only in patients with orchiectomy who receive ADT. This might show that an abrupt decrease in serum testosterone levels induces the upregulation of AR. Furthermore, there are many known mechanisms of AR changes, including gene amplification and mutation, which have also been reported in patients with ADT > 12 months [8–10]. However, this study examined only protein expression and did not further evaluate the other AR changes, namely, AR amplification and AR mutation.

PCa cell growth is promoted by androgens, especially DHT [12]. This study found that 5α-reductase isoenzymes, which regulate the conversion of T to DHT [11, 12], were increased in ADT-treated PCa patients. Similar to other studies, SRD5A1 [14, 24] and SRD5A3 [14, 25] were upregulated in ADT-PCa patients compared with ADT-naïve PCa patients, and SRD5A2 was downregulated [14, 24, 26]. However, until now, there has been very limited information on whether the isozyme is involved in the process of androgen biosynthesis. Interestingly, this study found that SRD5A was the only steroidogenic enzyme that was upregulated in the ADT ≤12 months group. This SRD5A upregulation was also related to AR upregulation. This suggests that PCa cells upregulate the expression of SRD5A, which is the primary enzyme responsible for the conversion of T to DHT expression, after or at the same time as AR expression is upregulated [14]. Thus, developing a new strategy or compound that targets SRD5A can reduce the risk of early resistance.

Among the PCa-ADT patients with ADT durations of less than 12 months, three patients showed upregulation of genes with increased protein expression. Three of four patients showed upregulation of AR, with one patient showing upregulation AR and SRD5A1, 2, and 3; one showing upregulation of AR, SRD5A1 and SRD5A2; and one showing only AR upregulation. These findings are novel, as no one has ever investigated below the cut-off of 12 months. This study suggests the possible upregulation of AR and steroidogenesis enzymes (namely, SRD5A1, SRD5A2, and SRD5A3) as a compensatory mechanism for the low testosterone level due to ADT [14]. Our study showed that patients whose SRD5A1, 2, or 3 level becomes upregulated have increased expression of the proteins later (at 7–9 months of ADT) than those with upregulated AR (at 3–7 months of ADT). This suggests that the increase in AR is the first compensatory mechanism, followed by the increases SRD5A1, 2, and 3. However, further studies with more patients are needed to validate this compensatory response.

Many studies have shown that there is a shift to adrenal androgen usage for maintaining DHT levels via upregulation of AKR1C3 expression [10–14]. This study showed that AKR1C3 can only be found in patients treated with ADT for more than 12 months, which is in accordance with other studies [27]. The next question is why AKR1C3 is not upregulated in the early state. Based on the steroidogenic pathway, AKR1C3 is an upstream enzyme that converts adrenal androgen to downstream androgens, which are needed as a source of DHT [12–14]. To support the previous statement, we hypothesize that in PCa cells, AKR1C3 expression is increased after AR and SRD5A upregulation. However, it has been shown that there are many variations in AKR1C3, SRD5A and AR expression among patients in the ADT > 12 months group. This might be due to the dynamic process of steroidogenesis. The AR or steroidogenesis enzymes are regulated based on 'real-time' conditions as needed by PCa cells.

The main limitation of our study is the small sample size. However, this is the first study that tried to evaluate AR signaling pathway changes during ADT in human prostate tissues. This study also revealed an important finding in which PCa cells may adapt to low androgen levels caused by ADT before PSA levels rise. This finding is not the first significant one with interesting information that is limited by a low sample size. One study performed by Alsinnawi M et al. contributed significant prognostic information in which high expression of the SLCO gene may result in worse disease-free survival (DFS), with only 11 samples included in the study [28]. Although the sample size was small, the results of the mentioned study were in concordance with the results of Terakawa T et al.'s team, who examine similar outcomes but with more patients included ($n = 494$) [29]. Similar studies had similarly small sample sizes yet showed significance in practice. With only a few samples, Tiwari et al. showed that AR and its transcriptional corepressor REST modulate SPINK1 expression and that SPINK1 plays a plausible role in the progression of neuroendocrine prostate cancer [30]. Another study by Cheung et al., using only 11 samples per group, found that Actin alpha cardiac muscle 1 (ACTC1) gene expression plays a role in compensating ADT administration for PCa as a response to ADT-induced muscle loss [31].

In addition to the sample size, other limitations of our study include the limited number samples available due to some nonutilizable old specimens unsuitable for RNA extraction and protein expression evaluation. Another limitation of this study is its use of the median expression level of each gene in BPH tissues as the cut-off for defining upregulation in other samples. This was the only available method, as there is currently no official validated cut-off to define upregulation of AR or steroidogenic genes in immunohistochemistry staining.

In conclusion, AR and steroidogenic enzymes are upregulated in PCa patients who are treated with ADT. Early AR and SRD5A upregulation can be found at 3 months in ADT patients. This indicates that the early evaluation of AR and SRD5A expression in intraprostatic tissue should be done. Further strategic treatment should target AR and the SRD5A enzyme to overcome early resistance to ADT.

## Conclusion

AR and steroidogenic enzymes are upregulated in ADT-PCa patients as early as 3 months without PSA elevation. Steroidogenic enzymes, especially SRD5A3 expression, were also upregulated before PSA rose.

## Supplementary information

**Additional file 1: Supplementary Table 1.** Description of Antibodies used in the Study. **Supplementary Table 2.** H-score of the included samples.

### Abbreviations

ACTC1: Actin alpha cardiac muscle 1; ADT: Androgen-Deprivation Therapy; AR: Androgen receptor; ARVs: Androgen receptor variants; BPH: Benign Prostatic Hyperplasia; CRPC: Castration resistant prostate cancer; DHT: Dihydrotestosterone; DFS: Disease-free survival; FFPE: Formalin Fixed Paraffin embedded; HIER: Heat induced Epitope retrieval; PCa: Prostate cancer; PSA: Prostate Specific Antigen

**Acknowledgments**
The Authors would like to thank Universitas Indonesia for providing support in facilities and fund in the whole process of this research.

**Authors' contributions**
ARAHH: Protocol/project development; Manuscript writing/editing. HWKP: Manuscript writing/editing; Data analysis. NPS: Protocol/project development; Data collection or management. PD: Data collection or management; Data analysis. SSS: Manuscript writing; Data analysis. EN: Data collection or management. FLG: Data collection or management. MS: Protocol/project development; Supervising. BT: Protocol/project development; Supervising. A: Protocol/project development; Supervising. RU: Protocol/project development; Supervising. CAM: Protocol/project development; Supervising. All authors contributing this papers has read and approved the manuscript. All participating authors has also consented for publication.

**Author details**
[1]Department of Urology, CiptoMangunkusumo Hospital - Faculty of Medicine Universitas Indonesia, Jl. Diponegoro No.71, RW.5, Kenari, Senen, RW.5, Kenari, Senen, Kota Jakarta Pusat, Daerah Khusus Ibukota Jakarta 10430, Indonesia. [2]Department of Biology, CiptoMangunkusumo Hospital - Faculty of Medicine Universitas Indonesia, Jl. Diponegoro No.71, RW.5, Kenari, Senen, RW.5, Kenari, Senen, Kota Jakarta Pusat, Daerah Khusus Ibukota Jakarta, Indonesia. [3]Department of Pathology Anatomy, CiptoMangunkusumo Hospital - Faculty of Medicine Universitas Indonesia, Jl. Diponegoro No.71, RW.5, Kenari, Senen, RW.5, Kenari, Senen, Kota Jakarta Pusat, Daerah Khusus Ibukota Jakarta, Indonesia.

**References**

1. Shariat SF, Kattan MW, Vickers AJ, Karakiewicz PI, Scardino PT. Critical review of prostate Cancer predictive tools. Future Oncol. 2009;5(10):1555–84. https://doi.org/10.2217/fon.09.121.
2. Lee DJ, Cha EK, Dubin JM, et al. Novel therapeutics for the Management of Castration-Resistant Prostate Cancer (CRPC). BJU Int. 2012;109(7):968–85. https://doi.org/10.1111/j.1464-410X.2011.10643.
3. Harzstak AL, Small EJ. Castrate-resistant prostate Cancer: therapeutic strategies. Expert Opin Pharmacother. 2010;11(6):937–45. https://doi.org/10.1517/14656561003677382.
4. Karantanos T, Corn PG, Thompson TC. Prostate Cancer progression after androgen deprivation therapy: mechanisms of castrate-resistance and novel therapeutic approaches. Oncogene. 2013;32(49):5501–11.
5. Titus MA, Schell MJ, Lih FB, Tomer KB, Mohler JL. Testosterone and dihydrotestosterone tissue levels in recurrent prostate cancer. Clin Cancer Res. 2005;11:4653–7.
6. Zarour L, Alumkai J. Emerging therapies in castrate-resistant prostate Cancer. Curr Urol Rep. 2010;11(3):152–8. https://doi.org/10.1007/s11934-010-0104-x.
7. Scher HI, Steineck G, Kelly WK. Hormone-refractory (D3) prostate cancer: refining the concept. Urology. 1995;46(2):142–8.
8. Tilki D, Schaeffer ME, Evans CP. Understanding mechanism of resistance in metastatic castration-resistant prostate cancer: the role of the androgen receptor. Eur Urol Focus. 2016;2:499–505.
9. Yuan X, Cai C, Chen S, Chen S, Yu Z, Balk SP. Androgen receptor functions in castration-resistant prostate Cancer and mechanisms of resistance to new agents targeting the androgen Axis. Oncogene. 2013;33:1–11. https://doi.org/10.1038/onc.2013.235.
10. Chandrasekar T, Yang JC, Gao AC, Evans CP. Mechanism of resistance in castration-resistant prostate Cancer (CRPC). Transl Androl Urol. 2015;4(3): 365–80.
11. Mostagher EA. Steroid hormone synthetic pathways in prostate Cancer. Transl Androl Urol. 2013;2(3):212–27. https://doi.org/10.3978/j.issn.2223-4683.2013.09.16.
12. Armandari I, Hamid AR, Verhaegh G, Schalken J. Intratumoral Steroidogenesis in castration-resistant prostate Cancer: a target for therapy. Prostate Int. 2014;2(3):105–13.
13. Lonergen PE, Tindall DJ. Androgen receptor signaling in prostate Cancer development and progression. J Carcinog. 2011;10:20. https://doi.org/10.4103/1477-3163.83937.
14. Li J, Ding Z, Wang Z, et al. Androgen regulation of 5α-Reductase Isoenzymes in prostate Cancer: implications for prostate Cancer prevention. PLoS One. 2011;6(12):e28840. https://doi.org/10.1371/journal.pone.0028840.
15. Sigma Aldrich. Product. Life science: Antibodies. [Available from: https://www.sigmaaldrich.com/life-science/cell-biology/antibodies.html].
16. Vander Griend DJ, Litvinov IV, Isaacs JT. Conversion of androgen receptor signaling from a growth suppressor in normal prostate epithelial cells to an oncogene in prostate cancer cells involves a gain of function in c-Myc regulation. Int J Biol Sci. 2014;10(6):627–42.
17. Lam HM, Ouyang B, Chen J, Ying J, Wang J, Wu CL, et al. Targeting GPR30 with G-1: a new therapeutic target for castration-resistant prostate cancer. Endocr Relat Cancer. 2014;21(6):903–14.
18. Liu C, Lou W, Zhu Y, Yang JC, Nadiminty N, Gaikwad NW, et al. Intracrine androgens and AKR1C3 activation confer resistance to Enzalutamide in prostate Cancer. Cancer Res. 2015;75(7):1413–22.
19. He M, Liu H, Cao J, et al. Predicting Castration-resistant prostate cancer after combined androgen blockade. Oncotarget. 2017;8(62):105458–62. https://doi.org/10.18632/oncotarget.22246.
20. Cornford P, Bellmunt J, Colla M, et al. EAU-ESTRO-SIOG Guidelines on Prostate Cancer. Part II: Treatment of Relapsing, Metastatic, and Castration-Resistant Prostate Cancer. Eur Urol. 2017;71(4):630–42.
21. Chen CD, Welsbie DS, Tran C, et al. Molecular determinants of resistance to antiandrogen therapy. Nat Med. 2004;10:33–9.
22. Koivisto P, Kononen J, Palmberg C, et al. Androgen receptor gene amplification: a possible molecular mechanism for androgen deprivation therapy failure in prostate cancer. Cancer Res. 1997;57:314–9.
23. Visakorpi T, Hyytinen E, Koivisto P, et al. In vivo amplification of the androgen receptor gene and progression of human prostate cancer. Nat Genet. 1995;9:401–6.
24. Shibata Y, Suzuki K, Arai S, et al. Impact of pre-treatment prostate tissue androgen content on the prediction of castration-resistant prostate cancer development in patients treated with primary androgen deprivation therapy. Andrology. 2013;1:505–11.
25. Godoy A, Kawinski E, Li Y, et al. 5alpha-reductase type 3 expression in human benign and malignant tissues: a comparative analysis during prostate cancer progression. Prostate. 2011;71:1033–46.
26. Luo J, Dunn TA, Ewing CM, et al. Decreased gene expression of steroid 5 alpha-reductase 2 in human prostate cancer: Implications for finasteride therapy of prostate carcinoma. Prostate. 2003;57(2):134–9.
27. Hamid AR, Pfeiffer MJ, et al. AKR1C3 is a biomarker and therapeutic target for Castration Resistant Prostate Cancer. Mol Med. 2013;18:1449–55.
28. Alsinnawi M, Zhang A, Bianchi-Frias D, Burns J, Cho E, Zhang X, et al. Association of prostate cancer *SLCO* gene expression with Gleason grade and alteration following androgen deprivation therapy. Prostate Cancer Prostatic Dis. 2019;22(4):560–8.
29. Terakawa T, Kastsuta E, Yan L, Turaga N, McDonald KA, Fujisawa M, et al. High expression of SLCO2B1 is asociated with prostate cancer recurrence after radical prostatectomy. Oncotarget. 2018;9(18):14207–18.
30. Tiwari R, Manzar N, Bhatia V, Yadav A, Nengroo MA, Datta D, et al. Androgen deprivation upregulates SPINK1 expression and potentiates cellular plasticity in prostate cancer. Nat Commun. 2020;11:384.
31. Cheung AS, de Rooy C, Lebinger I, Rana K, Clarke MV, How JM, et al. Actin alpha cardiac muscle 1 gene expression is upregulated in the skeletal muscle of men undergoing androgen deprivation therapy for prostate cancer. J Steroid Biochem Mol Biol. 2017;174:56–64.

9

# Physician preferences for non-metastatic castration-resistant prostate cancer treatment

Sandy Srinivas[1*], Ateesha F. Mohamed[2], Sreevalsa Appukkuttan[2], Marc Botteman[3], Xinyi Ng[3], Namita Joshi[3], Erica Horodniceanu[3], A. Reginald Waldeck[2] and Stacey J Simmons[2]

**Abstract**

**Background:** Recent approvals of second-generation androgen receptor inhibitors (SGARIs) have changed the treatment landscape for non-metastatic castration-resistant prostate cancer (nmCRPC). These SGARIs have similar efficacy but differ in safety profiles. We used a discrete choice experiment to explore how United States physicians make treatment decisions between adverse events (AEs) and survival gains in nmCRPC, a largely asymptomatic disease.

**Methods:** Treating physicians ($n = 149$) participated in an online survey that included 14 treatment choice questions, each comparing 2 hypothetical treatment profiles, which varied in terms of 5 safety and 2 efficacy attributes. We described safety attributes (fatigue, skin rash, cognitive problems, falls, and fractures) in terms of severity and frequency, and efficacy attributes (overall survival [OS] and time to pain progression) in terms of duration of effect. We used a random parameters logit model to estimate preference weights and importance scores for each attribute. We also estimated the amount of survival gain physicians were willing to trade for a reduction in specific AEs between treatment options.

**Results:** Physicians placed more importance on survival than on time to pain progression, and viewed a reduction in cognitive problems from severe to none, a reduction in risk of a serious fracture from 8% to none, and a reduction in fatigue from severe to none as the most important safety attributes. Physicians were willing to forego 9.1 and 6.6 months of OS, respectively, to reduce cognitive problems and fatigue from severe to mild-to-moderate. To reduce the risk of a serious fracture from 8 to 5% and 5% to none, physicians were willing to trade 3.9 and 5.3 months of OS, respectively.

**Conclusions:** Physicians were willing to trade substantial amounts of survival to avoid AEs between hypothetical treatments. These results emphasize the importance of carefully balancing therapies' benefits and risks to ultimately optimize the overall quality of nmCRPC patients' survival. Nonetheless, it is noted that the results from the study sample of 149 physicans may not be representative of the viewpoints of all nmCRPC-treating physicians.

**Keywords:** Prostatic neoplasms, Castration-resistant, Choice behavior, Risk assessment, Physicians

* Correspondence: sandysri@stanford.edu
[1]Stanford University Medical Center, Palo Alto, California, USA
Full list of author information is available at the end of the article

## Background

Non-metastatic castration-resistant prostate cancer (nmCRPC) is characterized by biochemical progression (i.e., rising prostate-specific antigen [PSA] after androgen deprivation therapy (ADT) without evidence of detectable disease on conventional imaging [1]. Patients with nmCRPC are in a critical period within the disease's clinical spectrum, as therapeutic interventions can prevent progression to metastatic disease, in which metastases to the bone, soft tissues, or viscera are associated with higher morbidity and mortality [2, 3]. Patients with nmCRPC are typically asymptomatic [1, 4]. Therefore, another therapeutic goal is to minimize treatment-related adverse events (AEs), which can adversely impact patients' daily activities or lead to treatment discontinuation. Until recently, the treatment of nmCRPC patients consisted of continued ADT, with or without second-line hormonal treatment or active surveillance using PSA doubling time and imaging [5]. The relative lack of evidence on these strategies' benefits presents a challenge to clinicians making treatment recommendations [5]. This can be further complicated by patients requesting treatment upon experiencing anxiety due to rising PSA levels [6, 7].

Recent approvals of second-generation androgen receptor inhibitors (SGARIs) have changed the nmCRPC treatment landscape. Large phase 3 randomized clinical trials have demonstrated SGARIs' benefits, notably their ability to prolong metastasis-free survival (MFS) [8–10]. However, SGARIs may be associated with various AEs and trial evidence suggests that different agents exhibit different safety profiles [8–10]. For example, 3 trials in nmCRPC patients reported rates of fatigue (a common AE among SGARIs) ranging from 12 to 33% [8–10].

In this context, nmCRPC patients, their caregivers, and physicians must balance efficacy with AEs when making treatment decisions. Several studies have elicited prostate cancer patients' benefit-risk preferences [11–17]. Hauber et al. demonstrated that most patients were willing to trade ≥3 months of survival to avoid bone complications [17]. A more recent study in localized prostate cancer also demonstrated that patients trade between survival and AEs [18]. While the patient perspective is paramount, prostate cancer patients' treatment decisions are often heavily influenced by physician recommendations [19]. To our knowledge, no study has examined physician preferences for nmCRPC treatment. Therefore, by using a formal discrete choice experiment (DCE) approach following recommended practices [20, 21], we aimed to quantify the benefit-risk preferences that United States (US) practicing physicians associate with nmCRPC and SGARI therapy, and examine the extent to which physicians are willing to trade their nmCRPC patients' overall survival (OS), to minimize or avoid AEs of interest.

## Methods

### Survey development

The DCE is a common approach used in healthcare research to elicit preferences for treatment characteristics (i.e., attributes) and the willingness to accept trade-offs among these attributes [22]. In a DCE, respondents are presented with a series of recurring questions in which they choose a preferred option from sets of hypothetical medication profiles with systematic variations in the levels of attributes. The attributes included in this DCE (Table 1) were selected based on a literature search and qualitative interviews. The literature search focused on preferences and/or outcomes studies and clinical trials of SGARIs [8–17, 23]. Using the preliminary list of search-identified attributes, individual phone interviews were conducted with 5 nmCRPC-treating physicians, 5 nmCRPC patients, and 5 caregivers of nmCRPC patients to evaluate the relevance from all perspectives. During the interviews, respondents were asked to look at a list of preliminary attributes and levels, rate their importance, and comment on their relevance, meaningfulness and comprehensibility. Verbatim quotes were noted and analyzed qualitatively. Based on the feedback from the interviews and discussion with the clinical experts, a final list of attributes and levels were derived and comprised 2 efficacy-related attributes (OS and time to pain progression [TPP]) and 5 AE-related attributes (frequency or severity of fatigue, skin rash, cognitive problems, risk of serious fall, and risk of serious fracture). This research focused on OS instead of MFS (the primary endpoint in the recent SGARI clinical trials) because the MFS definition varies slightly between trials and is a fairly recent endpoint, whereas OS is assumed to be universally understood by most physicians. The qualitative interviews also verified that physicians, patients and caregivers viewed OS as the most important efficacy attribute.

To create the alternative choices (i.e., medication profiles), a widely used algorithm (in SAS 9.4) was adapted to create a design that maximized statistical efficiency [24]. The final design was composed of 4 survey versions, each with 14 medication choice questions (i.e., pairs of hypothetical medication profiles; see example in Fig. 1). Each respondent was randomized to 1 of the versions. The survey proceeded as follows: sociodemographic and practice characteristics, treatment attribute descriptions, and 14 medication choice questions. An additional question was added whereby one medication profile was dominant over the other (i.e., higher levels of efficacy and lower levels of AEs) to assess whether respondents were paying attention. Attribute descriptions

**Table 1** Attributes, Attribute Labels and Levels included in the DCE

| Attributes | Attribute Labels | Levels |
|---|---|---|
| Overall Survival | Prolonging life | • 4 years and an additional 12 months |
| | | • 4 years and an additional 6 months |
| | | • 4 years and an additional 3 months |
| Time to Pain Progression | Delay in time until pain progresses (develops or worsens) | • 3 years and an additional 12 months |
| | | • 3 years and an additional 6 months |
| | | • 3 years and an additional 3 months |
| Fatigue | Fatigue (lack of energy) | • None |
| | | • Mild-to-moderate (may affect daily activities) |
| | | • Severe (affects self-care) |
| Skin Rash | Skin rash | • None |
| | | • Mild-to-moderate (30% of the body or less, may affect daily activities) |
| | | • Severe (more than 30% of the body, requires treatment and affects self-care) |
| Cognitive Problems | Cognitive problems | • None |
| | | • Mild-to-moderate (may affect daily activities) |
| | | • Severe (affects self-care) |
| Serious Fall | Risk of a serious fall | • None |
| | | • 5% (5 out of 100 people) |
| | | • 8% (8 out of 100 people) |
| Serious Fracture | Risk of a serious fracture | • None |
| | | • 5% (5 out of 100 people) |
| | | • 8% (8 out of 100 people) |

(appendix Tables 1 and 2, [additional files 1 and 2]) were included before the choice questions to ensure uniformity of interpretation by physicians. Descriptions of AEs and their respective severity levels were adapted from the common terminology criteria for adverse events (CTCAE) [25]. Severe AEs were based on CTCAE grade 3 and above, and mild-to-moderate AEs were based on CTCAE grades 1 and 2. In general, a severe AE affects self-care and a mild-to-moderate AE may affect ability to maintain daily activities.

The initial survey draft was pre-tested via phone interviews with 5 physicians (2 urologists, 3 oncologists) to assess clarity of survey instructions, comprehensibility of attribute descriptions, and whether physicians were willing to make trade-offs amongst attributes. Based on the pre-testing feedback, minor wording changes were made for clarity, and the ranges of levels for 4 attributes (OS, TPP, serious fall, serious fracture) were slightly expanded.

### Study sample

Published preference-related studies in prostate cancer have included sample sizes of 65 to 285 respondents [11, 13–16], and the target sample size of 150 completed responses in this study followed recommendations in DCEs (additional file 3) [26]. The survey was administered online in January 2019 to a convenience sample targeting 75 urologists and 75 oncologists recruited from existing online panels which update their member profiles annually. Eligible respondents were required to have experience treating patients with nmCRPC, be a urologist or oncologist, be ≥18 years of age, and practice within the US. Physicians were excluded if they had participated in an online survey on nmCRPC within the prior 6 weeks, or if they were unwilling to provide consent. All study procedures and materials were reviewed and approved by a centralized US Institutional Review Board.

### Statistical analysis

Descriptive statistics were used to analyze sociodemographic and practice characteristics. Quality checks for DCE responses were evaluated by checking for variability in responses (i.e., respondents who always chose the same medication, such as 'medication A', across all 14 choice questions) and assessing the dominance test. Respondents who failed both checks were excluded.

Effects-coded random parameter logit (RPL) models were used to analyze the DCE responses [27]. The RPL model yields a preference weight (i.e., coefficient) for

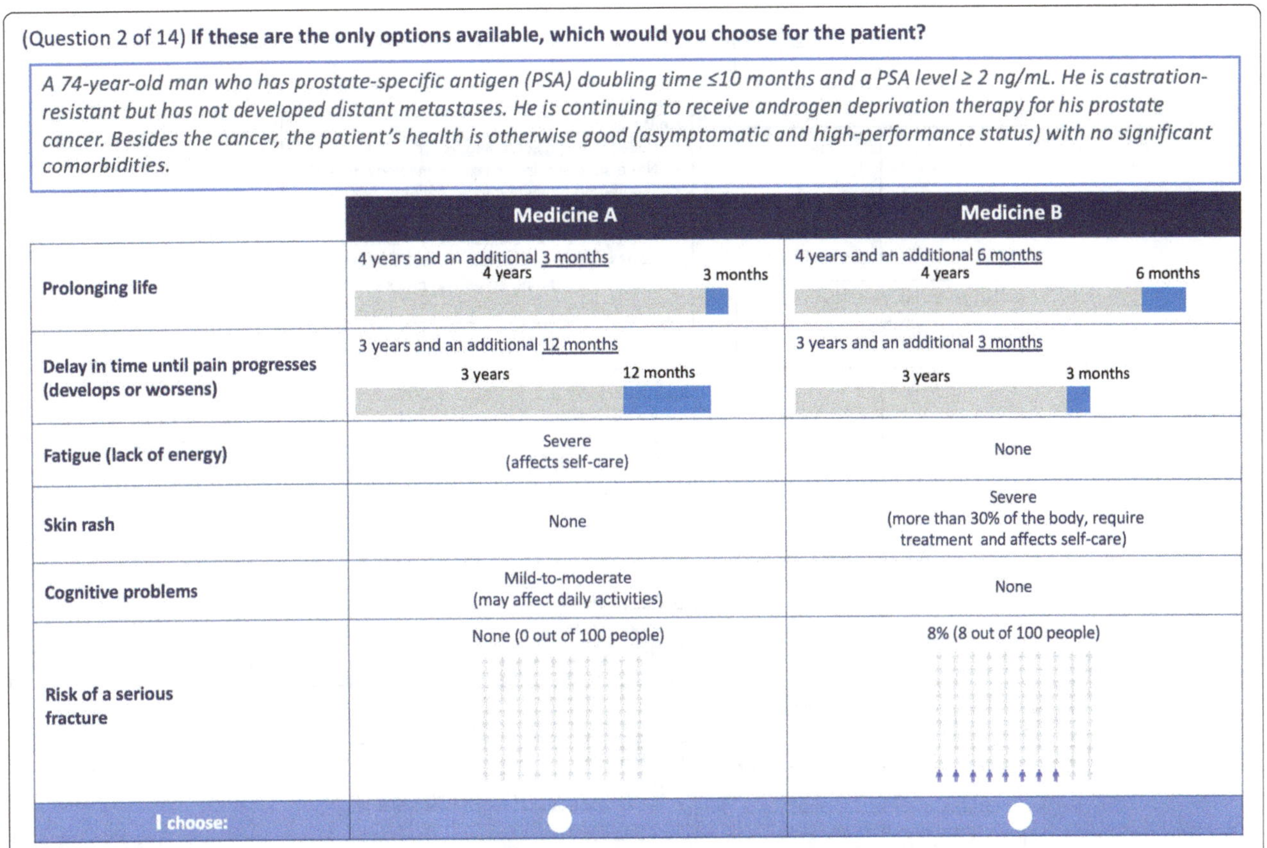


**Fig. 1** Example of a treatment choice question in the DCE. Note that falls and fractures are correlated and should not be included in the same choice questions. Therefore, risk of a serious fracture was shown in 50% of choice tasks and risk of a serious fall was shown in the other half

each attribute level, which can be interpreted as the relative preference strength for each attribute level; a greater preference weight indicates a stronger preference [27]. The difference between highest and lowest preference weights (i.e., vertical distance between an attribute's best and worst levels) is also a measure of the attribute's overall relative importance over the ranges represented in the DCE [27]. Relative attribute importance scores were also calculated by expressing this vertical distance as a percentage of the total variance observed (i.e., summation of vertical distances across all attributes). The estimated preference weights were used to calculate the rate at which physicians trade between efficacy and treatment risks (i.e., the marginal rate of substitution [MRS]). Specifically, we looked at the amount of OS that physicians would be willing to forego to achieve a given reduction in AE risk or severity. The MRS was calculated as the change in preference weights from a given improvement in AE that could be offset by the change in preference weights from a reduction in OS. In the MRS calculation, we specified OS as a continuous variable, as this was supported by model fit statistics. Separate models were estimated for each physician specialty to examine if there are differences in willingness to trade OS for AE risk/severity reductions. All DCE analyses used STATA/IC 14.2 and R Studio 3.5.0.

## Results

### Sample characteristics

Of the 150 physicians who completed the study survey, 1 oncologist was excluded from the analysis due to failing both quality checks (Fig. 2). Respondents' sociodemographic and practice characteristics are summarized in Table 2. Compared to oncologists, urologists were slightly older and had a higher proportion of males ($P < 0.05$). Among all physicians, the average time in practice was about 17.9 years. The most frequently reported medications prescribed for nmCRPC were enzalutamide (70.5%), leuprolide (67.1%), and bicalutamide (47.0%).

### Physician preferences and relative importance of attributes

The estimated preference weights and relative importance scores are presented in Fig. 3. Physicians' preferences were naturally and logically ordered (i.e., higher efficacy was preferred over lower efficacy, and lower risks were preferred over higher risks). The difference in preference weights of adjacent levels indicates the relative impact of

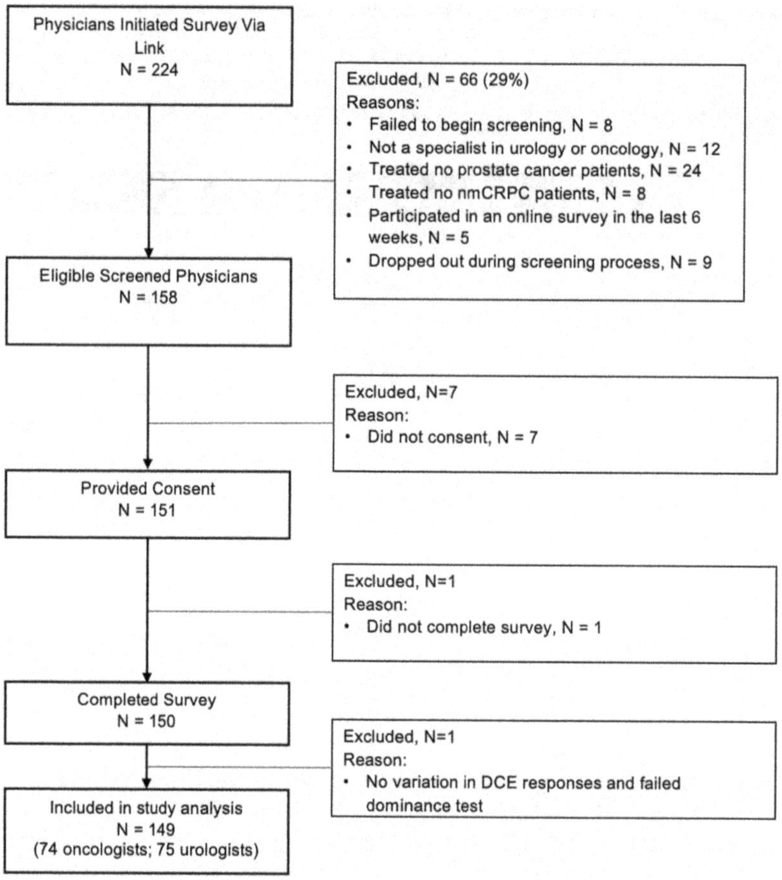


**Fig. 2** Flowchart of Physician Survey Respondent Selection. Note that the physician who dropped out of the survey dropped out immediately after the first question so no other information was collected. nmCRPC = non-metastatic castration-resistant prostate cancer

shifting from one level to the next, where a larger difference signifies a greater impact on treatment choices. The bar graphs in Fig. 3 represent the each attribute's relative importance to physicians' treatment choices. Of the efficacy attributes, physicians placed more importance on a 9-month improvement in OS compared to a 9-month improvement in TPP. Physicians viewed the risk attributes in the following order of importance: a reduction in cognitive problems from severe to none; a reduction in risk of a serious fracture from 8% to none; a reduction in fatigue from severe to none; a reduction in risk of a serious fall from 8% to none; and a reduction in rash from severe to none. Of note, physicians valued a reduction in cognitive problems (from severe to none) and serious fractures (from 8% to none) more than a 9-month improvement in OS. For the same amount of risk reduction, physicians placed more importance on avoiding serious fractures compared to serious falls.

### Trade-offs between OS and AEs

Table 3 presents the amount of OS that physicians were willing to forego for various improvements in the other 6 attributes. Specifically, physicians were willing to trade more OS months for AE reductions that they viewed as more important (i.e., cognitive problems, serious fracture, and fatigue). For cognitive problems and fatigue, physicians were on average willing to trade 9.1 and 6.6 months, respectively, to reduce the AEs from severe to mild-to-moderate. To reduce these AEs from mild-to-moderate to none, physicians were willing to trade 2.5 and 0.8 months of OS for cognitive problems and fatigue, respectively, between hypothetical medication profiles. Physicians were willing to trade 3.9 months and 5.3 months of OS, respectively, to reduce the risk of a serious fracture from 8 to 5% and 5% to none. They were also willing to trade 2.9 months of OS to reduce risk of a serious fall from 8 to 5%, and 2.3 months of OS to reduce the risk from 5% to none.

The amount of OS that urologists and oncologists were willing to forego, for their patients, in return for reduction in AEs were similar (95% confidence interval [CI] overlap) except with respect to rash (Table 3). Specifically, urologists placed relatively more importance on

**Table 2** Characteristics of Physicians and Their Practices by Specialty

| Variable | All Physicians ($N = 149$) | Urologists ($N = 75$) | Oncologists ($N = 74$) | $P$ value |
|---|---|---|---|---|
| Age, years | | | | |
| Mean (SD) | 51.27 (10.68) | 53.91 (11.27) | 48.59 (9.39) | 0.004 |
| Gender, n (%)[a] | | | | |
| Female | 15 (10.1) | 3 (4.0) | 12 (16.2) | 0.007 |
| Male | 132 (88.6) | 72 (96.0) | 60 (81.1) | |
| Race, n (%)[a] | | | | |
| White | 100 (67.1) | 54 (72.0) | 46 (62.2) | 0.474 |
| Black | 1 (0.7) | 0 (0.0) | 1 (1.4) | |
| Asian | 33 (22.1) | 13 (17.3) | 20 (27.0) | |
| Middle Eastern or North African | 3 (2.0) | 2 (2.7) | 1 (1.4) | |
| Native Hawaiian or Other Pacific Islander | 1 (0.7) | 0 (0.0) | 1 (1.4) | |
| Ethnicity, n (%)[a] | | | | |
| Hispanic | 7 (4.7) | 1 (1.3) | 6 (8.1) | 0.175 |
| Not Hispanic | 133 (89.3) | 69 (92.0) | 64 (86.5) | |
| Years in practice | | | | |
| Mean (SD) | 17.87 (8.45) | 19.52 (8.84) | 16.20 (7.75) | 0.025 |
| Median (Q1 to Q3) | 16.0 (11.0 to 25.0) | 19.0 (13.0 to 26.0) | 15.0 (10.0 to 21.0) | |
| Practice type, n (%) | | | | |
| Office-based private practice | 103 (69.1) | 55 (73.3) | 48 (64.9) | 0.291 |
| Hospital-based private practice | 18 (12.1) | 6 (8.0) | 12 (16.2) | |
| Academic hospital-based | 28 (18.8) | 14 (18.7) | 14 (18.9) | |
| No. of nmCRPC patients seen/physician/month | | | | |
| Mean (SD) | 26.21 (32.17) | 24.08 (29.21) | 28.38 (34.98) | 0.102 |
| Median (Q1 to Q3) | 15.0 (5.0 to 30.0) | 12.0 (5.0 to 30.0) | 20.0 (6.0 to 35.0) | |
| Most frequent medications prescribed to treat nmCRPC, n (%)[b] | | | | |
| Enzalutamide | 105 (70.5) | 56 (74.7) | 49 (66.2) | 0.258 |
| Leuprolide | 100 (67.1) | 61 (81.3) | 39 (52.7) | < 0.001 |
| Bicalutamide | 70 (47.0) | 38 (50.7) | 32 (43.2) | 0.364 |
| Abiraterone | 62 (41.6) | 23 (30.7) | 39 (52.7) | 0.006 |
| Apalutamide | 49 (32.9) | 28 (37.3) | 21 (28.4) | 0.245 |
| Goserelin | 18 (12.1) | 3 (4.0) | 15 (20.3) | 0.002 |
| Flutamide | 15 (10.1) | 3 (4.0) | 12 (16.2) | 0.015 |
| Nilutamide | 10 (6.7) | 0 (0.0) | 10 (13.5) | < 0.001 |
| Triptorelin | 6 (4.0) | 3 (4.0) | 3 (4.1) | > 0.999 |
| Ketoconazole | 3 (2.0) | 2 (2.7) | 1 (1.4) | > 0.999 |
| Histrelin | 1 (0.7) | 1 (1.3) | 0 (0.0) | > 0.999 |
| Others | 5 (3.4) | 4 (5.3) | 1 (1.4) | 0.367 |

[a] Two (1.3%), 11 (7.4%), and 9 (6.0%) physicians declined to answer questions on gender, race, and ethnicity, respectively
[b] Physicians were asked to select the 3 most frequent medications that they use to treat nmCRPC patients

avoiding rash compared to oncologists, and were willing to forego about 7.0 months of OS (95% CI: 4.3–11.0) to reduce rash from severe to none, whereas oncologists were not significantly willing to trade OS (CIs cross 0) to reduce rash (Table 3).

## Discussion

This is the first study that systematically evaluates how physicians weigh the benefits versus risks of nmCRPC treatments in the US, focusing on AEs of special interest. New SGARIs, which have

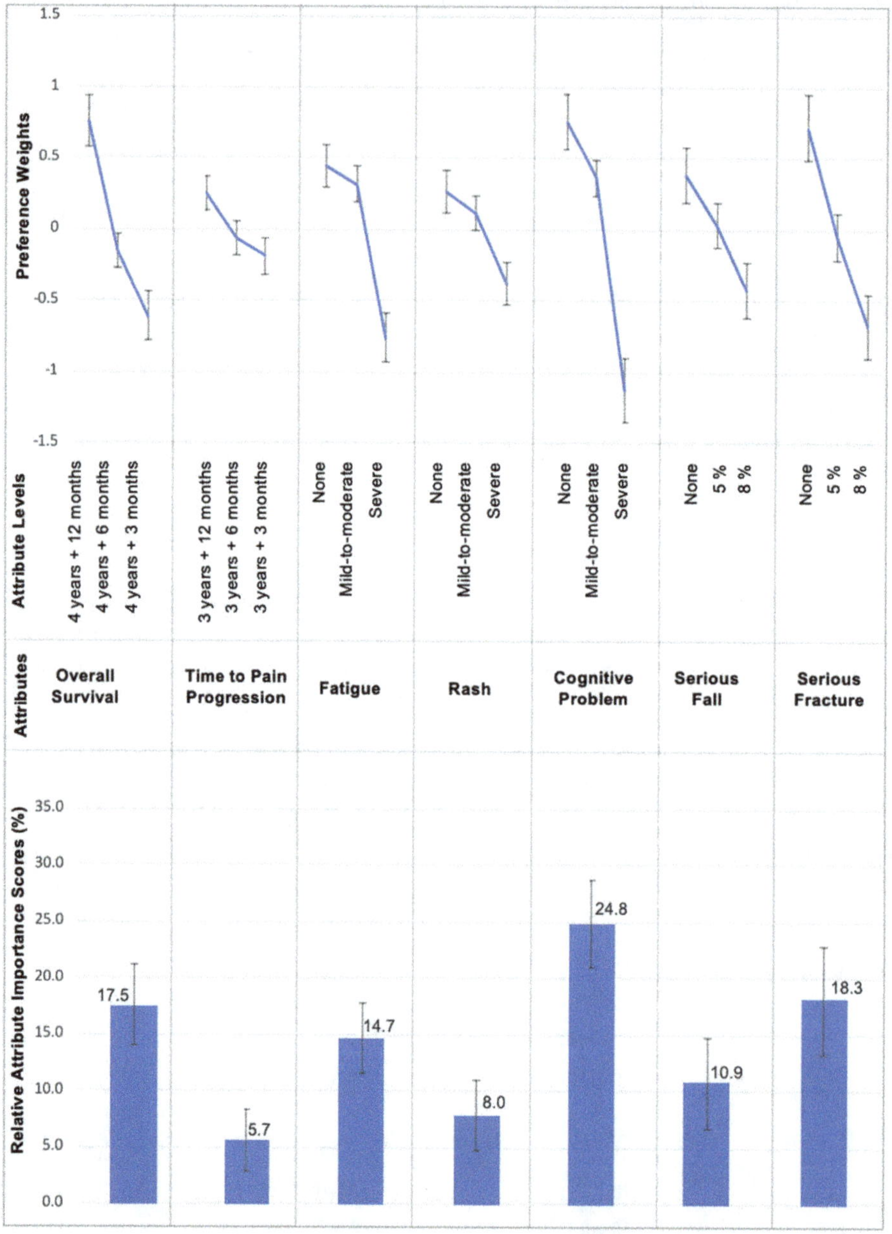


**Fig. 3** Preference Weights and Relative Importance of Attributes. The line graphs at the top of the figure represent preference weights estimates of each attribute level with 95% confidence intervals (CIs). A more positive preference weight indicates a stronger preference for the level. For example, physicians preferred no fatigue to severe fatigue. The vertical distance between an attribute's best and worst levels is a measure of the relative importance of the attribute. Relative attribute importance scores (with 95% CI) presented at the bottom of the figure were calculated by expressing this vertical distance as a percentage of the sum of vertical distances across all attributes. The larger the score, the greater the impact that variations in the attribute levels had on treatment choices

demonstrated similar efficacy in terms of delaying metastases, differ in their risk of AEs, which may impact patients' daily activities and the overall quality of their survival. Our study fills an important gap by considering the types of AEs physicians consider most important, and the extent to which physicians were willing to trade between these AEs and their patients' OS.

Several key findings emerged from this study. First, we demonstrated that treatment-related AEs greatly influenced physicians' treatment choices. In fact, physicians appeared to place more importance on avoiding certain AEs (e.g., severe cognitive problems and serious fracture) than improving survival (i.e., 9-month improvement in OS). Although OS is an important treatment goal, physicians were also concerned with minimizing AEs,

**Table 3** Number of Months of Overall Survival That Physicians Were Willing to Trade In Return for an Improvement in Other Attributes

| | All Physicians | | Urologists | | Oncologists | |
|---|---|---|---|---|---|---|
| | Reduction, months | 95% CI | Reduction, months | 95% CI | Reduction, months | 95% CI |
| **Time to pain progression** | | | | | | |
| Delay progression from 3 to 12 months | 3.0 | (1.6, 4.7) | 4.1 | (1.8, 7.0) | 1.5 | (−0.4, 3.8) |
| Delay progression from 6 to 12 months | 2.1 | (0.8, 3.6) | 3.7 | (1.6, 6.6) | 0.6 | (−1.2, 2.6) |
| Delay progression from 3 to 6 months | 0.9 | (− 0.5, 2.3) | 0.3 | (−1.8, 2.5) | 0.8 | (−1.1, 3.1) |
| **Fatigue** | | | | | | |
| Severe to none | 7.5 | (5.5, 10.1) | 10.6[a] | (7.0, 15.9) | 6.2 | (3.8, 10.4) |
| Severe to mild-to-moderate | 6.6 | (4.9, 9.1) | 9.2[a] | (6.3, 13.9) | 5.7 | (3.3, 9.9) |
| Mild-to-moderate to none | 0.8 | (−0.6, 2.3) | 1.4 | (−1.2, 3.8) | 0.5 | (− 1.5, 2.4) |
| **Skin rash** | | | | | | |
| Severe to none | 4.0 | (2.3, 6.0) | 7.0 | (4.3, 11.0) | 1.2 | (−1.1, 3.9) |
| Severe to mild-to-moderate | 3.0 | (1.7, 4.7) | 6.0 | (3.5, 9.6) | 0.7 | (−1.2, 2.8) |
| Mild-to-moderate to none | 0.9 | (−0.6, 2.5) | 1.0 | (−1.3, 3.7) | 0.5 | (−1.5, 2.7) |
| **Cognitive problems** | | | | | | |
| Severe to none | 11.6[a] | (8.9, 15.4) | 14.5[a] | (10.2, 21.2) | 10.5[a] | (6.7, 17.5) |
| Severe to mild-to-moderate | 9.1[a] | (6.9, 12.1) | 12.2[a] | (8.8, 18.0) | 7.3 | (4.3, 12.5) |
| Mild-to-moderate to none | 2.5 | (1.0, 4.2) | 2.2 | (−0.1, 4.8) | 3.2 | (0.9, 6.5) |
| **Serious fall** | | | | | | |
| 8% to none | 5.2 | (2.9, 7.9) | 4.3 | (1.2, 8.2) | 6.4 | (2.7, 12.1) |
| 8 to 5% | 2.9 | (1.0, 5.1) | 2.4 | (−0.5, 5.9) | 3.4 | (0.7, 7.4) |
| 5% to none | 2.3 | (0.4, 4.4) | 1.8 | (−1.0, 5.1) | 3.0 | (0.2, 6.6) |
| **Serious fracture** | | | | | | |
| 8% to none | 9.2[a] | (6.4, 12.7) | 7.7 | (3.7, 12.7) | 10.3[a] | (5.9, 17.7) |
| 8 to 5% | 3.9 | (1.8, 6.3) | 3.7 | (0.3, 7.4) | 4.6 | (1.5, 9.0) |
| 5% to none | 5.3 | (3.1, 7.8) | 4.0 | (0.7, 7.7) | 5.7 | (2.7, 10.5) |

CI = confidence interval
95% CIs are estimated by simulating 10,000 draws from a multivariate normal distribution defined by the variance-covariance matrix
[a]Estimated months are beyond the range (> 9 months) included in the discrete choice experiment and should be interpreted with caution as it assumes extrapolation beyond the ranges studied

presumably because nmCRPC patients are largely asymptomatic. Physicians viewed the examined AEs in the following order of importance (most to least): cognitive problems, serious fracture, fatigue, serious fall, and rash. These views were also reflected during the qualitative interviews and pre-tests. Prostate cancer patients are often elderly with multiple comorbidities [28]; as a result, the consequences of increased cognitive problems, fractures, and fatigue can be serious. Understanding how physicians value different treatment attributes (i.e., different AEs and OS) can potentially help them select treatments for a given patient based on the underlying risk for cognitive decline and the treatment's impact on other important AEs (e.g., fatigue, fractures). These study findings can also potentially inform outcomes for future trials in nmCRPC or decision aids.

Our study also estimated the amount of patient-survival gains that physicians were willing to forego to reduce the risk of treatment-related AEs, particularly those viewed as more problematic. Urologists and oncologists appeared to have different views on the importance of AEs, in particular towards treatment-related rash. Urologists placed more importance on avoiding severe rash and were willing to trade a significant amount OS to avoid rash, as compared to oncologists. However, the study was not designed or powered to detect statistical differences in subgroups, hence these differences should be interpreted cautiously. Other studies have also observed substantial trade-offs between survival and AEs among cancer patients. Bridges et al. found that patients with advanced non-small cell lung cancer require an additional 7.3 months of progression-free survival (PFS) (with mild disease symptoms) to accept an increase in fatigue from none to moderate [29]. Wong et al. found that patients with renal cell carcinoma were willing to trade 4.4 months of PFS to avoid fatigue increasing from mild-to-moderate to severe [30]. Lastly, Uemura et al. observed that patients with castration-resistant prostate cancer prioritized a reduction in fatigue over increasing OS, and de Freitas et al. noted that treatment-related risks were important to patients with biochemical-recurrent prostate cancer [15, 31]. Taken together, these studies further highlight the importance of carefully balancing the goal of extending survival with the introduction of treatment-related AEs.

This study examines treatment preferences in nmCRPC from the physician's perspective. Understanding physicians' preferences for treatment choices is important given that treatment decisions in prostate cancer are often heavily influenced by physician recommendations [19]. Undoubtedly, examining benefit-risk preferences from the patient perspective is crucial. A similar DCE has been conducted which showed that nmCRPC patients and caregivers were most concerned with reducing the risks of serious fractures and falls, and the severity of cognitive problems, which is fairly similar with the findings from this physician study [32].

This study is subject to some limitations, one of which is inherent to the nature of DCEs, in that respondents must evaluate hypothetical profiles. However, qualitative work and pre-testing were undertaken to ensure that the treatment profiles were clinically relevant. One other limitation is the inclusion of 5 patients, 5 caregivers and 5 physicians in the qualitative interviews, which may not be representative of viewpoints of all nmCRPC patients and physicians in attribute selection; however, feedback from the interviews were consistent across respondents. The use of online panels for physician recruitment may have also limited the results' generalizability to the wider nmCRPC-treating physician population, as physicians who participate in online panels may differ from those who do not. In addition, the majority of participating physicians had a private office-based practice and we cannot ascertain if physicians with an academic-based practice would have different preferences. Lastly, the majority of the participating physicians were non-Hispanic white and thus, results might not be generalizable to physicians of other race and ethnicity as benefit-risks preferences can potentially be influenced by cultural background.

## Conclusions

Physicians making treatment decisions for largely asymptomatic patients with nmCRPC were willing to trade substantial amounts of survival to avoid treatment-related AEs of special interest to nmCRPC and SGARI therapy. Physicians were most concerned with minimizing severe cognitive problems, severe fatigue, and serious fractures. However, avoiding lower grade AEs, especially cognitive problems, within nmCRPC is also of clinical relevance. These results underscore the importance of carefully balancing the benefit-risk profiles between newer SGARI therapies when treating this asymptomatic patient population.

## Supplementary information

**Additional file 1: Appendix Table 1**. Labels and Descriptions Used for Efficacy Attributes and Levels

**Additional file 2: Appendix Table 2**. Labels and Descriptions Used for Risk (Adverse Event) Attributes and Levels

**Additional file 3.** Sample Size Considerations in Discrete Choice Experiments

### Abbreviations

ADT: Androgen deprivation therapy; AE: Adverse event; CI: Confidence interval; CTCAE: Common terminology criteria for adverse events; DCE: Discrete choice experiment; MFS: Metastasis-free survival; MRS: Marginal rate of substitution; nmCRPC: Non-metastatic castration-resistant prostate cancer; OS: Overall survival; PFS: Progression-free survival; PSA: Prostate-specific antigen; RPL: Random parameter logit; SGARI: Second-generation androgen receptor inhibitor; TPP: Time to pain progression; US: United States

### Acknowledgements

The authors would like to thank Marion Rahard and Sonia López from Global Perspectives for their contribution towards physician recruitment, as well as all the physicians who have participated in this research. The authors would also like to thank Catherine Mirvis at Pharmerit International for editorial assistance in the preparation of this manuscript.

### Authors' contributions

SSr contributed to the study design, results interpretation and manuscript writing. AFM contributed to the study design, results interpretation and manuscript writing. SA contributed to the study design, results interpretation and manuscript writing. MB contributed to the study design, results interpretation and manuscript writing. XN contributed to the study design, data collection, data analysis, results interpretation and manuscript writing. NJ contributed to the study design, data collection, data analysis, results interpretation and manuscript writing. EH contributed to the study design, data collection and manuscript writing. ARW contributed to the study design, results interpretation and manuscript writing. SSi contributed to the study design, results interpretation and manuscript writing. All authors read and approved the final manuscript.

### Author details

[1]Stanford University Medical Center, Palo Alto, California, USA. [2]Bayer U.S. LLC, Whippany, NJ, USA. [3]Pharmerit International, Bethesda, MD, USA.

### References

1. Cookson MS, Roth BJ, Dahm P, et al. Castration-resistant prostate Cancer: AUA guideline. J Urol. 2013;190(2):429–38.
2. Halabi S, Kelly WK, Ma H, et al. Meta-analysis evaluating the impact of site of metastasis on overall survival in men with castration-resistant prostate Cancer. Journal of clinical oncology : official journal of the American Society of Clinical Oncology. 2016;34(14):1652–9.
3. Xie W, Regan MM, Buyse M, et al. Metastasis-free survival is a strong surrogate of overall survival in localized prostate Cancer. Journal of clinical oncology : official journal of the American Society of Clinical Oncology. 2017;35(27):3097–104.
4. Smith MR, Kabbinavar F, Saad F, et al. Natural history of rising serum prostate-specific antigen in men with castrate nonmetastatic prostate Cancer. J Clin Oncol. 2005;23(13):2918–25.
5. Alpajaro SIR, Harris JAK, Evans CP. Non-metastatic castration resistant prostate cancer: a review of current and emerging medical therapies. Prostate Cancer Prostatic Dis. 2019;22(1):16–23.
6. Patel MI, DeConcini DT, Lopez-Corona E, Ohori M, Wheeler T, Scardino PT. An analysis of men with clinically localized prostate cancer who deferred definitive therapy. J Urol. 2004;171(4):1520–4.
7. Latini DM, Hart SL, Knight SJ, et al. The relationship between anxiety and time to treatment for patients with prostate Cancer on surveillance. J Urol. 2007;178(3):826–32.
8. Fizazi K, Shore N, Tammela TL, et al. Darolutamide in nonmetastatic, castration-resistant prostate Cancer. N Engl J Med. 2019;380:1235–46.

9. Hussain M, Fizazi K, Saad F, et al. Enzalutamide in men with nonmetastatic, castration-resistant prostate Cancer. N Engl J Med. 2018;378(26):2465–74.
10. Smith MR, Saad F, Chowdhury S, et al. Apalutamide treatment and metastasis-free survival in prostate Cancer. N Engl J Med. 2018;378(15): 1408–18.
11. de Bekker-Grob EW, Bliemer MC, Donkers B, et al. Patients' and urologists' preferences for prostate cancer treatment: a discrete choice experiment. Br J Cancer. 2013;109(3):633–40.
12. King MT, Viney R, Smith DP, et al. Survival gains needed to offset persistent adverse treatment effects in localised prostate cancer. Br J Cancer. 2012; 106(4):638–45.
13. Sculpher M, Bryan S, Fry P, de Winter P, Payne H, Emberton M. Patients' preferences for the management of non-metastatic prostate cancer: discrete choice experiment. *BMJ (Clinical research ed).* 2004;328(7436):382.
14. Lloyd A, Penson D, Dewilde S, Kleinman L. Eliciting patient preferences for hormonal therapy options in the treatment of metastatic prostate cancer. Prostate Cancer Prostatic Dis. 2008;11(2):153–9.
15. Uemura H, Matsubara N, Kimura G, et al. Patient preferences for treatment of castration-resistant prostate cancer in Japan: a discrete-choice experiment. BMC Urol. 2016;16(1):63.
16. Eliasson L, de Freitas HM, Dearden L, Calimlim B, Lloyd AJ. Patients' preferences for the treatment of metastatic castrate-resistant prostate Cancer: a discrete choice experiment. Clin Ther. 2017;39(4):723–37.
17. Hauber AB, Arellano J, Qian Y, et al. Patient preferences for treatments to delay bone metastases. Prostate. 2014;74(15):1488–97.
18. Ahmed HU, Watson V, McCartan N, et al. Evaluating the trade-offs men with localised prostate cancer make between the risks and benefits of treatments: the COMPARE study 2018; http://abstracts.ncri.org.uk/abstract/evaluating-the-trade-offs-men-with-localised-prostate-cancer-make-between-the-risks-and-benefits-of-treatments-the-compare-study/.
19. Scherr KA, Fagerlin A, Hofer T, et al. Physician recommendations trump patient preferences in prostate Cancer treatment decisions. Medical decision making : an international journal of the Society for Medical Decision Making. 2017;37(1):56–69.
20. Bridges JF, Hauber AB, Marshall D, et al. Conjoint analysis applications in health—a checklist: a report of the ISPOR good research practices for conjoint analysis task force. Value Health. 2011;14(4):403–13.
21. Johnson FR, Lancsar E, Marshall D, et al. Constructing experimental designs for discrete-choice experiments: report of the ISPOR conjoint analysis experimental design good research practices task force. Value Health. 2013; 16(1):3–13.
22. Clark MD, Determann D, Petrou S, Moro D, de Bekker-Grob EW. Discrete choice experiments in health economics: a review of the literature. PharmacoEconomics. 2014;32(9):883–902.
23. Jenkins V, Fallowfield L, Edginton T, Payne H, Hamilton E. Preferences of healthy men for two different endocrine treatment options offered for locally advanced prostate cancer. Curr Med Res Opin. 2005;21(9):1329–35.
24. Kuhfeld WF. Marketing Research Methods in SAS: Experimental Design, Choice, Conjoint, and Graphical Techniques. http://support.sas.com/techsup/technote/mr2010.pdf. .
25. National Cancer Institute Division of Cancer Treatment and Diagnosis. Cancer Therapy Evaluation Program. Common Terminology Criteria for Adverse Events (CTCAE). https://ctep.cancer.gov/protocolDevelopment/electronic_applications/ctc.htm#ctc_50. Accessed June 11, 2018.
26. de Bekker-Grob EW, Donkers B, Jonker MF, Stolk EA. Sample size requirements for discrete-choice experiments in healthcare: a practical guide. The Patient-Patient-Centered Outcomes Research. 2015;8(5):373–84.
27. Hauber AB, Gonzalez JM, Groothuis-Oudshoorn CG, et al. Statistical methods for the analysis of discrete choice experiments: a report of the ISPOR conjoint analysis good research practices task force. Value in health : the journal of the International Society for Pharmacoeconomics and Outcomes Research. 2016;19(4):300–15.
28. Sternberg CN, Baskin-Bey ES, Watson M, Worsfold A, Rider A, Tombal B. Treatment patterns and characteristics of European patients with castration-resistant prostate cancer. BMC Urol. 2013;13(1):58.
29. Bridges JF, Mohamed AF, Finnern HW, Woehl A, Hauber AB. Patients' preferences for treatment outcomes for advanced non-small cell lung cancer: a conjoint analysis. *Lung cancer (Amsterdam, Netherlands).* 2012;77(1): 224–231.
30. Wong MK, Mohamed AF, Hauber AB, et al. Patients rank toxicity against progression free survival in second-line treatment of advanced renal cell carcinoma. J Med Econ. 2012;15(6):1139–48.
31. de Freitas HM, Ito T, Hadi M, et al. Patient preferences for metastatic hormone-sensitive prostate Cancer treatments: a discrete choice experiment among men in three European countries. Adv Ther. 2019;36(2):318–32.
32. Srinivas S, Mohamed AF, Appukkuttan S, et al. Patient and caregiver benefit-risk preferences for non-metastatic castration-resistant prostate Cancer treatment (nmCRPC). 2019; http://abstracts.asco.org/244/AbstView_244_274975.html.

# 10

# A double blind, placebo-controlled randomized comparative study on the efficacy of phytosterol-enriched and conventional saw palmetto oil in mitigating benign prostate hyperplasia and androgen deficiency

H. V. Sudeep[1,2*], Jestin V. Thomas[2] and K. Shyamprasad[1]

**Abstract**

**Background:** The present clinical trial was conducted to evaluate the efficacy and tolerability of a standardized saw palmetto oil containing 3% β-sitosterol in the treatment of benign prostate hyperplasia (BPH) and androgen deficiency.

**Methods:** Subjects aged 40–65 years with symptomatic BPH were randomized to 12-week double-blind treatment with 500 mg doses of β-sitosterol enriched saw palmetto oil, conventional saw palmetto oil and placebo orally in the form of capsules ($n = 33$ in each group). BPH severity was determined using the International Prostate Symptom Score (IPSS), uroflowmetry, serum measurement of prostate specific antigen (PSA), testosterone and 5α-reductase. During the trial, the androgen deficiency was evaluated using Aging Male Symptoms (AMS) scale, the Androgen Deficiency in the Aging Male (ADAM) questionnaire, serum levels of free testosterone.

**Results:** Subjects treated with β-sitosterol enriched saw palmetto oil showed significant decrease in IPSS, AMS and ADAM scores along with reduced postvoiding residual volume ($p < 0.001$), PSA ($p < 0.01$) and 5α-reductase from baseline to end of 12-week treatment as compared to placebo. There was also a significant increment in the maximum and average urine flow rate ($p < 0.001$), and serum free testosterone level of subjects treated with enriched saw palmetto oil as compared to placebo.

**Conclusion:** This study demonstrates the efficacy of β-sitosterol enriched saw palmetto oil superior to conventional oil thus extending the scope of effective BPH and androgen deficiency treatment with improved quality of life through the intake of functional ingredients.

**Keywords:** Saw palmetto oil, β-Sitosterol, Benign prostate hyperplasia, Androgen deficiency, Safety

* Correspondence: sudeepkashyap.82@gmail.com; research@vidyaherbs.com
[1]R&D Center for Excellence, Vidya Herbs Pvt. Ltd, #14A, Jigani I phase, Bangalore, Karnataka 560 105, India
[2]Leads Clinical Research and Bio services Private Ltd., Bangalore, India

## Background

Growing interest in the use of functional foods and dietary supplements for healthcare management has led to the availability of natural products in the market. However, development of nutraceuticals requires supportive evidence of efficacy and tolerability that must be clearly demonstrated with clinical trials [1]. *Serenoa repens* (saw palmetto) is one of the most studied plants for the treatment of lower urinary tract diseases (LUTS), especially mild to moderate prostatic diseases. Major bioactive principles attributing to the medicinal use of saw palmetto oil are the phytosterols and fatty acids. Explored mechanisms of action for saw palmetto oil includes inhibition of 5α-reductase, cyclooxygenase (COX) and 5-lipoxygenase (LOX). In addition, it exhibits antiproliferative effect on prostatic epithelial cells and antiestrogenic activity [2]. Thus, the candidature of saw palmetto preparations as alternative medicine to treat benign prostate hyperplasia has been the subject of clinical research.

Saw palmetto (SP) has been clinically tested either alone or in combination with other alpha-blockers and 5α-reductase inhibitors (5-ARIs). Guilianelli et al. demonstrated in a multicentre clinical trial that the use of SP extract for 6 months showed significant improvement in International Prostate Symptom (IPSS) score and uroflowmetry in subjects with BPH [3]. Sinescu et al. have reported the long-term efficacy of SP extract in improving the LUTS, urinary flow, erectile dysfunction and quality of life (QoL) [4]. In a recent double-blind, placebo-controlled study Ye et al. reported the improvements in LUTS and male sexual function followed by treatment with SP extract [5]. SP extract demonstrated equivalent efficacy when compared to treatments with other alpha-blockers and 5-ARIs [6–8].

Phytoconstituents such as sterols, fatty acids and vitamin E together contribute to the efficacy of SP extract in mitigating the BPH complications [9, 10]. Conventionally SP oil contains 0.2–0.3% β-sitosterol in addition to fatty acids. Here we have used a 3% β-sitosterol-containing SP oil for the clinical evaluation of therapeutic potential, alongside comparing with the conventional SP oil in a placebo-controlled trial. Previously we have demonstrated the improved efficacy of β-sitosterol-enriched SP oil as compared to the conventional oil in testosterone-induced BPH model rats [11]. Here we have provided the first ever clinical evidence on the improved efficacy of β-sitosterol-enriched SP extract superior to the conventional SP.

## Methods

### Investigational product

The investigational product was a standardized saw palmetto extract containing 3% β-sitosterol (VISPO™). VISPO and the conventional saw palmetto oil (SPO, 0.2% β-sitosterol) were prepared in-house from the berries (Florida, USA) using the supercritical fluid extraction method. The higher percentage of β-sitosterol in VISPO was achieved by column chromatography. The β-sitosterol content was quantified using LCMS analysis (Fig. 1). The extracts were then formulated into powder form with maltodextrin as excipient and filled in capsules (500 mg in weight). Each capsule contained 200 mg of extract. Placebo capsules consisted of maltodextrin only.

### Ethics, consent and permissions

The Institutional Ethics Committee of Aman Hospital and Research Center, Vadodara, India approved the study protocol and informed consent form (AHRC/IEC/026/2018). This clinical study was registered in Clinical Trials Registry – India (CTRI/2018/12/016724 dated 19/12/2018).

### Subjects

Ninety-nine male subjects aged 40–65 years, having mild-to-moderate BPH symptoms were enrolled into this clinical trial. Before enrolment, subjects were explained the study protocol approved by the Institutional Ethics Committee, and informed consent and consent to publish were obtained. The subjects having IPSS score > 7, Aging Male Symptoms (AMS) score ≥ 27, and responding positively to question 1 or 7 or any other three questions of the Androgen Deficiency in the Aging Male (ADAM) questionnaire, were included in the trial. Subjects with neurogenic bladder dysfunction, prostatic cancer, prostatitis, haematuria diabetes or any other chronic illness were excluded from the study.

### Study design

This study was conducted in compliance with ICH-GCP (International Conference on Harmonization of Technical Requirements for Registration of Pharmaceuticals for Human Use –Good Clinical Practice) guidelines and Helsinki Declaration Standards. This clinical study adheres to the CONSORT guidelines.

The study was performed at Aman Hospital and Research Center, Vadodara, India. The trial was designed as a double-blind, placebo-controlled, single-centered study including 99 male subjects randomised to three treatment arms: VISPO, SPO and placebo, on 1:1:1 ratio ($n = 33$ in each group). Block randomization was implemented for groupwise allocation of subjects wherein the participants received a xx-digit randomization number. The investigator and subjects were blinded of the interventions. The study medications were dispensed by the unblinded pharmacist at the site.

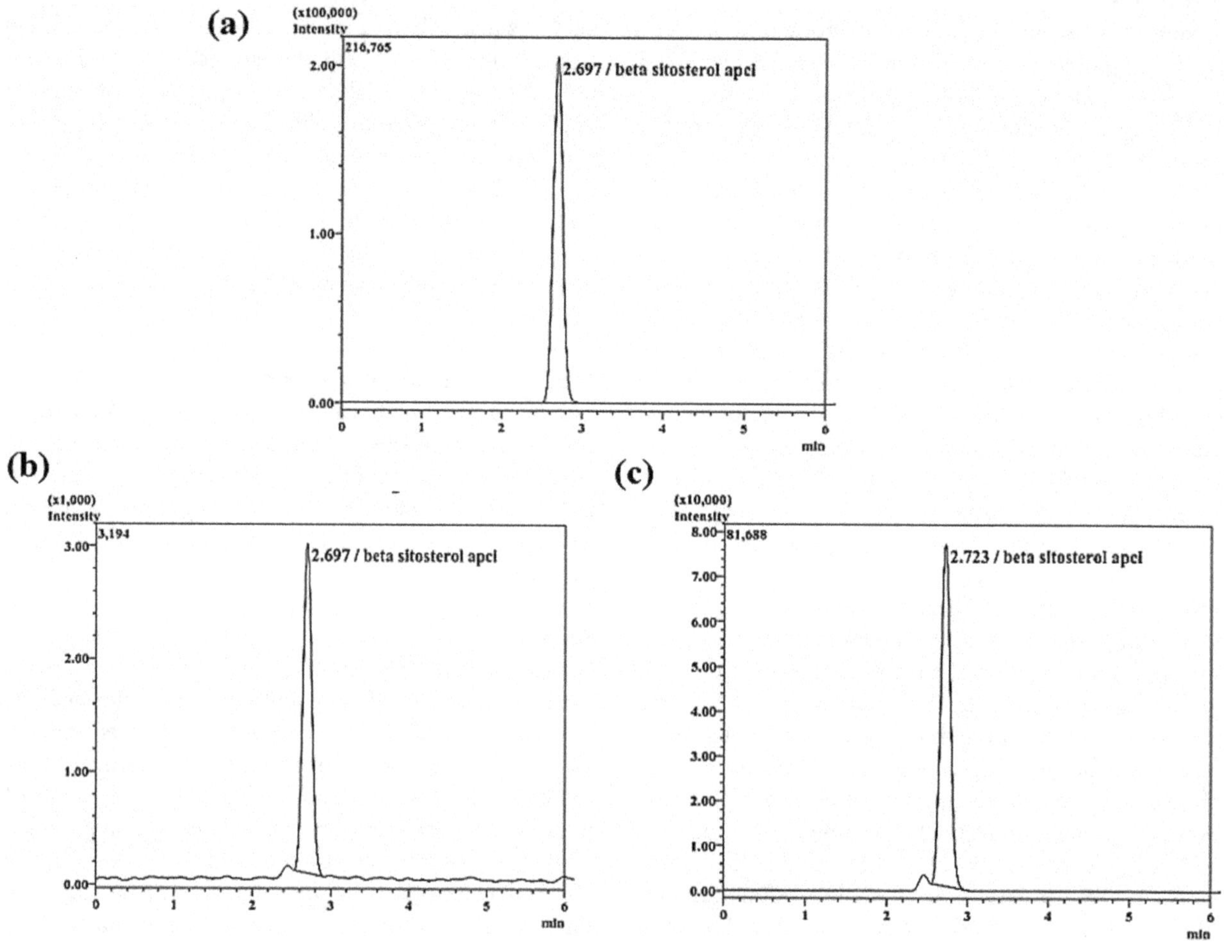


**Fig. 1** LCMS chromatograms of reference compound β-sitosterol (95%) (**a**), SPO (**b**) and VISPO (**c**)

The subjects received oral doses of 500 mg capsules twice daily (after breakfast and dinner) for 12 weeks. The study treatment details are provided in Table 1. Following baseline visit, during the intervention period there were two visits at study site every 6 weeks. The details of study procedures scheduled at each visit are provided in **supplementary file 1**. The treatment compliance was monitored during the trial using subject diary.

### Sample size

A sample size of 99 subjects (33 per group), was considered enough to detect a clinically important difference

**Table 1** Details of study treatments

| Group | Intervention (VISPO) | Comparator (SPO) | Placebo |
|---|---|---|---|
| Treatment | Saw palmetto oil (3% β-sitosterol) | Saw palmetto oil (0.2% β-sitosterol) | Maltodextrin |
| Dosage Form | Capsules | Capsules | Capsules |
| Composition | Capsule weight – 500 mg<br>Saw palmetto oil – 200 mg<br>Maltodextrin – 300 mg | Capsule weight – 500 mg<br>Saw palmetto oil – 200 mg<br>Maltodextrin – 300 mg | Capsule weight – 500 mg<br>Maltodextrin – 500 mg |
| Batch No. | VH/SPO/F18716 | VH/SPO/F18717 | VH/MD/F18612 |
| Route | Oral | | |
| Dose | 500 mg capsule two times a day; 400 mg/day of saw palmetto oil in active treatment groups. | | |
| Dosing Regimen | Twice a day after food | | |
| Treatment duration | 84 days | | |

between groups with 80% power and a 5% level of significance. Considering an estimated potential dropout rate of 12%, the sample size was finalized as 99 (33 per group). For the sample size calculation IPSS and maximum urine flowrates were considered with a delta value of 2.35 (**Supplementary file 2**).

### Study outcomes

The primary endpoints were determined as changes in IPSS, ADAM and AMS scores (subjective assessments). Objective assessment was based on post-void residual urine volume as measured by ultrasonography, and uroflowmetric determination of the maximum (Qmax) urine flowrate. The serum levels of prostate specific antigen (PSA), 5α-reductase and testosterone were measured at baseline and after 12 weeks of treatment using commercial kits. The general health status of subjects was assessed using the 12-tem Short Form Survey (SF-12) quality of life questionnaire. In SF-12, the questions are combined, scored, and weighted to create two scales that provide glimpses into mental and physical functioning and overall health-related-quality of life. Physical (PCS-12) and Mental Health Composite Scores (MCS-12) are computed using the scores of twelve questions and range from 0 to 100, where a zero score indicates the lowest level of health measured by the scales and 100 indicates the highest level of health. The questionnaires used in the study are detailed in **supplementary file 3**.

The safety assessments included physical examination, vital signs, biochemical and hematological parameters (Aspartate aminotransferase (AST), alanine aminotransferase (ALT), serum creatinine, blood urea nitrogen (BUN) and complete blood count).

### Statistical analysis

The general characteristics of the study subjects are summarized as mean ± standard deviation (SD) for continuous data. ANOVA was performed when equal variances were assumed to test between groups. Kruskal-Wallis test was performed when equal variances are not assumed. Paired t test was performed to test variables within groups.

## Results

A total of 118 human volunteers were screened of which 99 subjects meeting the inclusion criteria were enrolled in the study. Of the 99 subjects randomized to three treatment groups ($n = 33$ in each group), 91 subjects completed the study. There were 8 dropouts in the study (reason: lost to follow up). The intention-to-treat (ITT) analysis was used to assess the outcome of the study. The participant flow through the study is presented in Fig. 2. The demographic characteristics of subjects between the groups were not significantly different (Table 2). The efficacy and safety analysis were performed using ITT population.

The comparative efficacy of VISPO against the conventional saw palmetto oil was evaluated primarily using IPSS, ADAM and AMS scores assessed at visit 1 (baseline), visit 2 (6 weeks) and visit 3 (12 weeks) of the study.

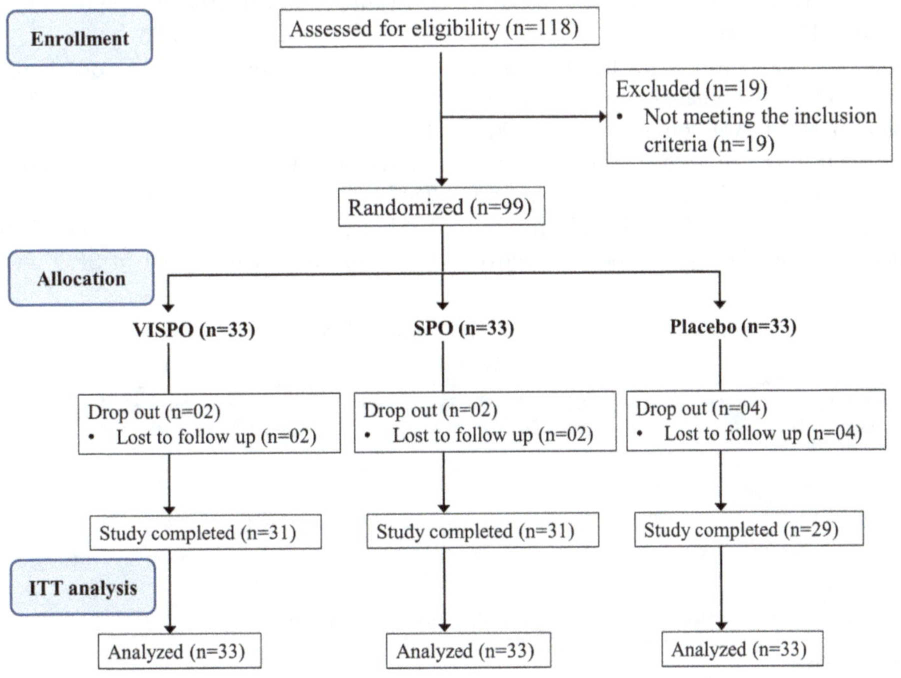


**Fig. 2** Subject participant flow chart

**Table 2** Demographic characteristics of subjects

| Variable | Intervention (VISPO) ($n$ = 33) | Comparator (SPO) ($n$ = 33) | Placebo ($n$ = 33) | $p$-value* |
|---|---|---|---|---|
| Age (Years) | 57.76 ± 7.25 | 57.48 ± 7.04 | 55.18 ± 8.56 | 0.327 |
| Weight (kg) | 61.09 ± 5.80 | 58.99 ± 4.89 | 60.87 ± 5.18 | 0.213 |
| Height (cm) | 158.94 ± 3.63 | 157.82 ± 4.16 | 157.82 ± 4.55 | 0.448 |
| BMI (kg/m$^2$) | 24.18 ± 2.12 | 23.69 ± 1.78 | 24.46 ± 2.10 | 0.290 |

*N* No of subjects; *BMI* Body Mass Index; Date presented as: Mean ± Standard deviation
*$p$ values were derived from ANOVA

At baseline there was no significant difference in the IPSS score between the groups while the values were decreased in VISPO and SPO groups during the study (Table 3). There was a significant decrease in the IPSS score from baseline value of 20.00 ± 4.41 to 18.06 ± 4.14 at visit 2 ($p < 0.001$) and 16.82 ± 4.03 at visit 3 ($p < 0.001$). The values were not significant for SPO group. In the placebo group there was a slight increase in IPSS score during the intervention period. The change in IPSS value from baseline to the end of treatment (visit 3) was significant in saw palmetto oil treated groups as compared to placebo ($p < 0.001$).

In the present study ADAM questionnaire was used to screen for the severity of androgen deficiency in men (Table 4). The ITT population analysis revealed that VISPO group subjects showed a significant reduction of ADAM score from baseline (4.33 ± 1.67) to the end of study (3.73 ± 1.74) ($p < 0.001$) while SPO and placebo groups showed an increase in the mean ADAM score. The change in the score from baseline to visit 3 of VISPO group (− 0.61 ± 1.06) was significant ($p < 0.01$) compared to placebo (0.15 ± 0.94).

Further AMS scale was used to assess the symptoms of ageing and to measure the changes in severity of symptoms pre- and post-intervention (Table 5). AMS scale has three dimensions (sub-scales) i.e., psychological, somatic, and sexual subscale. The composite scores for each of the three sub-scales is based on adding up the scores of the items of the respective dimensions. The AMS total score from baseline to end of treatment decreased considerably in VISPO group ($p < 0.001$). SPO group showed non-significant reduction in the mean score. The change in total AMS score from baseline to visit 3 of VISPO (− 3.64 ± 4.76) and SPO (− 1.12 ± 4.14) groups were significant ($p < 0.001$) when compared to placebo (1.70 ± 3.37). Similar trend was observed in the AMS subscale analyses (Table 6). Importantly, there was a significant reduction ($p < 0.001$) in the AMS sexual subscale from baseline to the end of treatment in VISPO (− 1.24 ± 1.84) and SPO (− 0.12 ± 1.47) groups as compared to placebo (0.73 ± 1.26).

Table 7 shows the urodynamic measurements obtained before and after the intervention period. The residual urine volume decreased significantly ($p < 0.001$) in VISPO group (from 112.55 ± 36.19 mL to 99.79 ± 29.27 mL) after the 12-week treatment. SPO group showed a slight improvement in residual urine volume, though not to a significant extent (110.12 ± 34.71 mL to 108.24 ± 33.22 mL). A significant improvement ($p < 0.001$) of Qmax was observed in the VISPO group (from 11.85 ± 2.06 mL/s to 14.27 ± 2.54 mL/s). In the SPO group a non-significant increase in the Qmax was recorded from 12.33 ± 1.61 mL/s to 12.82 ± 1.72 mL/s.

Assessment of serum BPH markers are presented in Table 8. Serum levels of PSA was decreased in the VISPO group from 2.77 ± 0.56 ng/mL to 2.70 ± 0.59 ng/mL while it was increased in SPO and placebo groups

**Table 3** Summary of International Prostate Symptom Score (IPSS) by visit and treatment

| Visit | Observed value | | | | Change from baseline | | | | | | |
|---|---|---|---|---|---|---|---|---|---|---|---|
| | Intervention (VISPO) $n = 33$ | Comparator (SPO) $n = 33$ | Placebo $n = 33$ | $p$-value** | Intervention (VISPO) $n = 33$ | $p$-value* | Comparator (SPO) $n = 33$ | $p$-value* | Placebo $n = 33$ | $p$-value* | $p$-value** |
| Visit 1 | 20.00 ± 4.41 | 19.45 ± 3.82 | 20.00 ± 3.74 | 0.815$^{(1)}$ | | | | | | | |
| Visit 2 | 18.06 ± 4.14$^{a}$ | 19.09 ± 3.89$^{ab}$ | 20.70 ± 3.37$^{b}$ | 0.021$^{(1)}$ | −1.94 ± 1.85$^{a}$ | < 0.001 | −0.36 ± 1.98$^{b}$ | 0.300 | 0.70 ± 1.38$^{b}$ | 0.007 | < 0.001$^{(1)}$ |
| Visit 3 | 16.82 ± 4.03$^{a}$ | 18.55 ± 4.22$^{ab}$ | 20.73 ± 4.87$^{b}$ | 0.002$^{(1)}$ | −3.18 ± 3.14$^{a}$ | < 0.001 | −0.91 ± 3.34$^{ab}$ | 0.128 | 0.73 ± 5.01$^{b}$ | 0.410 | < 0.001$^{(1)}$ |

Data are presented as Mean ± SD; $n$ = No of subjects
$^{a\text{-}b}$ values within a row with different superscript letters differ ($p < 0.05$), as analysed by one-way ANOVA
*$p$ values were compared within each group from baseline using paired t test
**$p$ values were compared between groups
$^{1)}$ $P$ values were derived from ANOVA, and Scheffe test was used to post hoc test

**Table 4** Summary of Androgen deficiency in the aging male (ADAM) scoring by visit and treatment

| Visit | Observed value | | | | Change from baseline | | | | | | |
|---|---|---|---|---|---|---|---|---|---|---|---|
| | Intervention (VISPO) $n = 33$ | Comparator (SPO) $n = 33$ | Placebo $n = 33$ | *p*-value** | Intervention (VISPO) $n = 33$ | *p*-value* | Comparator (SPO) $n = 33$ | *p*-value* | Placebo $n = 33$ | *p*-value* | *p*-value** |
| Visit 1 | 4.33 ± 1.67 | 4.15 ± 1.68 | 4.30 ± 1.76 | $0.898^{(1)}$ | | | | | | | |
| Visit 2 | 3.97 ± 1.74 | 4.12 ± 1.69 | 4.48 ± 1.73 | $0.461^{(1)}$ | $-0.36 \pm 0.70^{a}$ | 0.005 | $-0.03 \pm 0.53^{ab}$ | 0.744 | $0.18 \pm 0.68^{b}$ | 0.136 | $0.007^{(2)}$ |
| Visit 3 | 3.73 ± 1.74 | 4.21 ± 1.43 | 4.45 ± 1.64 | $0.179^{(1)}$ | $-0.61 \pm 1.06^{a}$ | 0.002 | $0.06 \pm 0.90^{b}$ | 0.701 | $0.15 \pm 0.94^{b}$ | 0.361 | $0.003^{(1)}$ |

Data are presented as Mean ± SD; *n* = No of subjects
a-b values within a row with different superscript letters differ ($p < 0.05$), as analysed by one-way ANOVA
*p values were compared within each group from baseline using paired t test
**p values were compared between groups
1) P values were derived from ANOVA, and Scheffe test was used to post hoc test
2) P values were derived from Kruskal-Wallis test, and Dunnett T3 test was used to post hoc test

after the treatment. The subjects in VISPO group showed an increase in free testosterone levels (6.23 ± 1.16 to 6.46 ± 1.43) after treatment ($p < 0.05$). On the contrary there was a reduction of serum levels of free testosterone in SPO and placebo groups. The change in free testosterone from baseline to end of treatment was significant in VISPO group as compared to placebo ($p < 0.05$). There was a reduction in total testosterone noted in all the treatment groups. However, the data were not significant. 5α-reductase activity was non-significantly reduced in VISPO group from baseline to the end of 12-week treatment (445.90 ± 105.40 ng/L to 438.24 ± 98.56). However, it was noticed that unexpectedly, the enzyme activity was increased in SPO group towards the end of study.

The Short-Form Health Survey (SF-12) is one of the most widely used questionnaire for assessing self-reported health-related quality of life. VISPO group subjects demonstrated a significant improvement ($p < 0.001$) in the quality of life as evident from the increase in the mean total score. Comparatively, SPO group showed moderate increase in the SF-12 total score. Both VISPO and SPO groups showed significant change in mean score from visit 1 to visit 3 as compared to placebo. The subset analysis revealed that VISPO group also showed significant improvement in PCS-12 and MCS-12 scores after 12-week treatment ($p < 0.001$), Fig. 3 shows the change in SF-12 scores from baseline to the end of treatment.

No serious adverse events (SAEs) were recorded during the study. The investigational products were well tolerated among the subjects. There were no significant alterations in the biochemical and haematological parameters among the subjects during the intervention period. The results of safety assessment are provided in **supplementary file 4**.

## Discussion

SP extracts used extensively for treatment of LUTS in traditional medicine have been clinically validated for improving the conditions such as BPH [12]. These medicinal attributes of SP extracts are due to the synergistic effect of phytosterols and fatty acids [13]. Previously, we have demonstrated the improved efficacy of SP oil containing 3% β-sitosterol (VISPO) compared to the conventional oil in alleviating the symptoms of BPH in rats [11]. Results from preclinical studies prompted us to conduct the clinical trial to further confirm the effectiveness of VISPO.

Here we have clinically evaluated the efficacy of VISPO in comparison with conventional SP oil (SPO).

**Table 5** Summary of total Aging male symptoms (AMS) score by visit and treatment

| Visit | Observed value | | | | Change from baseline | | | | | | |
|---|---|---|---|---|---|---|---|---|---|---|---|
| | Intervention (VISPO) $n = 33$ | Comparator (SPO) $n = 33$ | Placebo $n = 33$ | *p*-value** | Intervention (VISPO) $n = 33$ | *p*-value* | Comparator (SPO) $n = 33$ | *p*-value* | Placebo $n = 33$ | *p*-value* | *p*-value** |
| Visit 1 | 45.06 ± 9.28 | 44.64 ± 9.05 | 45.42 ± 10.39 | $0.946^{1)}$ | | | | | | | |
| Visit 2 | 43.52 ± 8.61 | 43.97 ± 9.01 | 46.06 ± 9.66 | $0.483^{1)}$ | $-1.55 \pm 2.18^{a}$ | < 0.001 | $-0.67 \pm 1.80^{a}$ | 0.041 | $0.64 \pm 1.71^{b}$ | 0.040 | $< 0.001^{2)}$ |
| Visit 3 | $41.42 \pm 7.52^{a}$ | $43.52 \pm 8.76^{ab}$ | $47.12 \pm 9.73^{b}$ | $0.031^{1)}$ | $-3.64 \pm 4.76^{a}$ | < 0.001 | $-1.12 \pm 4.14^{a}$ | 0.129 | $1.70 \pm 3.37^{b}$ | 0.007 | $< 0.001^{2)}$ |

Data are presented as Mean ± SD; *n* = No of subjects
a-b values within a row with different superscript letters differ ($p < 0.05$), as analysed by one-way ANOVA
*p values were compared within each group from baseline using paired t test
**p values were compared between groups
1) P values were derived from ANOVA, and Scheffe test was used to post hoc test
2) P values were derived from Kruskal-Wallis test, and Dunnett T3 test was used to post hoc test

**Table 6** Summary of Aging male symptoms (AMS) subscale analysis

| **AMS psychological score** | | | | | | | | | | | |
|---|---|---|---|---|---|---|---|---|---|---|---|
| Visit | **Observed value** | | | | **Change from baseline** | | | | | | |
| | Intervention (VISPO) $n = 33$ | Comparator (SPO) $n = 33$ | Placebo $n = 33$ | *p*-value** | Intervention (VISPO) $n = 33$ | *p*-value* | Comparator (SPO) $n = 33$ | *p*-value* | Placebo $n = 33$ | *p*-value* | *p*-value** |
| Visit 1 | 12.64 ± 4.08 | 12.97 ± 3.58 | 13.79 ± 4.92 | $0.559^{2)}$ | | | | | | | |
| Visit 2 | 12.58 ± 3.75 | 12.82 ± 3.40 | 13.79 ± 4.72 | $0.510^{2)}$ | − 0.06 ± 0.75 | 0.645 | − 0.15 ± 0.83 | 0.304 | 0.00 ± 0.50 | 1.000 | $0.683^{1)}$ |
| Visit 3 | 12.58 ± 3.67 | 12.73 ± 3.31 | 14.06 ± 4.39 | $0.351^{2)}$ | − 0.06 ± 1.00 | 0.730 | −0.24 ± 1.25 | 0.274 | 0.27 ± 1.04 | 0.141 | $0.162^{1)}$ |
| **AMS somatic score** | | | | | | | | | | | |
| Visit 1 | 19.27 ± 3.88 | 19.85 ± 4.43 | 20.67 ± 4.26 | $0.403^{1)}$ | | | | | | | |
| Visit 2 | 18.39 ± 3.64 | $19.45 \pm 4.37^{ab}$ | $20.85 \pm 3.97^{b}$ | $0.049^{1)}$ | $-0.88 \pm 1.14^{a}$ | < 0.001 | $- 0.39 \pm 0.90^{a}$ | 0.017 | $0.18 \pm 0.58^{b}$ | .083 | $< 0.001^{2)}$ |
| Visit 3 | $16.97 \pm 3.10^{a}$ | $19.12 \pm 4.52^{ab}$ | $20.79 \pm 3.90^{b}$ | $0.001^{2)}$ | $-2.30 \pm 2.65^{a}$ | < 0.001 | $-0.73 \pm 2.30^{b}$ | 0.078 | $0.12 \pm 2.06^{b}$ | .737 | $< 0.001^{1)}$ |
| **AMS sexual score** | | | | | | | | | | | |
| Visit 1 | $13.15 \pm 3.28^{a}$ | $11.82 \pm 2.48^{ab}$ | $10.97 \pm 2.89^{b}$ | $0.011^{1)}$ | | | | | | | |
| Visit 2 | 12.55 ± 3.10 | 11.70 ± 2.64 | 11.42 ± 2.69 | $0.247^{1)}$ | $-0.61 \pm 0.97^{a}$ | 0.001 | $-0.12 \pm 0.82^{ab}$ | 0.402 | $0.45 \pm 1.06^{b}$ | .020 | $< 0.001^{1)}$ |
| Visit 3 | 11.91 ± 2.96 | 11.70 ± 2.48 | 11.70 ± 2.65 | $0.935^{1)}$ | $-1.24 \pm 1.84^{a}$ | <.001 | $-0.12 \pm 1.47^{b}$ | 0.640 | $0.73 \pm 1.26^{C}$ | .002 | $< 0.001^{2)}$ |

Data are presented as Mean ± SD; *n* = No of subjects

[a-b] values within a row with different superscript letters differ (*p < 0.05*), as analysed by one-way ANOVA

**p* values were compared within each group from baseline using paired t test

***p* values were compared between groups

[1)] *P* values were derived from ANOVA, and Scheffe test was used to post hoc test

[2)] *P* values were derived from Kruskal-Wallis test, and Dunnett T3 test was used to post hoc test

Considering the prevalence of mild to moderate BPH symptoms in men from the age of 40 to 60 and above [14–16], subjects aged 40–65 years were included in the trial. This study was primarily focused on the changes in BPH symptoms assessed subjectively using the validated questionnaires. IPSS score is a convenient tool for the assessment of BPH-specific symptoms in order to evaluate the treatment outcomes [17, 18]. There was a significant decrease in the IPSS score from baseline (visit 1) to the end of treatment in VISPO and SPO groups indicating amelioration of BPH symptoms. Further we have used AMS scale and ADAM score as subjective measures of androgen deficiency. The age-related androgen deficiency associated with BPH must be considered for an effective therapeutic strategy [19]. The mean scores were markedly reduced in VISPO group following the treatment. It was interesting to note that the AMS sexual score was significantly reduced in VISPO group as compared to placebo. Several treatment strategies and surgical therapies for BPH have been associated with

**Table 7** Summary of urodynamic measurements by visit and treatment

| **Residual urine volume (mL)** | | | | | | | | | | | |
|---|---|---|---|---|---|---|---|---|---|---|---|
| Visit | Observed value | | | | Change from baseline | | | | | | |
| | Intervention (VISPO) $n = 33$ | Comparator (SPO) $n = 33$ | Placebo $n = 33$ | *p*-value** | Intervention (VISPO) $n = 33$ | *p*-value* | Comparator (SPO) $n = 33$ | *p*-value* | Placebo $n = 33$ | *p*-value* | *p*-value** |
| Visit 1 | 112.55 ± 36.19 | 110.12 ± 34.71 | 114.17 ± 30.67 | $0.888^{(1)}$ | $-12.76 \pm 14.44^{a}$ | < 0.001 | $-1.88 \pm 10.93^{b}$ | 0.331 | $1.11 \pm 13.89^{b}$ | 0.649 | $< 0.001^{(1)}$ |
| Visit 3 | 99.79 ± 29.27 | 108.24 ± 33.22 | 115.28 ± 33.25 | $0.149^{(1)}$ | | | | | | | |
| **Qmax (mL/s)** | | | | | | | | | | | |
| Visit | Observed value | | | | Change from baseline | | | | | | |
| | Intervention (VISPO) $n = 33$ | Comparator (SPO) $n = 33$ | Placebo $n = 33$ | *p*-value** | Intervention (VISPO) $n = 33$ | *p*-value* | Comparator (SPO) $n = 33$ | *p*-value* | Placebo $n = 33$ | *p*-value* | *p*-value** |
| Visit 1 | 11.85 ± 2.06 | 12.33 ± 1.61 | 12.27 ± 1.92 | $0.522^{(1)}$ | $2.42 \pm 2.61^{a}$ | < 0.001 | $0.48 \pm 1.56^{b}$ | 0.084 | $-0.64 \pm 2.28^{b}$ | 0.118 | $< 0.001^{(1)}$ |
| Visit 3 | $14.27 \pm 2.54^{a}$ | $12.82 \pm 1.72^{b}$ | $11.64 \pm 1.41^{c}$ | $< 0.001^{(2)}$ | | | | | | | |

Data are presented as Mean ± SD; *n* = No of subjects

[a-b] values within a row with different superscript letters differ (*p < 0.05*), as analysed by one-way ANOVA

**p* values were compared within each group from baseline using paired t test

***p* values were compared between groups

[1)] *P* values were derived from ANOVA, and Scheffe test was used to post hoc test

[2)] *P* values were derived from Kruskal-Wallis test, and Dunnett T3 test was used to post hoc test

**Table 8** Summary of BPH marker analysis

| Variable | Observed value | | | | Change from baseline | | | | | | |
|---|---|---|---|---|---|---|---|---|---|---|---|
| | Intervention (VISPO) $n = 33$ | Comparator (SPO) $n = 33$ | Placebo $n = 33$ | *p*-value** | Intervention (VISPO) $n = 33$ | *p*-value* | Comparator (SPO) $n = 33$ | *p*-value* | Placebo $n = 33$ | *p*-value* | *p*-value** |
| **Prostate specific antigen (PSA) (ng/ml)** | | | | | | | | | | | |
| Visit 1 | 2.77 ± 0.56 | 2.80 ± 0.72 | 2.83 ± 0.52 | 0.931$^{(1)}$ | | | | | | | |
| Visit 3 | 2.70 ± 0.59 | 2.99 ± 0.66 | 3.01 ± 0.54 | 0.072$^{(1)}$ | −0.07 ± 0.032$^{a}$ | 0.233 | 0.19 ± 0.40$^{b}$ | 0.011 | 0.18 ± 0.40$^{b}$ | 0.013 | 0.008$^{(1)}$ |
| **5α-reductase (ng/L)** | | | | | | | | | | | |
| Visit 1 | 445.90 ± 105.40 | 434.32 ± 93.76 | 441.31 ± 96.32 | 0.891$^{(1)}$ | | | | | | | |
| Visit 3 | 438.24 ± 98.56 | 440.40 ± 101.24 | 444.08 ± 138.16 | 0.978$^{(1)}$ | −7.66 ± 60.60 | 0.473 | 6.08 ± 51.46 | 0.502 | 2.77 ± 95.49 | 0.868 | 0.720$^{(1)}$ |
| **Total testosterone (ng/L)** | | | | | | | | | | | |
| Visit 1 | 459.62 ± 131.80 | 490.54 ± 166.66 | 433.50 ± 138.80 | 0.290$^{(1)}$ | | | | | | | |
| Visit 3 | 454.86 ± 137.31 | 481.02 ± 151.57 | 408.44 ± 140.43 | 0.119$^{(1)}$ | −4.76 ± 56.96 | 0.634 | −9.52 ± 52.69 | 0.307 | −25.07 ± 37.86 | 0.001 | 0.229$^{(1)}$ |
| **Free testosterone (ng/dL)** | | | | | | | | | | | |
| Visit 1 | 6.23 ± 1.16 | 6.26 ± 1.73 | 5.83 ± 1.31 | 0.394$^{(1)}$ | | | | | | | |
| Visit 3 | 6.46 ± 1.43 | 6.15 ± 1.62 | 5.64 ± 1.30 | 0.075$^{(1)}$ | 0.23 ± 0.77$^{a}$ | 0.093 | −0.11 ± 0.60$^{ab}$ | 0.294 | −0.19 ± 0.43$^{b}$ | 0.015 | 0.015$^{(1)}$ |

Data presented as: Mean ± SD; $N$ = No of subjects; $^{a-c}$ values within a row with different superscript letters differ ($p < 0.05$), as analyzed by one-way ANOVA

*$p$ values were compared within each group from baseline using paired t test;

**$p$ values were compared between groups

$^{1)}$ $P$ values were derived from ANOVA, and Scheffe test was used to post hoc test

$^{2)}$$P$ values were derived from Kruskal-Wallis test, and Dunnett T3 test was used to post hoc test

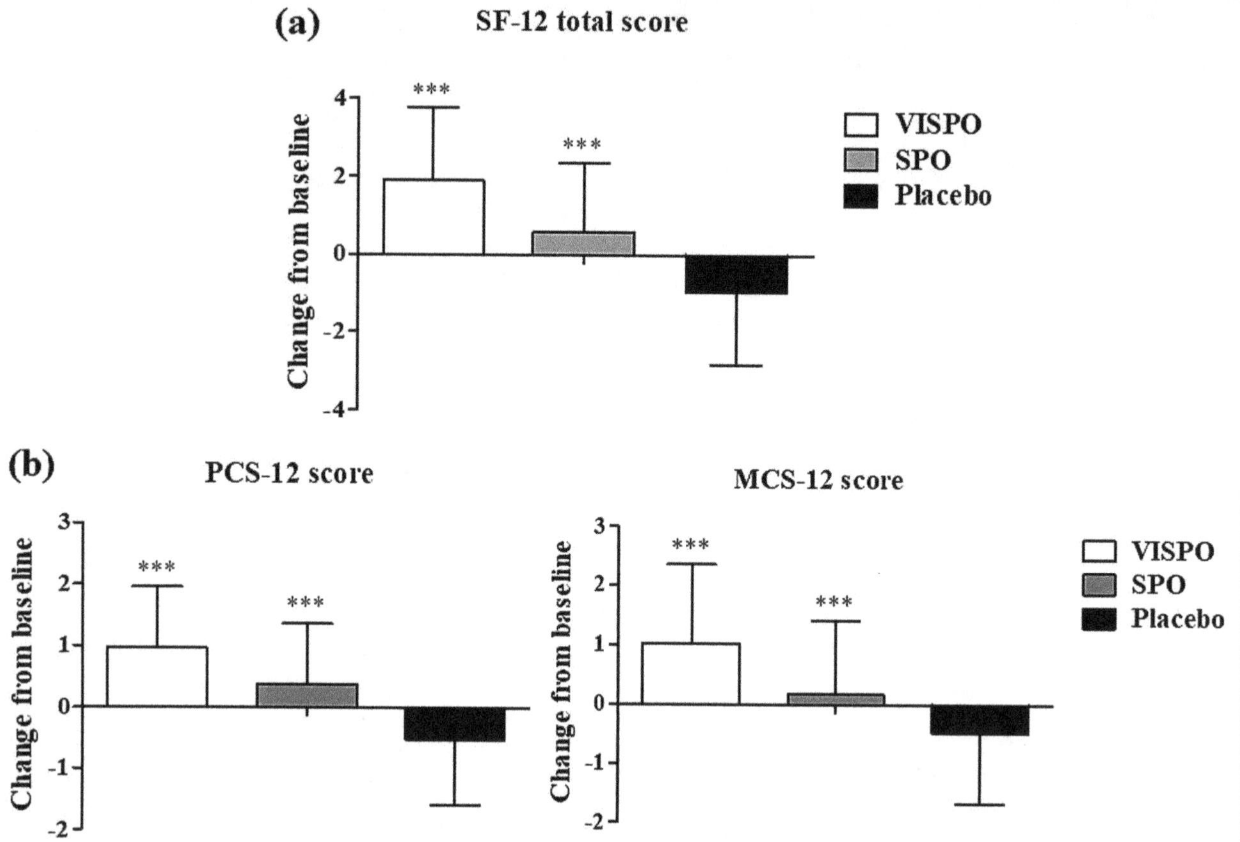


**Fig. 3** Mean change in SF-12 score of the study participants. The changes from baseline (visit 1) to the end of treatment (visit 3) in SF-12 total score (**a**), physical health composite (PCS-12) score and mental health composite (MCS-12) score (**b**) . The values are represented as mean ± SD ($n = 33$ in each group). The data were analysed by one way ANOVA followed by Scheffe test. ***$p < 0.001$ vs. placebo

sexual side effects [20]. It is an important observation from our study that a 12-week ingestion of β-sitosterol enriched SP oil could markedly improve the sexual function among the subjects while the conventional SP oil exerted the moderate efficacy. In accordance with the subjective measurements, the urodynamic parameters such as PVR and Qmax were significantly improved in VISPO group as compared to placebo. The mean changes from baseline to the end of treatment were appreciable in VISPO group than SPO group. Previously, Oki et al., have demonstrated that SP extract could significantly improve the urodynamic symptoms and micturition reflex in rats [21].

One of the important age-related symptoms is the testosterone deficiency which may subsequently lead to the adverse effects on androgen-responsive organ functions [22, 23]. Longitudinal studies have found dramatic reduction in free testosterone levels in aging men [24, 25]. In the present study, treatment with VISPO showed slight increase in the free testosterone and was significantly better as compared to SPO treated group.

Interestingly, there was an insignificant reduction in the 5α-reductase activity in VISPO group from baseline to the end of treatment. Our findings suggest that VISPO could exert its efficacy through other mechanisms such as alpha-adrenergic or muscarinic receptor blockage. Previously, SP extract was shown to reduce the bladder muscarinic and purinergic receptors and micturition frequency in a rat model of cystitis [26]. Suzuki et al., reported significant binding activity of SP extract on autonomic receptors in rats [27]. Studies from Aebi et al. reported oleic acid, lauric acid, myristic acid and linoleic acid as major fatty acids in SP extract having potential binding activity with alpha-adrenergic or muscarinic receptors in addition to 5α-reductase inhibitory activity [9, 28]. In accordance with these reports and the results of present study, a synergistic effect of fatty acids and β-sitosterol could contribute to the improved functional attributes of VISPO possibly with multiple mode of action. Other explanatory mechanisms of action include the anti-inflammatory and apoptotic effects [29]. In a multicentered pilot study, Vela Navarrete et al., reported that a 3-month treatment with 160 mg SP extract (Permixon®) could significantly reduce the IPSS score alongside the inflammatory parameters IL-1β and TNF-α in prostate tissues of BPH patients [30]. In another study, Permixon treatment significantly reduced the cell number and proliferative indices in BPH tissues indicating the role of SP extract in the induction of apoptosis in BPH [31]. We have previously demonstrated the anti-inflammatory and anti-proliferative effects of VISPO in preclinical model of BPH [11].

In this double-blind placebo-controlled study, we have demonstrated the improvement in BPH symptoms and androgen deficiency as a function of higher β-sitosterol content in VISPO. β-sitosterol has been previously reported to have profound influence on the prostate health [32]. Berges et al. have published their research findings on β-sitosterol wherein a 6-month administration of 20 mg of the compound significantly reduced the prostate size, increased the urine flow rate, and improved the mean voiding time and quality of life score in BPH patients [33]. In another multicentric, placebo-controlled, double-blind study daily intake of β-sitosterol markedly reduced the IPSS score with an increased Qmax and decreased post-void residual urine volume among BPH patients [34]. β-sitosterol was previously shown to inhibit the 5α-reductase activity in hamster prostate [35]. Our results are in line with these literature as ingestion of 400 mg/day VISPO, the SP extract with higher β-sitosterol content showed superior efficacy compared to conventional SP oil. The overall increment in efficacy parameters observed in VISPO group could be due to the synergistic effect of higher β-sitosterol content and the conventionally present fatty acids in saw palmetto extract. Collectively, the different constituents in the extract may contribute to the efficacy of the extract via multiple mode of action [36].

## Conclusion

The present study provides first ever clinical evidence on the improved efficacy of saw palmetto oil due to the enriched content of β-sitosterol. This comparative study clearly recommends the use of a phytosterol-enriched saw palmetto oil as a functional ingredient in dietary supplements for effective management of symptomatic BPH.

## Supplementary information

**Additional file 1: Supplementary file 1.** Schedule of study procedures

**Additional file 2: Supplementary file 2.** Sample size calculation

**Additional file 3: Supplementary file 3.** Questionnaires used in the study (Subjective assessment)

**Additional file 4: Supplementary file 4.** Safety evaluation data

### Abbreviations

BPH: Benign prostate hyperplasia; SF-12: The 12-item short form survey; PSA: Prostate specific antigen; SP: Saw palmetto; IPSS: International prostate symptom score; AMS scale: Aging males' symptoms scale; ADAM: Androgen deficiency in aging males; LUTS: Lower urinary tract symptoms; PCS-12: Physical health composite score; MCS-12: Mental health composite score; ITT: Intention-to-treat; ANOVA: Analysis of variance; AST: Aspartate aminotransferase; ALT: Alanine aminotransferase; BUN: Blood urea nitrogen; Qmax: Maximum urine flowrate; 5ARIs: 5α-Reductase inhibitors

### Acknowledgements

The authors thank Dr. Gouthamchandra K., and staff members of Biomedicinal Research Laboratory, R&D Center, Vidya Herbs Pvt. Ltd., for their technical support.

### Authors' contributions

All the authors have read and approved the manuscript. Conceptualization, KS; Protocol design, HVS and JVT; Study supervision, JVT; Study monitoring and coordination, HVS; writing – original draft preparation, HVS and JVT; review and editing, HVS and KS.

### References

1. Cicero AF, Petrini O, Prasad C. Clinical studies with nutraceuticals and how to carry them out. Curr Top Nutraceut R. 2017;15:63–6.
2. Governa P, Giachetti D, Biagi M, et al. Hypothesis on *Serenoa repens* (Bartram) small extract inhibition of prostatic 5α-reductase through an *in silico* approach on 5α-reductase x-ray structure. Peer J. 2016;4:e2698.
3. Giulianelli R, Pecoraro S, Sepe G, Leonardi R, Gentile BC, Albanesi L, et al. Multicentre study on the efficacy and tolerability of an extract of Serenoa repens in patients with chronic benign prostate conditions associated with inflammation. Arch Ital Urol Androl. 2012;84(2):94–8.
4. Sinescu I, Geavlete P, Multescu R, et al. Long-term efficacy of Serenoa repens treatment in patients with mild and moderate symptomatic benign prostatic hyperplasia. Urol Int. 2011;86:284–9.
5. Ye Z, Huang J, Zhou L, Chen S, Wang Z, Ma L, et al. Efficacy and safety of Serenoa repens extract among patients with benign prostatic hyperplasia in China: a multicenter, randomized, double-blind, placebo-controlled trial. Urology. 2019;129:172–9.
6. Alcaraz A, Carballido-Rodríguez J, Unda-Urzaiz M, Medina-López R, Ruiz-Cerdá JL, Rodríguez-Rubio F, et al. Quality of life in patients with lower urinary tract symptoms associated with BPH: change over time in real-life practice according to treatment--the QUALIPROST study. Int Urol Nephrol. 2016;48(5):645–56.
7. IuA P', Lopatkin NA, Gorilovskiĭ LM, Vinarov AZ, Sivkov AV, Medvedev AA. The results of long-term permixon treatment in patients with symptoms of lower urinary tracts dysfunction due to benign prostatic hyperplasia. Urologiia. 2004;(2):3–7.
8. Pytel YA, Vinarov A, Lopatkin N, Sivkov A, Gorilovsky L, Raynaud JP. Long-term clinical and biologic effects of the lipidosterolic extract of *Serenoa repens* in patients with symptomatic benign prostatic hyperplasia. Adv Ther. 2002;19(6):297–306.
9. Abe M, Ito Y, Oyunzul L, Oki-Fujino T, Yamada S. Pharmacologically relevant receptor binding characteristics and 5alpha-reductase inhibitory activity of free fatty acids contained in saw palmetto extract. Biol Pharm Bull. 2009; 32(4):646–50.
10. Cabeza M, Bratoeff E, Heuze I, Ramírez E, Sánchez M. Flores E effect of beta-sitosterol as inhibitor of 5 alpha-reductase in hamster prostate. Proc West Pharmacol Soc. 2003;46:153–5.
11. Sudeep HV, Venkatakrishna K, Amrutharaj B, Anitha, Shyamprasad K. A phytosterol-enriched saw palmetto supercritical $CO_2$ extract ameliorates testosterone-induced benign prostatic hyperplasia by regulating the inflammatory and apoptotic proteins in a rat model. BMC Complement Altern Med. 2019;19(1):270.

12. Cicero AFG, Allkanjari O, Busetto GM, Cai T, Larganà G, Magri V, et al. Nutraceutical treatment and prevention of benign prostatic hyperplasia and prostate cancer. Arch Ital Urol Androl. 2019;91(3):139-52.
13. Opoku-Acheampong AB, Penugonda K, Lindshield BL. Effect of saw palmetto supplements on androgen-sensitive LNCaP human prostate Cancer cell number and Syrian hamster flank organ growth. Evid Based Complement Alternat Med. 2016;2016:8135135.
14. Safarinejad MR. Prevalence of benign prostatic hyperplasia in a population-based study in Iranian men 40 years old or older. Int Urol Nephrol. 2008; 40(4):921–31.
15. Chicharro-Molero JA, Burgos-Rodriguez R, Sanchez-Cruz JJ, del Rosal-Samaniego JM, Rodero-Carcia P, Rodriguez-Vallejo JM. Prevalence of benign prostatic hyperplasia in Spanish men 40 years old or older. J Urol. 1998; 159(3):878–82.
16. Arrighi HM, Metter EJ, Guess HA, Fozzard JL. Natural history of benign prostatic hyperplasia and risk of pros-tatectomy. The Baltimore longitudinal study of aging. Urology. 1991;38(1 suppl):4–8.
17. O'Leary MP, Wei JT, Roehrborn CG. Miner M; BPH registry and patient survey steering committee. Correlation of the international prostate symptom score bother question with the benign prostatic hyperplasia impact index in a clinical practice setting. BJU Int. 2008;101(12):1531–5.
18. Roy A, Singh A, Sidhu DS, Jindal RP, Malhotra M, Kaur H. New visual prostate symptom score versus international prostate symptom score in men with lower urinary tract symptoms: a prospective comparison in Indian rural population. Niger J Surg. 2016;22(2):111–7.
19. Martov AG, Ergakov DV. Age-related androgen deficiency and benign prostatic hyperplasia: how to improve the rehabilitation of patients after transurethral surgery? Urologiia. 2016;6:110–7.
20. Voznesensky I, Shaw E, DeLay KJ, Yafi F, Hellstrom WJG. Benign prostatic hyperplasia treatment options and their effects on sexual function. Sexual Med Rev. 2017;5(1):87–102.
21. Oki T, Suzuki M, Nishioka Y, Yasuda A, Umegaki K, Yamada S. Effects of saw palmetto extract on micturition reflex of rats and its autonomic receptor binding activity. J Urol. 2005;173(4):1395–9.
22. Cauley JA, Ewing SK, Taylor BC, Fink HA, Ensrud KE, Bauer DC, et al. Sex steroid hormones in older men: longitudinal associations with 4.5-year change in hip bone mineral density--the osteoporotic fractures in men study. J Clin Endocrinol Metab. 2010;95:4314–23.
23. Guralnik JM, Eisenstaedt RS, Ferrucci L, Klein HG, Woodman RC. Prevalence of anemia in persons 65 years and older in the United States: evidence for a high rate of unexplained anemia. Blood. 2004;104:2263–8.
24. Harman SM, Metter EJ, Tobin JD, Pearson J, Blackman MR. Baltimore longitudinal study of aging. Longitudinal effects of aging on serum total and free testosterone levels in healthy men. Baltimore longitudinal study of aging. J Clin Endocrinol Metab. 2001;86:724–31.
25. Feldman HA, Longcope C, Derby CA, Johannes CB, Araujo AB, Coviello AD, et al. Age trends in the level of serum testosterone and other hormones in middle-aged men: longitudinal results from the Massachusetts male aging study. J Clin Endocrinol Metab. 2002;87:589–98.
26. Nasrin S, Masuda E, Kugaya H, Osano A, Ito Y, Yamada S. Effects of saw palmetto extract on urodynamic parameters, bladder muscarinic and purinergic receptors and urinary cytokines in rats with cyclophosphamide-induced cystitis. Low Urin Tract Symptoms. 2014;6(1):57–63.
27. Suzuki M, Oki T, Sugiyama T, Umegaki K, Uchida S, Yamada S. Muscarinic and alpha 1-adrenergic receptor binding characteristics of saw palmetto extract in rat lower urinary tract. Urology. 2007;69:1216–20.
28. Abe M, Ito Y, Suzuki A, Onoue S, Noguchi H, Yamada S. Isolation and pharmacological characterization of fatty acids from saw palmetto extract. Anal Sci. 2009;25(4):553–7.
29. Suzuki M, Ito Y, Fujino T, et al. Pharmacological effects of saw palmetto extract in the lower urinary tract. Acta Pharmacol Sin. 2009;30(3):227–81.
30. Vela Navarrete R, Garcia Cardoso JV, Barat A, Manzarbeitia F, López FA. BPH and inflammation: pharmacological effects of Permixon on histological and molecular inflammatory markers. Results of a double-blind pilot clinical assay. Eur Urol. 2003;44(5):549–55.
31. Vacherot F, Azzouz M, Gil-Diez-de-Medina S, Colombel M, De La Taille A, Lefrere Belda MA, et al. Induction of apoptosis and inhibition of cell proliferation by the lipido-sterolic extract ofSerenoa repens (LSESr, Permixon®) in benign prostatic hyperplasia. Prostate. 2000;45(3):259–66.
32. Wilt T, Ishani A, MacDonald R, Stark G, Mulrow C, Lau J. Beta-sitosterols for benign prostatic hyperplasia. Cochrane Database Syst Rev. 2000;2:CD001043.
33. Berges R, Windeler J, Trampisch H, Senge T. Group β-SS. Randomised, placebo-controlled, double-blind clinical trial of β-sitosterol in patients with benign prostatic hyperplasia. Lancet. 1995;345:1529–32.
34. Klippel KF, Hiltl DM, Schipp B. A multicentric, placebo-controlled, double-blind clinical trial of beta-sitosterol (phytosterol) for the treatment of benign prostatic hyperplasia. German BPH-Phyto study group. Br J Urol. 1997;80(3): 427–32.
35. Cabeza M, Bratoeff E, Heuze I, Ramírez E, Sánchez M, Flores E. Effect of β-sitosterol as inhibitor of 5α-reductase in hamster prostate. Proc West Pharmacol Soc. 2003;46:153–5.
36. Kwon Y. Use of saw palmetto (*Serenoa repens*) extract for benign prostatic hyperplasia. Food Sci Biotechnol. 2019;28(6):1599–606.

# Contrast-enhanced transrectal ultrasound can reduce collection of unnecessary biopsies when diagnosing prostate cancer and is predictive of biochemical recurrence following a radical prostatectomy in patients with localized prostate cancer

Hong-wei Zhao[1,2], Jian Li[3], Jia-Zheng Cao[4], Juan Lin[5], Zhu Wang[6], Jian-yao Lv[6], Jin-huan Wei[2], Zhen-hua Chen[2], Hao-hua Yao[2], Yi-hui Pan[2], Zhen-li Gao[1], Jun-hang Luo[2], Wei Chen[2], Lei Shi[1*] and Yong Fang[2*]

**Abstract**

**Background:** To investigate the value of using contrast-enhanced transrectal ultrasound (CETRUS) to reduce unnecessary collection of biopsies during prostate cancer diagnosis and its utility in predicting biochemical recurrence in patients with localized prostate cancer.

**Methods:** This was a prospective study of suspected prostate cancer patients who were evaluated with CETRUS followed by a prostate biopsy. Prostate blood flow via CETRUS was graded using a 5-point scale. The relationship between CETRUS score and biopsy outcome was then analyzed for all patients; univariate and multi-variate analyses were used to determine the probable prognostic factors for biochemical recurrence in patients with localized prostate cancer that underwent a radical prostatectomy.

**Results:** A total of 347 patients were enrolled in the study. Prostate cancer was found in 164 patients. A significant positive correlation ($r = 0.69$, $p < 0.001$) was found between CETRUS scores and prostate cancer incidence. Using CETRUS scores ≥2 as the threshold for when to biopsy could have safely reduced the number of biopsies taken overall by 12.1% (42/347) and spared 23.0% (42/183) of patients from undergoing an unnecessary biopsy. 77 patients with localized prostate cancer underwent a radical prostatectomy. The median follow-up time was 30 months (range: 8–56 months) and 17 of these 77 patients exhibited biochemical recurrence during the follow-up period. 3-year biochemical recurrence-free survival rates were 86% for patients with low CETRUS scores (≤ 3) and 59% for patients with high scores (> 3; $p = 0.015$). Multivariate Cox regression analysis indicated that CETRUS score
(Continued on next page)

* Correspondence: shileiyhd@sina.com; fymartin@sina.com
Hong-wei Zhao, Jian Li, Jia-Zheng Cao, and Juan Lin are co-first authors
[1]Department of Urology, Affiliated Yantai Yuhuangding Hospital, Qingdao University, Yantai 264000, Shandong, P. R. China
[2]Department of Urology, First Affiliated Hospital, Sun Yat-Sen University, No.58 ZhongShan 2nd Road, Guangzhou 510080, Guangdong, P. R. China
Full list of author information is available at the end of the article

(Continued from previous page)
was an independent predictor of biochemical recurrence (HR: 7.02; 95% CI: 2.00–24.69; $p = 0.002$).

**Conclusions:** CETRUS scores may be a useful tool for reducing the collection unnecessary biopsy samples during prostate cancer diagnosis and are predictive of biochemical recurrence in patients with localized prostate cancer following a radical prostatectomy.

**Keywords:** Contrast-enhanced, Transrectal ultrasound, Prostate cancer, Unnecessary prostate biopsy, Biochemical recurrence

## Background

Prostate cancer is the most common solid neoplasm and the second leading cause of cancer death in men in the US [1]. Both incidence and mortality are increasing, with an estimated 60,300 new cases diagnosed and 26,600 prostate cancer-related deaths in China in 2015 [2]. Approximately one million prostate biopsies are conducted per year in the US. However, prostate-specific antigen (PSA) testing, the most widely used screening test for prostate cancer, leads to 750,000 unnecessary biopsies—and accompanying pain, inconvenience, financial burden, and risk of infection [3]. Therefore, one way to reduce the use of PSA testing and shift the ratio of benefit to harm in favor of patient benefit would be to improve alternate methods with predictive value and thereby reduce unnecessary biopsy collection [4].

About 15–40% of patients with localized prostate cancer will suffer recurrence following a radical prostatectomy [5]. Traditional clinicopathologic risk factors, such as serum PSA levels, pathological grading (Gleason score), and TNM staging are used to predict the probability of recurrence in prostate cancer patients, but these tools are not accurate for every patient [6]. Therefore, new tools are needed to complement the prognostic value of traditional risk factors. Such tools may help guide individual therapeutic management, improve patient counseling, and help optimize the design of clinical trials.

Previous studies have shown that contrast-enhanced transrectal ultrasound (CETRUS)-based blood flow grading is a reliable tool for predicting pathological outcomes of prostate-related diseases [7–11]. The diagnostic accuracy of CETRUS has continually improved with the development of new ultrasound contrast agents and equipment [12]. Although CETRUS is a very promising imaging tool, it is still not widely used to help diagnose or evaluate prostate cancer. In this study, we investigated whether CETRUS can reduce unnecessary biopsy collection during prostate cancer diagnosis. We also investigated whether CETRUS can predict biochemical recurrence following a radical prostatectomy in patients with localized prostate cancer.

## Methods

### Patient selection

Patients referred for a prostate biopsy based on elevated total serum PSA levels (> 4 ng/mL) or abnormal digital rectal examination (DRE) between Feb 2014 and Sep 2018 at our collaborator institutions (Yantai Yuhuangding Hospital, First Affiliated Hospital of Sun Yat-sen University and Cancer Center of Sun Yat-sen University) were included in the study. The exclusion criteria were as follows: (1) age > 80 years; (2) refusal of CETRUS screening; (3) patient had received a previous prostate biopsy; (4) patient had a severe cardiopulmonary disease. The study was approved by the ethics committee of the institutions involved. Written informed consent to participate in the study and for the publication of their individual data was obtained from each participant enrolled in the study.

### Procedures

CETRUS was performed for each patient before prostate biopsy collection. The ultrasound equipment used for CETRUS was an IU 22 system (Philips, Holland), and the contrast agent used was SonoVue (Bracco, Milan, Italy). Conventional and contrast-enhanced transrectal ultrasound examinations were performed by sonographers that had more than 5 years of experience in conducting contrast-enhanced ultrasounds; these sonographers were not involved in the analysis of ultrasound images. All patients were examined in the left lateral position. A bolus of SonoVue (2.4 mL) was injected intravenously, followed by a 5 mL saline flush to ensure no residual contrast agent remained in the intravenous catheter. A series of axial sweeps through the gland were obtained from base to apex, with each sweep having a duration of 20–30 s [13]. This process was continuously observed for at least 3 min. Repeated injections (2.4 mL) were performed in 16 patients when initial results were unsatisfactory. All examinations at a given center were performed by the same sonographers. All CETRUS images were simultaneously examined by two sonographers. All sonographers involved were blinded to the patients' clinical presentations and other imaging results.

Diagnostic confidence was scored on a five-point scale based on blood flow, according to previously published reports: [8, 13] score 1, definitely benign, minimal enhancement (capsular and periurethral flow only); score 2, probably benign, mild enhancement (symmetric radial flow from capsular branches); score 3, indeterminate, mildly increased enhancement (asymmetric/increased flow in the prostate); score 4, probably malignant, moderately increased enhancement (asymmetric/increased flow in the prostate); score 5, definitely malignant, substantially increased enhancement (asymmetric/increased flow in the prostate) (Additional Fig. 1).

After CETRUS examination, a systematic 12-core prostate biopsy was performed. The systematic biopsy strategy consisted of collection of 6 standard cores and an additional 3 cores positioned more laterally on each side. Each biopsy sample was reviewed by a urological pathologist and reported individually. Tumors were classified according to the 2002 TNM staging system and graded according to the Gleason grading system. High-grade cancer was defined as a Gleason score 8 or higher.

### Surgical management and follow-up

Patients with clinical stage T1 and T2 prostate cancer underwent a laparoscopic radical prostatectomy. Patients with pathologically diagnosed localized prostate cancer (T1/T2N0M0) were enrolled and followed up prospectively. Data collected from each patient included age at diagnosis, CETRUS score, tumor stage, Gleason score, body-mass index (BMI), Eastern Cooperative Oncology Group performance status (ECOG PS), and biochemical recurrence-free survival time. Postoperatively, patients were examined to obtain serum PSA measurements every 3 months for the first year following surgery and semi-annually from the second through the fifth years. Biochemical recurrence was defined as a PSA level $\geq 0.2$ ng/mL and rising, and recurrence date was assigned to the first instance of a PSA value $\geq 0.2$ ng/mL [6]. No patient received adjuvant therapy prior to development of biochemical recurrence. Biochemical recurrence-free survival was calculated from the date of surgery to the date of biochemical recurrence and was concluded at the date of death from other causes or the date of the last follow-up visit.

### Statistical analysis

The correlation between CETRUS blood flow grades and biopsy outcomes were analyzed using a Spearman correlation test. Two groups were compared using the chi-square test for categorical variables. Receiver operating characteristic (ROC) curves and area under the curve (AUC) determinations were employed to assess the diagnostic accuracy of CETRUS. Survival curves were estimated using the Kaplan-Meier method. The univariate Cox proportional regression hazard model was used to analyze the correlation between variables and clinical outcomes. Multivariate survival analysis was performed on all parameters that were significant by univariate analysis using the Cox regression model. The predictive accuracy of prognostic factors was determined using time-dependent ROC analysis, and the AUC at 3 years post-surgery were used to measure predictive accuracy. R software version 2.7.1 (R Foundation for Statistical Computing, Vienna, Austria) was used for time-dependent ROC analysis. SPSS software (SPSS Standard version 16.0; SPSS Inc., Chicago, IL, USA) was used for all other calculations. Statistical significance was indicated by $p < 0.05$.

## Results

### Patient characteristics

A total of 379 consecutive patients suspected of prostate cancer were referred for a prostate biopsy. Thirty-two patients were excluded. 347 patients were enrolled into the study and evaluated with CETRUS followed by collection of prostate biopsy samples. No adverse events related to the contrast agent were observed in any of the 347 patients. The mean patient age was 68.5 years (range: 53–79), mean prostate volume was 52.8 mL$^3$ (range: 18–136), and median the PSA level was 8.9 ng/mL (range: 1.9–382). The number of men with a PSA level < 4, 4–10, 10–20 and > 20 were 28, 160, 116, and 43, respectively. Prostate cancer was found in a total of 164 of 347 (47.3%) patients. The proportion of patients with Gleason scores ≤6, =7 and ≥ 8 were 22.6% (37), 43.3% (76), and 31.1% (51), respectively. Among the 164 patients, 91 patients underwent a laparoscopic radical prostatectomy. Seventeen patients were excluded. Finally, 74 patients with localized prostate cancer were enrolled and followed up as shown in Fig. 1. Of the patients treated with a radical prostatectomy, the proportion of patients with Gleason scores ≤6, =7 and ≥ 8 were 24.7% (19), 41.6% (32), and 33.7% (26), respectively.

### CETRUS is a useful tool for reducing the performance of unnecessary biopsies

The percentage of prostate cancer patients in CETRUS score groups 1–5 were 0% (0/42), 11.5% (6/52), 32.5% (40/123), 87.1% (61/70), and 95.0% (57/60), respectively. A significant positive correlation ($r = 0.69$, $p < 0.001$) was found between CETRUS scores and prostate cancer incidence. When cut off at 4 (≤ 3 as BPH and ≥ 4 as prostate cancer), the CETRUS score had an accuracy of 83.3% (289/347) in correctly diagnosing prostate cancer, with a sensitivity and specificity of 90.8% (118/130) and 78.8% (171/217), respectively. ROC analysis showed the AUC of the CETRUS score was 0.89 (95% CI: 0.85–0.92), indicating that patient CETRUS scores can be used to

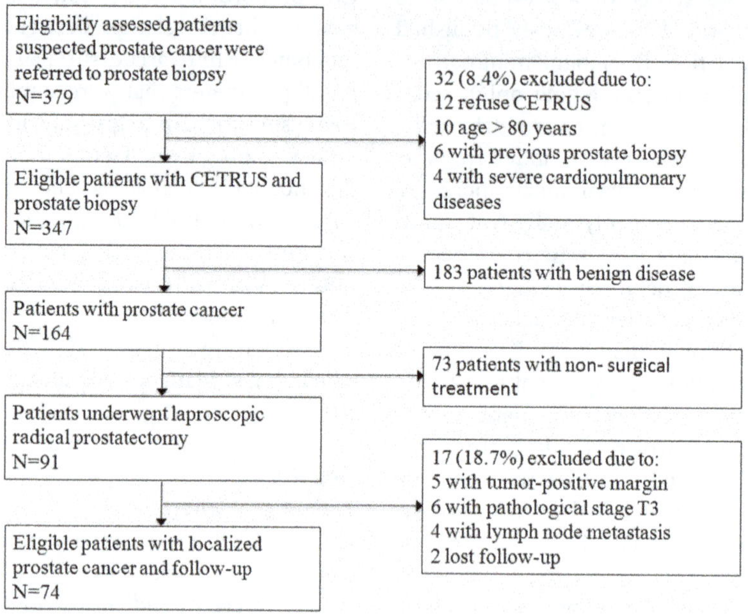


**Fig. 1** Flowchart for selection of patients for CETRUS examination and follow up

differentiate prostate cancer from benign prostatic hyperplasia (BPH) (Additional Table 1, Fig. 2). Moreover, when cut off at 2 (1 = BPH and ≥ 2 as prostate cancer), CETRUS scores demonstrated a specificity of 100% for differentiating prostate cancer from BPH, indicating that application of CETRUS using a cut-off score of 2 might be an effective tool for reducing the performance of unnecessary prostate biopsies. In this study, performing biopsy for cases with a CETRUS score ≥ 2 could have reduced the number of biopsies by 12.1% (42/347) without missing any cancer diagnoses and spared 23.0% (42/183) of men from undergoing an unnecessary biopsy (Table 1).

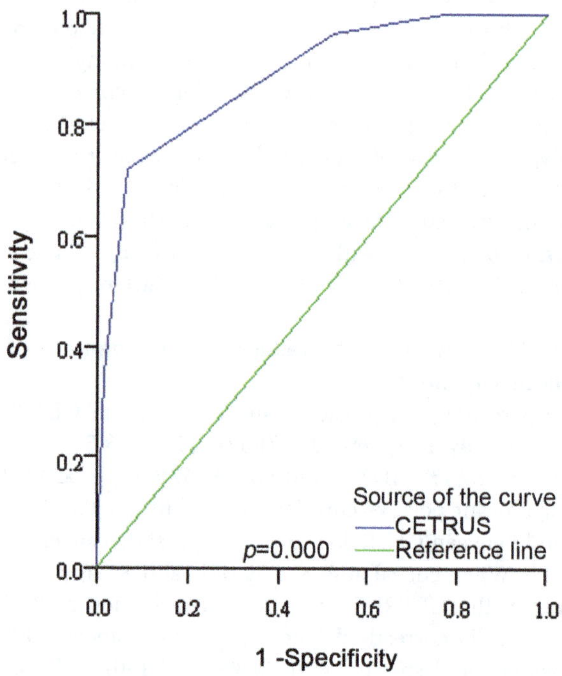


**Fig. 2** ROC curve using CETRUS scores to differentiate prostate cancer from benign disease. The AUC for the CETRUS scores was 0.89 (95% CI: 0.85–0.92, $p < 0.0001$)

### CETRUS can predict biochemical recurrence following a radical prostatectomy in patients with localized prostate cancer

The clinicopathologic characteristics of the 77 patients diagnosed with localized prostate cancer treated with a radical prostatectomy are summarized in Table 2. CETRUS score results were categorized in low score (≤ 3) and high score (> 3) groups. No significant correlation was found between CETRUS score and patient age, tumor stage, Gleason score, PSA level, BMI, or ECOG PS ($p > 0.05$, Table 2).

The median age of the 77 patients was 65.1 years (range: 49–74 years), and the median follow-up time after surgery was 30 months (range: 8–56 months). Biochemical recurrence was observed in 22% (17/77) of patients during the follow-up period. The 3-year biochemical recurrence-free survival rates were 86% (95% CI: 73–93%) for patients with low CETRUS scores and 59% (95% CI: 53–67%) for patients with high CETRUS scores (Fig. 3). Univariate Cox regression analysis revealed that CETRUS score, clinical stage, Gleason score, PSA level, and ECOG PS were significantly correlated with biochemical recurrence-free survival ($p$ = 0.015, 0.042, 0.011, 0.037 and 0.047, respectively,

**Table 1** Efficacy of CETRUS with a cut-off score of 2 in reducing unnecessary prostate biopsies

| Biopsy strategy | No. of biopsies | No. of necessary biopsies[a] | No. of unnecessary biopsies[a] |
|---|---|---|---|
| Conventional standard | 347 | 164 | 183 |
| Combining CETRUS score ≥ 2[b] | 305 | 164 | 141 |
| Reduction in the no. of biopsies | 42 | 0 | 42 |
| Proportion of the reduced biopsies | 12.1% (42/347)[c] | 0% (0/164) [c] | 23.0% (42/183) |

[a] Necessary biopsies: performed for malignant disease as confirmed by pathologic evaluation; Unnecessary biopsies: performed for benign disease as confirmed by pathologic evaluation

[b] Conventional standard of biopsy combining CETRUS blood flow scale score ≥ 2

[c] Proportion of reduced biopsies without missing cancer

Table 3), while other clinicopathologic variables, including age and BMI, were not ($p = 0.618$, 0.205, respectively, Table 3). Using multivariate analysis to further examine the parameters identified as significant by univariate analysis, we determined that patient CETRUS score at the time of diagnosis was an independent predictor of biochemical recurrence (HR: 7.02; 95% CI: 2.00–24.69; $p = 0.002$; Table 3).

To develop a more accurate prognostic tool, we used Cox proportional hazards regression to construct a prognostic model combining CETRUS scores with other clinicopathologic risk factors. A time-dependent ROC curve was used to compare the predictive accuracy of the combined model with the predictive accuracy of CETRUS scores alone or individual clinicopathologic factors alone. As shown in Fig. 4, the model combining patient CETRUS scores, Gleason scores, tumor stage, and PSA levels (AUC at 3 years: 0.886; 95% CI: 0.754–1.000) had a better prognostic value than relying on CETRUS scores alone (AUC at 3 years: 0.696; 95% CI: 0.520–0.890; $p = 0.006$), Gleason scores alone (AUC at 3 years: 0.679; 95% CI: 0.554–0.811; $p = 0.018$), tumor stage alone (AUC at 3 years: 0.620; 95% CI: 0.500–0.748; $p < 0.001$), or PSA levels alone (AUC at 3 years: 0.611; 95% CI: 0.500–0.792; $p = 0.004$). The Memorial Sloan Kettering Cancer Center (MSKCC) nomogram is currently the most commonly used predictor of biochemical recurrence and survival for prostate cancer. Therefore, we compared pre-radical prostatectomy CETRUS scores (0.696) and MSKCC nomograms (0.709) for 3-year AUC and found there was no significant difference between the two methods (Fig. 5). Therefore, CETRUS scores may add prognostic value to the clinicopathologic risk factors currently used in the context of localized prostate cancer.

**Table 2** Association of CETRUS scores with the clinicopathologic characteristics of 77 patients with localized prostate cancer who underwent radical prostatectomy

| Variables | No. | Low score (score ≤ 3) | High score (score > 3) | *p* |
|---|---|---|---|---|
| Age (years) | | | | 0.834 |
| ≤ 65 | 43 | 20 (46.5%) | 23 (53.5%) | |
| > 65 | 34 | 15 (44.1%) | 19 (55.9%) | |
| Tumor stage | | | | 0.756 |
| T1N0M0 | 25 | 12 (48.0%) | 13 (52.0%) | |
| T2N0M0 | 52 | 23 (44.2%) | 29 (55.8%) | |
| Gleason score | | | | 0.291 |
| ≤ 7 | 51 | 21 (41.2%) | 30 (58.8%) | |
| > 7 | 26 | 14 (53.8%) | 12 (46.2%) | |
| PSA (ng/mL) | | | | 0.611 |
| < 15 | 46 | 22 (47.8%) | 24 (52.2%) | |
| ≥ 15 | 31 | 13 (41.9%) | 18 (58.1%) | |
| BMI (kg/m$^2$) | | | | 0.802 |
| < 25 | 43 | 19 (44.2%) | 24 (55.8%) | |
| ≥ 25 | 34 | 16 (47.1%) | 18 (52.9%) | |
| ECOG PS | | | | 0.567 |
| 0 | 51 | 22 (43.1%) | 29 (56.9%) | |
| ≥ 1 | 26 | 13 (50.0%) | 13 (50.0%) | |
| Total | 77 | 35 (45.5%) | 42 (54.5%) | |

## Discussion

Our study shows that using CETRUS as a supplement to PSA-based diagnosis can reduce the performance of unnecessary prostate biopsies. We also found that CETRUS scores can independently predict biochemical recurrence of localized prostate cancer following a radical prostatectomy.

PSA testing is not limited to diagnosing prostate cancer. Other conditions, such as benign prostatic hyperplasia and prostatitis, also present with increased PSA levels. Therefore, it is necessary to design screening programs that maximize benefits and minimize morbidity and costs [14]. Angiogenesis, or the process of new blood vessel formation, is necessary for cancer progression. When compared with healthy tissue, the site of prostate cancer is generally characterized by an increased number of newly created blood vessels [15, 16]. However, most of these vessels have small diameters and may not have sufficient flow to be detected by a conventional Doppler transrectal ultrasound. The development of ultrasound contrast agents and contrast-specific

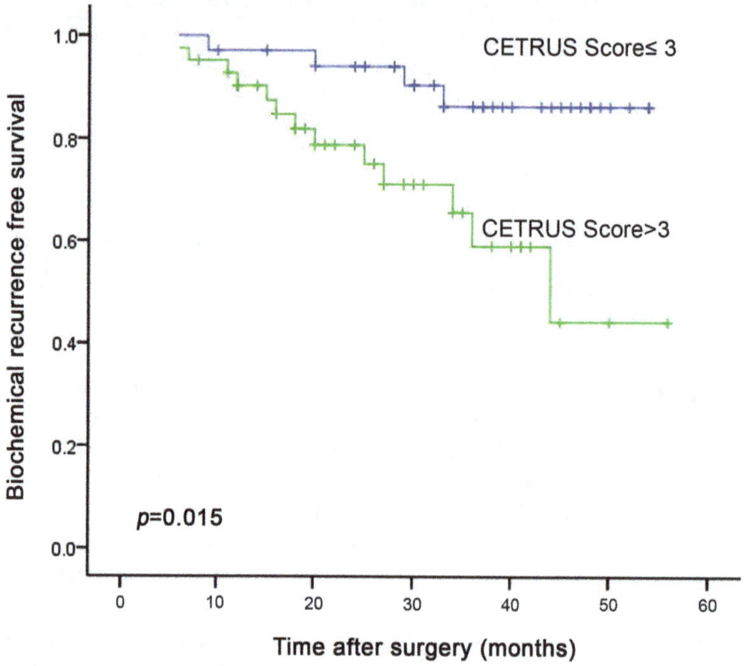


**Fig. 3** Kaplan-Meier biochemical recurrence-free survival analysis according to CETRUS scores for 77 patients with localized prostate cancer who underwent a radical prostatectomy ($p = 0.015$)

imaging techniques have facilitated introduction of CETRUS, a novel imaging modality for continuous visualization of neovascularity associated with prostate cancer [17]. Prostate cancer tissue is often characterized by increased microvessel density due to the proliferation of neovessels. In addition, the microvascular blood supply to prostate tissue is more uniform in malignant tissue than in benign tissue [18].

Multiparametric magnetic resonance imaging (mpMRI) is still the best method for diagnosing prostate cancer. The sensitivity of an MRI guided direct biopsy is as high as 89% of prostate cancer in clinical significance [19]. However, especially in developing countries, this method cannot be widely utilized in many clinics, so the relatively portable B-ultrasound has become another popular tool for diagnosis. Microbubble ultrasound contrast agents allow for the detection of microvessels below the resolution of a conventional transrectal ultrasound. Sedelaar et al. concluded in 2001 that CETRUS has the potential to reveal malignant prostate lesions with increased microvessel density, after finding that enhanced areas on CETRUS had a microvessel density 1.93 times higher than non-enhanced areas [20]. Ultrasound is a real-time, easily accessible, cost-effective, and non-invasive imaging modality. In addition, because ultrasound contrast agents have a low incidence of side effects and are not nephrotoxic, CETRUS can be used in patients with iodine allergies, impaired renal function, or other contraindications that may make them

**Table 3** Univariate and multivariate Cox regression analysis of the contribution of potential prognostic factors to biochemical recurrence-free survival of the 77 patients with localized prostate carcinoma who underwent radical prostatectomy

| Characteristics | Univariate Analysis | | Multivariate Analysis | |
|---|---|---|---|---|
| | HR (95% CI) | *p* | HR (95% CI) | *p* |
| Age (≤65 yrs. vs. > 65 yrs) | 1.28 (0.49–3.31) | 0.618 | – | – |
| CETRUS score (≤3 vs. > 3) | 4.11 (1.32–12.74) | **0.015** | 7.02 (2.00–24.69) | **0.002** |
| Tumor stage (T1 vs. T2) | 4.66 (1.06–20.53) | **0.042** | 5.30 (1.17–24.08) | **0.031** |
| Gleason score (≤7 vs. > 7) | 3.64 (1.35–9.84) | **0.011** | 6.38 (2.16–18.88) | **0.001** |
| PSA (≤15 ng/mL vs. > 15 ng/mL) | 2.81 (1.06–7.43) | **0.037** | 2.63 (0.74–9.32) | 0.135 |
| BMI (< 25 kg/m$^2$ vs. ≥25 kg/m$^2$) | 1.87 (0.71–4.93) | 0.205 | – | – |
| ECOG PS (0 vs. ≥1) | 2.67 (1.01–7.06) | **0.047** | 1.637 (0.46–5.78) | 0.444 |

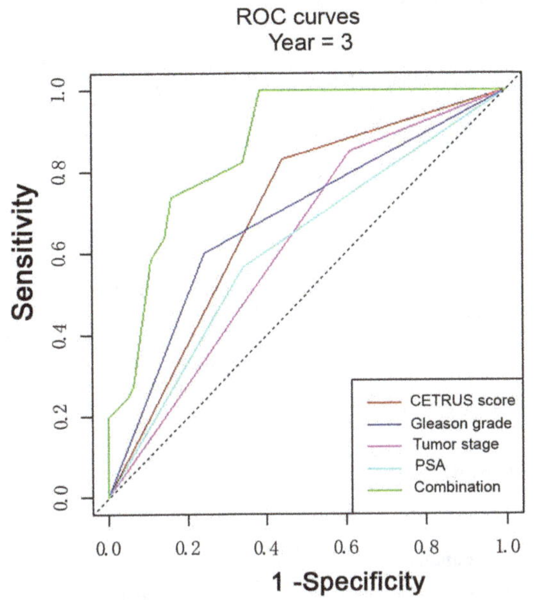


| | AUC at 3-yr (95% CI) | p value |
|---|---|---|
| Combination | 0.886 (0.766 - 1.000) | |
| CETRUS score | 0.696 ( 0.520 - 0.890) | 0.006 |
| Gleason grade | 0.679 (0.554- 0.811) | 0.018 |
| Tumor stage | 0.620 (0.500 - 0.748) | <0.001 |
| PSA | 0.611 (0.500 - 0.792 ) | 0.004 |

**Fig. 4** Comparison of the predictive accuracy of different models. *P* values showed the AUC for combined CETRUS score, Gleason grade, tumor stage, and PSA testing at the 3-year mark versus the AUC for CETRUS score alone at the 3-year mark, Gleason score alone, tumor stage alone, or PSA testing alone

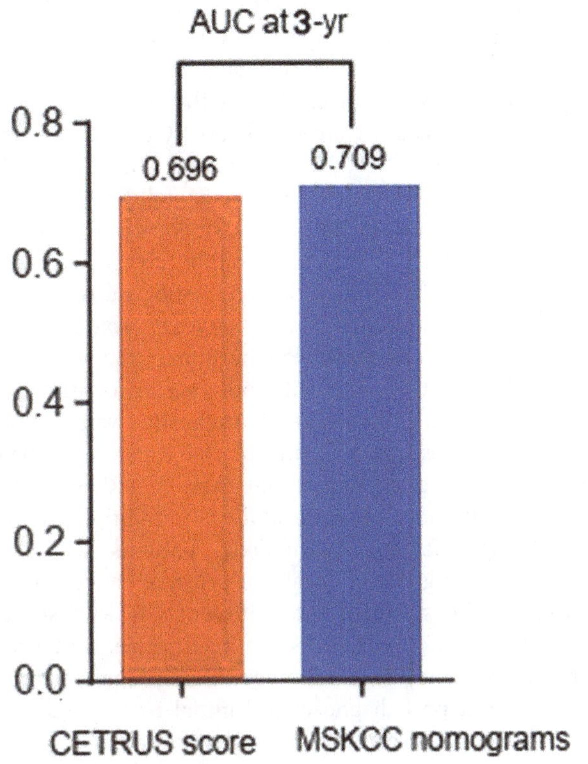


**Fig. 5** Comparison the 3-year AUC of pre-radical prostatectomy CETRUS scores (0.696) sand MSKCC nomogram (0.709) showed there was no significant difference

unsuitable for contrast-enhanced computed tomography or MRI [21]. Several studies have shown that the CETRUS-based blood flow grades significantly correlate with the histopathological outcome of biopsy samples. Thus, CETRUS can improve prostate cancer diagnosis, and performance of prostate biopsies based on CETRUS scores represents an innovative approach to detecting significant disease with fewer biopsy cores [8, 9, 22, 23]. With the development of new ultrasound contrast agents and equipment, the diagnostic accuracy of CETRUS is increasing, which will be helpful in eliminating unnecessary biopsy collection in patients without cancer [24]. However, at present, there is limited knowledge of the impact of CETRUS in reducing unnecessary biopsy collection in patients without prostate cancer. In the present study, a second generation contrast agent and low mechanical index were used to improve the survival of microbubbles in the circulation and facilitate real-time depiction of both macrocirculation and microcirculation. In addition, a low mechanical index was used to prolong the time of parenchymal enhancement [25]. The present study showed a strong correlation between CETRUS blood flow grade scores and histopathological findings. Asymmetrical, substantially increased enhancement of the prostate observed during CETRUS was more likely indicate the presence of malignant growth. On the contrary, minimal enhancement with only capsular and periurethral flow was more likely to be benign growth. We found that combining CETRUS scores with additional information besides PSA levels can help predict the result of biopsies in men with elevated PSA. Deciding to perform biopsies on the basis of a CETRUS score $\geq 2$ could have reduced the number of biopsies by 12% without missing cancer and spared 23% of men from undergoing an unnecessary biopsy.

Traditional clinicopathologic risk factors are inadequate for accurately predicting the prognosis of patients with localized prostate cancer following a radical prostatectomy. Therefore, additional tools for predicting prostate cancer recurrence may help to identify high-risk patients who might benefit from early intervention. Previous studies have shown that angiogenesis correlates with tumor recurrence following a radical prostatectomy [26–28]. Contrast-enhanced ultrasonography, which is useful for assessing microvessel density, has also been reported to have potential value in predicting the outcome of patients with prostate cancer [29, 30]. Our study demonstrated that CETRUS scores may be a reliable predictor of biochemical recurrence following a radical prostatectomy in patients with localized prostate cancer. CETRUS score successfully categorized patients into high-risk and low-risk subgroups with a significant difference in 3-year biochemical recurrence-free survival. Furthermore, the combination of CETRUS score with others clinicopathologic risk factors had a better prognostic value than CETRUS scores alone or any of the clinicopathologic risk factors alone, suggesting that CETRUS scores complement the prognostic ability of traditional clinicopathologic features. Ultimately, patients with the same stage or grade of localized prostate cancer could potentially be stratified into different CETRUS-score-defined risk groups for disease recurrence, and such stratification may lead to more effective personalized management post-diagnosis and initial treatment.

This study has several noteworthy limitations. First, a 12-core systematic biopsy scheme was used as the reference standard, and this approach may have missed significant tumors. Second, 46% of the men with PCa who underwent a radical prostatectomy had a CETRUS score of ≤3. These patients can easily be mistaken for benign or indeterminate diagnoses. Third, since our study was conducted across only three institutions, the results may not be universally generalizable. We acknowledge that prospective, large-scale, multicenter studies are necessary to confirm our results. With further clinical research confirming the reliability of our research results and improvements to the accuracy of B-ultrasound equipment, performance of B-ultrasounds can not only reduce the puncture rate of patients with localized prostate cancer following a radical surgery, but also reduce unnecessary prostate puncture and biopsy collection by improving the accuracy of prostate cancer screening.

## Conclusions

In summary, CETRUS-based blood flow grading is a reliable tool for reducing unnecessary collection of prostate biopsy samples for prostate cancer diagnosis. This CETRUS-based approach should also be considered to be a novel independent predictor for biochemical recurrence following radical prostatectomy in patients with localized prostate cancer. Our findings indicate that inclusion of CETRUS scores could in the current staging system could add significant prognostic value.

## Supplementary information

**Additional File 1: Table 1**: Diagnostic efficacy of CETRUS scores in differentiating prostate cancer from benign disease at different cut-off points.

**Additional File 2: Figure 1**: Baseline and CETRUS scores 1–5 are depicted in images a-e, respectively.

### Abbreviations

CETRUS: contrast-enhanced transrectal ultrasound; PSA: prostate-specific antigen; DRE: digital rectal examination; BMI: body-mass index; ECOG PS: Eastern Cooperative Oncology Group performance status; ROC: Receiver operating characteristic; AUC: area under the curve; BPH: benign prostatic hyperplasia; mpMRI: Multiparametric magnetic resonance imaging; MSKCC: Memorial Sloan Kettering Cancer Center.

### Acknowledgments

None.

### Authors' contributions

HW and YF: project development, data collection, study design, manuscript editing; JL, JZ, and JLin: manuscript writing, study design, data collection, statistical analysis; ZW, JY, and JH: manuscript editing, data collection; JH and ZH: data collection, statistical analysis; HH, YH, ZL, JH, WC, and LS: data collection, data interpretation. HW, JH, and JLperformed 12-core systematic prostate biopsies. All authors read and approved the final manuscript.

### Author details

[1]Department of Urology, Affiliated Yantai Yuhuangding Hospital, Qingdao University, Yantai 264000, Shandong, P. R. China. [2]Department of Urology, First Affiliated Hospital, Sun Yat-Sen University, No.58 ZhongShan 2nd Road, Guangzhou 510080, Guangdong, P. R. China. [3]State Key Laboratory of Oncology in South China, Department of Ultrasound, Sun Yat-Sen University Cancer Center, Guangzhou 510060, Guangdong, P. R. China. [4]Department of Urology, Jiangmen Hospital, Sun Yat-Sen University, Jiangmen 529000, Guangdong, P. R. China. [5]Department of Pediatrics, hird Affiliated Hospital of Sun Yat-sen University, Guangzhou 510630, Guangdong, P. R. China. [6]Department of Ultrasound, First Affiliated Hospital, Sun Yat-Sen University, Guangzhou 510080, Guangdong, P. R. China.

### References

1. Siegel RL, Miller KD, Jemal A. Cancer statistics, 2017. CA Cancer J Clin. 2017; 67:7–30.
2. Chen W, Zheng R, Baade PD, et al. Cancer statistics in China, 2015. CA Cancer J Clin. 2016;66:115–32.
3. Vickers AJ, Roobol MJ, Lilja H. Screening for prostate cancer: early detection or overdetection? Annu Rev Med. 2012;63:161–70.
4. Hayes JH, Barry MJ. Screening for prostate cancer with the prostate-specific antigen test: a review of current evidence. JAMA. 2014;311:1143–9.
5. Kotb AF, Elabbady AA. Prognostic factors for the development of biochemical recurrence after radical prostatectomy. Prostate Cancer. 2011; 2011:485189. https://doi.org/10.1155/2011/485189.
6. Blum DL, Koyama T, M'Koma AE, et al. Chemokine markers predict biochemical recurrence of prostate cancer following prostatectomy. Clin Cancer Res. 2008:7790–7.
7. Postema AW, Frinking PJ, Smeenge M, et al. Dynamic contrast-enhanced ultrasound. parametric imaging for the detection of prostate cancer. BJU Int. 2016;117:598–603.
8. Uemura H, Sano F, Nomiya A, et al. Usefulness of perflubutane microbubble-enhanced ultrasound in imaging and detection of prostate cancer: phase II multicenter clinical trial. World J Urol. 2013;31:1123–8.
9. Sano F, Uemura H. The utility and limitations of contrast-enhanced ultrasound for the diagnosis and treatment of prostate cancer. Sensors (Basel). 2015;15:4947–57.

10. Gao Y, Liao XH, Ma Y, et al. Prostate ultrasound imaging: evaluation of a two-step scoring system in the diagnosis of prostate cancer. Discov Med. 2017;24:295–303.
11. Trabulsi EJ, Sackett D, Gomella LG, et al. Enhanced transrectal ultrasound modalities in the diagnosis of prostate cancer. Urology. 2010;76:1025–33.
12. Halpern EJ. Contrast-enhanced ultrasound imaging of prostate cancer. Rev Urol. 2006;8(Suppl 1):29–37.
13. Li X, Pan Y, Huang Y, et al. Developing a model for forecasting Gleason score ≥7 in potential prostate cancer patients to reduce unnecessary prostate biopsies. Int Urol Nephrol. 2016;48:535–40.
14. Adesunloye BA, Karzai FH, Dahut WL. Angiogenesis inhibitors in the treatment of prostate cancer. Chem Immunol Allergy. 2014;99:197–215.
15. Grivas N, Goussia A, Stefanou D, et al. Microvascular density and immunohistochemical expression of VEGF, VEGFR-1 and VEGFR-2 in benign prostatic hyperplasia, high-grade prostate intraepithelial neoplasia and prostate cancer. Cent European J Urol. 2016;69:63–71.
16. Schalk SG, Demi L, Bouhouch N, et al. Contrast-enhanced ultrasound angiogenesis imaging by mutual information analysis for prostate Cancer localization. IEEE Trans Biomed Eng. 2017;64:661–70.
17. Kay PA, Robb RA, Bostwick DG. Prostate cancer microvessels: a novel method for three-dimensional reconstruction and analysis. Prostate. 1998;37:270–7.
18. Wulphert Venderink, Tim M Govers, Maarten de Rooij, Jurgen J Fütterer, J P Michiel Sedelaar (2015) Cost-Effectiveness Comparison of Imaging-Guided Prostate Biopsy Techniques: Systematic Transrectal Ultrasound, Direct In-Bore MRI, and Image Fusion. AJR Am J Roentgenol :208 (5), 1058–1063.
19. Sedelaar JP, van Leenders GJ, Hulsbergen-van de Kaa CA, et al. Microvessel density: correlation between contrast ultrasonography and histology of prostate cancer. Eur Urol. 2001;40:285–93.
20. Claudon M, Cosgrove D, Albrecht T, et al. Guidelines and good clinical practice recommendations for contrast enhanced ultrasound (CEUS) - update 2008. Ultraschall Med. 2008;29:28–44.
21. de Zordo T, Ladurner M, Horninger W, et al. New ultrasound technologies for the diagnostics of prostate cancer. Radiologe. 2011;51:940–6.
22. Sano F, Terao H, Kawahara T, et al. Contrast-enhanced ultrasonography of the prostate: various imaging findings that indicate prostate cancer. BJU Int. 2011;107:1404–10.
23. Aigner F, Mitterberger M, Rehder P, et al. Status of transrectal ultrasound imaging of the prostate. J Endourol. 2010;24:685–91.
24. Frauscher F, Klauser A, Halpern EJ, et al. Detection of prostate cancer with a microbubble ultrasound contrast agent. Lancet. 2001;357:1849–50.
25. Erbersdobler A, Isbarn H, Dix K, et al. Prognostic value of microvessel density in prostate cancer: a tissue microarray study. World J Urol. 2010;28:687–92.
26. Talagas M, Uguen A, Garlantezec R, et al. VEGFR1 and NRP1 endothelial expressions predict distant relapse after radical prostatectomy in clinically localized prostate cancer. Anticancer Res. 2013;33:2065–75.
27. Nordby Y, Andersen S, Richardsen E, et al. Stromal expression of VEGF-A and VEGFR-2 in prostate tissue is associated with biochemical and clinical recurrence after radical prostatectomy. Prostate. 2015;75:1682–93.
28. Xu G, Wu J, Yao MH, et al. Parameters of prostate Cancer at contrast-enhanced ultrasound: correlation with prostate cancer risk. Int J Clin Exp Med. 2015;8:2562–9.
29. Huang H, Zhu ZQ, Zhou ZG, et al. Contrast-enhanced transrectal ultrasound for prediction of prostate cancer aggressiveness: the role of normal peripheral zone time-intensity curves. Sci Rep. 2016. https://doi.org/10.1038/srep38643.
30. Mitterberger M, Aigner F, Pinggera GM, et al. Contrast-enhanced colour Doppler-targeted prostate biopsy: correlation of a subjective blood-flow rating scale with the histopathological outcome of the biopsy. BJU Int. 2010;106:1315–8.

# 12

# Skin rash following Administration of Apalutamide in Japanese patients with Advanced Prostate Cancer: An integrated analysis of the phase 3 SPARTAN and TITAN studies and a phase 1 open-label study

Hiroji Uemura[1], Yosuke Koroki[2*], Yuki Iwaki[3], Keiichiro Imanaka[4], Takeshi Kambara[5], Angela Lopez-Gitlitz[6], Andressa Smith[6] and Hirotsugu Uemura[7]

**Abstract**

**Background:** A higher incidence of apalutamide-related skin rash has been observed in Japanese patients with prostate cancer (PC).

**Methods:** This integrated analysis of data of Japanese patients from 2 global Phase 3 studies, SPARTAN (NCT01946204; patients with non-metastatic castration-resistant PC [nmCRPC]) and TITAN (NCT02489318; patients with metastatic castration-sensitive PC [mCSPC]), and the Phase 1 study 56021927PCR1008 (NCT02162836; patients with metastatic CRPC [mCRPC]), assessed clinical risk factors of apalutamide-related skin rash as well as the potential correlation with plasma exposure to apalutamide. Kaplan-Meier method was used for time-to-event analyses. Clinical risk factors for skin rash were assessed using odds ratio.

**Results:** Data from 68 patients (SPARTAN: $n = 34$, TITAN: $n = 28$, 56021927PCR1008: $n = 6$) receiving apalutamide 240 mg orally once-daily were analyzed. Rash (13 [19.1%]) and maculo-papular rash (11 [16.2%]) were the most frequently reported skin rash. All Grade and Grade 3 skin rash occurred in 35 (51.5%) and 10 (14.7%) patients, respectively. Most (85.7%) skin rash occurred within 4 months of apalutamide initiation and resolved in a median time of 1 month following the use of antihistamines, topical or systemic corticosteroids, with/without apalutamide dose interruptions/reductions. Median time-to-remission of first incidence of rash and maximum grade incidence of rash were 1.0 month (IQR: 0.36–1.81) and 1.0 month (IQR: 0.30–2.43), respectively. No significant clinical risk factors for the incidence of skin rash were observed. Areas under the curve (0–24 h) ($AUC_{0-24,\ ss}$) at steady-state of plasma apalutamide concentration were numerically slightly higher in patients with skin rash than those without.

(Continued on next page)

* Correspondence: ykoroki@its.jnj.com
[2]Medical Affairs, Janssen Pharmaceutical K.K., Tokyo, Japan
Full list of author information is available at the end of the article

(Continued from previous page)
**Conclusions:** No clinical risk factors for rash could be detected. There is a potential correlation between incidence of skin rash and plasma exposure to apalutamide. In general, apalutamide-related skin rash is easily managed, with appropriate treatment with or without dose adjustment.
**Keywords:** Apalutamide, Prostate cancer, Skin rash, Japanese

## Background

Apalutamide, an oral non-steroidal, second-generation, selective inhibitor of the androgen receptor (AR), binds directly to the ligand-binding domain of the AR, thereby preventing AR nuclear translocation and AR-mediated transcription, which in turn induces tumour cell death [1, 2]. Apalutamide is FDA-approved for the treatment of non-metastatic castration-resistant prostate cancer (nmCRPC) and metastatic castration-sensitive prostate cancer (mCSPC), based on data from two pivotal Phase 3 trials, SPARTAN (NCT01946204) and TITAN (NCT02489318), respectively. In the SPARTAN study, addition of 240 mg apalutamide once-daily (QD) to ongoing androgen-deprivation therapy (ADT) showed a significant increase in metastasis-free survival (MFS) (> 2 years) when compared to placebo, with an overall maintenance of health-related quality of life. However, the incidence of skin rash was higher in the apalutamide group compared to placebo (23.8% vs 5.5%) [3]. Similarly, in the TITAN study, skin rash was more frequently observed in the apalutamide group compared to placebo (27.1% vs 8.5%), although significant improvements in the dual primary endpoints of overall survival (OS) and radiographic progression-free survival (rPFS) were reported [4]. Rash is a grouped term that includes macular rash, maculo-papular rash, butterfly rash, erythematous rash, generalized rash, papules, papular rash, pruritic rash, pustular rash, systemic lupus erythematosus rash, erythema multiforme, stomatitis, and urticaria among others. It is important to note that the most commonly observed apalutamide-related rash is not graded based on severity but on body surface area (BSA) involved. Therefore, to be defined as a Grade 3 rash, it must cover > 30% BSA, regardless of concomitant symptoms, if any.

Interestingly, the subgroup analysis of Japanese patients in both the SPARTAN and TITAN studies showed that a greater proportion of patients treated with apalutamide developed skin rash compared with placebo (SPARTAN subgroup: 56.0% vs 0.0%; TITAN subgroup: 50.0% vs 8.7%) [5], [Uemura et al., *International Journal of Urology*, submitted], with the incidence in Japanese patients being nearly double the incidence observed in the global populations of the two studies. In a Phase 1 trial (56021927PCR1008, referred hereafter as PCR1008) conducted to study the safety, efficacy and pharmacokinetic (PK) profile of apalutamide in Japanese patients with metastatic CRPC (mCRPC) (NCT02162836) [6], skin rash was observed in 2/6 (33.3%) patients. Taken together, these data suggest that apalutamide-related skin rash is more frequently observed in Japanese patients. However, the relationship between patient characteristics and apalutamide-related skin rash is not clear. Moreover, the clinical risk factors for apalutamide-related skin rash and the relationship between apalutamide exposure and skin rash remains to be elucidated.

Therefore, we conducted an integrated analysis of data from Japanese patients in the SPARTAN and TITAN studies, along with data from the PCR1008 study primarily to investigate the incidence rate, types, severity and management of skin rash in Japanese subpopulation. Data from patients who developed skin rash were further analyzed to assess if the grade of skin rash had a correlation with the extent of exposure to apalutamide. In addition, various clinical risk factors, such as Gleason score and previous therapy were evaluated vis-à-vis their contribution to the incidence of skin rash.

## Methods

A pooled analysis of data from Japanese patients who were administered apalutamide in two global Phase 3 studies, SPARTAN and TITAN, and a Phase 1 study (PCR1008) was conducted. The study protocols and informed consent forms for the original trials had been reviewed and approved by their respective Independent Ethics Committee or Institutional Review Board. Studies were conducted in accordance with ethical principles outlined in the Declaration of Helsinki and were consistent with International Conference of Harmonization, Good Clinical Practices guidelines, and applicable regulatory requirements. Patients or their legally acceptable representatives provided written informed consent before enrollment. The original trials (SPARTAN, TITAN and PCR1008) were conducted and funded by Janssen Research & Development, LLC and Janssen Pharmaceuticals K.K.

The study design for each of the 3 studies is briefly presented below:

**SPARTAN**

A total of 1207 patients with nmCRPC, receiving ongoing ADT, were randomly assigned (2:1) to either apalutamide (240 mg, QD, orally) or matched placebo, and treated until disease progression, withdrawal of consent, unacceptable toxicity or death. The primary efficacy endpoint was MFS. Secondary efficacy endpoints were time to metastasis, PFS, time to symptomatic progression, time to initiation of cytotoxic chemotherapy and OS.

**TITAN**

A total of 1052 patients with mCSPC were randomized (1:1) to receive apalutamide (240 mg, QD, orally) plus ADT or placebo plus ADT, in this double-blind, Phase 3 trial. The dual primary endpoints were rPFS and OS. Secondary efficacy endpoints were time to cytotoxic chemotherapy, pain progression, chronic opioid use, and skeletal-related event.

***Population pharmacokinetic analysis in SPARTAN and TITAN***

A population PK analyses were performed using all available drug concentration data from SPARTAN and TITAN studies. The population PK model for plasma concentrations of apalutamide and its active metabolite, N-desmethyl apalutamide, was developed using nonlinear mixed-effects modeling. Individual exposure metrics i.e., areas under the curve after 24 h at steady-state ($AUC_{0-24,\ ss}$ [μg*h/mL]) of plasma concentration, for apalutamide and N-desmethyl apalutamide were derived using post-hoc estimates of the PK parameters. $AUC_{0-24,\ ss}$ was calculated based on an average dose up to time of the first rash event considering possible dose modifications. The details of the population PK model was reported in a separate article [7].

**PCR1008**

A total of 6 patients were included in this Phase 1, open-label, multi-center study to analyze the safety, tolerability, and PK profile of apalutamide (240 mg, QD, orally) in Japanese patients with mCRPC who were on ADT background therapy (either medical or surgical castration). Patients received a single apalutamide 240 mg dose on Day 1 of the PK week. Patients were reassessed for safety. If no safety signals were reported, patients received apalutamide 240 mg QD until disease progression, unacceptable toxicity, withdrawal of consent, or death, whichever occurred first. Safety was assessed. All adverse events (AEs) were graded according to National Cancer Institute Common Terminology Criteria for Adverse Events (NCI CTCAE), v4.0.3 in the SPARTAN and TITA N studies, while NCI CTCAE v4.0 was used in PCR1008.

***Analysis***

**Incidence rate, type of rash, severity, management** The incidence rate, type and grade of rash, along with the treatments for the management of rash in each of the 3 studies was analyzed.

**Time-to-event analysis** The time-to-event analysis for rash was performed using the Kaplan-Meier method. Kaplan-Meier curves were generated for time-to-rash (All Grade and Grade 3 or more) and time-to-remission (first incidence, All Grade; first incidence, Grade 3 or more; last incidence, All Grade; and last incidence, Grade 3 or more) using individual patient-level data.

**Clinical risk factors** Odds ratio and 95% confidence interval was used to assess whether factors including age; height; weight; body mass index; Eastern Cooperative Oncology Group Performance Status (ECOG PS); time from initial diagnosis to first dose, Gleason score at initial diagnosis; baseline prostate-specific antigen (PSA), alkaline phosphatase (ALP), hemoglobin, or lactate dehydrogenase levels; and previous local treatment, first-generation antiandrogens, or chemotherapy were related to the incidence of rash.

Pooled data for baseline characteristics, treatment duration, dose reduction, dose interruption, dose discontinuation, incidence of rash and management of rash are presented using descriptive statistics.

**Plasma exposure and incidence of rash** The relationships between the occurrence (by grade) of skin rash and the plasma exposure ($AUC_{0-24,\ ss}$) to apalutamide or N-desmethyl apalutamide were explored using boxplots. All exposure analyses were done based on data from the SPARTAN and TITAN studies.

## Results

In total, 1207 patients in SPARTAN and 1052 patients in TITAN were enrolled globally, of which 55 and 51 patients were Japanese, respectively. This integrated analysis included data from total 68 Japanese patients (SPARTAN: $n = 34$, TITAN: $n = 28$, PCR1008: $n = 6$) who had received apalutamide 240 mg QD orally (Fig. 1).

**Baseline characteristics**

Overall, the median age of patients was 77 years. Since the disease status at baseline was different in SPARTAN, TITAN, and PCR1008 studies, some of the baseline characteristics were not comparable between the three groups, with the median time from initial diagnosis, PSA levels, treatment durations, and ALP levels varying between the 3 patient populations. Median time from

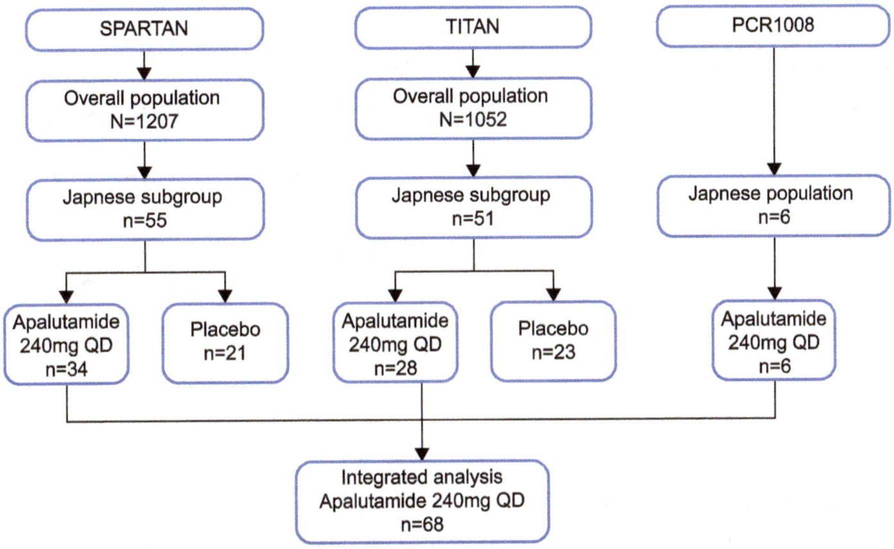


**Fig. 1** Flow diagram representing patient recruitment from SPARTAN, TITAN and PCR1008 studies

initial diagnosis to first dose was shortest in TITAN (2.19 months), followed by PCR1008 (68.89 months) and SPARTAN (87.10 months); with median PSA level [ng/mL] at baseline of 11.51, 54.42 and 4.35, respectively. All patients had received prior hormonal therapy (Table 1).

#### Incidence rate, types of rash, severity

In the global SPARTAN and TITAN studies, the overall incidence of skin rash in the apalutamide group was 191/803 (23.8%) and 142/524 (27.1%), respectively, with the combined incidence rates of the most commonly reported rash in the 2 studies, i.e., rash, generalized rash, and maculo-papular rash, being 167/1327 (12.6%), 53/1327 (4.0%), and 60/1327 (4.5%), respectively (Supplementary Table 1). In the present integrated analysis of Japanese patients from SPARTAN and TITAN, and PCR1008, skin rash was observed in 35/68 (51.5%) of the patients, and the incidence rates of rash (13/68 [19.1%]), generalized rash (11/68 [16.2%]), and maculo-papular rash (11/68 [16.2%]) (Table 2) were also higher than that observed in the global studies. Also, the incidence rate of the less commonly observed rash, erythema multiforme and stomatitis, were higher in Japanese patients (3/68 [4.4%], each) compared to their combined incidence rates in the global SPARTAN and TITAN studies (6/1327 [0.45%] and 10/1327 [0.75%], respectively) (Supplementary Table 1).

In the global SPARTAN and TITAN studies, the incidence of Grade 1 skin rash was 69/803 (8.6%) and 57/524 (10.9%), respectively, in the apalutamide group, while the corresponding values for Grade 2 events were 80/803 (10.0%) and 52/524 (9.9%), respectively (Supplementary Table 1). In the Japanese patients analyzed for this study, the incidence of Grade 1 rash was similar between the groups (SPARTAN: 4/34 [11.8%], TITAN: 4/28 [14.3%], PCR1008: 1/6 [16.7%]), with overall incidence being 9/68 (13.2%); Grade 2 rash were more frequently observed in the SPARTAN study (10/34 [29.4%]) compared to the TITAN (5/28 [17.9%]) and PCR1008 (1/6 [16.7%]) studies; while Grade 3 rash was observed only in the SPARTAN (5/34 [14.7%]) and TITAN (5/28 [17.9%]) studies. Overall, Grade 3 skin rash occurred in 10/68 (14.7%) patients in the current integrated analysis, compared to 42/803 (5.2%) and 33/524 (6.3%) patients in the SPARTAN and TITAN global studies, respectively. (Supplementary Table 1) There were no Grade 4 or 5 rashes due to the grading criteria used for reporting the types of rash observed.

#### Management of Rash

All Japanese patients with skin rash (35/68 [51.1%]) received supportive medications; topical corticosteroid was the most common (27/35 [77.1%]), followed by oral antihistamine and systemic corticosteroid (18/35 [51.4%] and 3/35 [8.6%], respectively) (Table 3). In comparison, in the global SPARTAN and TITAN studies, antihistamines were required in 67/191 (35.1%) and 54/142 (38.0%) patients, systemic corticosteroids in 33/191 (17.3%) and 29/142 (20.4%) patients, while topical corticosteroids were administered in 65/191 (34.0) and 61/142 (43.0%) patients, respectively (Supplementary Table 2).

Drug interruptions and dose reductions were required in 18/35 (51.4%) and 7/35 (20.0%) patients, respectively, with treatment discontinuation required in 5/35 (14.3%)

**Table 1** Baseline Characteristics (Safety Set)

| Categories | SPARTAN | TITAN | PCR1008 | Total |
|---|---|---|---|---|
| **Number of patients in safety analysis set, n** | 34 | 28 | 6 | 68 |
| **Median age, years (range)** | 79.00 (61–90) | 73.00 (47–89) | 78.00 (70–85) | 77.00 (47–90) |
| **Median weight, kg (range)** | 61.90 (45.5–84.0) | 63.55 (40.6–89.2) | 57.30 (49.8–62.6) | 61.80 (40.6–89.2) |
| **Median height, cm (range)**[a] | 163.50 (140.0–176.4) | 165.20 (151.7–172.8) | 163.55 (147.0–165.9) | 164.00 (140.0–176.4) |
| **ECOG PS**[a]**, n (%)** | | | | |
| 0 | 30 (88.24) | 25 (89.29) | 5 (83.33) | 60 (88.24) |
| 1 | 4 (11.76) | 3 (10.71) | 1 (16.67) | 8 (11.76) |
| **Median time from initial diagnosis to first dose, month (range)** | 87.10 (11.01–176.10) | 2.19 (1.28–74.15) | 68.89 (9.23–132.72) | 46.42 (1.28–176.10) |
| **GS at initial diagnosis, n (%)** | | | | |
| ≤ 7 | 9 (26.47) | 1 (3.57) | 2 (33.33) | 12 (17.65) |
| ≥ 8 | 25 (73.53) | 27 (96.43) | 4 (66.67) | 56 (82.35) |
| **Median PSA at baseline, ng/mL (range)** | 4.35 (0.45–21.71) | 11.51 (0.04–457.64) | 54.42 (8.92–310.11) | 5.73 (0.04–457.64) |
| **Median Hemoglobin at baseline, ng/mL (range)** | 12.95 (9.4–15.5) | 13.45 (10.2–15.9) | 11.95 (9.9–15.0) | 13.10 (9.4–15.9) |
| **Median LDH at baseline, U/L (range)** | – | 198.00 (123–272) | 192.00 (115–456) | 197.50 (115–456) |
| **Median ALP at baseline, U/L (range)** | 73.50 (33–137) | 104.50 (56–1149) | 204.50 (102–331) | 87.00 (33–1149) |
| **Disease status, n** | | | | |
| nmCRPC | 55 | – | – | 55 |
| mCSPC | – | 51 | – | 51 |
| mCRPC | – | – | 6 | 6 |
| **Tumor volume**[b]**, n (%)** | | | | |
| High | – | 18 (64.29) | – | 18 (64.29) |
| Low | – | 10 (35.71) | – | 10 (35.71) |
| **Previous treatment, n (%)** | | | | |
| *Local treatment* | 21 (61.76) | 1 (3.57) | 2 (33.33) | 24 (35.29) |
| RP | 5 (14.71) | 1 (3.57) | 1 (16.67) | 7 (10.29) |
| RT | 19 (55.88) | 1 (3.57) | 1 (16.67) | 21 (30.88) |
| *Hormonal treatment* | 34 (100.00) | 28 (100.00) | 6 (100.00) | 68 (100.00) |
| LHRHa | 34 (100.00) | 28 (100.00) | 5 (83.33) | 67 (98.53) |
| Orchiectomy | 1 (2.94) | 2 (7.14) | 1 (16.67) | 4 (5.88) |
| 1st generation AA | 33 (97.06) | 15 (53.57) | 6 (100.00) | 54 (79.41) |
| Other | 2 (5.88) | 0 (0.00) | 0 (0.00) | 2 (2.94) |
| *Chemotherapy* | 0 (0.00) | 0 (0.00) | 0 (0.00) | 0 (0.00) |
| *Other* | 3 (8.82) | 0 (0.00) | 2 (33.33) | 5 (7.35) |
| **Average dose of Apalutamide** | | | | |
| **Mean dose, mg (SD)** | 223.94 (28.91) | 214.07 (44.90) | 225.84 (25.76) | 220.04 (36.05) |
| **Median dose, mg (range)** | 236.55 (108.6–240.0) | 239.02 (90.6–240.0) | 236.10 (174.2–240.0) | 238.27 (90.6–240.0) |

*AA* Antiandrogen, *ALP* Alkaline phosphatase, *ECOG* Eastern Cooperative Oncology Group, *GS* Gleason score, *LDH* Lactate dehydrogenase LHRHa, hormone-releasing hormone antagonist, *nmCRPC* Non-metastatic castration resistant prostate cancer, *mCSPC* Metastatic castration sensitive prostate cancer, *mCRPC* Metastatic castration resistant prostate cancer, *PSA* Prostate-specific antigen, *RP* Radical prostatectomy, *RT* Radiotherapy, *SD* Standard deviation

[a]: count PCR1008 at screening

[b]: Denominator of proportion is TITAN's safety analysis set

patients. Among patients receiving apalutamide who developed skin rash in the global SPARTAN study, dose interruptions, does reductions, and treatment discontinuations were reported in 55/191 (28.8%), 22/191 (11.5%), and 19/191 (9.9%), patients, respectively, while the corresponding values in the global population from the TITAN study were 44/142 (31.0%), 28/142 (19.7%), and 12/142 (8.5%) (Supplementary Table 2).

**Table 2** Types of Skin Rash in Apalutamide-treated Patients

| Analysis Set (N = 68) | Total n (%) | Grade 1 n (%) | Grade 2 n (%) | Grade 3 n (%) |
|---|---|---|---|---|
| **Rash** | 35 (51.47) | 9 (13.23) | 16 (23.52) | 10 (14.70) |
| Rash | 13 (19.11) | 8 (11.76) | 4 (5.88) | 1 (1.47) |
| Rash maculo-papular | 11 (16.17) | 2 (2.94) | 6 (8.2) | 3 (4.41) |
| Rash generalised | 11 (16.17) | 1 (1.47) | 7 (10.29) | 3 (4.41) |
| Erythema multiforme | 3 (4.41) | 0 | 1 (1.47) | 2 (2.94) |
| Stomatitis | 3 (4.41) | 1 (1.47) | 2 (2.94) | 0 |
| Urticaria | 2 (2.94) | 2 (2.94) | 0 | 0 |
| Blister | 1 (1.47) | 1 (1.47) | 0 | 0 |
| Drug eruption | 1 (1.47) | 0 | 0 | 1 (1.47) |
| Rash macular | 1 (1.47) | 0 | 0 | 1 (1.47) |
| Skin erosion | 1 (1.47) | 1 (1.47) | 0 | 0 |
| Skin exfoliation | 1 (1.47) | 1 (1.47) | 0 | 0 |

### Time-to-event analyses

In the integrated analysis, the median time to onset of first incidence of rash of any grade in Japanese patients was 66 days, with time to incidence of first Grade 3 rash being 45 days and 9/10 (90.0%) Grade 3 events being reported in the first 4 months. The median time for first incidence of Grade 3 rash was 52 days and 38 days in the Japanese patients from SPARTAN and TITAN, respectively. In comparison, in the global population from the SPARTAN and TITAN studies, the median time to first incidence of skin rash were 82 days and 80.5 days, respectively (Supplementary Table 2). The median time for remission of first incidence of any grade in Japanese patients was 1.0 month (Interquartile range [IQR]: 0.36–1.81) (Fig. 2). In the global population of the SPARTAN study, skin rash of any grade resolved for 81% of the patients within 59.5 days, while the median time to resolution of skin rash of any grade in the TITAN study was 100 days (Supplementary Table 2). The time-to-remission of Grade 3 rash was 35 days and 17 days in the Japanese patients from SPARTAN and TITAN, respectively, with 1.0 month (IQR: 0.30–2.43) required for remission in the integrated analysis (Fig. 3). Some patients experienced skin rash more than once during apalutamide treatment. Even if patients resolved first incidence of rash, there was the potential for worsening in the second incidence of rash. Therefore, we assessed these two types of KM curves. KM figures for time-to-rash (All grade) (Supplementary Fig. 1), time-to-rash (≥Grade3) (Supplementary Fig. 2), time-to-remission of first incidence (≥Grade3) (Supplementary Fig. 3), and time-to-remission of maximum grade (≥Grade3) (Supplementary Fig. 4) are included in the supplementary files.

### Clinical risk factors

A number of clinical risk factors that could potentially affect the incidence of rash were assessed, including Eastern Cooperative Oncology Group Performance Status (ECOG PS), time from initial diagnosis to first dose, Gleason score, and previous treatments (Table 4). However, none of the factors were found to be significantly linked to the incidence of skin rash.

### Pharmacokinetic analysis

$AUC_{0-24,\ ss}$ of apalutamide were numerically slightly higher in patients with skin rash than those without; however, this did not significantly impact the grade of skin rash (Fig. 4a). No correlation was apparent with $AUC_{0-24,\ ss}$ of N-desmethyl apalutamide (Fig. 4b).

## Discussion

Apalutamide-related skin rash has been observed in previous studies, with a higher incidence of skin rash observed in the Japanese subpopulation compared to overall global population. In the global SPARTAN and TITAN studies, and the Japanese subpopulation analysis from these studies [5], [Uemura et al., *International Journal of Urology*, submitted], Grade 3 rash (covering > 30% of the body

**Table 3** Rash Management

| Analysis Set (N = 68) | SPARTAN | TITAN | PCR1008 | Total |
|---|---|---|---|---|
| **Number of patients in safety analysis set, n** | 34 | 28 | 6 | 68 |
| Rash, n (%) | 19 (55.88) | 14 (50.00) | 2 (33.33) | 35 (51.47) |
| **Patients who received supportive care for rash, n (%)** | | | | |
| Oral antihistamine | 11 (57.89) | 6 (42.86) | 1 (50.00) | 18 (51.43) |
| Systemic corticosteroid | 0 (0.00) | 3 (21.43) | 0 (0.00) | 3 (8.57) |
| Topical corticosteroid | 13 (68.42) | 13 (92.86) | 1 (50.00) | 27 (77.14) |
| Drug interruption | 11 (57.89) | 6 (42.86) | 1 (50.00) | 18 (51.43) |
| Dose reduction | 4 (21.05) | 3 (21.43) | 0 (0.00) | 7 (20.00) |
| Drug discontinuation | 3 (15.79) | 2 (14.29) | 0 (0.00) | 5 (14.29) |
| Other | 2 (10.53) | 1 (7.14) | 0 (0.00) | 3 (8.57) |

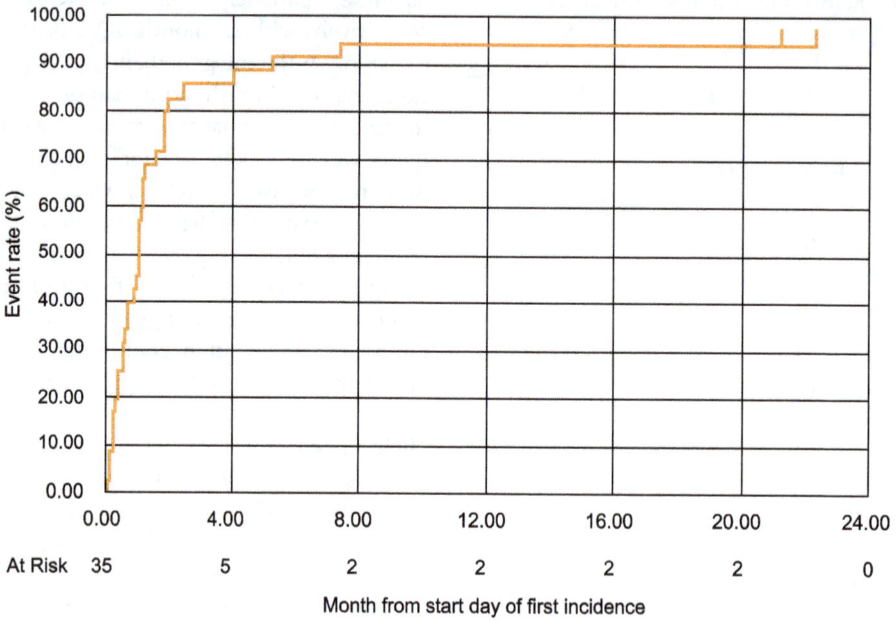


**Fig. 2** Kaplan-Meier plot for Time-to-Remission of First Incidence of rash (All Grade). Event: remission of first incidence of rash. Censor: not remission of first incidence of rash at the end of follow-up

surface) was observed more frequently with apalutamide [3, 4]. In the current integrated analysis, the incidence of Grade 3 rash (14.7%) was also higher than in the global SPAR TAN and TITAN studies (combined incidence, 5.7%). This suggests that both the frequency and grade of skin rash, across different disease status, are higher in Japanese patients compared to the global population with apalutamide treatment. Consequently, treatment discontinuation due to rash, which is recommended if oral corticosteroids are required for > 28 days, was required in 14.3% patients in the current integrated analysis compared with 2.3% patients in the global population [3, 4]. Most Grade 1/2 rash resolved following the use of oral antihistamines, topical or systemic corticosteroids, with or without apalutamide dose

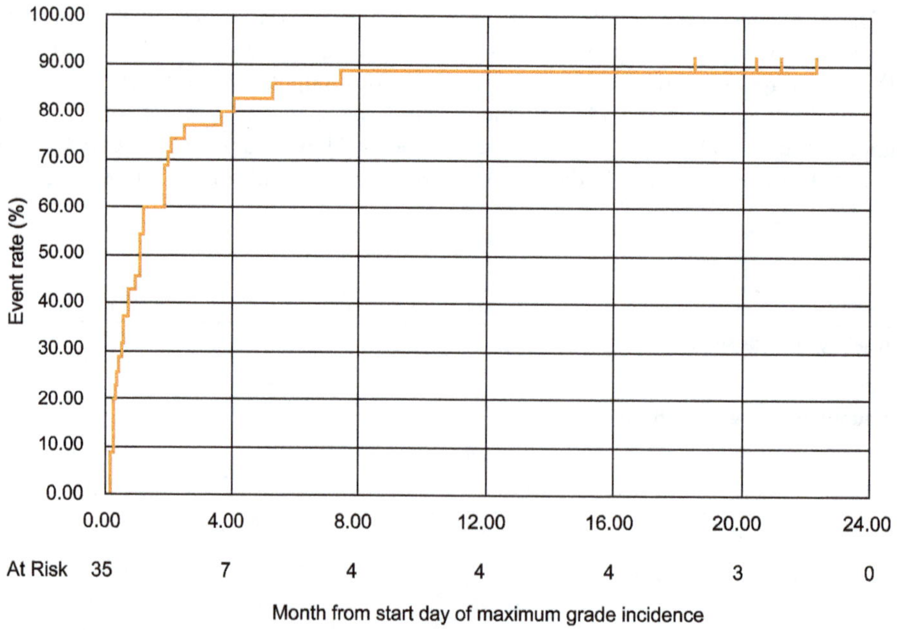


**Fig. 3** Kaplan-Meier plot for Time-to-Remission of Maximum Grade Incidence of rash (All grade). Event: remission of maximum Grade incidence of rash. Censor: not remission of maximum Grade incidence of rash at the end of follow-up

**Table 4** Odds Ratio (All Grade), Target Population: Safety

| Categories | | Number of Patients | Rash, n (%) Yes | No | 95% CI | Odds Ratio | p-value |
|---|---|---|---|---|---|---|---|
| **Number of patients in safety analysis set, n** | | 68 | 35 (51.47) | 33 (48.5) | | | |
| **Age class 1, year** | < 65 | 5 | 3 (60.00) | 2 (40.00) | | | |
| | ≥65 | 63 | 32 (50.79) | 31 (49.20) | 0.11–4.40 | 0.69 | 0.693 |
| **Age class 2, year** | < 75 | 28 | 13 (46.43) | 15 (53.57) | | | |
| | ≥75 | 40 | 22 (55.00) | 18 (45.00) | 0.53–3.72 | 1.41 | 0.487 |
| **Baseline weight** | < Median | 34 | 16 (47.06) | 18 (52.94) | | | |
| | ≥ Median | 34 | 19 (55.88) | 15 (44.12) | 0.55–3.70 | 1.43 | 0.467 |
| **Baseline height** | < Median | 34 | 15 (44.12) | 19 (55.88) | | | |
| | ≥ Median | 34 | 20 (58.82) | 14 (41.18) | 0.69–4.73 | 1.81 | 0.227 |
| **Body mass index (kg/m$^2$)** | < 25 | 48 | 22 (45.83) | 26 (54.17) | | | |
| | ≥25 | 20 | 13 (65.00) | 7 (35.00) | 0.75–6.46 | 2.19 | 0.154 |
| **ECOG PS** | 0 | 60 | 30 (50.00) | 30 (50.00) | | | |
| | 1 | 8 | 5 (62.50) | 3 (37.50) | 0.37–7.61 | 1.67 | 0.510 |
| **Time from initial diagnosis to first dose** | < Median | 34 | 14 (41.18) | 20 (58.82) | | | |
| | ≥ Median | 34 | 21 (61.76) | 13 (38.24) | 0.87–6.10 | 2.31 | 0.092 |
| **GS at initial diagnosis** | ≤ 7 | 12 | 9 (75.00) | 3 (25.00) | | | |
| | ≥ 8 | 56 | 26 (46.43) | 30 (53.57) | 0.07–1.18 | 0.29 | 0.084 |
| | Unknown | 0 | 0 | 0 | – | – | |
| **Baseline PSA** | < Median | 34 | 21 (61.76) | 13 (38.24) | | | |
| | ≥ Median | 34 | 14 (41.18) | 20 (58.82) | 0.16–1.15 | 0.43 | 0.092 |
| **Baseline Hemoglobin** | High | 68 | 35 (51.47) | 33 (48.53) | | | |
| | Normal or Low | 0 | 0 | 0 | – | – | – |
| **Baseline LDH** | High | 7 | 2 (28.57) | 5 (71.43) | | | 0.282 |
| | Normal or Low | 27 | 14 (51.85) | 13 (48.15) | 0.44–16.37 | 2.69 | |
| **Baseline ALP** | High | 13 | 4 (30.77) | 9 (69.23) | | | |
| | Normal or Low | 55 | 31 (56.36) | 24 (43.64) | 0.80–10.59 | 2.91 | 0.106 |
| **Previous local treatment** | No | 44 | 21 (47.73) | 23 (52.27) | | | |
| | Yes | 24 | 14 (58.33) | 10 (41.67) | 0.56–4.19 | 1.53 | 0.404 |
| **Previous 1st generation AA** | No | 14 | 9 (64.29) | 5 (35.71) | | | |
| | Yes | 54 | 26 (48.15) | 28 (51.85) | 0.15–1.74 | 0.52 | 0.286 |
| **Previous chemotherapy** | No | 68 | 35 (51.47) | 33 (48.53) | | | |
| | Yes | 0 | 0 | 0 | – | – | – |

*AA* Antiandrogen, *ALP* Alkaline phosphatase, *ECOG PS* Eastern Cooperative Oncology Group Performance Status, *GS* Gleason score, *LDH* Lactate dehydrogenase, *PSA* Prostate-specific antigen, *CI* Confidence interval

interruption or reduction, following which, patients were able to continue apalutamide treatment. Based on the current analysis, it is difficult to conclude whether supportive treatment or dose interruption was more effective in resolving the different grades of skin rash.

In our study, the median time to first incidence of rash was 66 days, and it resolved in a median time of 1.0 month. When compared to SPARTAN, both the onset and resolution of rash were faster in Japanese patients. These data require further investigation since the overall incidence of skin rashes was higher in the Japanese patients, yet their time to incidence and resolution was faster. Interestingly, in our study, the median time to first remission was 1.0 month, but the median time-to-remission of last incidence was 3.6 months, suggesting that some patients experienced several incidents of skin rash. However, the median time-to-remission of the worst grade (Grade 3) of skin rash was 1.0 month. Therefore, even if some patients experienced several incidents of skin rash, the worst grade of skin rash remitted within 1.0

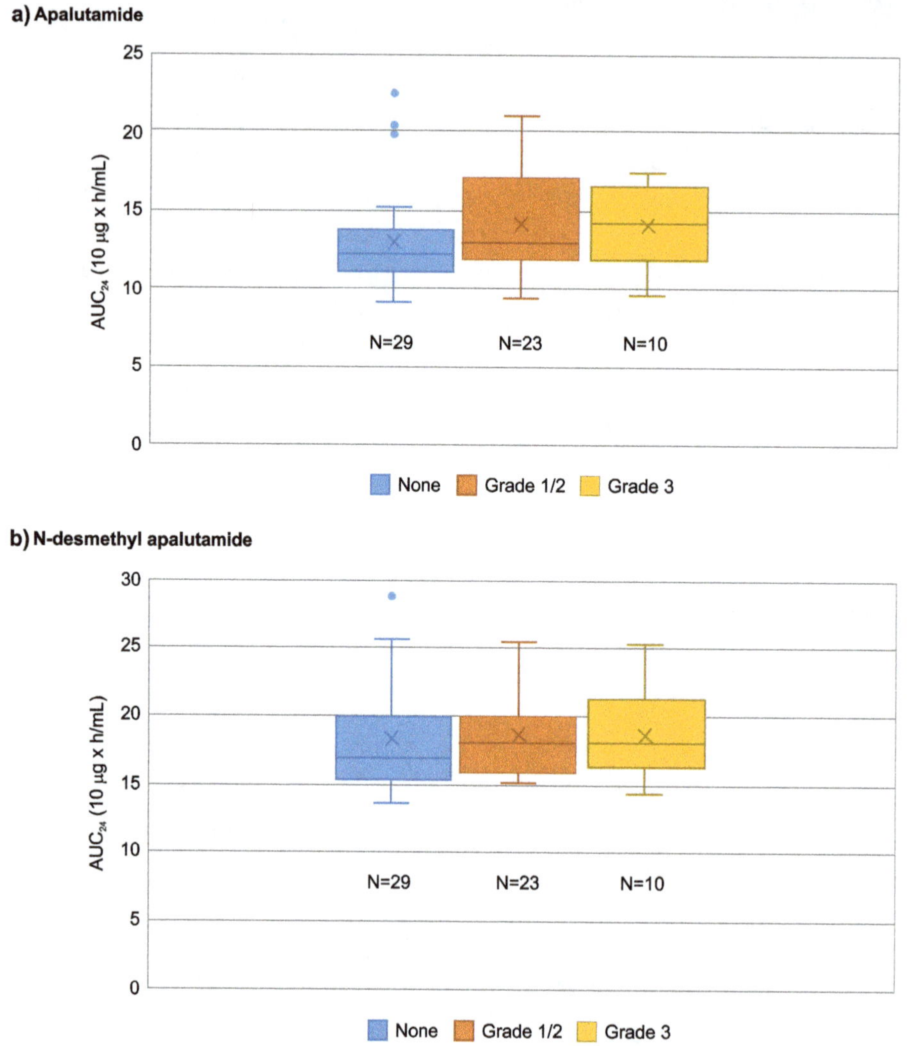


**Fig. 4** Plasma-Exposure and Incidence of Rash: Pooled results of Japanese patients from SPARTAN and TITAN studies. **a**) Apalutamide, **b**) N-desmethyl apalutamide. Relationships between incidence of rash (by grade) and the plasma exposure ($AUC_{0-24,\ ss}$) to apalutamide or N-desmethyl apalutamide were explored using boxplots

month following appropriate management by physicians. This could be attributed to the more frequent use of topical corticosteroids (77.1%) and oral antihistamines (51.4%) as supportive medication among Japanese patients when compared with patients in the global studies (combined data from SPARTAN and TITAN: topical corticosteroids, 37.8%; antihistamines, 36.3%.

Apalutamide and N-desmethyl apalutamide are two major pharmacologically active components detected in the systemic circulation at steady-state [8, 9]. The current integrated analysis showed that there was a possible correlation between plasma exposure to apalutamide and incidence of skin rash, but it did not significantly impact the grade of skin rash. However, the results should be interpreted with caution due to the limited sample size. The exposure-response modeling analysis for SPARTAN study based on whole study population was reported in a separate article [10].

Recently, the National Comprehensive Cancer Network (NCCN) guidelines were updated to recommend apalutamide or enzalutamide, another second-generation antiandrogen, in patients with nmCRPC with background ADT therapy [11]. Skin rash was not observed to be an adverse drug reaction (ADR) in Phase 3 trials, either in nmCRPC or mCRPC patients [12, 13] with enzalutamide, although a case report of enzalutamide-induced acute generalized exanthematous pustulosis was recently reported and the USPI includes rash as an ADR observed in post-marketing [14]. Skin rash has also been reported with the first-generation oral non-steroidal antiandrogen drug bicalutamide and other new-generation oral antiandrogen drugs such as darolutamide [15–18]. It remains to be elucidated if skin rash is a class-effect, particularly in Japanese patients.

There is evidence to suggest that ethnic difference and genotypic heterogeneity between the Japanese and Caucasian populations could have an impact on treatment responses in patients with PC [19–21]. The correlation of human leukocyte antigen (HLA) typing with serious drug-induced skin rash e.g., Stevens-Johnson syndrome or toxic epidermal necrosis, is well established. However, further studies to explore the correlation of HLA typing with apalutamide-related skin rash are needed. Interestingly, Japanese men have been observed to respond better to hormonal therapy compared to their Caucasian counterparts [22, 23]. With reports of skin rashes being disproportionately higher in the Japanese subset of SPARTAN and TITAN studies and no clinical risk factors identified in the current study, further studies are needed to understand the basis of the high incidence observed.

To assess the clinical risk factors associated with commonly administered PC drugs, an analysis of AEs among nmCRPC patients treated with abiraterone (a synthetic, steroidal CYP17A1 inhibitor recently approved in the treatment of PC), enzalutamide, or bicalutamide, was carried out in the real-world setting. Baseline AEs, Charlson comorbidity index, surgical castration, and older age were found to be significant predictors of AEs [24]. However, in our study, which was conducted based on registration trials, no clinical risk factors of skin rash were identified following apalutamide treatment. Therefore, it is important to analyze clinical risk factors of skin rash using real-world evidence.

A recent study assessed important safety factors that physicians considered in making treatment decisions for patients with nmCRPC. Among the safety attributes analyzed, which included incidence of skin rash, physicians were most concerned regarding cognitive problems, fractures, and fatigue. In fact, physicians regarded reduction in cognitive problems (from severe to none) to have a 36.0% higher importance in comparison to improving OS by 12 months instead of 3 months. Therefore, even though an important adverse event, skin rash was not a major determinant in physicians' choice of treatment for PC, reiterating the need to assess the benefit-risk ratio to determine the best treatment for a particular patient with PC [24, 25].

Some of the baseline characteristics were not comparable between SPARTAN, TITAN and PCR1008 groups, with the median time from initial diagnosis, PSA levels, treatment durations, and ALP levels varying between these patient populations, since these were inherently different patient populations with different disease status at baseline. Although the cohorts were relatively dissimilar, the overall apalutamide regimens were similar amongst different disease populations in three studies. There may be an observer bias in an open-label Phase 1 study, however, it was included in the pooled analysis since the treatment dose (240 mg/day) and the incidence of skin rash were similar to those in Phase 3 studies. In current research, we focussed on Japanese subpopulation for incidence of apalutamide-related skin rash. Most of skin rash occurred in the first 4 months after apalutamide initiation and it would be difficult to evaluate time to skin rash stratified by covariates since the patients' number is small. In order to conduct time-to-event analysis, larger apalutamide treatment data is warranted in the real-world settings.

The generalizability of the findings in this study is limited by the small number of patients analyzed ($N = 68$), its unplanned retrospective design, and the fact that the integrated analysis was done on different disease populations (nmCRPC, mCSPC and mCRPC). However, the results of this study underscore the need to undertake a prospective analysis of apalutamide-related skin rash in the Japanese population.

## Conclusions

The incidence of apalutamide-related skin rash was higher in Japanese patients with PC compared to patients from the rest of the world. Although there is a potential correlation between incidence of skin rash and plasma exposure to apalutamide, it did not significantly impact the grade of skin rash. Moreover, no clinical risk factors associated with skin rash were identified. Most skin rash is observed within 120 days of treatment initiation and close monitoring of the skin rash, dose reductions/interruptions and treatment with oral antihistamines and topical and systemic corticosteroids led to resolution of the majority of skin rash observed in Japanese patients within 30 days.

## Supplementary information

**Additional file 1. Supplementary Fig. 1.** Kaplan-Meier plot for Time-to-Rash (All Grade).

**Additional file 2. Supplementary Fig. 2.** Kaplan-Meier plot for Time-to-Rash (≥ Grade 3).

**Additional file 3. Supplementary Fig. 3.** Kaplan-Meier plot for Time-to-Remission of First Incidence of rash (≥ Grade 3).

**Additional file 4. Supplementary Fig. 4.** Kaplan-Meier plot for Time-to-Remission of Maximum Grade Incidence of rash (≥ Grade 3).

**Additional file 5. Supplementary Table 1.** Incidence of Rash in SPAR TAN and TITAN.

**Additional file 6. Supplementary Table 2.** Time to Incidence of Rash, Rash Management, and Resolution of Rash in SPARTAN and TITAN.

### Abbreviations

ADR: Adverse drug reaction; ADT: Androgen-deprivation therapy; ALP: Alkaline phosphatase; AR: Androgen receptor; BSA: Body surface area; CI: Confidence interval; ECOG PS: Eastern Cooperative Oncology Group Performance Status; HLA: Human leukocyte antigen; mCSPC: Metastatic castration-sensitive prostate cancer; mCRPC: Metastatic castration-resistant prostate cancer; MFS: Metastasis-free survival; NCCN: National Comprehensive Cancer Network; NCI CTCAE: National Cancer Institute Common Terminology Criteria for Adverse Events; nmCRPC: Non-metastatic castration-resistant prostate cancer; OS: Overall survival; PFS: Progression-free survival; PK: Pharmacokinetic; PSA: Prostate-specific antigen; QD: Once-daily; SD: Standard deviation

### Acknowledgements

Anupama Singh, M. Tech, ISMPP, CMPP™ and Akshada Deshpande, PhD provided medical writing assistance and Sangita Patil, PhD, ISMPP, CMPP™ (all from SIRO Clinpharm Pvt. Ltd) provided additional editorial support for this manuscript.

### Authors' contributions

HU1 was an investigator for SPARTAN, TITAN and PCR1008; HU2 was an investigator for SPARTAN and TITAN; both were involved in data collection for this study. YK and YI were involved in the design and analysis of this study. ALG and AS had a primary role in the study design and data interpretation for SPARTAN. KI and YI contributed to conception and design of PCR1008 study. All authors were involved in data interpretation, development, and critical revision of the manuscript for intellectual content. All authors met ICMJE criteria and all those who fulfilled those criteria are listed as authors. All authors had access to the study data and made the final decision about where to publish these data and approved submission to this journal.

### Competing interests

Dr. Hiroji Uemura received research grants from Janssen Pharmaceutical (during the conduct of the study) and lecture fees/subsidies from Bayer Yakuhin, Limited, Takeda Pharmaceutical Company Limited, AstraZeneca K.K., TAIHO Pharmaceutical Company Limited, Astellas Pharma Inc. and Pfizer Inc.
Dr. Takeshi Kambara has no competing interests.
Dr. Hirotsugu Uemura received lecture fee from Pfizer Japan Inc., Ono pharmaceutical Co., Ltd., Bayer Yakuhin, Limited, Bristol-Myers Squibb, MSD K.K., research fee or grants from TAIHO Pharmaceutical Company Limited, Janssen Pharmaceutical K.K., Mebix, Inc., MSD K.K., Astellas Pharma Inc., Covence, Bayer Yakuhin, Limited, Prexel International Inc., Pfizer Japan Inc. ICON Japan K.K., Ono pharmaceutical Co., Ltd., Daiichi Ssankyo Company Limited, AstraZeneca K. K, EPS Corporation, Green Peptide, PPD-SNBL K.K., Takeda Pharmaceutical Company Limited, Chugai Pharmaceutical Co. Ltd., IQVIA, Mediscience Planning Inc., Osaka Urology Research Foundation, scholarship/encouragement donations from Asahi Kasei Corporation, Kissei Pharmaceutical Co., Ltd., Novartis Pharmaceutical, Pfizer Japan Inc., Astellas Pharma Inc., Ono pharmaceutical Co., Ltd., Takeda Pharmaceutical Company Limited, Sanofi K.K., Daiichi Sankyo Co., Ltd.
The following authors are full-time employees of Janssen Pharmaceutical K.K. of Johnson & Johnson: Yosuke Koroki, Yuki Iwaki, and Keiichiro Imanaka; and Janssen Research and Development: Andressa Smith and Angela Lopez-Gitlitz.

### Author details

[1]Department of Urology and Renal Transplantation, Yokohama City University Medical Center, Yokohama, Japan. [2]Medical Affairs, Janssen Pharmaceutical K.K., Tokyo, Japan. [3]Clinical Pharmacology, Janssen Pharmaceutical K.K, Tokyo, Japan. [4]Clinical Science, Janssen Pharmaceutical K.K, Tokyo, Japan. [5]Department of Dermatology, Yokohama City University Medical Center, Yokohama, Japan. [6]Janssen Global Research & Development, Spring House, PA, USA. [7]Department of Urology, Kindai University Faculty of Medicine, Osaka, Japan.

### References

1. Clegg NJ, Wongvipat J, Joseph JD, et al. ARN-509: a novel antiandrogen for prostate cancer treatment. Cancer Res. 2012;72:1494–503.
2. Rice MA, Malhotra SV, Stoyanova T. Second-generation antiandrogens: from discovery to standard of Care in Castration Resistant Prostate Cancer. Front Oncol. 2019;9:801.
3. Smith MR, Saad F, Chowdhury S, et al. Apalutamide treatment and metastasis-free survival in prostate cancer. N Engl J Med. 2018;378:1408–18.
4. Chi KN, Agarwal N, Bjartell A, et al. Apalutamide for metastatic, castration-sensitive prostate cancer. N Engl J Med. 2019;381:13–24.
5. Uemura H, Satoh T, Tsumura H et al. Efficacy and safety of apalutamide in Japanese patients with non-metastatic castration-resistant prostate cancer: A subgroup analysis of a randomized, double-blind, placebo-controlled, phase 3 study. Prostate Int. 2020. https://doi.org/10.1016/j.prnil.2020.05.002.
6. Tsuchiya T, Imanaka K, Iwaki Y, et al. An open-label, phase 1 study of androgen receptor antagonist, apalutamide in Japanese patients with metastatic castration-resistant prostate cancer. Int J Clin Oncol. 2019;24: 1596–604.
7. Pérez-Ruixo C, Pérez-Blanco JS, Chien C, et al. Population pharmacokinetics of apalutamide and its active metabolite N-desmethyl-apalutamide in healthy and castration-resistant prostate cancer subjects. Clin Pharmacokinet. 2020;59:229–44.
8. Rathkopf DE, Morris MJ, Fox JJ, et al. Phase I study of ARN-509, a novel antiandrogen, in the treatment of castration-resistant prostate cancer. J Clin Oncol. 2013;31:3525–30.
9. Alkhudair NA. Apalutamide: emerging therapy for non-metastatic castration-resistant prostate cancer. Saudi Pharm J. 2019;27:368–72.
10. Perez-Ruixo C, Ackaert O, Ouellet D et al. Efficacy and safety exposure-response relationships of apalutamide in patients with non-metastatic castration-resistant prostate cancer. Clin Cancer Res. 2020. https://doi.org/10.1158/1078-0432.CCR-20-10412020.
11. NCCN. Prostate Cancer. https://www.nccn.org/patients/guidelines/content/PDF/prostate-patient.pdf. Accessed on 10 Oct 2019.
12. Hussain M, Fizazi K, Saad F, et al. Enzalutamide in men with nonmetastatic, castration-resistant prostate cancer. N Engl J Med. 2018;378:2465–74.
13. Beer TM, Armstrong AJ, Rathkopf DE, et al. Enzalutamide in metastatic prostate cancer before chemotherapy. N Engl J Med. 2014;371:424–33.
14. Alberto C, Konstantinou MP, Martinage C, et al. Enzalutamide induced acute generalized exanthematous pustulosis. J Dermatol Case Rep. 2016;10:35–8.
15. Lee S, Chung YJ, Kim BH, et al. Comparative pharmacokinetic evaluation of two formulations of bicalutamide 50-mg tablets: an open-label, randomized-sequence, single-dose, two-period crossover study in healthy Korean male volunteers. Clin Ther. 2009;31:3000–8.
16. Chodak G, Sharifi R, Kasimis B, et al. Single-agent therapy with bicalutamide: a comparison with medical or surgical castration in the treatment of advanced prostate carcinoma. Urology. 1995;46:849–55.
17. Kolvenbag GJCM, Blackledge GRP. Worldwide activity and safety of bicalutamide: a summary review. Urology. 1996;47:70–9.
18. Fizazi K, Shore N, Tammela TL, et al. Darolutamide in nonmetastatic, castration-resistant prostate cancer. N Engl J Med. 2019;380:1235–46.
19. Irvine RA, Yu MC, Ross RK, Coetzee GA. The CAG and GGC microsatellites of the androgen receptor gene are in linkage disequilibrium in men with prostate cancer. Cancer Res. 1995;55:1937–40.
20. Suzuki H, Akakura K, Komiya A, et al. CAG polymorphic repeat lengths in androgen receptor gene among Japanese prostate cancer patients: potential predictor of prognosis after endocrine therapy. Prostate. 2002;51: 219–24.
21. Sartor O, Zheng Q, Eastham JA. Androgen receptor gene CAG repeat length varies in a race-specific fashion in men without prostate cancer. Urology. 1999;53:378–80.
22. Fukagai T, Namiki TS, Carlile RG, et al. Comparison of the clinical outcome after hormonal therapy for prostate cancer between Japanese and Caucasian men. BJU Int. 2006;97:1190–3.
23. Namiki M, Ueno S, Kitagawa Y. Role of hormonal therapy for prostate cancer: perspective from Japanese experiences. Transl Androl Urol. 2012;1:160–72.
24. Shah A, Hussain A, Shah R, et al. Predictors and rates of adverse events (AEs) among non-metastatic prostate cancer (nmPC) patients (pts) treated with bicalutamide, abiraterone, or enzalutamide following surgical/medical castration. J Clin Oncol. 2019;37:e16556.
25. Mateo J, Fizazi K, Gillessen S, et al. Managing nonmetastatic castration-resistant prostate cancer. Eur Urol. 2019;75:285–93.

13

# Efficacy and safety of transurethral split of prostate for benign prostatic hyperplasia

Yiyu Huang[1], Jiaxin LI[2], Shan Yang[3], Daozhang Yuan[1*] and Shusheng Wang[4*]

**Abstract**

**Background:** Transurethral resection of the prostate (TURP) is the first choice for the treatment of benign prostatic hyperplasia. However, Transurethral split of prostate (TUSP) also seems to have clear clinical efficacy and clinical promotion value. To better clarify the potential and limitations of this treatment of prostate hyperplasia. This study objectively evaluated the clinical efficacy and safety of TUSP.

**Methods:** The Pubmed, Cochrane Library, Embase, China National Knowledge Infrastructure (CNKI), Database for Chinese Technical Periodicals (VIP), Wanfang (Wanfang data), and SinoMed databases were searched for relevant studies. We then used Revman Manager 5.3 to perform a meta-analysis of all randomized controlled trials that evaluated the efficacy and safety of TUSP versus the classic surgical procedures commonly used in the clinic.

**Results:** A total of 7 studies involving 592 patients were included. The combined data showed that TUSP can shorten the operation time [MD: -33.68; 95% CI: − 38.45 to − 28.91; $P < 0.001$], reduce intraoperative blood loss [MD: -56.06; 95% CI: − 62.68 to − 49.43; $P < 0.001$], shorten the time of indwelling catheter [MD: -1.83; 95% CI: − 1.99 to − 1.67; $P < 0.001$], shorten the postoperative hospital stay length [MD: -1.61; 95% CI: − 1.90 to − 1.32; $P < 0.001$] and improved postoperative quality of life score (QOL) [MD: 0.16; 95% CI: 0.02 to 0.29; $P = 0.02$] compared to traditional surgical approaches. There were no statistically significant differences in international prostate symptom score (IPSS), maximum urinary flow rate (Qmax), residual urine volume (RUV), or complications between TUSP and traditional approached.

**Conclusion:** TUSP can be an effective alternative for clinical treatment of benign prostatic hyperplasia. Given the limitations of the included studies, more high-quality randomized controlled trials are needed in the future to validate or update the results of this analysis.

**Keywords:** Transurethral split of prostate, TUSP, Benign prostatic hyperplasia, BPH, Meta-analysis

* Correspondence: t18819158987@163.com; W15625982171@126.com
[1]Department of Urology, GuangDong Second Traditional Chinese Medicine Hospital, No.212, Luogang Road Street, Luogang District, Guangzhou 510700, Guangdong, China
[4]Department of Urology, Guangdong Provincial Hospital of Chinese Medicine, No.261, Datong Road, Yuexiu District, Guangzhou 510030, Guangdong, China
Full list of author information is available at the end of the article

## Background

Benign prostatic hyperplasia (BPH) is one of the most common benign diseases in middle-aged men. The incidence of the disease is positively correlated with age. According to statistics, the histological prevalence rates is approximately 10% for men aged 30–40, 20% for men aged 41–50, 50 to 60% for men aged 60–70, and 80 to 90% for men aged 70–90. Lower urinary tract symptoms (LUTS), such as frequent urination, urgency, and dysuria, are the main pathological features of BPH [1]. Extremely high morbidity and the resultant LUTS have brought much pain to the lives of male patients. If the treatment is not appropriate or timely, it may also be complicated with upper urinary tract damage or even affect dual renal function [2]. Currently, transurethral resection of the prostate (TURP) is the clinically preferred treatment [3, 4]. However, there are still complications such as hemorrhage, transurethral resection syndrome (TURS) and retrograde ejaculation [5]. New surgical methods, such as bipolar transurethral electrovaporization of the prostate (TUPKP) and transurethral plasmakinetic enucleation of the prostate (TUKEP), have emerged and have been shown to have relatively few complications. However, these methods also have the problem of expensive equipment and high technical requirements for doctors, which is not conducive to clinical promotion [6]. Therefore, it is necessary to find an effective, relatively safe and inexpensive surgical method. Professor Guo Yinglu from the First Hospital of Peking University, China, has been working on the transurethral split of prostate (TUSP) method for many years and finally developed a variety of models of double-chambered water balloon expansion catheters. They standardized the surgical procedure, making the surgery more mature in the treatment of BPH, and proved that the operation is safe and effective through related research [7, 8].

Although some Chinese scholars have conducted randomized controlled trials (RCTs) on using TUSP to treat BPH and found that it has relatively clear clinical efficacy and clinical promotion value, small sample size made it is impossible to provide a comprehensive evaluation. To date, there has been no systematic review and meta-analysis of the efficacy and safety of TUSP in the treatment of BPH. Therefore, we systematically searched and analyzed existing literature to assess the efficacy and potential advantages of TUSP.

## Methods

This meta-analysis were following the Cochrane Handbook of Systematic Reviews of Interventions and was conducted in accordance with the Preferred Reporting Items for Systematic Reviews and Meta-Analyses guidelines [9, 10].

### Search strategy

To obtain the relevant research, we comprehensively searched the Pubmed, Cochrane Library, Embase, China National Knowledge Infrastructure (CNKI), Database for Chinese Technical Periodicals (VIP), Wanfang (Wanfang data), and SinoMed database from inception until April 2019. The combined search used the Medical Subject Heading (MeSH) terms and non-MeSH terms, such as "prostatic hyperplasia", "BPH", "transurethral prostate division", "TUSP", and "randomized controlled trial". All articles were viewed and read independently by two authors (YYH and JXL), and any objections were submitted to another investigator (SSW) who was not involved in the initial process. References were also manually searched for additional studies in the relevant original and commentary articles.

The inclusion criteria were as follows: (1) randomized control design; (2) full-text content and related data can be obtained; (3) the study provides accurate data that can be analyzed, including the total number of subjects and the valuable results of each indicator. In addition, the exclusion criteria were as follows: (1) duplicate studies, case reports, conference abstracts, animal experiments, editorial opinions; (2) insufficient data for research, such as a lack of means and standard deviations; (3) case-control study or cohort study; and (4) lack of parallel control.

### Study selection and data extraction

Two investigators independently screened the literature based on the inclusion and exclusion criteria, and if there were differences, discussed the resolution or resolved it by consulting a third party. The extracted data included the first author's name, research characteristics (publication year, duration, and design), participant characteristics (mean age and sample size), baseline status, interventions, outcome measures, and adverse events.

### Assessment of risk of Bias in included studies

The RCT bias risk assessment tool of the Cochrane Collaboration was used to evaluate the quality of the included studies. Specific items included selection bias (random sequence generation, allocation concealment), implementation bias (blind method of implementers and participants), measurement Bias (blindness in outcome assessment), incomplete outcome data, publication bias (selective reporting), and other biases. The reviewers evaluated each item as "low risk of bias", "high risk of bias" or "unclear of bias" based on the specific details of the study. Disagreements in quality evaluation were resolved through discussions between researchers.

### Statistical analysis

Meta-analysis of the data was performed using RevMan 5.3 (Cochrane Collaboration, Oxford, UK) [11] provided by the Cochrane Collaboration. The relative risk (risk ratio, RR) and the 95% confidence interval (95% CI) were used to calculate the effect size of the dichotomous data. The effect sizes for continuous variable were presented as the mean difference (MD) and 95% CI. Heterogeneity test was assessed by the chi-square test, and the test efficiency was set to $\alpha = 0.05$. When the heterogeneity test result was not statistically significant ($P > 0.05$, $I^2 < 50\%$), the fixed effect model (FEM) was used. When the heterogeneity test results were statistically significant ($P < 0.05$, $I^2 > 50\%$), a random effects model (REM) was used. Sensitivity analysis was used if necessary to find the sources of heterogeneity, and subgroup analyses were used to reduce heterogeneity.

## Results

### Description of studies

Figure 1 shows the flow chart for the search process and study selection. Through a comprehensive search, a total of 318 articles were obtained. After excluding 163 duplicate articles, 155 articles were included. After screening the titles and abstract, 145 articles were excluded because they did not meet the inclusion criteria for the following reasons: retrospective analysis (60), non-clinical studies (3), and irrelevant studies (76). Finally, we carefully read the full text of the remaining 10 articles, and 3 articles were excluded because they did not use random assignment.

### Study characteristics and quality of evidence

A total of 7 studies involving 592 patients were included in the meta-analysis [12–18]. Table 1 describes the basic characteristics of the included studies. These studies

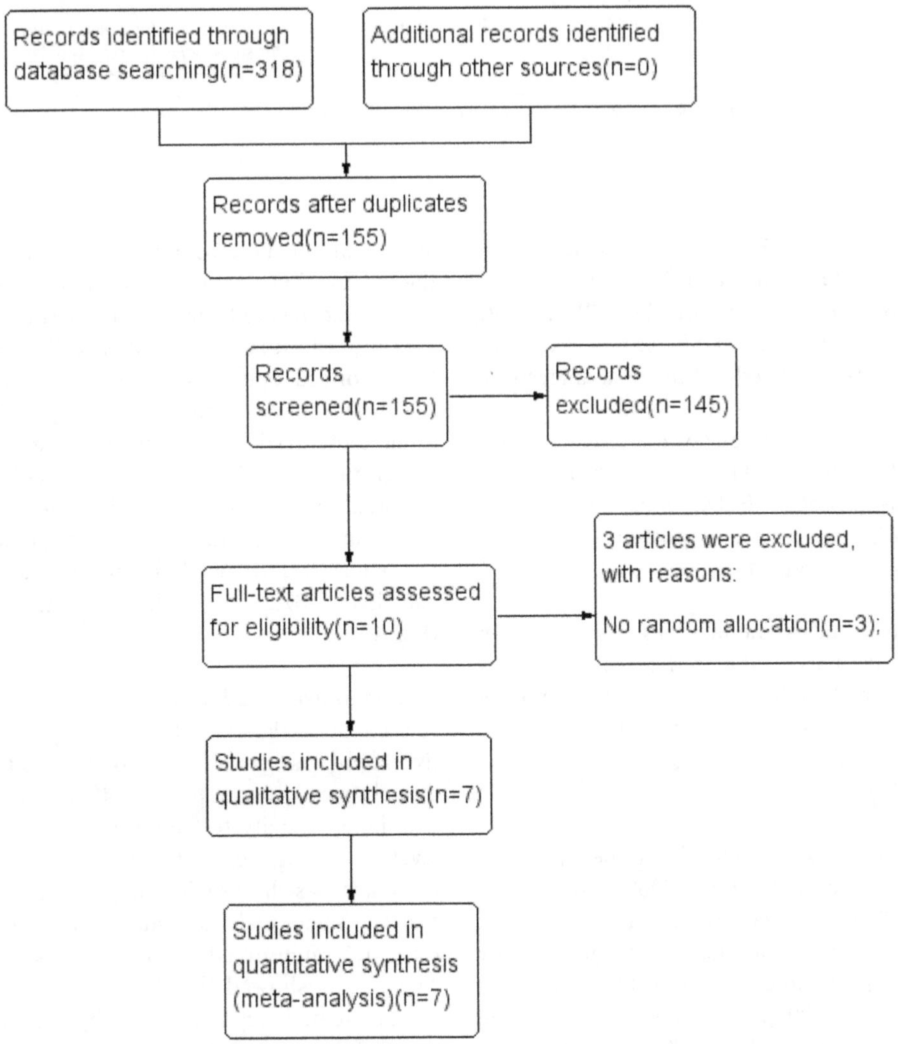


**Fig. 1** Flow diagram of literature searches according to the Preferred Reporting Items for Systematic Reviews and Meta-Analyses statement

**Table 1** Characteristics of the included studies

| Author | Year | Sample size (EG/CG) | Age(Y) | | Intervention methods | | Follow-times | outcomes |
|---|---|---|---|---|---|---|---|---|
| | | | EG | CG | EG | CG | | |
| Kong Min [12] | 2017 | 40/40 | NA | NA | TUSP | TUKEP | 3 months | Operation time (min); Intraoperative blood loss (ml); IPSS; Qmax; |
| Wang Qi [13] | 2017 | 50/50 | 74.4 ± 9.8 | 73.1 ± 9.4 | TUSP | TUPKP | 3 months | Operation time (min); Intraoperative blood loss (ml); Postoperative indwelling catheter time(d); Postoperative hospital stay length(d); IPSS; Qmax; QOL; RUV; Complications |
| Zhou Jin [14] | 2018 | 30/30 | 79.21 ± 15.37 | 78.86 ± 15.25 | TUSP | TUPKP | NA | Operation time (min); Intraoperative blood loss (ml); Complications |
| Kong Qingkuo [15] | 2018 | 107/103 | NA | NA | TUSP | TURP | 3 months | Operation time (min); Postoperative indwelling catheter time(d); Postoperative hospital stay length(d); IPSS; Qmax; QOL; RUV; Complications |
| Li Hong [16] | 2018 | 15/15 | 67.4 ± 10.1 | 69.1 ± 10.5 | TUSP | TUPKP | 3 months | Operation time (min); Intraoperative blood loss (ml); Postoperative indwelling catheter time(d); Postoperative hospital stay length(d); IPSS; Qmax; QOL; RUV; Complications |
| Liu Shuzhi [17] | 2018 | 10/10 | 72.58 ± 12.42 | 74.85 ± 12.28 | TUSP | TUPKP | 12 months | Operation time (min); Intraoperative blood loss (ml); Postoperative indwelling catheter time(d); Postoperative hospital stay length(d); |
| Wang Bo [18] | 2019 | 46/46 | 69.3 ± 3.8 | 69.8 ± 3.7 | TUSP | TUKEP | 3 months | Postoperative indwelling catheter time(d); Postoperative hospital stay length(d);IPSS; Qmax; Complications |

*Qmax* maximum urinary flow rate, *RUV* residual urine volume, *IPSS* international prostate symptom score, *QOL* quality of life

were published between 2017 and 2019. Four of the studies compared TUSP with TUPKP [13, 14, 16, 17], two of studies compared TUSP with TUKEP [12, 18], and another study compared TUSP with TURP [15]. The outcome measures involved in this meta-analysis included operation time, intraoperative blood loss, postoperative indwelling catheter time, postoperative hospital stay length, IPSS score at 3 months postoperatively, QOL at 3 months postoperatively, Qmax at 3 months postoperatively, RUV at 3 months postoperatively and complications. All of these tests were conducted in China.

For the included 7 studies, the bias was largely unclear. Figure 2 shows a summary of the methodological quality of each of the included studies. The judgment of the reviewers for each item of risk of bias tool is shown in Fig. 3 as a percentage.

### Operation time

A total of 6 trials [12–17] reported on the operation time, involving a total of 510 patients (259 in the observation group and 251 in the control group). The results showed that TUSP required a shorter time for surgery than traditional clinical surgery [MD:-33.68; 95% CI: −38.45 to −28.91; $P < 0.001$], but there was a large amount of heterogeneity ($P < 0.001$, $I^2 = 88\%$). We performed a sensitivity analysis, which revealed that the source of the heterogeneity may have been trials conducted by Kong Min [12]. By reading the full text, we found that the study group underwent endoscopic observation of the surgical field after TUSP treatment, leading to prolonged operation time in the observation group, which may have resulted in heterogeneity. After eliminating these trials, we found no heterogeneity between the groups ($P = 0.71$, $I^2 = 0\%$), so a fixed effect model was adopted for the meta-analysis. The time required for TUSP in the treatment of benign prostatic hyperplasia was shorter, and the difference was statistically significant [MD: -37.21; 95% CI: −38.77 to −35.65; $P < 0.001$) (Fig. 4).

### Intraoperative blood loss

A total of 5 trials [12–14, 16, 17] described intraoperative blood loss, involving a total of 300 patients (152 in the observation group and 148 in the control group). The heterogeneity test indicated that the data had high level of heterogeneity ($P = 0.005$, $I^2 = 73\%$), but the sensitivity analysis did not find any sources of heterogeneity, and the meta-analysis results were more stable. Therefore, the random effects model was used for analysis. The results showed that the amount of bleeding in the treatment of benign prostatic hyperplasia was lower in the TUSP group, and the difference was statistically significant [MD: -56.06; 95% CI: −62.68 to −49.43; $P <$

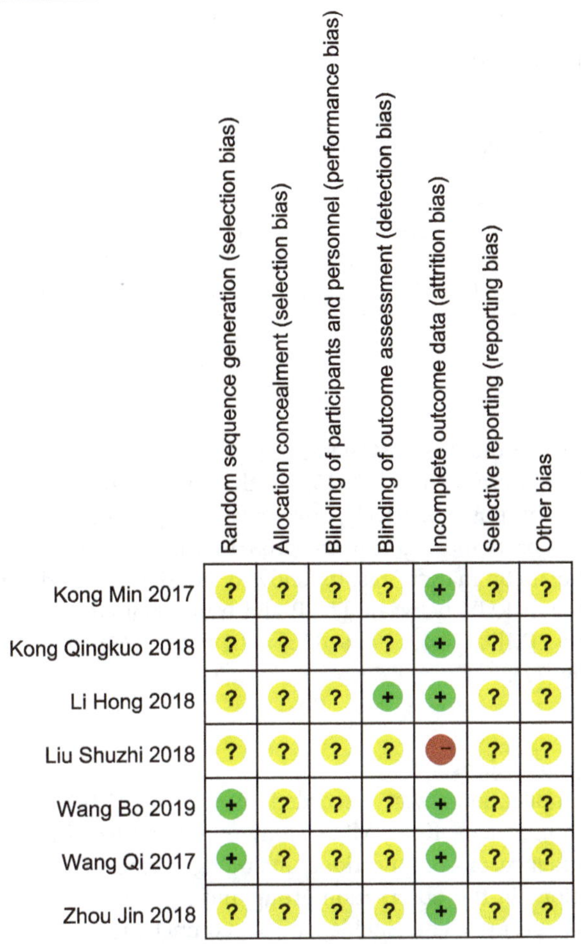


**Fig. 2** Risk of bias summary of included studies

0.001]. Subgroup analysis based on the different surgical methods of the control group showed that TUSP can reduce intraoperative blood loss compared with TUPKP or TUKEP (Fig. 5).

### Postoperative indwelling catheter time

A total of 5 trials [13, 15–18] recorded postoperative urinary catheter indwelling time, including 228 patients in the observation group and 224 patients in the control group. The meta-analysis showed that compared with traditional clinical surgery, the time of indwelling catheter after TUSP was shorter, and the difference was statistically significant [MD: -1.83; 95% CI: – 1.99 to – 1.67; $P < 0.001$) (Fig. 6). There was no heterogeneity among the studies ($P = 0.93$, $I^2 = 0\%$).

### Postoperative hospital stay length

A total of 5 trials [13,15–18] reported on postoperative hospital stay length, involving a total of 452 patients (228 in the observation group and 224 in the control group). The final results showed that compared with traditional clinical surgical treatment, patients with benign prostatic hyperplasia after TUSP treatment had a significantly shorter postoperative hospital stay length [MD: -1.61; 95% CI: – 1.90 to – 1.32; $P < 0.001$] (Fig. 7). There was no heterogeneity between the studies ($P = 0.88$, $I^2 = 0\%$).

### IPSS score at 3 months postoperatively

Five of the included trials [12, 13, 15, 16, 18] recorded the patient's IPSS score at 3 months postoperatively, involving a total of 512 patients. The results showed that there was no significant difference in the IPSS score between TUSP and traditional clinical surgery at 3 months

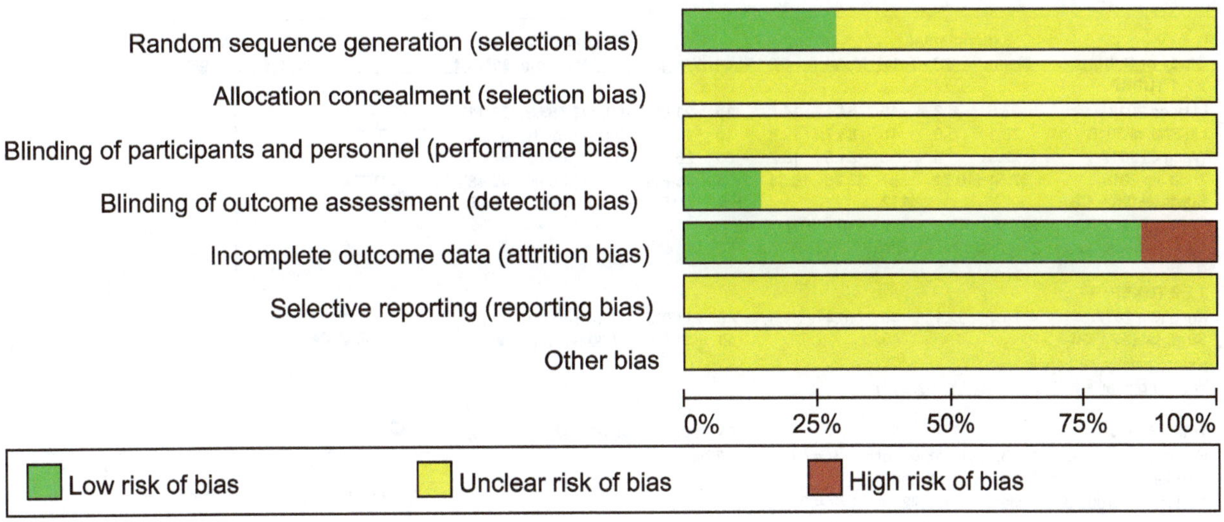


**Fig. 3** Evaluation for bias risk of included studies

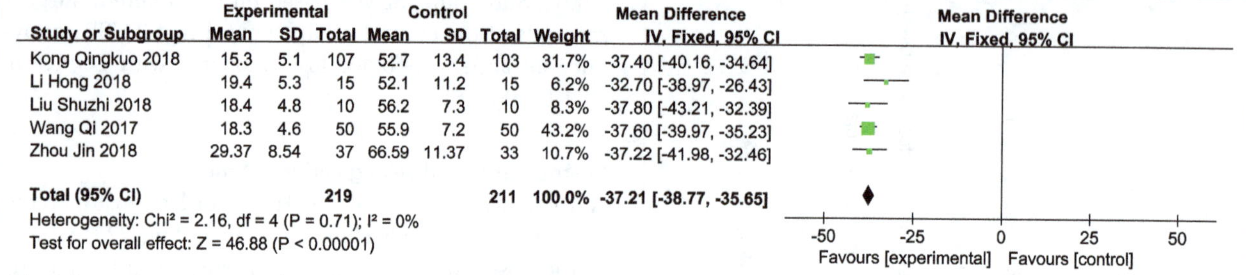


**Fig. 4** Forest plot and meta-analysis of Operation time (min). Experimental: the group of TUSP; Control: the group of traditional clinical surgery

postoperatively [MD: -2.01; 95% CI: − 4.16 to − 0.14; $P$ = 0.07) (Fig. 8).

### Qmax at 3 months postoperatively

A total of 5 trials [12, 13, 15, 16, 18] compared the patient's Qmax at 3 months postoperatively, with 258 patients in the observation group and 254 patients in the control group. There was no significant difference in the Qmax between TUSP and traditional clinical surgery at 3 months postoperatively [MD: 3.59; 95% CI: − 2.38 to 9.56; $P = 0.24$] (Fig. 9).

### QOL scores at 3 months postoperatively

There were 3 trials [13, 15, 16] that examined the QOL scores at 3 months postoperatively, involving 340 patients (172 in the observation group and 168 in the control group). The meta-analysis showed that the QOL scores of patients after TUSP were higher, and the difference was statistically significant [MD: 0.16; 95% CI: 0.02 to 0.29; $P = 0.02$] (Fig. 10). There was no heterogeneity between the studies ($P = 0.55$, $I^2 = 0\%$).

### RUV at 3 months postoperatively

There were 3 trials [13, 15, 16] that examined RUV at 3 months postoperatively, involving 340 patients (172 in the observation group and 168 in the control group). The meta-analysis results showed no significant difference in RUV between TUSP and traditional clinical surgery [MD: -0.42; 95% CI: − 3.49 to 2.65; $P = 0.79$) (Fig. 11).

### Complications

Complications were recorded in 6 trials [12–16, 18]. Among them, Kong Min's study only recorded the total incidence of complications, including 1 case of complications in the observation group and 7 cases in the control group. The incidence of complications in the treatment group was significantly lower than that of the control group. Figure 12 shows an analysis of the complications in the other five trials. The results showed that there were no statistical differences between the two types of temporary urinary incontinence, urinary

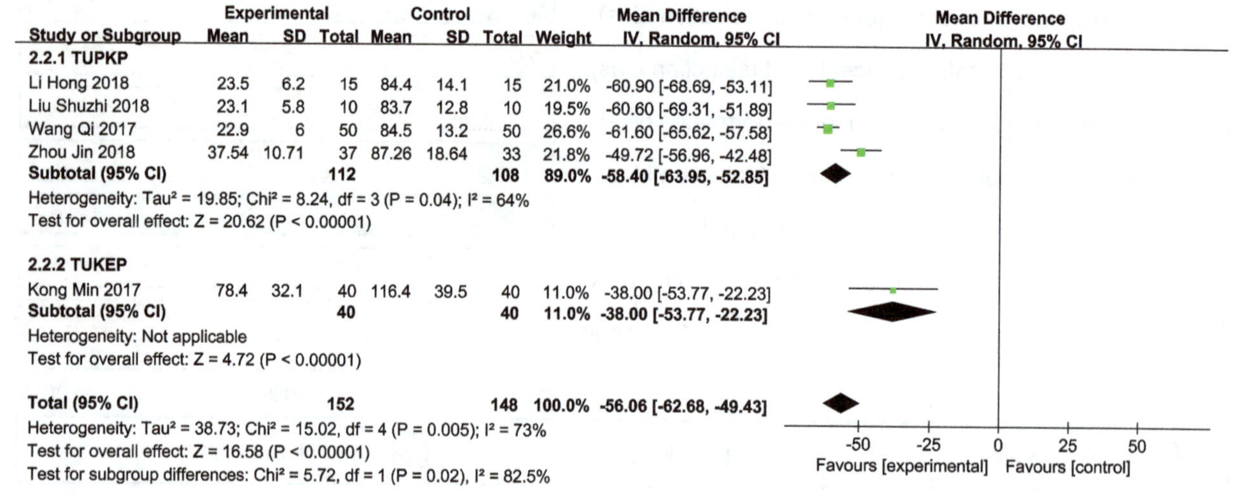


**Fig. 5** Forest plot and meta-analysis of Intraoperative blood loss (ml). Experimental: the group of TUSP

| Study or Subgroup | Experimental Mean | SD | Total | Control Mean | SD | Total | Weight | Mean Difference IV, Fixed, 95% CI |
|---|---|---|---|---|---|---|---|---|
| Kong Qingkuo 2018 | 2.1 | 0.6 | 107 | 3.9 | 0.9 | 103 | 59.4% | -1.80 [-2.01, -1.59] |
| Li Hong 2018 | 2.1 | 0.3 | 15 | 4.1 | 0.8 | 15 | 13.7% | -2.00 [-2.43, -1.57] |
| Liu Shuzhi 2018 | 3.4 | 1.1 | 10 | 5.1 | 2.2 | 10 | 1.1% | -1.70 [-3.22, -0.18] |
| Wang Bo 2019 | 2.2 | 0.56 | 46 | 4.03 | 1.12 | 46 | 19.6% | -1.83 [-2.19, -1.47] |
| Wang Qi 2017 | 3.5 | 1.3 | 50 | 5.2 | 1.9 | 50 | 6.3% | -1.70 [-2.34, -1.06] |
| **Total (95% CI)** | | | **228** | | | **224** | **100.0%** | **-1.83 [-1.99, -1.67]** |

Heterogeneity: $Chi^2 = 0.86$, df = 4 (P = 0.93); $I^2 = 0\%$
Test for overall effect: Z = 22.36 (P < 0.00001)

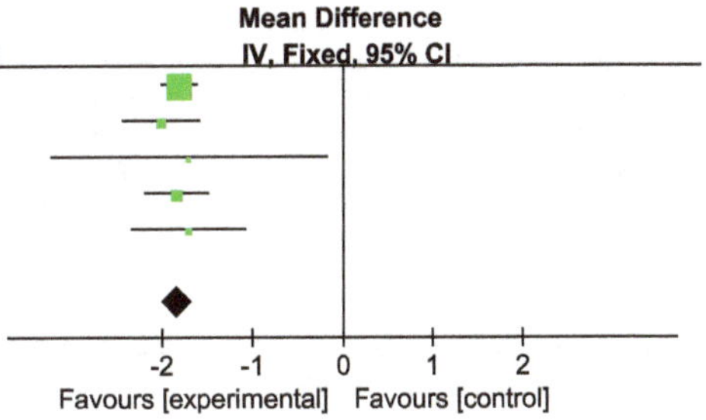


**Fig. 6** Forest plot and meta-analysis of Postoperative indwelling catheter time(d). Experimental: the group of TUSP; Control: the group of traditional clinical surgery

retention, bladder neck contracture, urethral stricture and secondary bleeding.

### Publication Bias analysis

We used the Egger test of Stata 15.1 to assess the possibility of publication bias. Egger's test of QOL indicated that there was significant publication bias ($P = 0.011$) and the other outcome indicators have no significant publication bias.

## Discussion

Benign prostatic hyperplasia is one of the most common diseases in middle-aged men. The clinical manifestations of prostate enlargement and lower urinary tract symptoms are extremely troublesome for the patient's life and work. As the global population ages, the incidence of this disease is increasing [19, 20]. At present, it is difficult to achieve satisfactory results using simple drug treatments; surgery is the most effective way to treat BPH, and traditional transurethral resection of the prostate is considered the gold standard for the treatment of BPH [21]. However, traditional clinical surgery is highly invasive, and it has shortcomings such as long operation time, large amounts of intraoperative blood loss, TURS and high treatment costs [22], so it is difficult to be widely used in developing countries. Therefore, we urgently need a safer and cheaper surgical method to treat BPH.

In 1984, with the development of interventional radiology, Burhenne et al. used arteriographic balloon catheters to perform prostate balloon dilatation on 10 male cadavers, which proved that the procedure can increase the diameter of the prostatic urethra. Additionally, the author used this method to perform TUDP to himself, verifying the potential value of TUDP [23]. In 1987, Castaneda performed prostate balloon dilatation on 12 BPH patients and achieved satisfactory results. The application of this surgical procedure was reported for the first time [24]. Because of the simplicity and convenience of this operation, the complications are relatively few. This has been positively received by most clinicians, prompting a large number of doctors to conduct more research on this technology [25]. Unfortunately, Gill [26] and McLoughlin [27] did not achieve satisfactory results in clinical studies of TUDP. Lepor [28] compared TUDP and cystoscopy and found that they have the same effect on symptom responses. Further clinical studies have shown that, since the therapeutic effect of TUDP on BPH is uncertain, even with a low incidence of complications, TURP is still the best choice for BPH [29]. This has led doctors and patients to gradually lose confidence in TUDP.

| Study or Subgroup | Experimental Mean | SD | Total | Control Mean | SD | Total | Weight | Mean Difference IV, Fixed, 95% CI |
|---|---|---|---|---|---|---|---|---|
| Kong Qingkuo 2018 | 4.2 | 1.1 | 107 | 5.7 | 1.7 | 103 | 56.1% | -1.50 [-1.89, -1.11] |
| Li Hong 2018 | 4.1 | 1.2 | 15 | 6.1 | 1.4 | 15 | 9.7% | -2.00 [-2.93, -1.07] |
| Liu Shuzhi 2018 | 4 | 1.6 | 10 | 5.6 | 1.8 | 10 | 3.8% | -1.60 [-3.09, -0.11] |
| Wang Bo 2019 | 4.1 | 1.21 | 46 | 5.89 | 2.3 | 46 | 15.0% | -1.79 [-2.54, -1.04] |
| Wang Qi 2017 | 4.1 | 1.8 | 50 | 5.7 | 2 | 50 | 15.3% | -1.60 [-2.35, -0.85] |
| **Total (95% CI)** | | | **228** | | | **224** | **100.0%** | **-1.61 [-1.90, -1.32]** |

Heterogeneity: $Chi^2 = 1.20$, df = 4 (P = 0.88); $I^2 = 0\%$
Test for overall effect: Z = 10.84 (P < 0.00001)

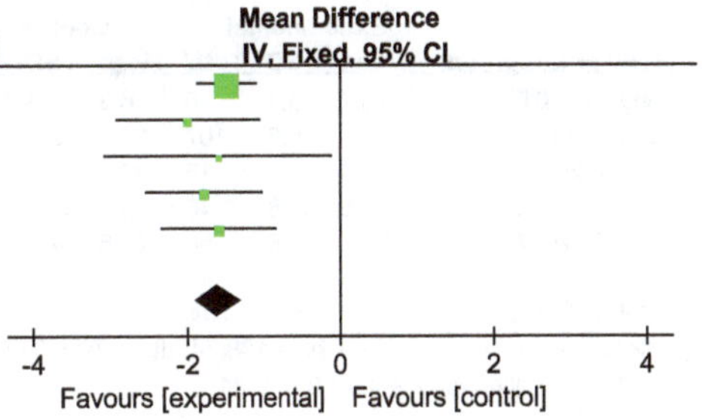


**Fig. 7** Forest plot and meta-analysis of Postoperative hospital stay length(d). Experimental: the group of TUSP; Control: the group of traditional clinical surgery

| Study or Subgroup | Experimental Mean | SD | Total | Control Mean | SD | Total | Weight | Mean Difference IV, Random, 95% CI |
|---|---|---|---|---|---|---|---|---|
| Kong Min 2017 | 17.5 | 4.2 | 40 | 24.4 | 3.8 | 40 | 19.3% | -6.90 [-8.66, -5.14] |
| Kong Qingkuo 2018 | 8.3 | 1.9 | 107 | 8.3 | 2 | 103 | 21.9% | 0.00 [-0.53, 0.53] |
| Li Hong 2018 | 8.5 | 2.1 | 15 | 8.4 | 2 | 15 | 20.1% | 0.10 [-1.37, 1.57] |
| Wang Bo 2019 | 7.58 | 5.98 | 46 | 12.03 | 5.55 | 46 | 17.5% | -4.45 [-6.81, -2.09] |
| Wang Qi 2017 | 6.7 | 2.3 | 50 | 6.3 | 2.5 | 50 | 21.3% | 0.40 [-0.54, 1.34] |
| **Total (95% CI)** | | | **258** | | | **254** | **100.0%** | **-2.01 [-4.16, 0.14]** |

Heterogeneity: Tau² = 5.43; Chi² = 69.39, df = 4 (P < 0.00001); I² = 94%
Test for overall effect: Z = 1.83 (P = 0.07)

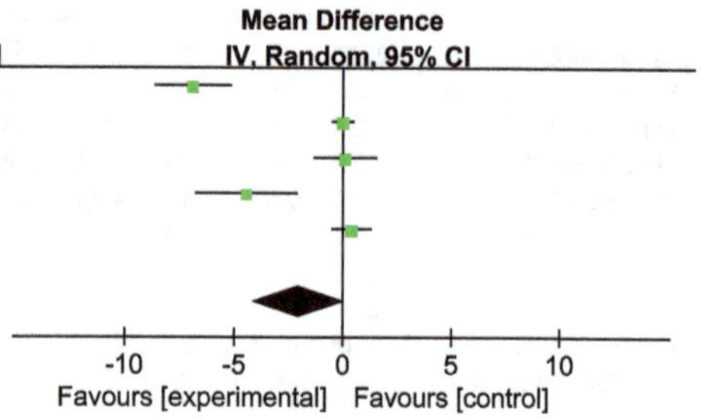


**Fig. 8** Forest plot and meta-analysis of IPSS scores at 3 months postoperatively. Experimental: the group of TUSP; Control: the group of traditional clinical surgery

However, because this surgical method is relatively inexpensive and suitable for use in developing countries such as China, Huang [7, 8] has improved TUDP and redesigned the balloon catheter. The new operation can crack the prostate capsule. Therefore, it was named transurethral split of the prostate (TUSP), and the efficacy and safety of TUSP were verified in animal experiments and clinical trials.

The main principle of TUSP is to expand the prostatic capsule at the 12 o'clock position of the apex of the prostate through the internal balloon to reduce the urethral closure pressure. Then, the external balloon continues to expand the entire dorsal capsule. Finally, a wide "U"-shaped urethra extending to the 12 o'clock position is formed, which reduces the tension of the urethral wall [30]. To obtain a better curative effect, there are certain requirements. First, the appropriate catheter type should be selected strictly according to the prostate volume before operation. If necessary, surgeons should observe the prostate shape and size with and endoscope first to accurately determine the type. Second, the catheter should be stabilized to prevent slippage during the operation. The inner balloon is fixed to the membranous part, and the external balloon is fixed to the prostatic urethra [7]. Some Chinese scholars use ultrasound-guided TUSP surgery, which greatly improves the accuracy of positioning and the success rate of surgery [31]. Finally, it is advisable to stabilize the pressure of the internal and external balloon of the catheter at 0.3 MPa.

TUSP simply dilates the obstructed urethral prostate on the basis of preserving the prostate organs, and it has less trauma and simple operation. It is especially suitable for patients who require the preservation of sexual function, are accompanied by a variety of underlying diseases, are poorly tolerated by anesthesia, or are elderly. However, there are still some limitations. First, TUSP can cause mechanical laceration of the prostate urethra, which may cause bleeding during the operation. The catheter has no hemostatic function, so electrocoagulation hemostasis may be needed during the operation. Secondly, TUSP is unavailable for viewable operation [8], which may require further research and development of visual and automatic instruments. Finally, it is impossible to collect prostate tissue for histological examination because TUSP operation is performed while preserving prostate function [8].

After 328 patients were followed up for 38–99 months, Huang [8] found only 2 cases of recurrent dysuria, which

| Study or Subgroup | Experimental Mean | SD | Total | Control Mean | SD | Total | Weight | Mean Difference IV, Random, 95% CI |
|---|---|---|---|---|---|---|---|---|
| Kong Min 2017 | 18.1 | 3.1 | 40 | 6.3 | 1.6 | 40 | 20.9% | 11.80 [10.72, 12.88] |
| Kong Qingkuo 2018 | 31.9 | 10.6 | 107 | 30.6 | 6.9 | 103 | 20.4% | 1.30 [-1.11, 3.71] |
| Li Hong 2018 | 31.9 | 10.2 | 15 | 30.3 | 6.3 | 15 | 17.3% | 1.60 [-4.47, 7.67] |
| Wang Bo 2019 | 15.86 | 3.88 | 46 | 12.26 | 5.27 | 46 | 20.6% | 3.60 [1.71, 5.49] |
| Wang Qi 2017 | 22.8 | 4.6 | 50 | 23.6 | 4.3 | 50 | 20.7% | -0.80 [-2.55, 0.95] |
| **Total (95% CI)** | | | **258** | | | **254** | **100.0%** | **3.59 [-2.38, 9.56]** |

Heterogeneity: Tau² = 44.02; Chi² = 188.74, df = 4 (P < 0.00001); I² = 98%
Test for overall effect: Z = 1.18 (P = 0.24)

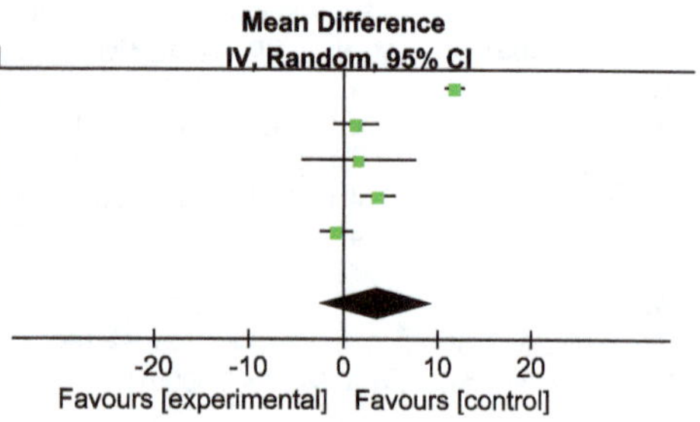


**Fig. 9** Forest plot and meta-analysis of Qmax at 3 months postoperatively. Experimental: the group of TUSP; Control: the group of traditional clinical surgery

| Study or Subgroup | Experimental Mean | SD | Total | Control Mean | SD | Total | Weight | Mean Difference IV, Fixed, 95% CI |
|---|---|---|---|---|---|---|---|---|
| Kong Qingkuo 2018 | 1.9 | 0.6 | 107 | 1.8 | 0.7 | 103 | 57.2% | 0.10 [-0.08, 0.28] |
| Li Hong 2018 | 2.1 | 0.6 | 15 | 1.8 | 0.3 | 15 | 15.5% | 0.30 [-0.04, 0.64] |
| Wang Qi 2017 | 2.1 | 0.7 | 50 | 1.9 | 0.6 | 50 | 27.3% | 0.20 [-0.06, 0.46] |
| **Total (95% CI)** | | | **172** | | | **168** | **100.0%** | **0.16 [0.02, 0.29]** |

Heterogeneity: Chi² = 1.19, df = 2 (P = 0.55); I² = 0%
Test for overall effect: Z = 2.32 (P = 0.02)

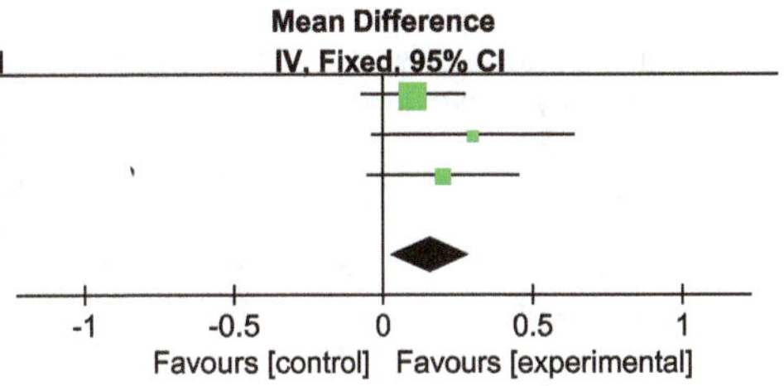


**Fig. 10** Forest plot and meta-analysis of QOL scores at 3 months postoperatively. Experimental: the group of TUSP; Control: the group of traditional clinical surgery

showed that TUSP had a good long-term curative effect. However, due to the limited amount of literature, it is expected that more research on long-term linkages will be published in the future.

The successful application of TUSP in the treatment of patients with BPH may be associated with a significant reduction in inflammatory infiltration and collagen content in the bladder neck, prostatic urethra and urethra. Bianchi-Frias [32] and Huang [7] found in experiments on mice and dogs that the inflammatory infiltration and collagen content in the ageing prostate is very rich. When the dog is subjected to TUSP, inflammatory infiltration and collagen in the bladder neck, prostatic urethra and urethra are significantly reduced. These factors may weaken the contraction of the prostate tissue and expand the urethra. However, the mechanism remains to be confirmed by further research.

The purpose of this review is to analyze the efficacy and safety of TUSP in the treatment of benign prostatic hyperplasia. We searched the existing literature and included 7 randomized controlled trials of TUSP in the treatment of BPH. The results of the analysis showed that compared with the traditional surgical approach, TUSP can shorten the operation time, reduce the amount of intraoperative blood loss, shorten the time of indwelling catheter and speed up the postoperative recovery. At the same time, we also compared IPSS, Qmax, RUV, QOL and complications at 3 months after the operation. The results showed that except for the higher QOL score after TURP, the IPSS, Qmax, RUV and complications of the two treatments were not statistically significant. Therefore, from a clinical point of view, TUSP leads to less trauma, can shorten the operation time, and has relatively high safety. It is suitable for patients who are intolerant or unwilling to undergo surgical resection of the prostate, such as elderly or physically weak patients.

Although this review included a systematically search and analysis, there are still some limitations. First, the sample size was small, and not all outcomes are reported in each of the included studies, which may affect the accuracy of the results. Second, due to the insufficient number of articles included in the literature, this study classified TURP, TUPKP and TUKEP into the traditional clinical surgery approach as a control group, which may lead to the emergence of heterogeneity. We hope that more research can be carried out in the future. Third, only one study had a follow-up period of 12 months, while other studies had a follow-up period of 3 months. Therefore, the long-term effectiveness and safety of TUSP could not be evaluated. It is strongly recommended that future studies use longer follow-up periods. Fourth, due to the particularity of the surgery, the surgical approach requires the consent of the patient and the family, so the included studies were not double-blind. Finally, the included studies were all from China, so the evaluation of TUSP in this review may only be applicable to Chinese people. We look forward to future clinical research in more countries.

| Study or Subgroup | Experimental Mean | SD | Total | Control Mean | SD | Total | Weight | Mean Difference IV, Fixed, 95% CI |
|---|---|---|---|---|---|---|---|---|
| Kong Qingkuo 2018 | 51.3 | 10.7 | 107 | 52.4 | 15.8 | 103 | 70.3% | -1.10 [-4.76, 2.56] |
| Li Hong 2018 | 51.4 | 11.1 | 15 | 52.3 | 15.3 | 15 | 10.3% | -0.90 [-10.47, 8.67] |
| Wang Qi 2017 | 46.3 | 18.2 | 50 | 44 | 17.4 | 50 | 19.4% | 2.30 [-4.68, 9.28] |
| **Total (95% CI)** | | | **172** | | | **168** | **100.0%** | **-0.42 [-3.49, 2.65]** |

Heterogeneity: Chi² = 0.73, df = 2 (P = 0.70); I² = 0%
Test for overall effect: Z = 0.27 (P = 0.79)

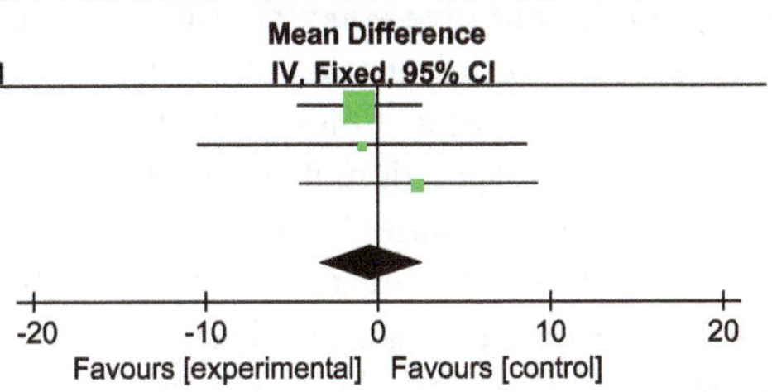


**Fig. 11** Forest plot and meta-analysis of RUV at 3 months postoperatively. Experimental: the group of TUSP; Control: the group of traditional clinical surgery

| Study or Subgroup | Experimental Events | Experimental Total | Control Events | Control Total | Weight | Risk Ratio M-H, Fixed, 95% CI |
|---|---|---|---|---|---|---|
| **9.1.1 temporary urinary incontinence** | | | | | | |
| Kong Qingkuo 2018 | 1 | 107 | 1 | 103 | 12.0% | 0.96 [0.06, 15.19] |
| Li Hong 2018 | 1 | 15 | 2 | 15 | 23.5% | 0.50 [0.05, 4.94] |
| Wang Bo 2019 | 0 | 46 | 3 | 46 | 41.1% | 0.14 [0.01, 2.69] |
| Wang Qi 2017 | 4 | 50 | 2 | 50 | 23.5% | 2.00 [0.38, 10.43] |
| **Subtotal (95% CI)** | | **218** | | **214** | **100.0%** | **0.76 [0.28, 2.06]** |
| Total events | 6 | | 8 | | | |
| Heterogeneity: Chi² = 2.72, df = 3 (P = 0.44); I² = 0% | | | | | | |
| Test for overall effect: Z = 0.54 (P = 0.59) | | | | | | |
| **9.1.2 urinary retention** | | | | | | |
| Kong Qingkuo 2018 | 0 | 107 | 2 | 103 | 38.9% | 0.19 [0.01, 3.96] |
| Li Hong 2018 | 1 | 15 | 2 | 15 | 30.5% | 0.50 [0.05, 4.94] |
| Wang Bo 2019 | 1 | 46 | 2 | 46 | 30.5% | 0.50 [0.05, 5.32] |
| **Subtotal (95% CI)** | | **168** | | **164** | **100.0%** | **0.38 [0.09, 1.58]** |
| Total events | 2 | | 6 | | | |
| Heterogeneity: Chi² = 0.30, df = 2 (P = 0.86); I² = 0% | | | | | | |
| Test for overall effect: Z = 1.33 (P = 0.18) | | | | | | |
| **9.1.3 bladder neck contracture** | | | | | | |
| Kong Qingkuo 2018 | 0 | 107 | 1 | 103 | 37.9% | 0.32 [0.01, 7.79] |
| Wang Qi 2017 | 0 | 50 | 2 | 50 | 62.1% | 0.20 [0.01, 4.06] |
| **Subtotal (95% CI)** | | **157** | | **153** | **100.0%** | **0.25 [0.03, 2.18]** |
| Total events | 0 | | 3 | | | |
| Heterogeneity: Chi² = 0.04, df = 1 (P = 0.83); I² = 0% | | | | | | |
| Test for overall effect: Z = 1.26 (P = 0.21) | | | | | | |
| **9.1.4 urethral stricture** | | | | | | |
| Kong Qingkuo 2018 | 0 | 107 | 1 | 103 | 27.4% | 0.32 [0.01, 7.79] |
| Wang Qi 2017 | 1 | 50 | 3 | 50 | 53.7% | 0.33 [0.04, 3.10] |
| Zhou Jin 2018 | 4 | 37 | 1 | 33 | 18.9% | 3.57 [0.42, 30.34] |
| **Subtotal (95% CI)** | | **194** | | **186** | **100.0%** | **0.94 [0.29, 3.06]** |
| Total events | 5 | | 5 | | | |
| Heterogeneity: Chi² = 2.76, df = 2 (P = 0.25); I² = 28% | | | | | | |
| Test for overall effect: Z = 0.10 (P = 0.92) | | | | | | |
| **9.1.5 bleeding** | | | | | | |
| Kong Qingkuo 2018 | 0 | 107 | 1 | 103 | 50.5% | 0.32 [0.01, 7.79] |
| Li Hong 2018 | 0 | 15 | 1 | 15 | 49.5% | 0.33 [0.01, 7.58] |
| Wang Qi 2017 | 2 | 50 | 3 | 0 | | Not estimable |
| **Subtotal (95% CI)** | | **172** | | **118** | **100.0%** | **0.33 [0.04, 3.05]** |
| Total events | 2 | | 5 | | | |
| Heterogeneity: Chi² = 0.00, df = 1 (P = 0.99); I² = 0% | | | | | | |
| Test for overall effect: Z = 0.98 (P = 0.33) | | | | | | |

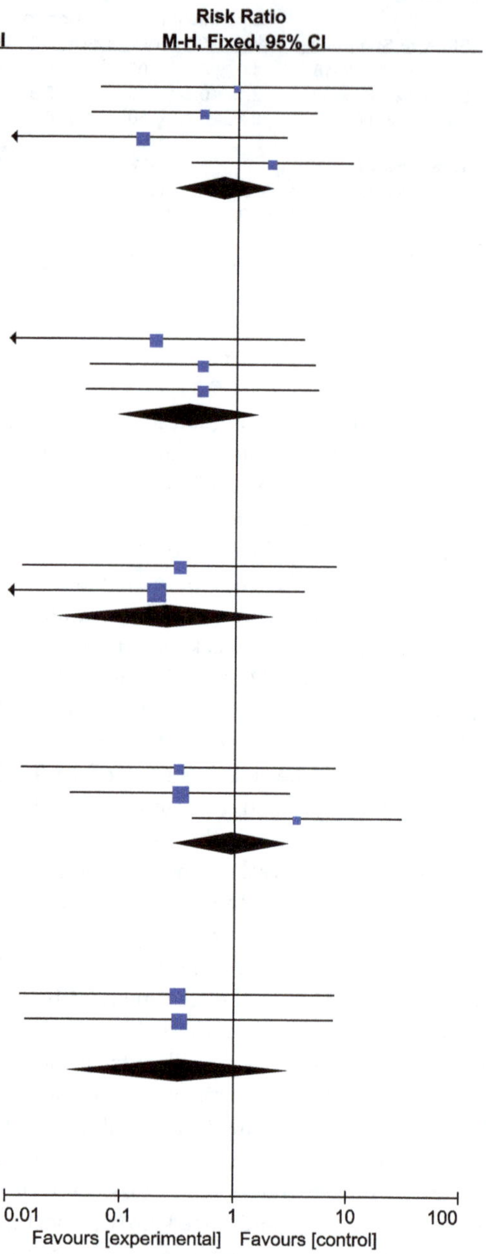


**Fig. 12** Forest plot and meta-analysis of Complications. Experimental: the group of TUSP; Control: the group of traditional clinical surgery

## Conclusions

Compared with traditional prostatectomy, TUSP may have a similar curative effect on BPH, and it has the advantages of reduced trauma, less intraoperative blood loss, shorter operation times and shorter hospital stays. In the Chinese population, it is an effective and safe surgical procedure for patients who are old or weak and unable to tolerate prostatectomy. It is worth promoting. However, given the small number of studies included in this meta-analysis and the low quality, this conclusion requires further validation from more high-quality clinical randomized controlled trials.

### Abbreviations

BPH: Benign prostatic hyperplasia; TUSP: Transurethral split of prostate; TURP: Transurethral resection of the prostate; TUPKP: Bipolar transurethral electrovaporization of the prostate; TUKEP: Transurethral plasmakinetic enucleation of the prostate; TURS: Transurethral resection syndrome; QOL: Quality of life score; IPSS: International prostate symptom score; Qmax: Maximum urinary flow rate; RUV: Residual urine volume; MD: Mean difference; RR: Risk ratio; CI: Confidence interval; RCTs: Randomized controlled trials

### Acknowledgments

We wish to thank Daozhang Yuan for his suggestions on manuscript revision and thank American Journal Experts (AJE) for its linguistic assistance during the preparation of this manuscript.

## Authors' contributions

YYH and SY drafted the study and conducted the analyses. YYH and JXL performed the data extraction, carried out the meta analysis and drafted the manuscript. SSW and DZY reviewed and revised the manuscript. All authors approved the final version of the manuscript.

## Author details

[1]Department of Urology, GuangDong Second Traditional Chinese Medicine Hospital, No.212, Luogang Road Street, Luogang District, Guangzhou 510700, Guangdong, China. [2]Department of Colorectal Surgery, The Sixth Affiliated Hospital, Sun Yat-Sen University, Guangzhou 510655, China. [3]Department of Emergency, Guangdong Provincial Hospital of Chinese Medicine, Guangzhou 510120, China. [4]Department of Urology, Guangdong Provincial Hospital of Chinese Medicine, No.261, Datong Road, Yuexiu District, Guangzhou 510030, Guangdong, China.

## References

1. Bushman W. Etiology, epidemiology, and natural history. Urol Clin N Am. 2009;36(4):403–15.
2. Rule AD, Lieber MM, Jacobsen SJ, et al. Is benign prostatic hyperplasia a risk facto r for chronic renal failure? J Urol. 2005;173(3):691–6.
3. Peyronnet B, Pradere B, Brichart N, et al. Complications associated with Photoselective vaporization of the prostate: categorization by a panel of GreenLight users according to Clavien score and report of a single-center experience. Urology. 2014;84(3):657–64.
4. Oelke M, Bachmann A, Descazeaud A, et al. EAU guidelines on the treatment and follow-up of non-neurogenic male lower urinary tract symptoms including benign prostatic obstruction. Eur Urol. 2013;64(1):118–40.
5. Mamoulakis C, de la Rosette, Jean J.M.C.H (2015) Bipolar transurethral resection of the prostate: Darwinian evolution of an instrumental technique. Urology 85(5):1143–1150.
6. Mebust WK (2003) Transurethral surgery. In: Walsh PC, Retok AB, Vaughan ED, Wein AJ (eds) Campbell' s urology, Vol 2.8th (ed) Philadelphia: Saunders, pp 1479–1505.
7. Huang W, Guo Y, Xiao G, et al. Treatment of benign prostatic hyperplasia using transurethral Split of the prostate with a columnar balloon catheter. J Endourol. 2015;29(3):344–50.
8. Huang W, Huang Z, Xiao G, et al. Effect of transurethral split of the prostate using a double-columnar balloon catheter for benign prostatic hyperplasia. Medicine. 2016;95(40):e4657.
9. Higgins JPT, Green S (2011) Cochrane handbook for systematic reviews of interventions, version 5.1.0. The Cochrane collaboration. www.cochrane-handbook.org.
10. Moher D, Liberati A, Tetzlaff J, et al. Preferred reporting items for systematic reviews and meta-analyses: the PRISMA statement. BMJ. 2009:339.
11. DerSimonian R, Laird N. Meta-analysis in clinical trials. Control Clin Trials. 1986;7(3):177–88.
12. Min KONG, Jun CHEN, Wu-zhen YUAN, et al. Efficacy of modified transurethral split of prostate enlargement for the treatment of benign prostatic hyperplasia. Contemp Med. 2017;23(29):55–6.
13. Qi WANG, Chaokun LI, Liang HUANG. Efficacy of transurethral columnar balloon dilation of prostate in treatment of benign prostatic hyperplasia in high risk elderly patients. Chin J Multip Organ Dis Elderly. 2017;16(06):423–7.
14. Jin Z. Analysis of the application effect of transurethral split of prostate enlargement in patients with benign prostatic hyperplasia. Zhejiang J Traumatic Surg. 2018;23(05):930–1.
15. Kong Q, Jingwei S, Bin L, et al. Effect of transurethral split of the prostate for the treatment of prostatic hyperplasia in the elderly. Chin J Exp Surg. 2018; 35(2):361–2.
16. Hong L. Cylindrical water balloon prostate expansion catheter for the treatment of benign prostatic hyperplasia. Zhejiang J Traumatic Surg. 2018; 23(05):904–5.
17. Shuzhi L, Jingren Z, Bao Z, et al. Clinical study of columnar water sac in the treatment of benign prostatic hyperplasia with neurogenic bladder. Health Guide. 2018;48:326.
18. Wang B. Clinical effect of transurethral split of prostate in the treatment of benign prostatic hyperplasia. Clin Res Pract. 2019;4(10):83–5.
19. Sivarajan G, Borofsky MS, Shah O, et al. The role of minimally invasive surgical techniques in the Management of Large-gland Benign Prostatic Hypertrophy. Rev Urol. 2015;17(3):140–9.
20. Woodard TJ, Manigault KR, Mcburrows NN, et al. Management of Benign Prostatic Hyperplasia in older adults. Consult Pharm. 2016;31(8):412–24.
21. Blankstein U, Van AB, Elterman DS. BPH update: medical versus interventional management. Canadian. J Urol. 2016;23(1S1):10.
22. Reich O, Gratzke C, Bachmann A, et al. Morbidity, mortality and early outcome of transurethral resection of the prostate: a prospective multicenter evaluation of 10,654 patients. J Urol. 2008;180(1):246–9.
23. Burhenne HJ, Chisholm RJ, Quenville NF. Prostatic hyperplasia: radiological intervention. Work in progress. Radiology. 1984;152(3):655–7.
24. Castaneda F, Letourneau JG, Reddy P, et al. Alternative treatment of prostatic urethral obstruction secondary to benign prostatic hypertrophy. Non-surg Ball Catheter Prost Dilatation RoFo. 1987;147:426–9.
25. Wasserman NF, Reddy PK, Zhang G, et al. Experimental treatment of benign prostatic hyperplasia with transurethral balloon dilation of the prostate: preliminary study in 73 humans. Radiology. 1990;177(2):485–94.
26. Gill KP, Machan LS, Allison DJ, et al. Bladder outflow tract obstruction from benign prostatic hypertrophy treated by balloon dilatation. Br J Urol. 1989; 64:618–22.
27. Mcloughlin J, Keane PF, Jager R, et al. Dilatation of the prostatic urethra with 35 mm balloon. BJU Int. 1991;67(2):177–81.
28. Lepor H, Sypherd D, Machi G, et al. Randomized double blind study comparing the effectiveness of balloon dilation of the prostate and cystoscopy for the treatment of symptomatic benign prostatic hyperplasia. J Urol. 1992;147(3):639–42.
29. Vale JA. Balloon dilation of the prostate-should it have a place in the urologist's armamentarium? J R Soc Med. 1993;86(2):83–6.
30. Weizhen B, Wang X, Wang D, et al. The application of endoscopic assisted direct vision in transurethral columnar balloon dilation of the prostate. Chin J Endourol. 2019;13(03):198–202.
31. Wang C, Xiaolin M, Wenfeng L, et al. Transurethral columnar balloon dilation of prostate under ultrasound guidance for treatment of benign prostatic hyperplasia. J Minim Invasive Urol. 2018;7(04):263–6.
32. Daniella BF, Funda VL, Coleman IM, et al. The effects of aging on the molecular and cellular composition of the prostate microenvironment. PLoS One. 2010;5(9):e12501.

# 14

# A urine-based Exosomal gene expression test stratifies risk of high-grade prostate Cancer in men with prior negative prostate biopsy undergoing repeat biopsy

James McKiernan[1], Mikkel Noerholm[2], Vasisht Tadigotla[2], Sonia Kumar[2], Phillipp Torkler[2], Grannum Sant[2], Jason Alter[2], Michael J. Donovan[2,3*] and Johan Skog[2]

## Abstract

**Background:** Initial prostate biopsy often fails to identify prostate cancer resulting in patient anxiety, especially when clinical features such as prostate specific antigen (PSA) remain elevated, leading to the need for repeat biopsies. Prostate biomarker tests, such as the ExoDx™ Prostate *(IntelliScore)*, or EPI test, have been shown to provide individualized risk assessment of clinically significant prostate cancer at initial biopsy; however, the performance in the repeat biopsy setting is not well established.

**Methods:** As part of a previous prospective clinical validation study evaluating the performance of the EPI test, we collected first-catch, non-DRE urine samples across 22 sites from men with at least one prior negative biopsy scheduled to undergo a repeat prostate biopsy to rule out prostate cancer. All men were 50 years or older with a PSA 2–10 ng/mL. Exosomal mRNA was extracted and expression of three genomic markers, PCA3, ERG and SPDEF was measured. The resulting EPI score was correlated with biopsy results.

**Results:** 229 men with a prior negative biopsy underwent repeat biopsies. ExoDx Prostate demonstrated good performance ruling out high-grade (Grade group 2, GG2, or higher) prostate cancer (HGPCa) using the previously validated 15.6 cut point in the initial biopsy setting. The EPI test yielded an NPV of 92% independent of other clinical features and would have avoided 26% of unnecessary biopsies while missing only five patients with HGPCa (2.1%). Furthermore, the EPI test provided additional information at a cut-point of 20 and 29.6 with an NPV of 94%, potentially delaying 35 and 61% of unnecessary biopsies, respectively. AUC curves and Net Health Benefit Analyses demonstrated superior performance of ExoDx Prostate over PSA and clinical only risk calculators, i.e. ERSPC.

**Conclusions:** The EPI test provided good performance using the 15.6 cut-point for ruling out HGPCa / GG2 or higher in men undergoing a repeat prostate biopsy with a PSA of 2–10 ng/ml. Furthermore, the test utilizes gene expression data independent of clinical features to predict the likelihood of HGPCa / GG2 on a subsequent needle biopsy.

**Keywords:** Prostate Cancer, Exosomes, Urine, Early detection, Prostate biopsy

* Correspondence: Mjdonovan54@gmail.com
[2]Exosome Diagnostics, a Bio-Techne Brand, Waltham, MA, USA
[3]Icahn School of Medicine at Mt. Sinai, New York City, NY, USA
Full list of author information is available at the end of the article

## Background

Prostate cancer (PCa) is a leading cause of cancer death among men in the United States, with more than 3.6 million men living with prostate cancer. It is estimated that 174,650 newly diagnosed cases occurred in 2019 [1]. Prostate needle biopsies are typically recommended for men with elevated serum PSA levels and/or a suspicious digital rectal exam (DRE) with added considerations based on family history, age, and race. The anxiety, pain, and potential complications associated with prostate biopsy are well documented [2–6]. Furthermore, a large percentage of newly diagnosed prostate cancers are indolent, clinically insignificant, and with low metastatic potential. These cancers typically do not require definitive treatment and may be managed most effectively with Active Surveillance (AS). The low specificity of PSA which contributes to the high frequency of newly-diagnosed low-risk PCa suggests that 60–70% of men may be able to avoid biopsy [7–10]. Compounding the challenge, the majority of initial biopsy tests do not find cancer [11]. For each negative initial biopsy, it is unknown whether elevated PSA levels and/or a suspicious DRE facilitated the biopsy decision or if the biopsy simply missed a cancerous lesion due to sampling error, tumor heterogeneity and multifocality [12].

The European Randomized Study of Screening for Prostate Cancer (ERSPC) demonstrated that the overdiagnosis and overtreatment of PCa resulting from current practice requires more contemporary and improved methods to identify high-grade disease [13, 14]. Novel diagnostics such as the current test that provide additional clinical value to risk stratify high-grade PCa (Gleason Grade, or GG ≥2) have been developed with a primary objective to avoid biopsies for patients with an increased likelihood of having benign or non-aggressive (GG ≤1) disease [15–17].

The ExoDx Prostate assay relies on the isolation and analysis of urinary exosomes, which are small lipid bilayer membrane extra-cellular microvesicles (typically 30–200 nm in diameter) that are secreted from all living cells. Exosomes contain RNA, DNA, and protein, and have been identified in a variety of biofluids such as blood, cerebrospinal fluid, and urine. They are particularly promising for RNA expression profiling given their protected microanatomic environment [18–21]. The ExoDx Prostate (EPI) test has been extensively validated in two prospective multi-center US studies for biopsy naive patients and the signature is generated from quantitative analysis of PCA3 (prostate cancer antigen 3), ERG (V-ets erythroblastosis virus E26 oncogene homologs) and SPDEF RNA [16, 17].

The present analysis was designed to evaluate the performance of the ExoDx Prostate gene signature in a cohort of men with a history of prior negative biopsy and now presenting for a repeat biopsy.

## Methods

### Study population

First-catch, non-DRE urine samples were collected at 22 clinical sites (academic and community) in the USA from men with a prior negative prostate biopsy scheduled for a repeat biopsy between June 2014 and April 2015. The men were prostate cancer free, 50 years or older, and undergoing repeat biopsy for either a suspicious DRE and/or PSA level between 2 and 10 ng/mL. Men with a history of invasive treatment for benign prostatic hyperplasia within 6 months or taking medications that affect serum PSA levels within 3–6 months were excluded. The prostate biopsies were reported by the local hospital/practice pathologist who was blinded to ExoDx Prostate results. The study protocol was approved by the Western Institutional Review Board, Olympia, WA and individual academic institutional review boards (Johns Hopkins Hospital, University of Michigan); all study participants provided written informed consent and were not compensated for participating in the study.

### Sample collection and processing

First catch urine samples (25–50 mL) were stored at 4 °C for up to 14 days before shipment on ice to the central laboratory (Exosome Diagnostic Laboratory, Waltham, MA). At the Exosome Diagnostics CLIA Laboratory, samples were filtered (0.8um) and stored at -80 °C until further processing which included exosome isolation and concentration by ultrafiltration centrifugation.

For each sample, exosomal RNA was extracted, and the RNA copy numbers of ERG, PCA3, and SPDEF determined. The methodology for urinary exosome isolation, primer generation, RNA extraction and normalization as well as reverse transcriptase polymerase chain reaction have been previously reported in an original analytic and technical feasibility study by Donovan et al., 2015 [14] and in two subsequent independent validation studies [15, 16] of which the McKiernan et al., 2016 [15] provided the prior negative patients included in the current analysis. The test result is calculated based on the relative gene expression of these three genes, without inclusion of other clinical parameters, and provides a risk score (scale 0–100) that predicts the presence of HGPCa (≥GG2). Men with a score ≥ 15.6 (or 20) are at increased risk for having HGPCa on a subsequent biopsy.

### Statistical analysis

Evaluate ability of the EPI assay to predict GG 2 or higher prostate cancer (PCa) on repeat biopsy in men with a history of a prior negative biopsy and a PSA level 2–10 ng/mL. Area under the Receiver operating characteristics (AUC-ROC) curves for PSA vs. the EPI test are utilized as a measure of clinical performance. A well-established risk calculator (RC), The European Randomized Study of Screening for Prostate Cancer (ERSPC) RCs was utilized to further determine risk of GG2 or higher PCa using available clinical parameters [14, 22]. As prostate volume is not generally obtained, the ERSPC RC DRE is used as a surrogate for prostate volume [23]. Missing DRE results were imputed as nonsuspicious. The initial biopsy 15.6 cut point from two prior prospective studies [16, 17] was utilized in the repeat biopsy setting and compared to the EPI cut points of 20 (adjusted cutpoint from the first validation study [16] and 29.6 (adjusted cutpoint), using sensitivity, specificity, negative predictive value (NPV), and positive predictive value (PPV). EPI test was also assessed with a decision curve analysis to investigate the net health benefit for predicting GG2 or higher PCa [24]. The datasets analyzed during the current study may be available from the corresponding author on reasonable request.

## Results

### Study population and biopsy outcome

Between June 2014 and April 2015, non-DRE, first catch urine samples were collected from 1563 participants enrolled in a prospective validation study of the ExoDx Prostate test for men undergoing initial diagnostic prostate biopsy with a PSA between 2 and 10 ng/mL. The enrollment included patients with a prior negative biopsy however they were excluded in the validation analysis by design. Here we show the outcome in the population that had at least one prior negative biopsy. Urine samples from subjects who had incomplete data and/or > 49 ml were excluded of which all were initial biopsy patients. There were no patients excluded from the prior negative biopsy cohort. 229 patients met the criteria for the 'Intended Use Population': a prior negative biopsy and "gray zone" serum PSA levels (2–10 ng/mL). The median age was 65 years, and median pre-biopsy serum PSA was 6.1 ng/mL (Table 1). Most subjects had no family history of PCa (75.1%) and 66.4% had a nonsuspicious DRE with 71.6% of subjects of Caucasian descent and 14.4% African American. Of the 229 patients, 90% underwent a 12-core, transrectal ultrasound-guided prostate needle biopsy using a standard template with diagnosis performed at site affiliated pathology practices without a central pathology review. The total positive biopsy rate was 31% ($n = 72$): 19% ($n = 44$) GG1 and 12% ($n = 28$) ≥ GG2 with 69% benign biopsies.

**Table 1** Demographic and clinical characteristics of prior negative biopsy cohort

| | |
|---|---|
| Total Cohort, N | 229 |
| Median Age (IQR) | 65 (60–70) |
| Median PSA ng/mL (IQR) | 6.1 (4.71–7.5) |
| Family History, N (%) | 172 (75.1%) |
| Ethnicity, N (%) | |
| African Americans | 33 (14.4%) |
| Asian/Pacific Islander | 4 (1.7%) |
| Caucasian | 164 (71.6%) |
| Hispanic | 17 (7.4%) |
| Other | 11 (4.8%) |
| DRE non-suspicious, N (%) | 152 (66.4%) |
| Grade Groups, N (%) | |
| Benign | 157 (68.6%) |
| GG1 | 44 (19.2%) |
| GG2 | 17 (7.4%) |
| GG3 | 6 (2.6%) |
| GG4 | 4 (1.4%) |
| GG5 | 1 (0.4%) |

### EPI PERFORMANCE IN PREDICTING ≥GG2 PCa

In 229 men undergoing repeat biopsy for a prior negative biopsy, the ExoDx Prostate test with the prior validated cut point of 15.6 (for the initial biopsy) demonstrated good performance in discriminating HGPCa, GG2 or higher from low-grade prostate cancer (Gleason 6, GG1) and benign disease on biopsy. The assay performance in the prior negative patients showed an NPV and sensitivity of 92% (95%CI, 0.81–0.97) 82%, respectively. An EPI score less than or equal to 15.6 would have avoided 26% of all biopsies (i.e. 59 of 229) or 27% of unnecessary biopsies (i.e. true negative or specificity) and delayed detection of ≥ GG2 disease in 5 men (2.1%) (Table 2). Importantly, only 3 men with GG3 or higher (1%) would have delayed detection in the repeat biopsy setting. Using an EPI score of ≤20 or ≤ 29.6 would have avoided biopsies in 35% (i.e. 80 of 229) and 61% (i.e. 140 of 229) or 37 and 65%, respectively of unnecessary biopsies, thereby reducing anxiety and potential complications associated with an unnecessary biopsy. It is important to keep in mind that with the cut-point adjustments other measures of accuracy and performance will change, notably applying a cut-point of 29.6 will decrease the sensitivity to 68% while using either the 15.6 or 20 will yield comparable NPV and sensitivity while increasing the number of unnecessary biopsies from 26%^ to 37% with the 20 cut-point.

On comparing the performance of the EPI test (AUC 0.66, 95%CI: 0.55–0.78) with alternative models, the EPI test was superior to PSA only (AUC 0.54, 95%CI: 43–66), and the ERSPC-RC (AUC 0.47, 95%CI: 0.36–0.58), for predicting ≥GG2 PCa, (Fig. 1a).

We also investigated the clinical value of the EPI test relative to alternative models using a decision curve analysis (Fig. 1b). EPI's performance was superior (highest net benefit) to all models tested, including PSA and ERSPC-RC.

**Table 2** Projected impact of the validated EPI 15.6 and adjusted cut-points 20 and 29.6 (with presumed 100% compliance) on expected biopsies performed and avoided

| EPI cut point | Expected Biopsies Performed | Expected Biopsies Avoided | Delayed GG2 | Delayed ≥GG3 | NPV | Sensitivity | Specificity |
|---|---|---|---|---|---|---|---|
| 15.6 | 170 (74%) | 59 (26%) | 2 | 3 | 91.5 (81.3–97.2) | 82.1 (63.1–93.9) | 26.9 (20.9–33.6) |
| 20 | 149 (65%) | 80 (35%) | 2 | 3 | 93.8 (86.0–97.9) | 82.1 (63.1–93.9) | 37.3 (30.6–44.4) |
| 29.6 | 89 (39%) | 140 (61%) | 2 | 6 | 93.6 (88.1–97.0) | 67.9 (47.6–84.1) | 65.2 (58.2–71.7) |

## Discussion

Over 1 million transrectal ultrasonography guided (TRUS) prostate biopsies are performed annually in the US and Europe [6]. Although clinical information such as age, race, family history, or a suspicious DRE are triggers, most TRUS biopsies are driven by PSA screening. Biopsies are often associated with pain, bleeding, sepsis and, of significant concern, an increasing rate of antibiotic resistant infection [6, 25]. A significant number (approximately 70% of men) are not found to have prostate cancer on initial biopsy, and this leads to patient anxiety because of the false negative rate as a result of prostatectomy under-sampling and tumor heterogeneity/multifocality. These concerns drive many men to undergo repeat biopsy. In fact, the Surveillance, Epidemiology, and End Results (SEER) data indicates that ~ 12% of men with a prior negative biopsy have a repeat biopsy within 1 year and 44% of men younger than 70 years old have a repeat biopsy [26].

The ExoDx (EPI) Prostate test is a urine-based genomic assay which uses the expression levels of three genes (ERG, PCA3 and SPDEF) involved in PCa initiation and progression, to predict risk of HGPCa, independent of clinical features or standard of care (SOC) [27–33].. The test algorithm was developed and validated on the intended use cohort, i.e. men presenting for their initial biopsy with a PSA 2–10 ng/mL where it achieved an NPV of 91%, a sensitivity of 91 and 34% specificity [16]. A recent blinded control arm utility study demonstrated that the EPI test reduced the number of biopsies when the test was negative, and helped to identify 30% more high-grade prostate cancers compared to the control arm without the EPI test result [34]. It is well established in the literature that prevalence of prostate cancer is significantly lower in a prior negative biopsy population and that this clinical feature will favorably impact test performance when included in risk assessment models (and some commercial assays) [35, 36]. To address this issue, we evaluated the accuracy of EPI in the prior negative biopsy population using the AUC and compared results with PSA alone and a well-established risk calculator, the European Randomized

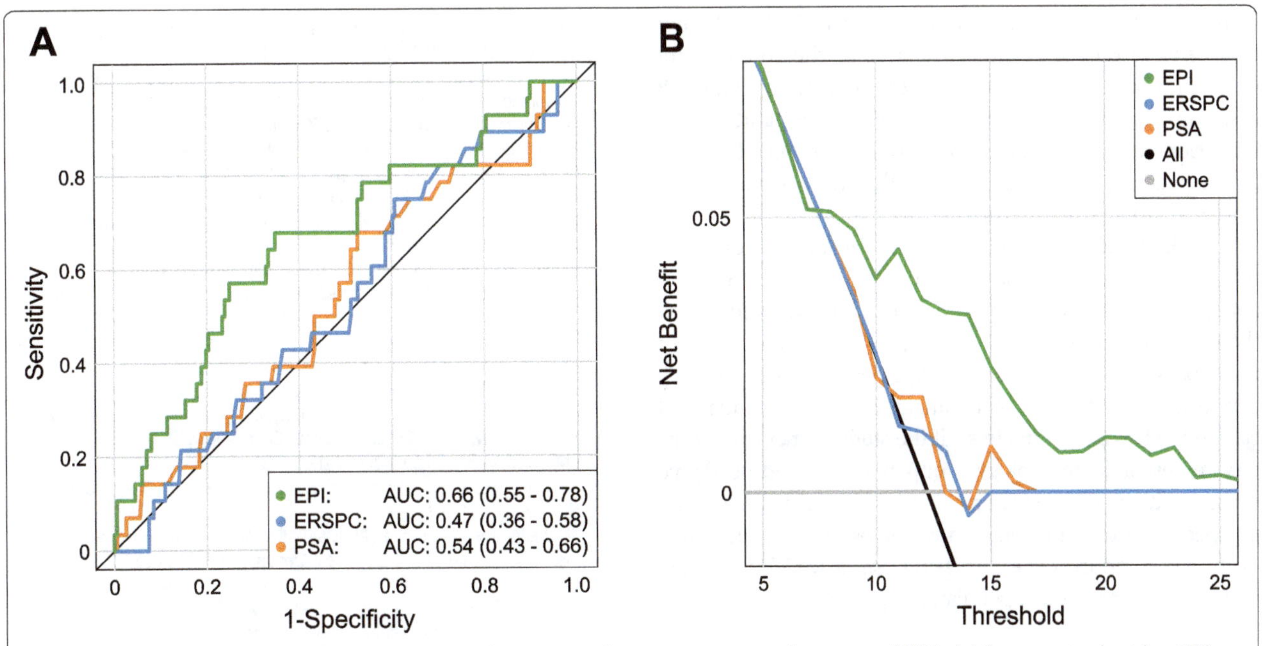


**Fig. 1** Area under receiver operating characteristic (AUC) curves are shown to compare performances of EPI in (**a**) the current cohort ($n = 229$) with the ERSPC, and PSA alone. The corresponding net benefit analysis for this cohort is shown in **b**. EPI = ExoDx Prostate (IntelliScore); ERSPC = European Randomized Study of Screening for prostate cancer (risk calculator); PSA = prostate-specific antigen

Study of Screening for Prostate Cancer (ERSPC) [13, 14]. EPI had a superior AUC of 0.66 vs PSA AUC 0.54, and ERSPC AUC 0.47. As EPI is independent of all clinical features it represents an independent biological assessment of prostate cancer risk.

In addition to the AUC we also employed a decision curve analysis which considers overall net health benefit of various biomarkers and risk assessment tools. When EPI was compared with PSA and clinical-only models such as the ERSPC, a higher net benefit was observed at a biopsy threshold probability of 10%, and maintained up to a maximum biopsy rate of 30%. In contemporary practice the decision to proceed with a biopsy is a delicate balance between the risk associated with the biopsy procedure vs. the risk of missing a potentially clinically significant cancer. The benefit for a test such as EPI is that the risk score is a biological construct independent of all clinical factors thereby allowing for combination with other variables such as race, family history and an underlying disease.

In the current prior negative biopsy population, an EPI risk score less than 15.6 would have potentially avoided biopsy in 26% of men based on total number of biopsies in the study (i.e. 229) and a score of less than 20 would have avoided a biopsy in 35% of men without missing additional GG2 or higher PCa. Furthermore, if we equate benign and Grade Group 6 biopsy outcomes as unnecessary biopsies, the < 15.6 and < 20 cut-points would represent 27 and 37% unnecessary biopsies, respectively. Furthermore, as per the 2020 NCCN Early Detection of Prostate Cancer Guidelines [37], it is clinically important to differentiate GG2 vs GG3 PCa which is relevant for the performance of EPI as only 3 patients with GG3 or higher disease were missed at either the 15.6 or the 20 cut-point vs. 6 individuals (3%) with the 29.6 cut-point. The EPI assay also generated a comparable NPV of 92 and 94% in the prior negative biopsy population (cut-points 15.6 and 20, respectively) vs. 91 and 89% in the two prior initial biopsy validation studies [16, 17].

Study limitations include the sample size and lack of a central pathology review, which may have introduced some variability, specifically when reporting small volume cancers and the fact that there were no men in the study who underwent multi-parametric MRI imaging pre-biopsy. During the study period (2014 and 2015), MRI imaging was not standard of care in the USA. Nevertheless, all the study participating centers represent large urology group practices and academic centers with highly experienced uropathologists. A second prospective study in prior negative biopsy men is underway in the US to address the increasing use of mpMRI imaging and fusion biopsy in this population.

## Conclusion

The ExoDx Prostate *(IntelliScore)* EPI test is a validated, non-invasive urine exosome gene expression assay that performs equally well for men at initial biopsy or with a history of at least one prior negative biopsy. The gene expression assay is more accurate than existing risk assessment methods, is not dependent on clinical features, and informs decision-making at both initial and or repeat biopsy time-points.

### Abbreviations

PCA3: Prostate cancer antigen 3; ERG: ETS (erythroblast transformation-specific) -related gene; SPDEF: SAM pointed domain-containing ETS transcription factor

### Acknowledgements

We would like to thank the various urology practices, investigators, and laboratory/support personnel for assisting in patient accrual, data collection and EPI report generation.

### Authors' contributions

JM, MD, VT, PT, SK had full access to all the data in the study and take responsibility for the integrity of the data and the accuracy of the data analysis. Drs JM, MD contributed equally to this research and article. Study concept and design: JM, MD, JK, PT, MN. Acquisition, analysis, or interpretation of data: JM, MD, JS, VT, PT, MN. Drafting of the manuscript: JA, VT, SK, MD, SK, PT, MN. Critical revision of the manuscript for important intellectual content: JA, MD, GS, SK, MN, PT, VT, JS. Statistical analysis: VT, PT, JS, MD. Obtained funding: Exosome Diagnostics. Administrative, technical, or material support: JM, SK. Study supervision: JM, MD, JS. All Authors have read and approved the manuscript.

### Author details

[1]Columbia University Medical Center, New York City, NY, USA. [2]Exosome Diagnostics, a Bio-Techne Brand, Waltham, MA, USA. [3]Icahn School of Medicine at Mt. Sinai, New York City, NY, USA.

### References

1. Miller KD, Nogueira L, Mariotto AB, et al. Cancer treatment and survivorship statistics, 2019. CA Cancer J Clin. 2019;69:363–85.
2. Bjurlin MA, Wysock JS, Taneja SS. Optimization of prostate biopsy: review of technique and complications. Urol Clin North Am. 2014;41:299–313.
3. Lundstrom KJ, Drevin L, Carlsson S, Garmo H, Loeb S, Stattin P, et al. Nationwide population-based study of infections after transrectal ultrasound-guided prostate biopsy. J Urol. 2014;192:1116–22.
4. Nam RK, Saskin R, Lee Y, Liu Y, Law C, Klotz LH, et al. Increasing hospital admission rates for urological complications after transrectal ultrasound-guided prostate biopsy. J Urol. 2010;183:963–8.
5. Bruyere F, Malavaud S, Bertrand P, Decock A, Cariou G, Doublet JD, et al. Prosbiotate: a multicenter, prospective analysis of infectious complications after prostate biopsy. J Urol. 2014;193:145–50.
6. Loeb S, Vellekoop A, Ahmed HU, Catto J, Emberton M, Nam R, et al. Systematic review of complications of prostate biopsy. Eur Urol. 2013;64:876–92..
7. Abouassaly R, Thompson IM Jr, Platz EA, Klein EA. Epidemiology, etiology, and prevention of prostate cancer. In: WS MD, Wein A, Kavoussi L, Novick AC, Partin AW, Peters CA, et al., editors. Campbell-Walsh Urology. 10th ed. Philadelphia: Elsevier Saunders; 2012.
8. Berman DM, Epstein JI. When is prostate cancer really cancer? Urol Clin North Am. 2014;41:339–46.
9. Klotz L. Active surveillance versus radical treatment for favorable-risk localized prostate cancer. Curr Treat Options in Oncol. 2006;7:355–62.
10. Getzenberg RH, Partin AW. Prostate cancer tumor markers. In: Wein AJ, Kavoussi LR, Novick AC, Partin AW, Peters CA, editors. Campbell-Walsh urology. 10th ed. Philadelphia: Elsevier Saunders; 2012.
11. Ahmed HU, El-Shater BA, Brown LC, Gabe R, Kaplan R, Parmar MK, et al. Diagnostic accuracy of multi-parametric MRI and TRUS biopsy in prostate cancer (PROMIS): a paired validating confirmatory study. Lancet. 2017; 389(10071):815–22.

12. Welch HG, Fisher ES, Gottlieb DJ, Barry MJ. Detection of prostate cancer via biopsy in the Medicare-SEER population during the PSA era. J Natl Cancer Inst. 2007;99:1395–400.
13. Schroder FH, Hugosson J, Roobol MJ, Tammela TL, Zappa M, Nelen V, et al. Screening and prostate cancer mortality: results of the European randomized study of screening for prostate cancer (ERSPC) at 13 years of follow-up. Lancet. 2014;384:2027–35.
14. Foley RW, Maweni RM, Gorman L, et al. European randomized study of screening for prostate cancer (ERSPC) risk calculators significantly outperform the Prostate Cancer Prevention Trial (PCPT) 2.0 in the prediction of prostate cancer: a multi-institutional study. BJU. 2016;118:706–13..
15. Donovan MJ, Noerholm M, Bentink S, et al. A molecular signature of PCA3 and ERG exosomal RNA from non-DRE urine is predictive of initial prostate biopsy result. PCPD. 2015;18:370–5.
16. McKiernan J, Donovan MJ, O'Neill V, et al. A novel urine exosome gene expression assay to predict high-grade prostate cancer at initial biopsy. JAMA Oncol. 2016;2(7):1–8.
17. McKiernan J, Donovan MJ, Margolis E, et al. A prospective adaptive utility trial to validate performance of a novel urine exosome gene expression assay to predict high-grade prostate cancer in patients with prostate-specific antigen 2-10 ng/mL at initial biopsy. Eur Urol. 2018;74:731–8.
18. van der Vos KE, Balaj L, Skog J, Breakefield XO. Brain tumor microvesicles: insights into intercellular communication in the nervous system. Cell Mol Neurobiol. 2011;31:949–59.
19. Nilsson J, Skog J, Nordstrand A, Baranov V, Mincheva-Nilsson L, Breakefield XO, et al. Prostate cancer-derived urine exosomes: a novel approach to biomarkers for prostate cancer. Br J Cancer. 2009;100:1603–7.
20. Skog J, Wurdinger T, van Rijn S, Meijer DH, Gainche L, Sena-Esteves M, et al. Glioblastoma microvesicles transport RNA and proteins that promote tumour growth and provide diagnostic biomarkers. Nat Cell Biol. 2008;10: 1470–6.
21. Valadi H, Ekstrom K, Bossios A, Sjostrand M, Lee JJ, Lotvall JO. Exosome-mediated transfer of mRNAs and microRNAs is a novel mechanism of genetic exchange between cells. Nat Cell Biol. 2007;9:654–9.
22. Ankerst DP, Hoefler J, Bock S, et al. Prostate cancer prevention trial risk calculator 2.0 for the prediction of low vs. high-grade prostate cancer. Urology. 2014;83:1362–7.
23. Roobol MJ, Schröder FH, Hugosson J, et al. Importance of prostate volume in the European randomised study of screening for prostate Cancer (ERSPC) risk calculators: results from the prostate biopsy collaborative group. World J Urol. 2012;30:149–55.
24. Vickers AJ, Elkin EB. Decision curve analysis: a novel method for evaluating prediction models. Med Decis Mak. 2006;26(6):565–74.
25. Feliciano J, Teper E, Ferrandino M, et al. The incidence of fluoroquinolone resistant infections after prostate biopsy--are fluoroquinolones still effective prophylaxis? J Urol. 2008;179(3):952–5.
26. Loeb S. When is a negative prostate biopsy really negative? Repeat biopsies in detection and active surveillance. J Urol. 2017;197:973–4.
27. Wei JT, Feng Z, Partin AW, et al. Can urinary PCA3 supplement PSA in the early detection of prostate cancer? J Clin Oncol. 2014;32(36):4066–72.
28. Gittelman MC, Hertzman B, Bailen J, et al. PCA3 molecular urine test as a predictor of repeat prostate biopsy outcome in men with previous negative biopsies: a prospective multicenter clinical study. J Urol. 2013;190(1):64–9.
29. Leyten GH, Hessels D, Jannink SA, et al. Prospective multicentre evaluation of PCA3 and TMPRSS2-ERG gene fusions as diagnostic and prognostic urinary biomarkers for prostate cancer. Eur Urol. 2014;65(3):534–42.
30. Cheng XH, Black M, Ustiyan V, et al. SPDEF Inhibits Prostate Carcinogenesis by Disrupting a Positive Feedback Loop in Regulation of the Foxm1 Oncogene. PLoS Genet 2014; 10(9): https://doi.org/10.1371/journal.pgen.1004656.
31. Haller AC, Tan W, Payne-Ondracek R, et al. High SPDEF may identify patients who will have a prolonged response to androgen deprivation therapy. Prostate. 2014;74(5):509–19.
32. St John J, Powell K, Conley-Lacomb MK, et al. TMPRSS2-ERG fusion gene expression in prostate tumor cells and its clinical and biological significance in prostate Cancer progression. J Cancer Sci Ther. 2012;4(4):94–101.
33. Hagen RM, Adamo P, Karamat S, et al. Quantitative analysis of ERG expression anz.D its splice isoforms in formalin-fixed, paraffin-embedded prostate cancer samples: association with seminal vesicle invasion and biochemical recurrence. Am J Clin Pathol. 2014;142(4):533–40.
34. Tutrone R, Donovan MJ, Torkler P, et al. Clinical utility of the exosome based ExoDx prostate (Intelliscore) EPI test in men presenting for initial biopsy with a PSA 2–10 ng/mL. Prostate cancer and Prostatic Diseases; 2020. https://doi.org/10.1038/s41391-020-0237.
35. Parekh DJ, Punnen S, Sjoberg SD, et al. A multi-institutional prospective trial in the USA confirms that the 4kscore accurately identifies men with high-grade prostate cancer. Eur Urol. 2015;68:464–70.
36. Neste LV, Hendriks RJ, Dijkstra S, et al. Detection of high-grade prostate cancer using a urinary molecular biomarker–based risk score. Eur Urol. 2016; 70(5):740–8.
37. Prostate Cancer Early Detection. National Comprehensive Cancer Network version 2.2020 – July 24, 2020.

15

# Studying the urine microbiome in superficial bladder cancer: Samples obtained by midstream voiding versus cystoscopy

Suchitra K. Hourigan[1,2*], Wei Zhu[2], Wendy S.W.Wong[2], Nicole C. Clemency[2], Marina Provenzano[2], Thierry Vilboux[2], John E. Niederhuber[2,3], John Deeken[2,3,4], Simon Chung[4,5], Kim McDaniel-Wiley[5] and Donald Trump[4]

**Abstract**

**Background:** Preliminary data suggest that the urinary microbiome may play a role in bladder cancer. Information regarding the most suitable method of collecting urine specimens is needed for the large population studies needed to address this. To compare microbiome metrics resulting from 16S ribosomal RNA gene sequencing between midstream, voided specimens and those obtained at cystoscopy.

**Methods:** Adults, with a history of superficial urothelial cell carcinoma (non-muscle invasive bladder cancer) being followed with periodic surveillance cystoscopy had a urine sample collected by a mid-stream, voided technique and then from the bladder at cystoscopy. Urine samples underwent 16S ribosomal RNA gene sequencing on the Illumina MiSeq platform.

**Results:** 22 subjects (8 female, 14 male) were included. There was no significant difference in beta diversity (diversity between samples) in all samples between collection methods. However, analysis by sex revealed a difference between voided and cystoscopy samples from the same individual in males ($p = 0.006$, Adonis test) but not in females ($p = 0.317$, Adonis test). No differences were seen by collection method in any alpha diversity (diversity within a sample) measurement or differential abundance of taxa.

**Conclusions:** Beta diversity of the urine microbiome did differ by collection method for males only. This suggests that the urinary microbiomes of the two collection methods are not equivalent to each other, at least in males, which is the sex that bladder cancer occurs most frequently in. Therefore, the same collection method within a given study should be used.

**Keywords:** Urine, Microbiome, Cystoscopy

## Background

It is increasingly clear that the urinary tract, once considered in healthy individuals to be a sterile body niche, on more specialized analysis maintains a microbial population. The role of these populations and the impact of changes in them in various genitourinary conditions is still being defined [1]. Changes in the urinary tract microbiome have been observed among individuals with urinary incontinence,, neurogenic bladder dysfunction, sexually transmitted infections, benign prostatic hyperplasia and lower urinary tract symptoms [2–7].

Urothelial carcinoma (UC) is a major health problem, accounting for approximately 75,000 new cases annually and resulting in 16,000 cancer deaths each year in the Unites States [8]. Muscle invading bladder cancer, which accounts for approximately 30% of new cases of UC each year is by far the most dangerous form of UC, with a 50% mortality rate at 5 years. Superficial UC, which is usually not life threatening, has a substantial risk to

* Correspondence: suchihourigan@gmail.com
[1]Inova Children's Hospital, 3300 Gallows Road, Falls Church, VA 22042, USA
[2]Inova Translational Medicine Institute, 3300 Gallows Road, Falls Church, VA 22042, USA
Full list of author information is available at the end of the article

recur after initial treatment and hence requires regular surveillance cystoscopy and often retreatment markedly increasing the inconvenience, risk and cost. It is plausible to hypothesize that changes or differences in the urinary microbiome could be associated with different risk of superficial or muscle-invading cancer as well as the risk of recurrence of superficial disease. Many studies have examined the relationship between the host microbiome and cancer susceptibility in systems other than the urinary tract [9]. Many studies have focused on the association of intestinal microbiota and cancers of the gastrointestinal tract. There are, however, few studies of the urinary microbiome in individuals with UC and the role of the urinary microbiome in bladder cancer has not yet been elucidated. Nevertheless, there are intriguing potential relationships between urinary tract microorganisms and UC: (i) schistosomal infection is clearly associated with an increased risk of UC, intriguingly most often of squamous histology, a relatively uncommon histology among all individuals with UC [10] (ii) carcinogen exposure of the urinary epithelium is clearly a cause of UC in experimental and human studies; it is plausible that there may be a role of bacterial communities in the urinary tract influencing the metabolism of carcinogenic compounds and increasing or decreasing the risk of UC [11, 12] and (iii) the role of Bacillus Calmette-Guerin, an attenuated *Mycobacterium tuberculosis* in the treatment of superficial UC may not be just from inducing inflammation [13]; local microbiota may directly inactivate BCG in the bladder or modulate urothelial sensitivity to BCG [14]. Overall the bladder microbiome may also promote or inhibit UC pathogenesis and progression [14]. Xu and colleagues in a small study of patients with UC ($n = 8$) found differences in the urine microbiome compared to healthy individuals, such as enrichment of the genus *Streptococcus* in patients' urine [1]. Bao et al. reported differences in the urine microbiome among patients in whom superficial UC recurred compared to those in whom it did not [15].

Voided, mid-stream urine samples are traditionally thought to be representative of the bladder in both males and females minimizing distal urethral contamination and are relatively easy to collect for large epidemiological studies [16]. However, it has been shown voided samples contained genital tract bacteria in females, and more recently that catheterized samples contained fewer lower urinary tract microbes than voided samples in males [5, 17] However, in the bladder cancer population, it is unknown what the microbiome differences are in voided urine samples versus urine samples obtained directly from the bladder (i.e. obtained by urinary catheterization or at cystoscopy). Delineating the differences, if any, between these two methods of urine sampling will be important in designing studies of large numbers of individuals which will be necessary to elucidate the role of the urine microbiome in bladder cancer.

### Aim

To compare microbiome metrics resulting from 16S ribosomal (r) RNA gene sequencing between urine obtained from mid-stream urine (voided) and cystoscopy among a population of individuals undergoing regular surveillance cystoscopy because of a prior history of superficial UC.

## Methods

Informed written consent to obtain mid-stream voided urine specimens and immediately thereafter a urine specimen from the bladder at the time of cystoscopy was obtained individuals undergoing surveillance cystoscopy for a prior history of superficial UC defined as non-muscle invasive bladder cancer (IRB# 15–1986). Inclusion criteria were 1) History of non-muscle invasive bladder cancer undergoing routine surveillance cystoscopy; 2) > 180 days since last intravesical therapy; 3) > 180 days since last urethral instrumentation; 4) No current symptoms or signs of an active urinary tract infection; 5) > 18 years of age; 6) No history of urinary tract stones and 7) No nephrostomy or bladder catheter in place. Exclusion criteria were 1) Failure to satisfy inclusion criteria and 2) Inability to provide informed consent.

Standard technique for mid-stream collection was employed for men and women. Cystoscopy was then performed. Intraurethral lubricant jelly was used for all subjects for comfort and safety. No subject received periprocedural antibiotics. Immediately after insertion of the cystoscope a 20 cc aliquot of urine was removed. Urine samples were stored within 90 min of collection at − 80 °C until analysis. Clinical data was collected including demographics and recent antibiotic use.

Prior to DNA extraction, 1–1.5 ml of urine was thawed and centrifuged at 20,000 x g for 3 min. The supernatants were discarded and the pellets were resuspended in 400 μL of Buffer ATL (Qiagen, CA) and treated with 25 μL of lysozyme solution (50 mg/mL) (Sigma Aldridge, MO). Samples were heated for 5 min at 70 °C and cooled before loading on the EZ1 Advanced (Qiagen) for DNA extraction by using the EZ1 DSP Virus kit (Qiagen). Samples were then cleaned and concentrated using the DNeasy PowerClean Cleanup Kit (Qiagen). Sequencing was prepared using a Nextera XT kit according to the Illumina 16S Metagenomic Sequencing Library Preparation protocol for analysis of hypervariable regions V3-V4. The locus specific sequences (Illumina, CA) using standard IUPAC nucleotide nomenclature were: 16S Amplicon

PCR Forward Primer = 5′- GACTACHVGGGTATCTAATCC -3′, 16S Amplicon PCR Reverse Primer = 5′- CCTACGGGNGGCWGCAG - 3′.For normalization, each library was quantified with the KAPA Library Quantification Kit (Kapa Biosystems, MA). The libraries were sequenced on the Illumina MiSeq with paired-end 300 bp reads.

Three control samples were included; *Staphylococcus aureus* (Strain NCTC 8532, ATCC, VA), *Escherichia coli* (Strain NCTC 9001, ATCC, VA) and a "blank" control of 400 μL of buffer ATL which underwent the same DNA extraction process as above. Quantification of the library of the negative control was below the recommended concentration of 4 nM.

Qiime 1.9 was used to demultiplex fastq files, for open-reference Operational Taxonomic Unit (OTU) picking and building the phylogenetic tree using the open reference method [18]. The OTU table and the tree were then imported into R packages phyloseq [19] (version 1.19.1) and vegan (version 2.4–3) for analysis. Similar to our previous microbiome study, OTUs that were not seen more than three times in at least 20% of the samples were removed [20]. Samples with low read counts (< 5,000) and subjects with unpaired samples (i.e. not having both a voided and a cystoscopy sample) were removed. Rarefaction was performed on the remaining samples to be able to compare species richness.

Alpha diversity measures (i.e., observed species, Shannon, Simpson, Fisher) and beta diversity measures (unweighted UniFrac Distance, weighted UniFrac Distance, Bray-Curtis, and Jensen-Shannon divergence) were evaluated between voided samples and those collected by cystoscopy.

The 16S rRNA sequence data is deposited in NCBI Sequence Read Archive (SRA), PRJNA600265.

## Results

After sample filtering was applied (see methods), 8 samples were removed for low read counts (< 5000) and 5 for unmatched samples, leaving 22 subjects with paired samples (both voided and collected by cystoscopy) that were included. Clinical and demographic features of the study population are shown in Table 1. Females were younger than males (mean age female 68.5 years versus mean age male 76.8 years, $p = 0.004$). 4 subjects had antibiotic use within the three months prior to urine sample collection; these were all female.

Among all subjects there was no significant difference in any alpha diversity measure between collection methods (voided versus cystoscopy) or sex (Fig. 1).

When examining beta diversity in all samples (Fig. 2a), there were no significant differences between voided and cystoscopy samples. When split by sex (Fig. 2b), there was a difference in voided and cystoscopy samples from the same individual in males ($p = 0.006$, Adonis test) but not in females ($p = 0.317$, Adonis test). Samples from the same collection method did not cluster together more than samples from the same individual (Additional file 1: Figure S1).

**Table 1** Clinical and demographics features of subjects

| | Female | Male | P |
|---|---|---|---|
| Number | 8 | 14 | |
| Mean age in years (SD) | 68.5 (6.7) | 76.8 (5.2) | **0.004** |
| Smoking history – yes (%) | 5 (50) | 8 (57.1) | 1 |
| Mean body mass index, kg/m$^2$ (SD) | 27.1 (5.9) | 28.2 (3.3) | 0.602 |
| Antibiotic use in last 3 months –yes (%) | 4 (40) | 0 (0) | **0.024** |

The relative abundance between taxa in voided and cystoscopy samples was examined. Figure 3 shows the relative abundance at an order level. In this plot, most of the samples can be clustered into two groups and there is no enrichment of the sex or collection method between these two clusters ($p = 0.11$ for Collection and $p = 0.49$ for sex; Fisher's exact test), suggesting there is no particular pattern associated with sex or the collection approach in the overall relative abundance at the order level.

Even though there is no enrichment detected among the clustering, the plausibility that there is association between collection method or sex and the relative abundance of a particular OTU cannot be excluded. To address this, a mixed-effect regression model was applied for every OTU which has at least 0.1% abundance in at least one sample. Some differences were seen in different taxa between collection method and sex without multiple test correction (Additional file 2: Figure S2, Table 2). However, after multiple corrections with the Benjamini–Hochberg procedure, they did not remain statistically significant.

## Discussion

This study compared the urinary microbiome from urine samples from the same individual collected by mid-stream voiding and directly from the bladder, by cystoscopy, adding substantively to prior urine microbiome studies. Although there were no differences between collection methods for most microbiome metrics (alpha diversity measures (diversity within a sample) and relative abundance of taxa after multiple correction), beta diversity (diversity between samples) did differ by collection method but for males only.

A possible reason for the difference in beta diversity between collection methods for males only is the longer urethra length in male compared to females. The

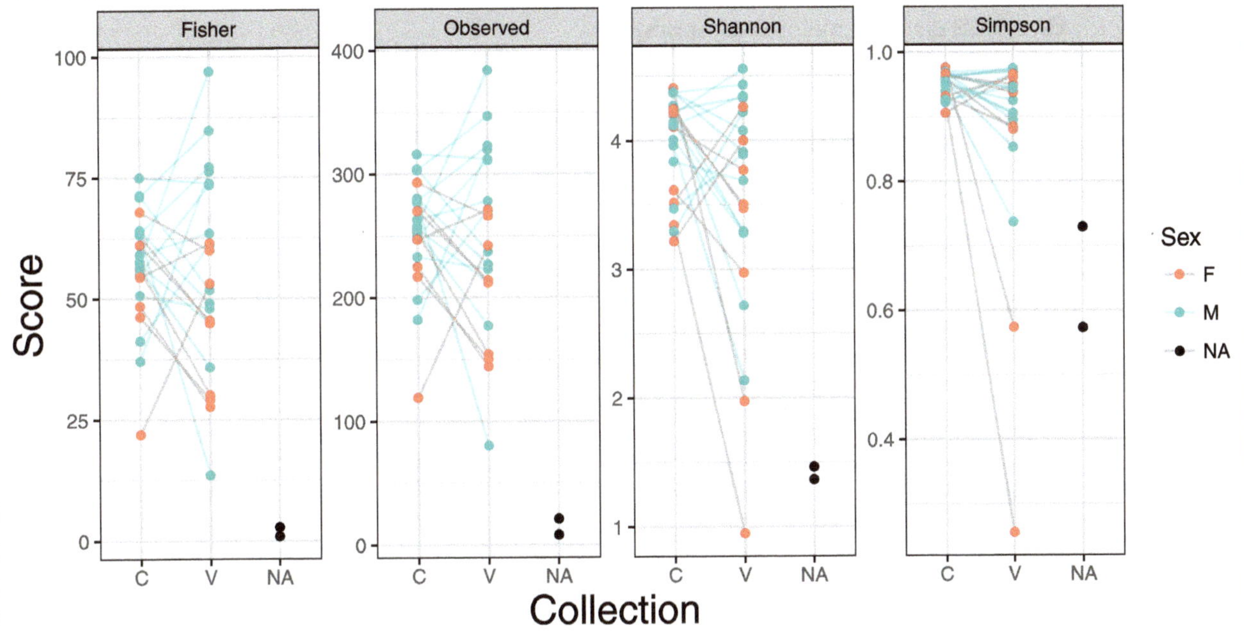


**Fig. 1** Alpha diversity of voided (V) versus cystoscopy (C) urine samples; lines connect samples from the same individual. NA represents control samples

average length of the male urethra is 20 cm compared with 4 cm in females [21]. Given the shorter length of urethra in females there may be more ascending bacteria entering the bladder, and hence the propensity for females to have urinary tract infections; therefore the urine microbiome of the bladder and urethra may be more similar in females compared with males. Indeed in males with lower urinary tract symptoms, voided specimens contained more lower urinary tract microbes than catheterized specimens [5]. Other sex specific factors to consider include hormonal and sexual activity differences. However, Wolfe et al examined urine samples from adult women only by 16 s rRNA gene sequencing and found that voided urine samples contained mixtures of urinary and genital tract bacteria whereas parallel urine samples collected by transurethral catheter and suprapubic aspirate were similar to each other [17].

Prior to multiple corrections, some differences in the relative abundance of taxa were seen between collection methods and sex. Lactobacillales was both increased in voided samples and in females; a predominance of the order Lactobacillales and genus *Lactobacillus* have been previously reported in the female urine microbiome [22]. However, after multiple corrections there was no statistical significance. Possible differences in taxa abundance between collection methods warrants further exploration in a larger sample size.

Large epidemiological studies are needed to investigate the role of the urinary microbiome in bladder cancer and hence the optimal method for collecting urine for these studies need to be understood. Although there were no statistically significant differences in most microbiome metrics in samples from the same individual collected by mid-stream voided urine and from the bladder by cystoscopy, there were differences in beta diversity in males. This suggests that the urinary microbiome of the two collection methods are not equivalent to each other, at least in males, which is the sex bladder cancer occurs most frequently, and therefore the same collection method should be used within a given study. It is currently unknown whether the urine microbiome from voided urine versus a sample obtained from the bladder would be better as a screening tool for bladder cancer. The urethral microbiome which is likely more reflected in a voided sample, could potentially play a pathogenic role too. For population based studies a voided urine specimen in much easier to collect and has lower associated risks, but the microbiome of this sample is not equivalent to a sample obtained directly from the bladder in males.

Although this is the largest study in bladder cancer of which we are aware that directly compared the urinary microbiome of urine from the samples collected by midstream voiding versus cystoscopy in both sexes, there were several limitations. While the sample size in this study is still relatively small, the ability to compare collection methods in the same individual does increase the strength of this study. In

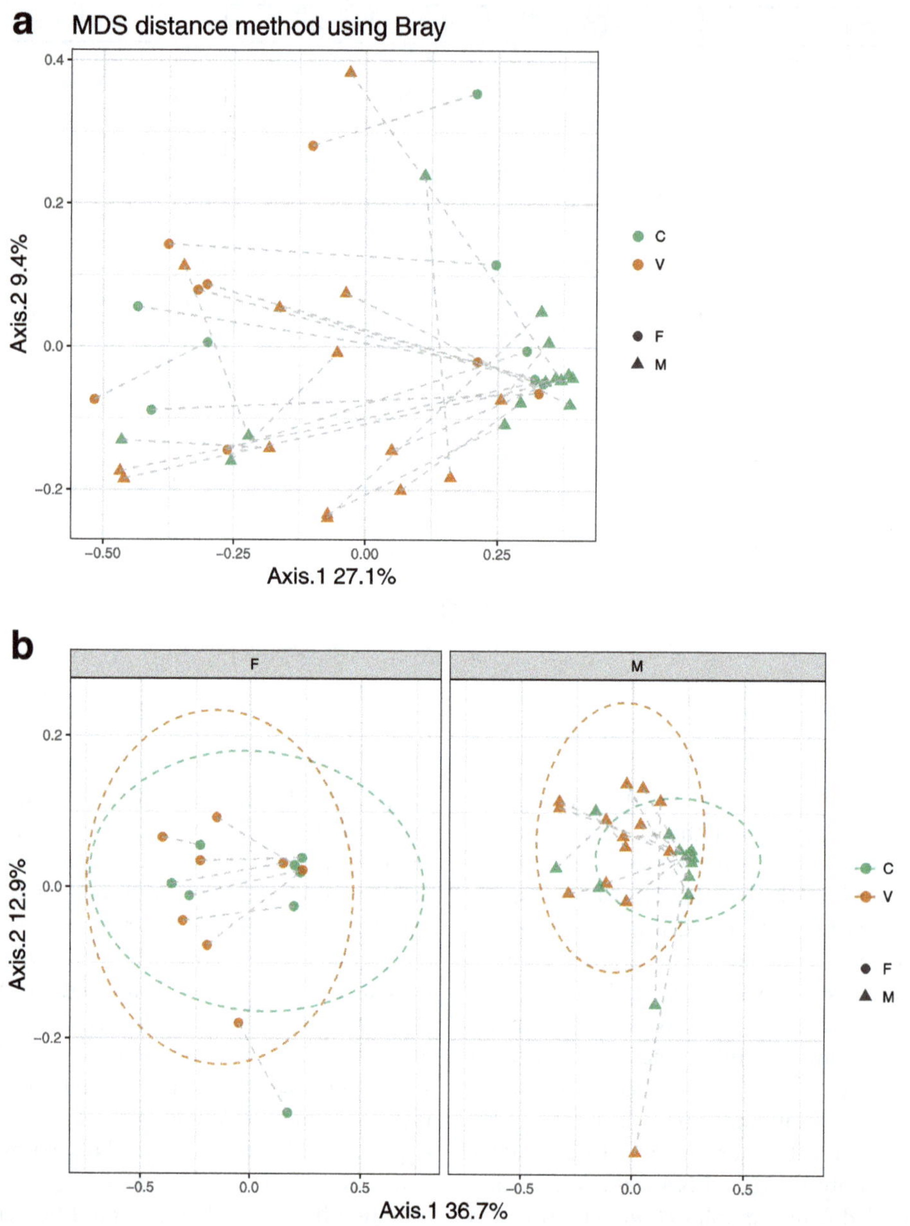


**Fig. 2 a** Principal Coordinate Analysis (PCoA) of urine microbiome composition with Bray-Curtis dissimilarity; lines connect urine samples from the same individual. C: cystoscopy; V: voided; F: female; M: male. **b** Principal Coordinate Analysis (PCoA) of urine microbiome composition with Bray-Curtis dissimilarity by sex; lines connect urine samples from the same individual. C: cystoscopy; V: voided; F: female; M: male

addition, urinary samples generally have a low abundance of bacteria and as with any low abundance microbiomes there is potential for contamination [23]. Our inclusion of both positive and negative controls serves to minimize this concern. While it was documented whether there was antibiotic use within three months of the collected urine sample, using stool microbiome as a reference with substantial recovery within this time period [24], it is unknown if more distant use of antibiotics can have a lasting more pervasive effect on the urine microbiome. Additionally intraurethral lubricant jelly was used on all subjects for cystoscopy; it could be hypothesized that this may transmit distal urethral microbes into the bladder in between voided urine specimen collection and cystoscopic specimen collection.

## Conclusion

There were no differences in urine microbiome metrics of alpha diversity measures and relative abundance of

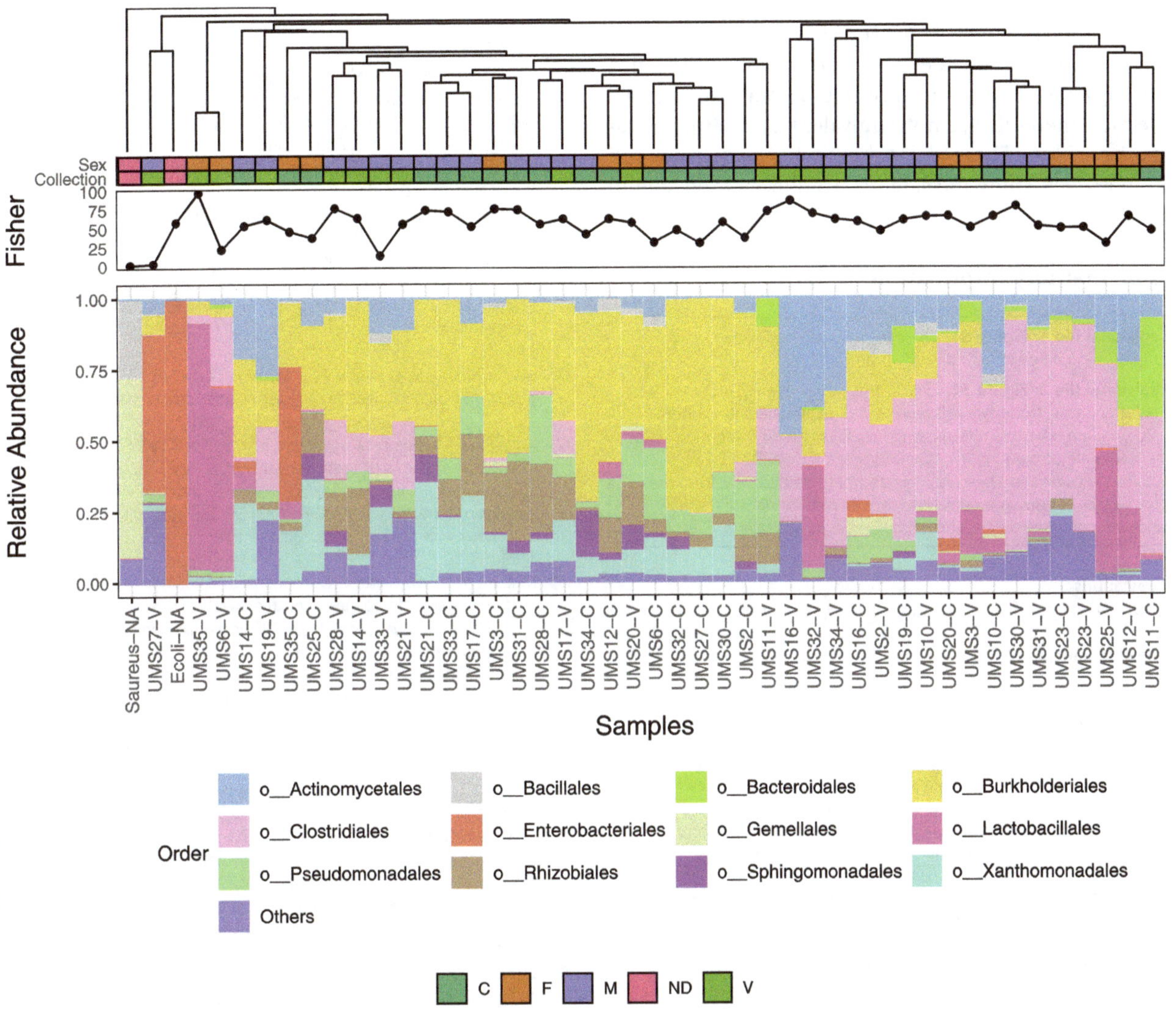


**Fig. 3** Relative abundance at an order level of samples. In this tree plot, most of the samples can clustered be clustered into two groups: cluster A (shaded in blue; $N = 22$) and cluster B (shaded in brown); $N = 17$). There is no enrichment of the sex or collection method between these two clusters ($p = 0.11$ for Collection, and $p$-value = 0.49 for sex; Fisher's exact test). Sex of the subject and sample collection approach are indicated by the colored tiles below the tree, where dark green represents for cystoscopy (C), light green for voided (V), orange for female (F), blue for male (M) and pink for not defined (ND, i.e. positive controls)

**Table 2** Differentially abundant taxa with a raw $p < 0.05$ for the covariates of collection method and sex from the mixed-effect regression model. Note that there is no statistically significance after multiple-testing correction

| | Phylum (p) | Class (p) | Order (p) | Family (p) | Genus (p) |
|---|---|---|---|---|---|
| Increased in voided samples | Firmicutes (0.012) | Bacilli (0.027) | Lactobacillales (0.037) | | |
| Increased in cystoscopy samples | | | Xanthomonadales (0.037) | Xanthomonadaceae (0.037) | *Stenotrophomonas* (0.035) |
| Increased in males | Proteobacteria (0.014) | Betaproteobacteria (0.008 | Burkholderiales (0.008) | Comamonadaceae (0.015) | *Tepidimonas* (0.009) |
| Decreased in males | | Bacilli (0.021) | Lactobacillales (0.011) | | |
| | | | | Prevotellaceae (0.006) | *Prevotella* (0.006) |
| | | | | | *Veillonella* (0.004) |

taxa, between specimens collected by midstream voiding versus cystoscopy-. However, there were differences in beta diversity by collection method for males only. This suggests that the urinary microbiomes of the two collection methods are not equivalent to each other, at least in males. These data should be confirmed and within a given study the same collection method should be used.

## Supplementary information

**Additional file 1: Figure S1.** Distances between and within urine samples using different beta diversity metrics.

**Additional file 2: Figure S2.** Circular tree plot of the OTUs with at least 0.1% abundance. Node symbols represent OTUs in different taxonomic rank: kingdom (k), phylum (p), class (c), order (o), family (f), and genus (g). The nodes are colored in pink, blue and green if the OTU has raw $p < 0.05$ for the covariates Collection, Sex, and both, respectively, from the mixed-effect regression model. Note that there is no statistical significance after multiple-testing correction. V: voided; M: male.

### Abbreviations

OTU: Operational Taxonomic Unit; UC: Urothelial carcinoma

### Acknowledgements

None.

### Authors' contributions

SH: Protocol development, Data analysis, Manuscript Writing, Read and approved final manuscript. WZ: Data analysis, Manuscript Writing, Read and approved final manuscript. SW: Data analysis, Manuscript Editing, Read and approved final manuscript. NCI: Data collection or management, Manuscript Writing, Read and approved final manuscript. MP: Data collection or management, Manuscript Writing, Read and approved final manuscript. TV: Data collection or management, Manuscript Editing, Read and approved final manuscript. JN: Protocol development, Manuscript Editing, Read and approved final manuscript. JD: Protocol development, Manuscript Editing, Read and approved final manuscript. SC: Data collection or management, Manuscript Editing, Read and approved final manuscript. KM: Data collection or management, Manuscript Editing, Read and approved final manuscript. DT: Protocol development, Manuscript Writing, Read and approved final manuscript

### Author details

[1]Inova Children's Hospital, 3300 Gallows Road, Falls Church, VA 22042, USA. [2]Inova Translational Medicine Institute, 3300 Gallows Road, Falls Church, VA 22042, USA. [3]Public Health Sciences, Center for Genomics in Public Health, School of Medicine, University of Virginia, Charlottesville, VA 22908, USA. [4]Inova Schar Cancer Institute, 3224 Gallows Road, Fairfax, VA 22031, USA. [5]Department of Urology, Inova Fairfax Medical Center, 3300 Gallows Road, Falls Church, VA 22042, USA.

### References

1. Aragón IM, Herrera-Imbroda B, Queipo-Ortuño MI, et al. The urinary tract microbiome in health and disease. Eur Urol Focus. 2016;1:128–38.
2. Thomas-White K, Kliethermes S, Rickey L, et al. Original research: evaluation of the urinary microbiota of women with uncomplicated stress urinary incontinence. Obstet Gynecol. 2017;216:55.
3. Karstens L, Asquith M, Davin S, et al. Does the urinary microbiome play a role in urgency urinary incontinence and its severity? Front Cell Infect Microbiol. 2016;6:78.
4. Pearce MM, Hilt EE, Rosenfeld AB, et al. The female urinary microbiome: a comparison of women with and without urgency urinary incontinence. MBio. 2014;4:e01283–14.
5. Bajic P, Van Kuiken ME, Burge BK, et al. Male bladder microbiome relates to lower urinary tract symptoms. Eur Urol Focus. 2018;21:S2405-4569(18)30220-7.
6. Groah SL, Pérez-Losada M, Caldovic L, et al. Redefining healthy urine: a cross-sectional exploratory metagenomic study of people with and without bladder dysfunction. J Urol. 2016;196(2):579–87.
7. Nelson DE, Van Der Pol B, Dong Q, et al. Characteristic male urine microbiomes associate with asymptomatic sexually transmitted infection. PLoS One. 2010;5(11):e14116.
8. Siegel R, Ma J, Zou Z, et al. Cancer statistics, 2014. CA Cancer J Clin. 2014;64:9–29.
9. Schwabe RF, Jobin C. The microbiome and cancer. Nat Rev Cancer. 2013;13:800–12.
10. Mostafa MH, Sheweita SA, O'Connor PJ. Relationship between schistosomiasis and bladder cancer. Clin Microbiol Rev. 1999;12(1):97–111.
11. Alfano M, Canducci F, Nebuloni M, et al. The interplay of extracellular matrix and microbiome in urothelial bladder cancer. Nat Rev Urol. 2016;13(2):77–90.
12. Xu W, Yang L, Lee P, et al. Mini-review: perspective of the microbiome in the pathogenesis of urothelial carcinoma. Am J Clin Exp Urol. 2014;2(1):57–61.
13. Redelman-Sidi G, Glickman MS, Bochner BH. The mechanism of action of BCG therapy for bladder cancer--a current perspective. Nat Rev Urol. 2014;11(3):153–62.
14. Bajic P, Wolfe AJ, Gupta GN. The urinary microbiome: implications in bladder Cancer pathogenesis and therapeutics. Urology. 2019;126:10–5.
15. Bao Y, Razvi H, Gloor G, et al. Mp88-19 urinary microbiome patterns appears to be correlative to intravesical recurrence of non-muscle invasive bladder cancer. J Urol. 2016;195:e1136.
16. Manoni F, Gessoni G, Alessio MG, et al. Mid-stream vs. first-voided urine collection by using automated analyzers for particle examination in healthy subjects: an Italian multicenter study. Clin Chem Lab Med. 2011;50(4):679–84.
17. Wolfe AJ, Toh E, Shibata N, et al. Evidence of uncultivated bacteria in the adult female bladder. J Clin Microbiol. 2012;50(4):1376–83.
18. Caporaso JG, Kuczynski J, Stombaugh J, et al. QIIME allows analysis of high-throughput community sequencing data. Nat Methods. 2010;7(5):335–6.
19. McMurdie PJ, Holmes S. Phyloseq: an R package for reproducible interactive analysis and graphics of microbiome census data. PLoS One. 2013;8(4):–e61217.
20. Wong WSW, Clemency N, Klein E, et al. Collection of non-meconium stool on fecal occult blood cards is an effective method for fecal microbiota studies in infants. Microbiome. 2017;5(1):114.
21. Basic human anatomy. O'Rahilly, Müller, Carpenter & Swenson. Chapter 33. 2008.
22. Fouts DE, Pieper R, Szpakowski S, et al. Integrated next-generation sequencing of 16S rDNA and metaproteomics differentiate the healthy urine microbiome from asymptomatic bacteriuria in neuropathic bladder associated with spinal cord injury. J Transl Med. 2012;10:174.
23. Bao Y, Al KF, Chanyi RM, Whiteside S, et al. Questions and challenges associated with studying the microbiome of the urinary tract. Ann Transl Med. 2017;5(2):33.
24. Dethlefsen L, Huse S, Sogin ML, Relman DA. The pervasive effects of an antibiotic on the human gut microbiota, as revealed by deep 16S rRNA sequencing. PLoS Biol. 2008;6(11):e280.

# An evaluation of the real world use and clinical utility of the Cxbladder Monitor assay in the follow-up of patients previously treated for bladder cancer

Madhusudan Koya[1], Sue Osborne[1*], Christophe Chemaslé[2], Sima Porten[3], Anne Schuckman[4] and Andrew Kennedy-Smith[5]

**Abstract**

**Background:** Surveilling recurrent urothelial carcinoma (UC) requires frequent cystoscopy, which is invasive, expensive and time-consuming. An accurate urinary biomarker has the potential to reduce the number of cystoscopies required during post-treatment surveillance.

**Objective:** To audit the clinical utility of a new surveillance protocol incorporating the Cxbladder Monitor (CxbM) test in real-world practice.

**Methods:** Three hospitals implemented a new surveillance protocol. Patients were risk stratified, and then provided urine samples for CxbM testing. Low-risk CxbM-positive patients and all high-risk patients had cystoscopy at 2–3 months. Low-risk CxbM-negative patients had cystoscopy at ~ 12 months.

**Results:** 443 CxbM tests were conducted on samples from 309 patients: 257 (83.2%) low-risk and 52 (16.8%) high-risk. No pathology-confirmed recurrences were seen in low-risk CxbM-negative patients ($n = 108$) during the first post-CxbM cystoscopy undertaken a mean ± SD 10.3 ± 3.9 months after testing. Three recurrences were detected during cystoscopy at 2.7 ± 3.4 months in 53 low-risk CxbM-positive patients. In 49 high-risk patients, 39 (79.6%) were CxbM-negative with no pathology-confirmed recurrences. Ten high-risk patients (20.4%) were CxbM-positive with four confirmed recurrences; 2 high-grade and 2 low-grade. The median time to first cystoscopy was 12.13 (95% CI: 11.97–12.4) months in patients with a CxbM-negative result versus 1.63 (95% CI: 1.13–2.3) months in patients with a CxbM-positive result ($p < 0.00001$). No positive cases were missed, no patients progressed to invasive or metastatic disease, and no patient died of cancer over 35 months of follow-up.

**Conclusions:** CxbM accurately identified a high proportion of patients (77.8%) who were safely managed with only one cystoscopy per year. Including CxbM in the protocol for patient surveillance provided clinical utility by reducing the average number of annual cystoscopies by approximately 39%, thereby sparing patients the potential discomfort and anxiety, without compromising detection rates. No advantage was observed for risk stratification prior to CxbM.

**Keywords:** Bladder cancer, Cystoscopy, Recurrence, Genomic rule-out test

* Correspondence: Sue.Osborne@waitematadhb.govt.nz
[1]Waitemata District Health Board, Auckland, New Zealand
Full list of author information is available at the end of the article

## Background

Most forms of urothelial carcinoma (UC) are cancers of the bladder. Although most cases of non-muscle-invasive UC can be treated, bladder cancer has a high rate of recurrence. Even patients with low-grade or low-risk UC require regular surveillance after treatment [1]. As a result, bladder cancer carries the highest per-lifetime, per-patient cost of any type of cancer [2], with 60% of the total cost attributable to surveillance and recurrence [3].

Major guidelines recommend risk-adjusted surveillance or active surveillance strategies for patients after treatment for UC, cystoscopy, cytology and imaging for diagnosis and monitoring in most cases [4–10]. The first cystoscopy should be at 3–4 months after the completion of treatment [10]. If this is negative, patients should undergo cystoscopies over longer time periods for low-risk vs intermediate vs high-risk categorizations [7, 10]. All patients with a recurrence start their evaluation sequence again. Costs rapidly accrue because cystoscopy is an invasive endoscopic procedure requiring local anesthesia, expensive equipment and expertise. Patients often find the procedure disagreeable and time-consuming, keeping them from work and life activities. Reluctance to undergo cystoscopy impacts patient compliance with guideline-recommended surveillance protocols [11], which may increase disease progression.

There is evidence to suggest that the benefit: risk equation for diagnostic and surveillance procedures does not necessarily favor current practices [12–14]. For example, American Urological Association (AUA) guidelines for the evaluation of hematuria recommend extensive and intensive use of tests and procedures, including CT imaging [10], impacting significantly on costs, compared with guidelines that recommend less intensive assessment [12]. Comparatively less intensive approaches miss more low-grade UCs, but with fewer adverse outcomes [12]. Moreover, studies specifically investigating the surveillance of patients after treatment for UC suggest that low-risk patients often undergo more frequent surveillance cystoscopies than is recommended by AUA guidelines [13, 14]. Such overuse is associated with increases in surgical procedures and total medical costs, without reducing risk of UC progression or death [14].

The level of diagnostic performance of the current generation of urinary biomarker tests means that they now successfully reduce the need for invasive and expensive cystoscopy assessments in patients being managed for bladder cancer. Recent real-world evidence has been published investigating a new protocol that combines imaging with Cxbladder Triage™, an algorithm combining urinary biomarker data with patient phenotypic data, for hematuria patients being evaluated for UC [15]. With the high negative predictive value (NPV) and high sensitivity of Cxbladder Triage, the new protocol provided a rule-out strategy that was able to safely identify patients without disease and avoid the need for cystoscopy in 32% of patients undergoing evaluation of hematuria [15].

The Cxbladder-Monitor (CxbM) test uses a similar 'rule-out strategy' to rule out the presence of UC among patients being evaluated for UC recurrence. CxbM quantifies urine mRNA levels of five cancer biomarkers [16, 17], and incorporates this information into a mathematical algorithm with clinical variables (primary versus recurrent UC and time since previous tumor resection) to derive a score with a binary outcome [16] (see Additional file 1). Prospective studies in patients undergoing surveillance for recurrent bladder cancer have reported sensitivity of between 91 to 95% for CxbM, and an NPV of 96 to 97% [16, 17].

Based on these published data, several of New Zealand's public healthcare providers (PHP) have integrated CxbM into their routine clinical surveillance of patients for recurrence of bladder cancer. The new clinical practice alternates the use of CxbM and cystoscopy during regular surveillance of low-risk patients.

This real-world audit describes the use and outcomes of cystoscopy at these PHPs over a 35-month period after the inclusion of CxbM into the surveillance protocol, and specifically the clinical utility and rule-out rate of CxbM when used in routine surveillance of patients at low or high risk of recurrent bladder cancer.

## Methods

### Design

This was a retrospective audit of cystoscopy patterns and results following the introduction of CxbM into the real-world surveillance of all patients being evaluated for UC recurrence.

Three PHPs in New Zealand (Waitemata, Mid-Central, Capital & Coast) implemented a new surveillance protocol. All patients (newly treated for UC and those being surveilled for recurrence) consented to a clinical work-up for identifying UC recurrence using the new protocol (Fig. 1). First, patients underwent clinical assessment of recurrence risk based on previous bladder cancer history, where patients with low-grade Ta cancers were considered to be at low risk of recurrence and patients with carcinoma in situ (Cis) or any high-grade tumor were considered to be at high risk for recurrence. All patients provided a urine sample, which was analyzed using the commercial CxbM test [16, 17]. The first CxbM result defined subsequent management of low-risk patients as follows: CxbM-negative patients were considered to be at low risk for recurrence, and underwent flexible cystoscopy only at the next scheduled assessment approximately 12 months later (unless their

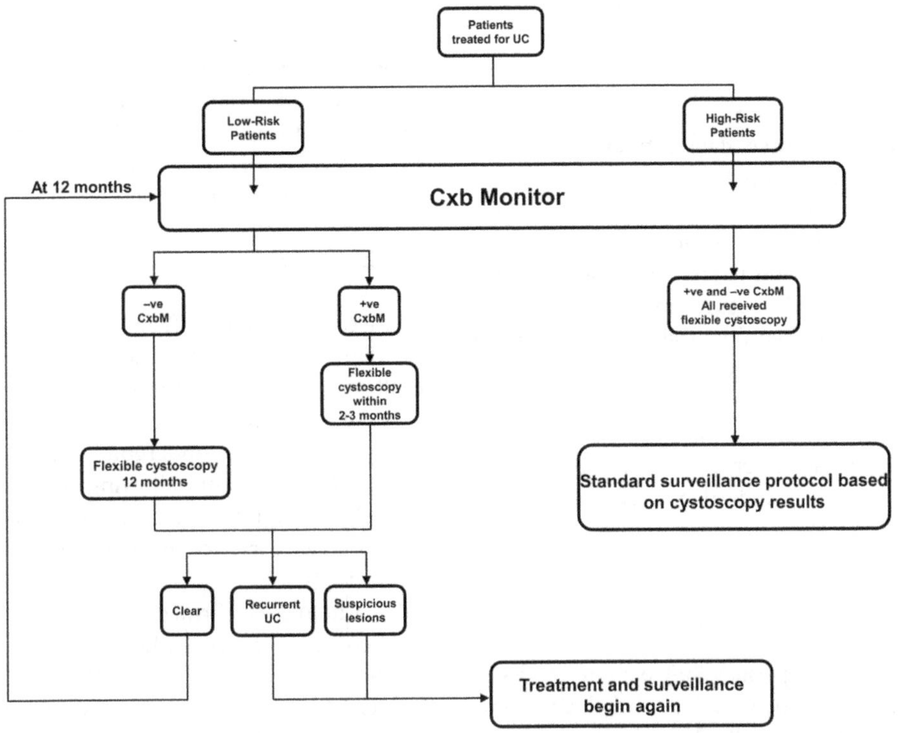


**Fig. 1** Protocol using Cxbladder-Monitor for surveillance of recurrent bladder cancer. –ve, negative; +ve, positive; CxbM, Cxbladder-Monitor; UC, urothelial carcinoma

treating physician chose to do otherwise). Subsequent annual surveillance alternated between flexible cystoscopy and CxbM testing while test results remained negative. Low-risk patients who had a positive first CxbM result were considered to be at higher risk of having a recurrence and were scheduled for cystoscopy (Fig. 1). When a low-risk patient returned a CxbM-positive or cystoscopy-positive result, the patient was then treated and the surveillance schedule continued according to whether the patient was assessed as low or high risk (see Additional file 2).

All high-risk patients had flexible cystoscopy within the normal scheduled follow-up time in accordance with the local guidelines' standard of care for these patients (Additional file 2). The CxbM result for high-risk patients did not affect this cystoscopy surveillance protocol (CxbM data was solely collected for retrospective analysis of patients who qualified as high-risk).

All patients who presented to the clinic for recurrence evaluation, including new patients and those who have had previous evaluations for recurrence, between 25th July 2016 and 5th July 2019 in the low-risk cohort and between 31st March 2017 and 5th July 2019 in the high-risk cohort (i.e. for the 35 months from the first CxbM test under the new protocol) were included in this audit. Data were included from all patients (regardless of risk stratification) who had undergone treatment for non-muscle invasive UC and who provided a urine sample for CxbM testing at that center.

### Outcomes

The clinical utility of CxbM was based on the number of cystoscopies avoided under the new protocol compared with the former surveillance protocol, in which all assessments were by cystoscopy. A second outcome was the number of patients who developed recurrent bladder cancer at the first post-CxbM cystoscopy and over the 35-month audit; recurrent tumors were those identified by cystoscopy and confirmed by pathology.

### Statistical analysis

Within each cohort of low- and high-risk patients, the number of recurrence events at the first cystoscopy was calculated as the number of patients with a pathology-confirmed recurrent UC diagnosis as a proportion of the total number of patients in that cohort. The timing of subsequent cystoscopies and the identification of recurrent tumors at those cystoscopies were calculated and demographic and clinical characteristics summarized using mean ± standard deviation (SD) used for continuous variables. Time between CxbM result and cystoscopy was calculated as median with 95% confidence intervals (CI), and compared between the CxbM-positive and -negative groups using log rank tests; a $p$-value of $< 0.05$ was considered significant.

### Ethics

The analysis used anonymized data extracted from patients' electronic medical records and was compliant with New Zealand national privacy regulations on the use of patient data. Patients provided verbal informed consent to CxbM testing, and to the surveillance protocol, following a written disclosure and in accordance with consent procedures used for local treatment protocols, and thus with appropriate local ethics oversight (and not requiring written informed consent). The Health and Disabilities Ethics Committee (HDEC) determined that the study was undertaken to assess diagnostic quality as part of the standard of care and did not require approval.

## Results

### Patients

Over the 35-month audit period, 309 patients had entered the surveillance protocol and provided 443 samples for CxbM testing. Overall, 257 (83.2%) low-risk patients provided 391 urine samples (Fig. 2), while 52 (16.8%) high-risk patients provided 52 urine samples (Fig. 2). At the time of data analysis, four low-risk patients had not provided a urine sample for CxbM, and three high-risk patients had provided a urine sample that was not available for analysis by CxbM, so 253 and 49 patients, respectively, in these groups had CxbM data available (Fig. 2). At the data cutoff, 208 patients ($n$ = 161 low-risk; $n = 47$ high-risk) had undergone at least one cystoscopy.

Low-risk patients ($n = 253$) had a mean age of 73.1 years; mean time since the primary bladder cancer was 6.5 years and time since last UC treatment was 3.7 years, irrespective of this being the primary event or most recent recurrence (Additional file 3: Table S1).

### Low-risk cohort

Overall, 196/253 (77.5%) low-risk patients had a CxbM-negative result and 57 (22.5%) had a CxbM-positive result (Fig. 3). Of the 196 patients with a CxbM-negative result, 108 underwent the first cystoscopy a mean ± SD of 10.3 ± 3.9 months after sample collection. The other 88 patients had not undergone follow-up cystoscopy by the cutoff date for the following reasons: cystoscopy was scheduled for a future date ($n = 60$), patients had moved, died or been removed from the list of those requiring follow-up ($n = 28$). At the first cystoscopy, no patients had pathology-confirmed UC, but 10 had equivocal cystoscopic findings without pathology confirmation. Follow-up (mean 3.2 ± 1.6 months) of the 10 (9.2%) low-risk CxbM-negative patients with suspicious lesions identified pathology-confirmed low-grade recurrent Ta tumors in three patients. Therefore, over 35 months, confirmed recurrence occurred in three of the 196 low-risk patients with a CxbM-negative result (1.5%; Additional file 4: Figure S1).

Of the 57 CxbM-positive patients, 53 underwent cystoscopy a mean ± SD of 2.7 ± 3.4 months after sample collection. The other four patients had not undergone follow-up cystoscopy; reasons were: scheduled for a

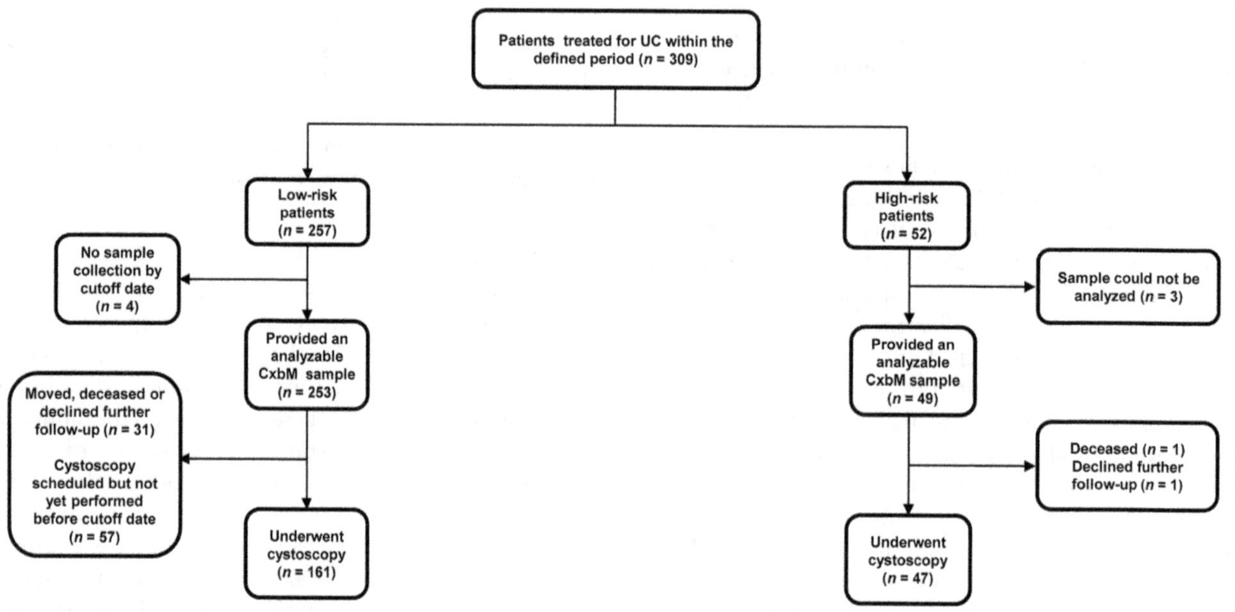


**Fig. 2** Patient flow chart for number of patients entering and completing the audit

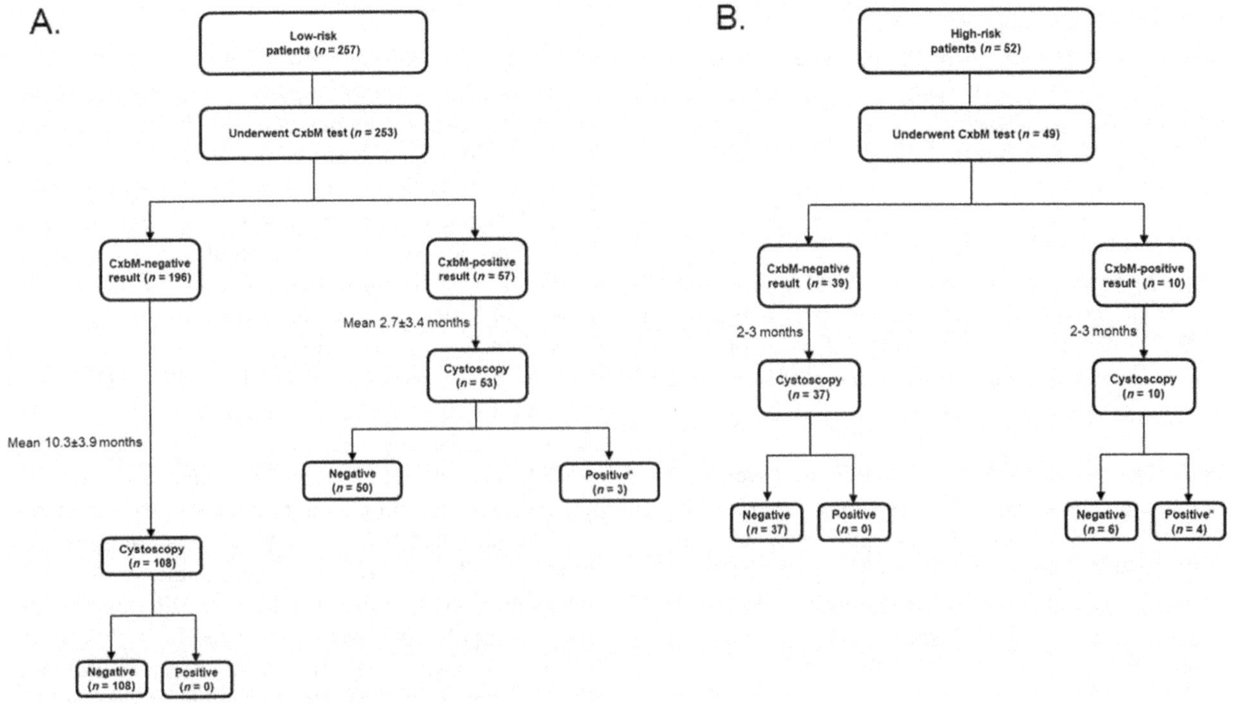


**Fig. 3** Patients completing the Cxbladder-Monitor test and flexible cystoscopy according to the protocol for (**a**) low-risk and (**b**) high-risk patients. Mean time to follow-up flexible cystoscopy is the time from the CxbM test. CxbM, Cxbladder-Monitor. *Patients proceeded to treatment for recurrent UC

future date, patient declined, or unknown reason. Fifty patients had a negative cystoscopy result and three had pathology-confirmed recurrent UC (Fig. 3a); all three were low-grade Ta tumors. Therefore, three confirmed recurrence events were identified in 57 CxbM-positive low-risk patients (5.3%), or in 3/53 (5.7%) when limiting the analysis to patients who had undergone cystoscopy at 2–3 months. Another 13 patients had (unconfirmed) suspicious lesions on cystoscopy (Additional file 5: Figure S2). Follow-up of these 13 low-risk CxbM-positive patients with suspicious lesions identified pathology-confirmed recurrence in six patients (4 low-grade Ta; 1 Cis; 1 papillary neoplasm of low malignant potential). Therefore, a total of nine patients who had originally been categorized as low-risk and who tested CxbM-positive had pathology-confirmed UC recurrence (9/57; 15.8%).

## High-risk cohort

Within the evaluable cohort of 49 high-risk patients, 39 (79.6%) had a CxbM-negative result and 10 (20.4%) had a CxbM-positive result (Fig. 3b). All 10 high-risk CxbM-positive patients and 37/39 high-risk CxbM-negative patients underwent cystoscopy less than 1 month after CxbM urine sample collection. The other two CxbM-negative patients were scheduled for cystoscopy but did not have the procedure (one patient declined and one deceased).

No pathology-confirmed cases of recurrence were identified in patients with a CxbM-negative result (Additional file 5: Figure S2). In high-risk patients with a CxbM-positive result, four had recurrent tumors (40%); two were high-grade and two were low-grade UCs. No patient had Cis.

## Both risk cohorts combined

Overall, 235 patients of the 302 tested returned CxbM-negative results (77.8%). None of these 235 had pathology-confirmed recurrence, with an overall pathology-confirmed recurrence rate at first cystoscopy of nil (0%) in patients testing CxbM-negative (regardless of the initial low- or high-risk categorization). Follow-up of patients with equivocal cystoscopic findings identified three more cases of pathology-confirmed recurrence in patients with an initial CxbM-negative result ($n = 3/253$; 1.2%).

Seven pathology-confirmed cases were identified at first cystoscopy in 67 patients who tested positive for CxbM, and an additional six were identified after follow-up of suspicious cystoscopies for a total of 13 confirmed recurrence events in CxbM-positive patients ($n = 13/67$; 19.4%). Therefore, there was 16.2-fold difference in the total number of confirmed recurrences between patients with CxbM-positive and -negative results.

During 35 months of follow-up, no patients progressed to invasive disease or metastases and there was no cancer-specific mortality.

### Time since last tumor

Figure 4 shows the time of cystoscopy relative to the time of the last tumor in all low-risk and high-risk patients, irrespective of CxbM result. CxbM identified all seven of the confirmed recurrence events identified on the first cystoscopy after CxbM introduction. Additional file 6: Figure S3 shows the same data but includes suspicious cystoscopy findings.

### Relationship between CxbM and time to cystoscopy

The median time to the first cystoscopy was 12.13 (95% CI: 11.97–12.4) months in patients with a CxbM-negative result compared with 1.63 (95% CI: 1.13–2.3) months in patients with a CxbM-positive result ($p <$ 0.00001; Additional file 4: Figure S1 and Additional file 5: Figure S2).

## Discussion

This audit demonstrated the real-world clinical utility of CxbM as a rule-out test for both low- and high-risk patients undergoing surveillance for recurrent UC. The data showed no advantage to patients being segregated on the basis of risk prior to the use of CxbM.

There were no incidences of pathology-confirmed recurrence at the post CxbM cystoscopy testing ~ 10 months later. Three patients with an equivocal cystoscopy finding were pathology confirmed at a subsequent follow-up ~ 3 months later. Overall, for low-risk and high-risk patients, a CxbM-positive result was associated with a 16.2-fold greater likelihood of confirmed UC on initial cystoscopy compared with CxbM-negative findings. High-grade tumors were seen in only two patients (0.79%) who had been initially categorized as being at high risk for recurrence. One additional low-risk patient progressed to a Cis. All three had a CxbM-positive result.

Previous studies have shown that CxbM has high sensitivity and NPV [16, 17], and the current audit demonstrates that CxbM provides tangible clinical utility when used as a rule-out test to identify patients at low risk of recurrence who do not need a cystoscopy and identify those at higher risk who would benefit from cystoscopy. The integration of CxbM into local practice guidelines identified a high proportion of patients (77.8%) who were safely managed by only one cystoscopy every 2 years. Reducing by half the number of cystoscopies in this portion of patients treated for UC would decrease the total number of annual cystoscopies needed by 39%, thereby significantly reducing long-term costs of UC surveillance, without compromising detection, and enabling resources to be focused on patients most in need.

CxbM incorporates risk factors in its validated algorithm, providing an objective, repeatable measure. The audit showed that use of CxbM as a rule-out test in all recurrence patients obviates the need for risk stratification because CxbM identifies those at high risk of recurrence, irrespective of their guideline-defined risk stratification.

Other noninvasive biomarker assays have been approved in the US for the diagnosis or monitoring of bladder cancer including an Enzyme-Linked Immunosorbent Assay (ELISA) test for Nuclear Matrix Protein 22 (NMP22) (BladderChek®; Matritech Inc., Newton, MA, USA [18, 19]), a multiprobe fluorescence in situ hybridization (FISH) test (UroVysion®; Abbott Molecular, Des Plaines, IL) and an immunocytologic fluorescent assay (ImmunoCyt™/uCyt™ Diagnocure; Quebec City, Quebec, Canada). However, it has been previously observed they provide low overall sensitivity [20]. A previous study compared CxbM with NMP22 ELISA assays and UroVysion FISH in patients previously diagnosed with UC undergoing monitoring for recurrence [17]. CxbM provided significantly better sensitivity and NPV than BladderCheck (91% vs. 11% and 96% vs. 86%,

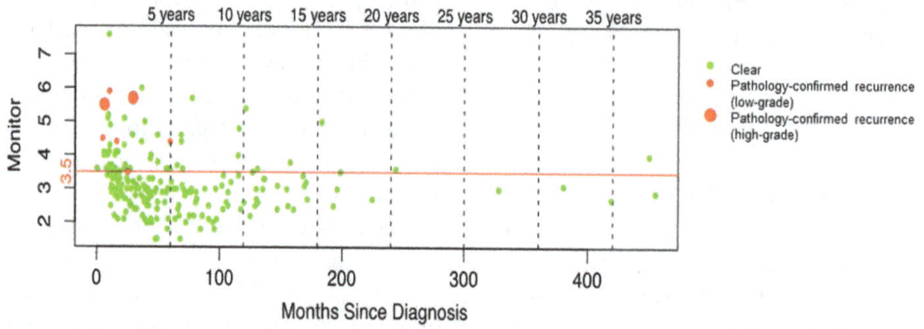


**Fig. 4** Time since last tumor recurrence in all patients with Cxbladder-Monitor-positive results. The red line indicates the CxbM score threshold for defining positive (≥3.5) and negative (< 3.5). CxbM, Cxbladder-Monitor

respectively), and in a smaller patient sample, showed a similar advantage over UroVysion FISH (sensitivity 33%, NPV 92%) [17]. These data suggest that the NMP22 point-of-care test is likely to miss a substantial number of patients with recurrence, whereas CxbM does not.

Currently, there are limited data on the clinical value of introducing urinary biomarkers into the surveillance protocol for recurrent UC, and most studies have used the early generation, single biomarker tests with low performance [21, 22]. To our knowledge, this study is the first to have investigated the impact of incorporating a multi-biomarker urine test into a routine clinical surveillance protocol in a real-world setting. Further longer-term studies should be conducted to confirm our findings.

Collection of a urine sample carries a significantly lower burden for patients compared with cystoscopy in terms of time away from work, anxiety, pain and discomfort during the procedure, and painful micturition afterwards and is likely to lead to an increase in patient compliance with physician recommendation [11]. The results of in-office cystoscopy may be available sooner than the results of some out-sourced biomarker tests, which may limit patient anxiety compared with waiting for a result [23, 24]. However, not all cystoscopies provide a clear result, and patients may need to undergo further testing if cystoscopy is equivocal or cytology atypical [25].

Adding urine biomarker testing to a standard regimen of cystoscopy may not be cost effective when added to the standard tests and procedures for each scheduled assessment [26, 27]; however reducing the frequency of cystoscopy would significantly reduce the cost of post-treatment UC surveillance in low-risk patients [28]. The more sensitive and accurate the urine biomarker test is, the more cost-effective it is in the surveillance of recurrent UC [26], and the more acceptable it becomes to patients as an alternative to routine cystoscopy [29].

Our data have clinical implications for the surveillance of UC patients after treatment. First, because of the high sensitivity (91–95%) and NPV (96–97%) of the CxbM test, a voided urine sample can be used to rule out a substantial number of both high- and low-risk patients who are very unlikely to have recurrent UC and can safely miss one of the recommended cystoscopies, saving money and sparing patients the discomfort and anxiety. Our study also showed that CxbM effectively identified patients at higher risk of recurrence regardless of the time since the original UC diagnosis, and therefore can be implemented at any time during the post-treatment course of the disease. All three centers included in this audit now use the CxbM test in their clinical protocols to rule-out low risk patients and prioritize UC patients for follow-up cystoscopy.

This audit is not without limitations. Because this was a real-world analysis of clinical practice, a complete dataset was not available for each patient, no data were available of treatments received, and some patients were lost to follow-up through real-world events such as moving, change of contact details, or death from co-morbidities. Some patients had both CxbM and cystoscopy simultaneously, reflecting patient-specific variation in the implementation of the new standard protocols. Variability in the timing of the first post-CxbM cystoscopies and differences in data availability existed between the low- and high-risk groups (e.g. 391 urine samples vs. 52 urine samples, respectively), and some low-risk patients had more than one cystoscopy and recurrence, which impacted on the comparison of recurrence rates between the CxbM-positive and -negative patient groups over time. The difference in the number of urine samples between the low-risk and high-risk patients was partly an artefact of the new surveillance protocol, where high-risk patients underwent frequent surveillance by cystoscopy, rather than by CxbM, whereas low-risk patients had an alternating surveillance regimen (CxbM then cystoscopy, then CxbM and so on). Finally, low-risk CxbM-negative patients did not undergo any conventional follow-up until the 12-month cystoscopy, so we are unable to confirm whether the 12-month equivocal cystoscopy events were developed after CxbM testing. Any comparison between CxbM and cystoscopy results in the low-risk patient group is similarly limited by missing data, as a consequence of adopting this alternating CxbM to cystoscopy protocol.

Strengths of this study are that we included a large sample of patient data collected over a 35-month audit period, during real-world clinical practice, in which clinical decisions were made based on the results of the CxbM molecular test.

## Conclusion

When integrated into the evaluation of all patients under surveillance for bladder cancer recurrence, CxbM accurately ruled out patients who did not have recurrent UC. This enabled all low-risk patients to safely undergo cystoscopy at a longer-than-recommended interval, thereby reducing the cystoscopy burden, and sparing patients the potential discomfort and anxiety associated with the procedure. CxbM missed no high grade tumors or failed to identify high-risk patients and the rate of pathology-confirmed UC recurrence was 16.2-fold lower in CxbM-negative than CxbM-positive patients. The current study results indicate that CxbM provides an objective and repeatable measure of recurrence, obviating the need for risk stratification based on clinical parameters.

## Supplementary information

**Additional file 1.** Cxbladder Monitor description and validation results.

**Additional file 2.** Flexible cystoscopy surveillance protocols.

**Additional file 3: Table S1.** Patient demographic and clinical characteristics.

**Additional file 4: Figure S1.** Time from initial Cxbladder-Monitor (CxbM) test to cystoscopy in all low-risk patients anchored on first CxbM result.

**Additional file 5: Figure S2.** Time from initial Cxbladder-Monitor (CxbM) test to cystoscopy in all high-risk patients anchored on first CxbM result.

**Additional file 6: Figure S3.** Time from last tumor recurrence to the first cystoscopy after Cxbladder Monitor (CxbM) introduction in all patients with CxbM results. The red line indicates the CxbM score threshold for defining positive (≥3.5) and negative (< 3.5). CxbM, Cxbladder-Monitor.

### Abbreviations

AUA: American Urological Association; CI: Confidence interval; Cis: Carcinoma in situ; CxbM: Cxbladder Monitor; ELISA: Enzyme-linked immunosorbent assay; FISH: Fluorescence in situ hybridization; HDEC: Health and Disabilities Ethics Committee; NMP22: Nuclear Matrix Protein 22; NPV: Negative predictive value; PHP: Public healthcare provider; SD: Standard deviation; UC: Urothelial carcinoma

### Acknowledgments

We would like to thank Shelly de Boer of Capital & Coast District Health Board and Karen Nistor of Mid-Central District Health Board for data collection and review, and Catherine Rees and Tracy Harrison of Springer Healthcare Communications who wrote the outline of the manuscript and helped edit revisions subsequent to peer review, respectively. This medical writing assistance was funded by Pacific Edge Ltd.

### Authors' contributions

MK, SO, and AKS were involved in study design, patient enrolment and consent, data collection, data analysis, and manuscript preparation. CC was involved in study design, patient enrolment and consent, data collection, and data analysis. SP and AS contributed to study design and helped to draft the manuscript. All authors reviewed the manuscript for important content and approved the final draft for submission.

### Author details

[1]Waitemata District Health Board, Auckland, New Zealand. [2]Mid Central District Health Board, Palmerston North, New Zealand. [3]University of California San Francisco, San Francisco, CA, USA. [4]USC Institute of Urology, USC/Norris Comprehensive Cancer Center, University of Southern California, Los Angeles, CA, USA. [5]Capital & Coast District Health Board, Wellington, New Zealand.

### References

1. National Cancer Institute. Bladder cancer treatment (PDQ) - health professional version. 2018. https://www.cancer.gov/types/bladder/hp/bladder-treatment-pdq. Accessed 3 Sept 2018.
2. Yeung C, Dinh T, Lee J. The health economics of bladder cancer: an updated review of the published literature. Pharmacoeconomics. 2014; 32(11):1093–104.
3. Avritscher EB, Cooksley CD, Grossman HB, et al. Clinical model of lifetime cost of treating bladder cancer and associated complications. Urology. 2006; 68(3):549–53.
4. Woldu SL, Bagrodia A, Lotan Y. Guideline of guidelines: non-muscle-invasive bladder cancer. BJU Int. 2017;119(3):371–80.
5. Babjuk M, Bohle A, Burger M, et al. EAU guidelines on non-muscle-invasive Urothelial carcinoma of the bladder: update 2016. Eur Urol. 2017;71(3):447–61.
6. Linder BJ, Bass EJ, Mostafid H, Boorjian SA. Guideline of guidelines: asymptomatic microscopic haematuria. BJU Int. 2018;121(2):176–83.
7. National Comprehensive Cancer Network. NCCN Clinical Practice Guidelines in Oncology (NCCN Guidelines): Bladder cancer. Version 4.2019. 2019.
8. Committee for Establishment of the Clinical Practice Guidelines for the Management of Bladder Cancer and the Japanese Urological Association. Evidence-based clinical practice guidelines for bladder cancer (summary - JUA 2009 Edition). Int J Urol. 2010;17(2):102–24.
9. Chang SS, Bochner BH, Chou R, et al. Treatment of non-metastatic muscle-invasive bladder Cancer: AUA/ASCO/ASTRO/SUO guideline. J Urol. 2017; 198(3):552–9.
10. Chang SS, Boorjian SA, Chou R, et al. Diagnosis and treatment of non-muscle invasive bladder Cancer: AUA/SUO guideline. J Urol. 2016;196(4): 1021–9.
11. Daneshmand S. Survey reveals factors in bladder Ca surveillance non-compliance. Urology Times. 2018; Available from: https://www.urologytimes.com/genitourinary-cancers/survey-reveals-factors-bladder-ca-surveillance-non-compliance.
12. Georgieva MV, Wheeler SB, Erim D, et al. Comparison of the harms, advantages, and costs associated with alternative guidelines for the evaluation of hematuria. JAMA Intern Med. 2019;179(10):1352–62.
13. Han DS, Lynch KE, Chang JW, et al. Overuse of Cystoscopic surveillance among patients with low-risk non-muscle-invasive bladder Cancer - a National Study of patient, provider, and facility factors. Urology. 2019;131: 112–9.
14. Schroeck FR, Lynch KE, Li Z, et al. The impact of frequent cystoscopy on surgical care and cancer outcomes among patients with low-risk, non-muscle-invasive bladder cancer. Cancer. 2019;125(18):3147–54.
15. Davidson PJ, McGeoch G, Shand B. Inclusion of a molecular marker of bladder cancer in a clinical pathway for investigation of haematuria may reduce the need for cystoscopy. N Z Med J. 2019;132(1497):55–64.
16. Kavalieris L, O'Sullivan P, Frampton C, et al. Performance characteristics of a multigene urine biomarker test for monitoring for recurrent Urothelial carcinoma in a multicenter study. J Urol. 2017;197(6):1419–26.
17. Lotan Y, O'Sullivan P, Raman JD, et al. Clinical comparison of noninvasive urine tests for ruling out recurrent urothelial carcinoma. Urol Oncol. 2017; 35(8):531 e15–22.
18. Caraway NP, Katz RL. A review on the current state of urine cytology emphasizing the role of fluorescence in situ hybridization as an adjunct to diagnosis. Cancer Cytopathol. 2010;118(4):175–83.
19. Grossman HB, Soloway M, Messing E, et al. Surveillance for recurrent bladder cancer using a point-of-care proteomic assay. JAMA. 2006;295(3): 299–305.
20. Chou R, Gore JL, Buckley D, et al. Urinary biomarkers for diagnosis of bladder Cancer: a systematic review and meta-analysis. Ann Intern Med. 2015;163(12):922–31.
21. Ku JH, Godoy G, Amiel GE, Lerner SP. Urine survivin as a diagnostic biomarker for bladder cancer: a systematic review. BJU Int. 2012;110(5):630–6.
22. Soria F, Droller MJ, Lotan Y, et al. An up-to-date catalog of available urinary biomarkers for the surveillance of non-muscle invasive bladder cancer. World J Urol. 2018;36(12):1981–95.
23. Koo K, Zubkoff L, Sirovich BE, et al. The burden of Cystoscopic bladder Cancer surveillance: anxiety, discomfort, and patient preferences for decision making. Urology. 2017;108:122–8.
24. van der Aa MN, Steyerberg EW, Sen EF, et al. Patients' perceived burden of cystoscopic and urinary surveillance of bladder cancer: a randomized comparison. BJU Int. 2008;101(9):1106–10.
25. Konety B, Shore N, Kader AK, et al. Evaluation of Cxbladder and Adjudication of Atypical Cytology and Equivocal Cystoscopy. Eur Urol. 2019; 76(2):238–43.
26. de Bekker-Grob EW, van der Aa MN, Zwarthoff EC, et al. Non-muscle-invasive bladder cancer surveillance for which cystoscopy is partly replaced by microsatellite analysis of urine: a cost-effective alternative? BJU Int. 2009; 104(1):41–7.
27. Kamat AM, Karam JA, Grossman HB, Kader AK, Munsell M, Dinney CP. Prospective trial to identify optimal bladder cancer surveillance protocol: reducing costs while maximizing sensitivity. BJU Int. 2011;108(7):1119–23.
28. Neiboer D, Lansorp-Vogelaar I, de Bekker-Grob EW, Nielsen ME. Evaluating the cost-effectiveness of surveillance schedules for recurrence in low-risk bladder cancer patients. J Urol. 2016;195(Suppl 4S):e620.
29. Yossepowitch O, Herr HW, Donat SM. Use of urinary biomarkers for bladder cancer surveillance: patient perspectives. J Urol. 2007;177(4):1277–82 discussion 82.

# 17

# Spontaneous vesicorectal fistula: A rare complication of neurogenic bladder

Weilin Fang[1], Lei Xu[1], Jiabei Sun[1], Jacques Corcos[2] and Jiayi Li[1*]

**Abstract**

**Background:** We report a rare case of spontaneous vesicorectal fistula.

**Case presentation:** A 13-year-old female spina bifida patient who complained of fecal and urinary incontinence was eventually diagnosed with a spontaneous vesicorectal fistula. We hypothesized that infection, neurogenic bowel and neurogenic bladder caused her vesicorectal fistula. The patient refused the operation, and she is currently in a delicate balance.

**Conclusions:** Early repair of the fistula is necessary. The treatment of neurogenic bladder after fistula repair is difficult and deserves further observation and follow-up.

**Keywords:** Vesicorectal fistula, Neurogenic bladder, Video urodynamic

## Background

Myelomeningocele is frequently associated with neurogenic bladder dysfunction. In these cases, tethered cords are a common finding. Age and height growth may worsen tethered cord syndrome, including symptoms of bladder and bowel dysfunction, pain, and lower limb malformation. In advanced cases, bladder and upper urinary tract distension as well as rectal distension may lead to severe complications. We report a rare case of spontaneous vesicorectal fistula.

## Case presentation

In 2017, we managed a 13-year-old female spina bifida patient with fecal and urinary incontinence associated with recurrent urinary tract infections. Myelomeningocele repair was performed at 4 months after birth. At the age of 4, she began clean intermittent self-catheterization (CIC) due to weak bladder emptying and hydronephrosis. Further follow-up showed remission of hydronephrosis. Two years later, she stopped CIC on her own and was lost to follow-up. She is currently complaining of urinary incontinence, urinary dribbling, and stool incontinence.

Her postvoid residual urine and upper urinary tract ultrasound were normal. We performed a video urodynamic study (Fig. 1 (a) and Table 1). It showed decreased bladder compliance ($C = 2.12\ ml/cmH_2O$) and detrusor overactivity with no ureteral reflux. There was no detrusor contraction during the voiding phase, but abdominal straining assisted voiding. There was no voluntary voiding (most urine leaked slowly during the filling phase). At the end of the voiding phase, we noticed a concentration of contrast around the bladder. To explain this phenomenon, we performed another video urodynamic study. This time, in the filling phase, we noticed the following: 1. the patient's bladder compliance returned surprisingly to normal ($C = 31\ ml/cmH_2O$), and 2. leakage of contrast from the bladder to rectum was found on the lateral radiograph. Although a follow-up colonoscopy found no obvious abnormality, cystoscopy and a methylene blue test confirmed the existence of a 1 cm diameter fistula on the posterior wall of the bladder.

We speculate that this fistula existed initially but was blocked by substances in the bladder, which were washed out during the first urodynamic study, opening the fistula and causing the leakage of contrast around the bladder during the voiding phase. On the

* Correspondence: lijiayi0817@163.com
[1]Department of Urology, Renji Hospital, School of Medicine, Shanghai Jiaotong University, Shanghai, 200127, People's Republic of China
Full list of author information is available at the end of the article

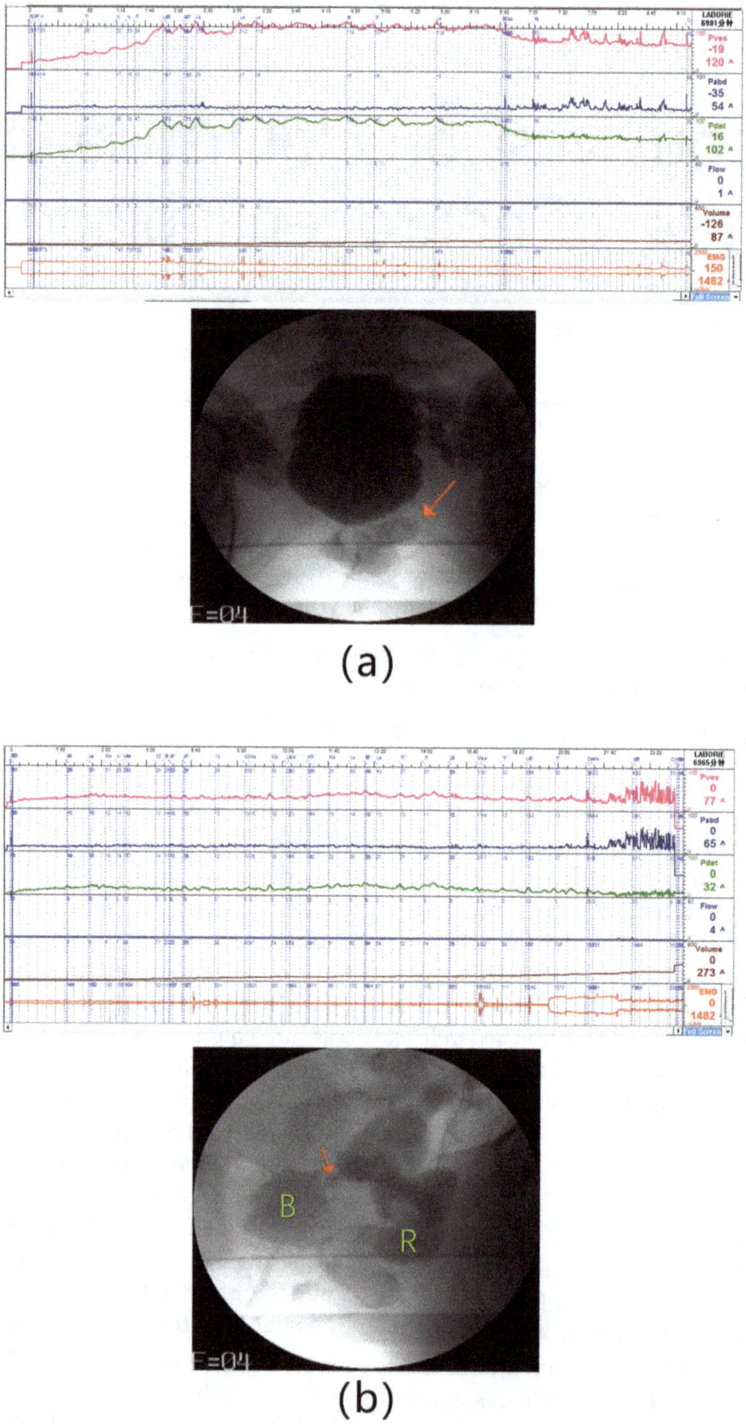


**Fig. 1** **a** Result and radiograph of patient's first video urodynamic. Bladder compliance significantly decreased during the filling phase(C = 2.12 ml/cmH2O). In the anteroposterior film, there is a suspicious concentration of contrast around the bladder (arrow). **b** Result and radiograph of patient's second video urodynamic. Bladder compliance was normal this time (C = 31). On oblique incidences, the contrast agent leaked into rectum from the bladder (B: bladder; R: rectum; arrow: fistula)

other hand, the opening of the fistula led to a decrease in the internal pressure of the bladder, which made the second bladder compliance result normal.

When the patient learned that she was going to start CIC again after the operation, she rejected our operation proposal to close the fistula. She believed that she had no

**Table 1** Results of two times urodynamic tests in this patient

| | Pdet.max (cmH2O) During Filling phase | Pves.max (cmH2O) During Filling phase | bladder compliance (ml/cmH2O) | DO | Ureteral reflux | detrusor contracts during urination | Qmax | PVR (ml) |
|---|---|---|---|---|---|---|---|---|
| 1st | 102 | 120 | 2.12 | Yes | No | No | No voluntary voiding | 18 |
| 2nd | 32 | 64 | 31 | Yes | No | No | No voluntary voiding | 16 |

Qmax: Maximal urinary flow, *Pdet.max* Maximal detrusor pressure, *Pves.max* Maximal vesical pressure, *PVR* Post-void residual

apparent symptoms other than anal leakage and incontinence and that surgery may make the situation worse. Because of the patient's attitude, she is currently under close follow-up observation.

## Discussion and conclusions

Most vesicorectal fistulas are caused by intestinal diseases, including diverticulitis, intestinal tumors, and Crohn's disease [1]. However, obstruction/high internal pressure in the adjacent lumen (e.g., biliary tract) of the intestine is also one of the causes of spontaneous intestinal fistula [2]. The patient had neurogenic bowel and neurogenic bladder. We hypothesized that infection and intravesical and intrarectal distension caused her vesicorectal fistula.

A vesicorectal fistula may induce many complications, including recurrent urinary tract infection, pelvic abscess, peritonitis, and intestinal obstruction. Surgical intervention is usually required, and choosing a single- or two-stage repair depends on the location of the fistula and general health [3]. Non-operative management is a viable option only in selected patients with intravenous total parenteral nutrition, bowel rest, and antibiotics [4].

Therefore, surgical closure of the fistula is undoubtedly necessary. The goal of operative management is to separate and close the involved organs with minimal anatomic disruption and normal long-term function of both systems. However, the greatest problem will be the management of the patient's bladder after the operation since high intravesical pressure and hydronephrosis will most likely reappear. A mixture of medication/botulinum toxin/surgery will be necessary to achieve a low-pressure storage system. Fistula repair combined with bladder enlargement may be a good option if the patient is willing to start CIC again.

Despite the disadvantages of being expensive and requiring expertise, the advantages of video urodynamic studies in the diagnosis of complex urinary dysfunction are still irreplaceable. In this case, it can be predicted that if we choose to initially give patients a conventional urodynamic study, the final diagnosis will greatly altered.

We believe that this is the first report of spontaneous vesicorectal fistula due to neurogenic bladder and neurogenic bowel. Although it resulted in the patient's firm rejection of the operation, the delicate balance of the patient at present is also worth discussing. Early repair of the fistula is still necessary. The treatment of neurogenic bladder after fistula repair will be difficult and deserves further observation and follow-up.

### Abbreviations

CIC: Clean intermittent self-catheterization; Pdet.max: Maximal detrusor pressure; Pves.max: Maximal vesical pressure; PVR: Post-void residual; Qmax: Maximal urinary flow

### Acknowledgments

Not applicable.

### Authors' contributions

WF collected the information, reviewed the literature, and wrote the report. LX operated the video-urodynamic test and analyzed the data. JS is responsible for contact and follow-up with patients. JC is responsible for providing advice on patients' treatment and revision of reports. JL is the patient's attending physician and planned the writing of this report. All authors read and approved the final manuscript.

### Author details

[1]Department of Urology, Renji Hospital, School of Medicine, Shanghai Jiaotong University, Shanghai, 200127, People's Republic of China.
[2]Department of Urology, Jewish General Hospital, 3755 Côte Ste Catherine Road, Suite E-945, Montreal,, QC, Canada.

### References

1. King RM, Beart RJ, Mcllrath DC. Colovesical and rectovesical fistulas. Arch Surg. 1982;117(5):680–3.
2. LeBlanc KA, Barr LH, Rush BM. Spontaneous biliary enteric fistulas. South Med J. 1983;76(10):1249–52. https://doi.org/10.1097/00007611-198310000-00013[1983-10-01].
3. Najjar SF, Jamal MK, Savas JF, et al. The spectrum of colovesical fistula and diagnostic paradigm. Am J Surg. 2004;188(5):617–21.
4. Dudrick SJ, Maharaj AR, McKelvey AA. Artificial nutritional support in patients with gastrointestinal fistulas. World J Surg. 1999;23(6):570–6.

18

# Clinical efficacy of submucosal injection of triamcinolone acetonide in the treatment of type II/III interstitial cystitis/bladder pain syndrome

Tao Jiang†, Xiaozhou Zhou†, Zhipeng Chen, Tailin Xiong, Jian Fu, Zhengchao Liu, Dishi Yan, Zhansong Zhou and Wenhao Shen*

**Abstract**

**Background:** To evaluate the efficacy of submucosal injection of triamcinolone acetonide for the treatment of type II/III interstitial cystitis/bladder pain syndrome.

**Methods:** A retrospective analysis of the clinical data of type II/III interstitial cystitis/bladder pain syndrome patients treated in our department from April 2016 to August 2018 was conducted, and changes in International Prostate Symptom Scores and the Pelvic Pain and Urgency/Frequency symptom scale after surgery were evaluated to explore factors that may affect patient outcomes.

**Results:** A total of 27 female patients and 8 male patients were enrolled, with type II patients accounting for 62.9% of the sample, and the median follow-up duration was 31 months (range: 12–40 months). Twenty-two patients (74.3%) had significantly improved questionnaire scores at 4 weeks postoperatively. Treatment efficacy was sustained for at least 1 year in 15 patients, and persistent effectiveness was noted in 10 (28.6%) patients. Patients with an advanced age ($p = 0.015$), high pain scores ($p = 0.040$), and higher International Prostate Symptom Scores ($p = 0.037$) and Pelvic Pain and Urgency/Frequency symptom scale scores ($p = 0.020$) were more likely to benefit from submucosal injection of triamcinolone acetonide. Gender, disease duration, and the presence of Hunner's lesions had no predictive value for treatment outcomes.

**Conclusion:** Submucosal injection of triamcinolone acetonide can improve the clinical symptoms and quality of life in both men and women with type II/III interstitial cystitis/bladder pain syndrome. Patients with an advanced age and more severe interstitial cystitis/bladder pain syndrome related symptoms may benefit more from triamcinolone acetonide injection.

**Keywords:** Bladder pain syndrome, Hunner's lesion, Interstitial cystitis, Triamcinolone

* Correspondence: chongqingswh@aliyun.com
†Tao Jiang and Xiaozhou Zhou contributed equally to this work.
Department of Urology, Urology Institute of PLA, Southwest Hospital, Third Military Medical University (Army Medical University), Gao Tanyan Street 29#, Sha Pingba, Chongqing 400038, China

## Background

Interstitial cystitis/bladder pain syndrome (IC/BPS) is a clinical syndrome with an unclear cause. It mainly manifests as pain in the suprapubic area or discomfort with bladder filling, which can be alleviated with urination. IC/BPS is often accompanied by frequent urination, urgency, and nocturia and is more common in middle-aged women. IC/BPS seriously affects the quality of life of patients [1]. The etiology and pathophysiology of this disease are still not fully understood, and readily available and effective treatment methods are currently lacking in clinical practice.

The European Society for the Study of Interstitial Cystitis (ESSIC) divided IC/BPS into the following three major types based on changes in the bladder mucosa after cystoscopy and/or bladder hydrodistention in IC/BPS patients: type I: normal bladder mucosa; type II: glomerulations in the bladder mucosa; and type III: visible Hunner's lesions in the bladder mucosa with or without glomerulations. Type II and type III account for 30 ~ 60% of all IC/BPS cases [2].The American Urological Association (AUA) IC/BPS guideline of recommends endoscopic laser ablation/ electrocauterization of Hunner's lesions or injection of triamcinolone acetonide (TA) into lesions as alternative treatments for Hunner's subtype of IC/BPS [3].

Cox and other researchers have reported treating female patients with type III IC/BPS with submucosal TA injection [4]. Whether this treatment is effective for male patients remains unclear, and no studies have reported treating type II IC/BPS using the same method [4, 5]. This study is the first to include male patients and type II IC/BPS patients. With at least 1 year of follow-up for each patient, this study showed the efficacy of TA for the treatment of IC/BPS patients with intravesical Hunner's lesions and/or submucosal hemorrhage in our center, and relevant factors that may affect the treatment efficacy were analyzed.

## Methods

The medical records of type II/III IC/BPS patients treated with submucosal TA injection in our hospital from April 2016 to August 2018 were retrospectively analyzed. IC/BPS was diagnosed using the "exclusive diagnosis" method and according to the AUA IC/BPS Guideline [3] and the IC/BPS diagnostic criteria of the ESSIC [2].All patients had a poor response to lifestyle modifications and conservative drug therapy with amitriptyline. Patients who voluntarily underwent cystoscopy and submucosal injection of TA signed an informed consent form. The Institutional Review Board of Southwest Hospital, The Third Military Medical University approved this investigation.

Endoscopic diagnosis and treatment were performed by an experienced specialist. After successful spinal anesthesia, bladder hydrodistention was performed with the patient in the lithotomy position at the pressure of 60 cm $H_2O$ for 5 min under cystoscopy. After venting, the bladder was filled again, and lesions in the bladder wall were observed and recorded in detail. For patients who did not show obvious abnormalities under cystoscopy, surgery was concluded. For type II/III IC/BPS patients, TA solution was injected into the submucosa at the bladder hemorrhage site and/or into the center of Hunner's lesions (0.5 ml, 40 mg/ml per point, up to 20 points). After ensuring the absence of active bleeding in the bladder, a 16 Fr double-lumen catheter was inserted. The catheter was removed the next day after surgery.

The patients were assessed with the International Prostate Symptom Score (IPSS) and the Pelvic Pain and Urgency/Frequency (PUF) symptom scale before surgery, and 4 weeks, 6, 12, and 18 months after surgery. If a patient's symptoms recurred, then he or she returned to the hospital for a timely follow-up.

The results are presented as the means ± standard deviation (SD). Comparisons were performed using the Wilcoxon rank-sum test to analyze scores before and after treatment The Mann-Whitney test was used to analyze factors influencing the treatment effect. Data with $p$ values of 0.05 or less was considered statistically significant. A Kaplan-Meier curve was plotted to depict the sustained efficacy duration after the first treatment; Patients for whom no repeat procedure occurred and exhibited persistent effectiveness at the last follow-up were censored. All of the statistical analyses were performed using the Statistical Package for Social Sciences, version 19, for Windows (SPSS, Chicago, IL).

## Results

A total of 35 patients were included in the study, with 8 males (22.9%) and 27 females (77.1%). The patients' ages ranged from 33 to 80 years, with an average age of 51.7 ± 12.0 years. The average disease duration was 5.2 ± 4.6 years. Twenty-two patients (62.9%) had type II IC/BPS, and 13 patients (37.1%) had type III IC/BPS. All patients were followed up for at least 1 year after the first submucosal injection, with a median follow-up duration of 31 months (range: 12–40 months).

IPSS and PUF scores at 4 weeks after surgery are shown in Table 1. At 4 weeks postoperatively, 26 (74.3%) patients had significant improvements in IC/BPS-related symptoms such as urinary frequency, urgency, and pain. Among these patients, quality of life (QOL) scores decreased by 3.6 points ($p < 0.0001$), IPSS decreased by 17.2 points ($p < 0.0001$), PUF symptom scores decreased by 8.9 points ($p < 0.0001$), and PUF bother scores decreased by 4.5 points ($p < 0.0001$).

**Table 1** Mean pre-procedure and post-procedure scores for individual questionnaire items and Wilcoxon rank-sum analysis of cohort responses (Wilcoxon rank-sum test)

| Question | | Pre-procedure Score Mean (SD) | Post-procedure Score Mean (SD) | *p*-value |
|---|---|---|---|---|
| IPSS | Incomplete Emptying | 4.5 (0.7) | 2.1 (1.3) | < 0.0001 |
| | Frequency | 4.5 (0.7) | 2.1 (1.5) | |
| | Intermittenc | 2.1 (2.0) | 0.9 (1.2) | |
| | Urgency | 4.4 (0.6) | 1.8 (1.4) | |
| | Weak Stream | 2.2 (1.9) | 1.0 (1.1) | |
| | Nocturia | 3.7 (0.7) | 2.3 (1.0) | |
| | QOL | 5.7 (0.5) | 2.1 (2.0) | |
| | Total Score | 31.4 (5.5) | 14.2 (9.1) | |
| PUF | Daytime Voids | 3.0 (1.0) | 1.0 (1.0) | |
| | Nighttime Voids | 3.7 (0.7) | 2.3 (1.0) | |
| | Pain in Bladder, Pelvis | 2.3 (0.9) | 0.9 (0.6) | |
| | Pain Scale | 2.1 (0.8) | 0.8 (0.7) | |
| | Urgency after Voiding | 2.2 (0.8) | 0.9 (0.9) | |
| | Urgency Scale | 2.4 (0.7) | 0.8 (1.0) | |
| | Total Bother Score | 7.5 (1.8) | 3.0 (3.5) | |
| | Total Symptom Score | 16.6 (3.3) | 7.7 (4.9) | |
| | Total PUF Score | 24.1 (4.8) | 10.7 (8.1) | |

*SD* Standard deviation, *IPSS* International Prostate Symptom Score, *PUF* Pelvic Pain and Urgency/Frequency, *QOL* Quality of life

We further analyzed the clinical characteristics of the patients with a positive therapeutic effect and nonresponsive patients (Table 2). Patients with an advanced age ($p = 0.015$), high pain scores ($p = 0.040$), and high IPSS ($p = 0.037$) and PUF scores ($p = 0.020$) were more likely to benefit from submucosal injection of TA. No difference in the response to treatment was noted for patients with Hunner's lesions ($p = 0.644$), and male patients had similar treatment response rates to those of female patients ($p = 0.959$). Disease duration had no

**Table 2** Patient demographics stratified by no response vs symptom relief with analysis of risk factors associated with clinical effect (Mann-Whitney U test)

| | No response | Symptom relief | *p*-value |
|---|---|---|---|
| No. patients (%) | 9 (25.7) | 26 (74.3) | |
| Age Mean ± SD | 41.0 (9.1) | 54.5 (11.8) | 0.015 |
| No. gender (%) | | | |
| Male | 2 (22) | 6 (23) | 0.959 |
| Female | 7 (78) | 20 (77) | |
| IC/BPS type (%) | | | |
| Type II | 6 (66.7) | 16 (61.5) | 0.644 |
| Type III | 3 (33.3) | 10 (38.5) | |
| Symptom history (years) Mean ± SD | 4.7 (2.2) | 5.4 (5.2) | 0.516 |
| Pain Scale Mean ± SD | 1.7 (0.5) | 2.3 (0.8) | 0.040 |
| QOL Mean ± SD | 5.4 (0.5) | 5.7 (0.5) | 0.124 |
| Total IPSS Score Mean ± SD | 22.8 (5.0) | 26.7 (5.0) | 0.037 |
| PUF Bother Score Mean ± SD | 6.6 (1.3) | 7.9 (1.8) | 0.065 |
| PUF Symptom Score Mean ± SD | 14.4 (2.4) | 17.3 (3.3) | 0.019 |
| Total PUF Score Mean ± SD | 21.0 (3.2) | 25.2 (4.8) | 0.020 |

*SD* Standard deviation, *IC/BPS* Interstitial cystitis/bladder pain syndrome, *IPSS* International Prostate Symptom Score, *PUF* Pelvic Pain and Urgency/Frequency, *QOL* Quality of life

significant predictive value for treatment efficacy ($p$ = 0.516).

Fifteen (42.9%) patients were satisfied with symptom control at 1 year after surgery. Their 1-year postoperative scores increased slightly compared with those at 4 weeks after surgery, but no significant difference was found (IPSS: $p = 0.46$, PUF symptom score: $p = 0.16$, and PUF bother score: $p = 0.60$).At the last follow-up, 10 (28.6%) patients had no significant worsening of symptoms. We further analyzed the factors that may have influenced the treatment efficacy for at least 1 year. No clinical parameters that clearly affected patients' treatment effect duration was found (Online resource Additional file 1: Table S1). The Kaplan-Meier curve shown in Fig. 1 demonstrates the sustained efficacy duration among patients with effective submucosal TA injection.

Seven patients with effective first-time treatment were retreated with submucosal TA injection after symptom recurred. The duration of symptom control after reinjection was basically the same as that with the first injection. No significant intraoperative and postoperative complications were observed in any patients.

## Discussion

IC/BPS is a complex and challenging clinical syndrome. No universally effective treatment is available for this disease. A treatment regimen based on bladder pathology changes is one of the therapeutic directions for IC/BPS. Glomerulations and Hunner's lesions of the bladder mucosa are typical pathological changes commonly observed with bladder hydrodistention under cystoscopy in patients with IC/BPS, which the ESSIC classifies as type II and III IC/BPS [2]. The IC/BPS guidelines of the AUA recommend surgical removal of ulcers in IC/BPS patients with Hunner's lesion subtypes [3]. According to studies reported by Payne et al., the average symptom score for IC/BPS patients improved by 76% [6] with electrocautery or removal of Hunner's lesions under cystoscopy. Some researchers have reported that for refractory IC/BPS patients without ulcers, transurethral electrocautery applied to hemorrhage sites after bladder hydrodistention can also effectively relieve clinical symptoms [7]. Surgical removal of bladder mucosal lesions often requires the lesions to be relatively limited. If the range of Hunter's lesions is greater than 25% of the bladder mucosal area, then surgical removal is not a suitable treatment option [8]. Regardless of whether electrical resection, electrocautery or laser ablation is performed, potential complications such as bladder perforation and digestive tract injuries may occur, and a larger range of bladder mucosal cauterization may also cause bladder contracture.

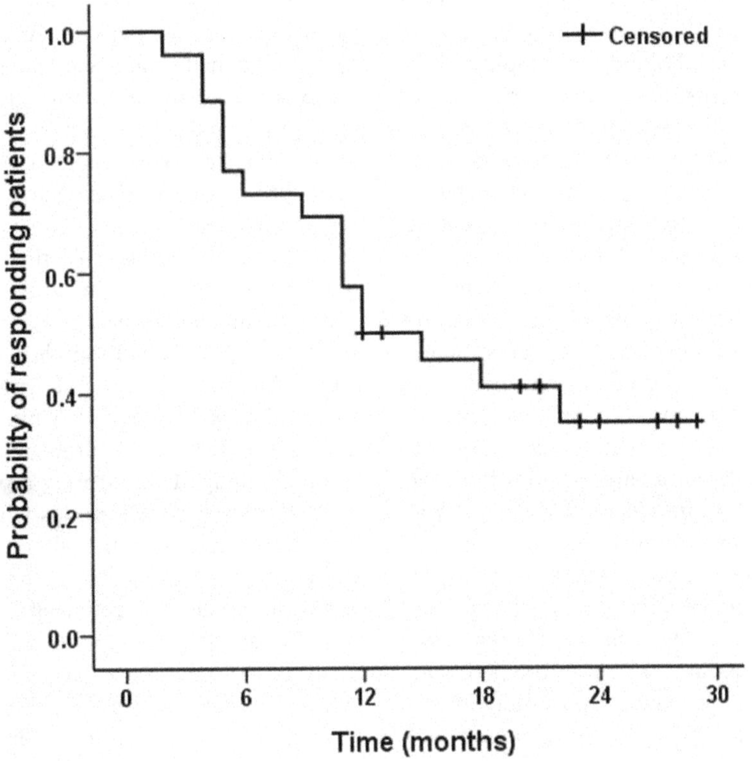


**Fig. 1** Kaplan-Meier curve shows maintenance time of clinical efficacy after single intramucosal triamcinolone acetonide injection

Although the etiology of IC/BPS is still unclear, autoimmunity is recognized as one of the main causes of IC/BPS [9]. Supporting evidence demonstrates similar gender and age distributions among IC/BPS patients to those of patients with known autoimmune diseases, and the clinical features of IC/BPS are similar to those of other established autoimmune diseases [10]. Immunosuppressive drugs routinely used to treat autoimmune diseases have yielded positive results in specific IC/BPS patients [11, 12], which also confirms that autoimmunity plays a key role in IC/BPS. Mast cell activation with the release of inflammatory mediators interacting with other inflammatory cells and nervous system also revealed an important role of inflammatory response in the pathogenesis of IC /BPS [2, 13, 14]. TA is a long-acting adrenal corticosteroid with anti-inflammatory, anti-itching and vasoconstricting effects. It has strong and long-lasting anti-inflammatory and anti-allergic effects but a weak water-sodium retention effect. TA is inexpensive and extremely well tolerated when used locally. Cox and other researchers pioneered the submucosal TA injection method for the treatment of refractory Hunner's lesion-subtype IC/BPS patients and reported satisfactory results[4]. A preliminary study by Rittenberg et al. on IC/BPS patients with Hunner's lesions and bladder mucosal fissures also showed that TA contributes to symptom control and improves the quality of life of IC/BPS patients [5].

Based on the positive efficacy of electrocautery or electrical resection of bladder mucosal lesions in patients with type II and type III IC/BPS and the significant alleviation of clinical symptoms observed among type III IC/BPS patients with TA injection, we speculate that this treatment is also suitable for type II IC/BPS patients. Although the incidence of IC/BPS is lower in men than in women, IC/BPS in men is not uncommon in clinical practice and is easily misdiagnosed and mistreated. All of the 8 male patients in our study had been diagnosed with chronic prostatitis/chronic pelvic pain syndrome (CP/CPPS) in the past and the therapeutic effect aimed at CP/CPPS with antibiotics, alpha-blockers and other phytotherapeutic agents was poor. For one patient with the symptom of dysuria, concomitant bladder-outlet obstruction was also considered. The maximum flow rate was 11 ml/s with urinary volume 95 ml and the obstruction was ruled out by pressure-flow study with normal result. These male patients complained with pelvic region pain during the urine storage period which could be relieved after urination. The pain is different from CP/CPPS pain, which is usually located in the perineum, penis, testicles or suprapubic region, and often worsens by urination or ejaculation. They were diagnosed with IC/BPS finally. Because the symptoms also could not be relieved by oral taken of amitriptyline. They were enrolled in the study. This study is the first to include male patients with type II IC/BPS, to demonstrate the efficacy of this therapy for Hunner's lesion-subtype IC/BPS and to explore the efficacy of this treatment in males and type II IC/BPS patients. The IPSS is mainly used to evaluate urinary symptoms, is easy to understand and manage, and can easily and intuitively reflect the negative impact of urinary symptoms on quality of life. By comparing the preoperative and postoperative IPSS and PUF scores, nearly 3/4 of the patients were found to have significant pain relief and reduced urinary tract symptoms at 4 weeks after surgery, and their quality of life improved significantly. No perioperative and long-term complications were noted, and the treatment efficacy was comparable to that reported by researchers such as Cox [4]. Furthermore, we found that submucosal injection of TA at hemorrhage sites can also control the symptoms of IC/BPS, and the efficacy was the same as that for type III IC/BPS. Significant effects can also be achieved in male patients. Among the factors influencing the efficacy outcome, patients with an advanced age and higher IPSS and PUF scores were more likely to experience a good response to treatment.

The current study shows that the duration of the treatment effect of simple bladder hydrodistention for IC/BPS is generally less than 6 months, and the duration of the treatment effect of submucosal injection of TA for IC/BPS is not clear. The longest follow-up time in the current study was only 3 months [5]. We performed a follow-up of all patients for at least 1 year, and 43% of the patients had a one-year remission period in terms of symptom control after this treatment. Patients with symptoms recurrence had a similar remission period after reinjection to that after the first injection. Ten patients still showed effectiveness at the time of the last follow-up, and 5 patients had sustained efficacy for more than 2 years. Whether this treatment can fully control IC/BPS symptoms remains to be further determined.

The main limitations of our study include the retrospective analysis, small sample size, and lack of a control group. Although the time of symptom relief we reported was obviously longer than simple bladder hydrodistention, the efficacy of hydrodistension can't be ignored. We are aiming at performing a prospective, randomized control study with the groups who will receive saline injections or only bladder hydrodistention at present. The study will reveal more information on the therapeutic effect of submucosal injection of TA for IC/BPS in the future. In addition, The Multidisciplinary Approach to the Study of Chronic Pelvic Pain (MAPP) Network findings [15, 16] indicate that specific clinical factors that are easy to measure – including the pain beyond the pelvis, the presence of nonurological chronic overlapping pain conditions (COPCs) and the severity of bladder-focused symptoms (particularly pain with bladder filling) – have a significant impact on symptom trajectories over time. All the enrolled patients in our study were excluded from COPCs including fibromyalgia, chronic fatigue syndrome and irritable bowel syndrome. However, two patients showed diffuse pain preoperatively and the duration of symptom relief was relatively short after the treatment. More detailed clarification of the location of pelvic pain and of possible concomitant non-urological-associated symptoms according to MAPP consensus should also be considered in the future research.

## Conclusions

Submucosal injection of TA has demonstrated an acceptable safety profile for treating IC/BPS. TA may be effective in controlling symptoms in type II as well as type III IC/BPS, and can improved symptoms and the quality of life of male IC/BPS patients. Patients with an advanced age and more severe IC/BPS-related symptoms may have greater benefits. Further investigation of submucosal injection of TA for the treatment of IC/BPS is warranted with a larger, longer, randomized and controlled trial.

## Supplementary information

**Additional file 1: Table S1.** Patient demographics stratified by the length of time (less than 1 year vs at least 1 year) of symptom relief with analysis of risk factors associated with clinical effect.

### Abbreviations

AUA: American Urological Association; ESSIC: European Society for the Study of Interstitial Cystitis; IC/BPS: Interstitial cystitis/bladder pain syndrome; IPSS: International Prostate Symptom Scores; PUF: Pelvic Pain and Urgency/Frequency; QOL: Quality of life; TA: Triamcinolone acetonide

### Acknowledgements

No.

### Authors' contributions

TJ: project development, manuscript writing. XZZ: project development, data analysis. ZPC: statistical analysis and manuscript editing. TLX, JF, ZCL and DSY: data collection and management. ZSZ: supervision and manuscript editing. WHS: project development, manuscript editing. All authors reviewed the results and approved the final version of the manuscript.

### References

1. Nickel JC, Tripp DA, Pontari M, Moldwin R, Mayer R, Carr LK, et al. Psychosocial Phenotyping in women with interstitial cystitis/painful bladder syndrome: a case control study. J Urol. 2010;183:167–72. https://doi.org/10.1016/j.juro.2009.08.133.
2. van de Merwe JP, Nordling J, Bouchelouche P, Bouchelouche K, Cervigni M, Daha LK, et al. Diagnostic criteria, classification, and nomenclature for painful bladder syndrome/interstitial cystitis: an ESSIC proposal. Eur Urol. 2008;53:60–7. https://doi.org/10.1016/j.eururo.2007.09.019.
3. Hanno PM, Erickson D, Moldwin R, Faraday MM. Diagnosis and treatment of interstitial cystitis/bladder pain syndrome: AUA guideline amendment. J Urol. 2015;193:1545–53. https://doi.org/10.1016/j.juro.2015.01.086.
4. Cox M, Klutke JJ, Klutke CG. Assessment of patient outcomes following submucosal injection of triamcinolone for treatment of Hunner's ulcer subtype interstitial cystitis. Can J Urol. 2009;16:4536–40.
5. Rittenberg L, Morrissey D, El-Khawand D, Whitmore K. Kenalog injection into Hunner's lesions as a treatment for interstitial cystitis/bladder pain syndrome. Curr Urol. 2017;10:154–6.
6. Bahlani S, Moldwin R. Endoscopic lysis of bladder scar associated with Hunner's lesions: a new technique. Asian J Urol. 2015;2:59–62. https://doi.org/10.1016/j.ajur.2015.04.008.
7. Yi T, Lv J, Fu Q, Jiang C, Li J, Lv T, et al. Efficacy and safety of transurethral cystoscopic fulguration in the treatment of refractory and non-ulcer interstitial cystitis/painful bladder syndrome. J Mod Urol. 2016;21:511–5.
8. Hillelsohn JH, Rais-Bahrami S, Friedlander JI, Okhunov Z, Kashan M, Rosen L, et al. Fulguration for Hunner ulcers: long-term clinical outcomes. J Urol. 2012;188:2238–41. https://doi.org/10.1016/j.juro.2012.08.013.
9. van de Merwe JP. Interstitial cystitis and systemic autoimmune diseases. Nat Clin Pract Urol. 2007;4:484–91. https://doi.org/10.1038/ncpuro0874.
10. Alagiri M, Chottiner S, Ratner V, Slade D, Hanno PM. Interstitial cystitis: unexplained associations with other chronic disease and pain syndromes. Urology. 1997;49:52–7. https://doi.org/10.1016/S0090-4295(99)80332-X.
11. Soucy F, Gregoire M. Efficacy of prednisone for severe refractory ulcerative interstitial cystitis. J Urol. 2005;173:841–3. https://doi.org/10.1097/01.ju.0000153612.14639.19.
12. Bosch PC. A randomized, double-blind, placebo-controlled trial of Certolizumab Pegol in women with refractory interstitial cystitis/bladder pain syndrome. Eur Urol. 2018;74:623–30. https://doi.org/10.1016/j.eururo.2018.07.026.
13. Theoharides TC, Kempuraj D, Sant GR. Mast cell involvement in interstitial cystitis: a review of human and experimental evidence. Urology. 2001;57:47–55. https://doi.org/10.1016/S0090-4295(01)01129-3.
14. Nordling J, Anjum F, Bade J, Bouchelouche K, Bouchelouche P, Cervigni M, et al. Primary evaluation of patients suspected of having interstitial cystitis (IC). Eur Urol. 2004;45:662–9. https://doi.org/10.1016/j.eururo.2003.11.021.
15. Clemens JQ, Mullins C, Ackerman AL, Bavendam T, van Bokhoven A, Ellingson BM, et al. Urologic chronic pelvic pain syndrome: insights from the MAPP research network. Nat Rev Urol. 2019;16(3):187–200.
16. Afari N, Buchwald D, Clauw D, Hong B, Hou X, Krieger JN, et al. A MAPP network case-control study of urological chronic pelvic pain compared with nonurological pain conditions. Clin J Pain. 2020;36:8–15.

19

# Characterizing relaxin receptor expression and exploring relaxin's effect on tissue remodeling/fibrosis in the human bladder

Edward C. Diaz[1,2*], Mason Briggs[1,3], Yan Wen[3], Guobing Zhuang[3], Shannon L. Wallace[3], Amy D. Dobberfuhl[1], Chia-Sui Kao[4] and Bertha C. Chen[3]

**Abstract**

**Background:** Relaxin is an endogenous protein that has been shown to have antifibrotic properties in various organ systems. There has been no characterization of relaxin's role in the human bladder. Our objective was to characterize relaxin receptor expression in the human bladder and assess relaxin's effect on tissue remodeling/fibrosis pathways in bladder smooth muscle cells.

**Methods:** Relaxin family peptide receptor 1 (RXFP1) and RXFP2 expression was assessed using quantitative reverse transcriptase-PCR (qRT-PCR) and immunohistochemistry (IHC) on primary bladder tissue. Primary human smooth muscle bladder cells were cultured and stimulated with various concentrations of relaxin. Western blot, qRTPCR, ELISA, and zymogram assays were used to analyze fibrosis/tissue remodeling pathway proteins.

**Results:** There was universal mRNA transcript detection and protein expression of relaxin receptors in primary bladder specimens. Immunohistochemistry demonstrated RXFP1 and RXFP2 localizing to both urothelial and smooth muscle cell layers of the bladder. 24 h of in vitro relaxin stimulation did not affect mRNA expression of selected proteins in human bladder smooth muscle cells. However, 48 h of in vitro relaxin stimulation resulted in upregulation of active ($p = 0.004$) and latent ($p = 0.027$) MMP-2 in cell lysate, and upregulation of active MMP-2 in supernatant ($p = 0.04$). There was a dose dependent relationship with increasing expression of MMP-2 with increasing relaxin concentration. Relaxin stimulation resulted in decreased levels of active and total TGF-β1 in supernatant and extracellular matrix ($p < 0.005$ with 100 ng/mL relaxin stimulation).

**Conclusions:** In the human bladder, relaxin receptors are expressed at the dome and trigone and localize to the urothelium and smooth muscle cell layers. Stimulation of human bladder SMCs with relaxin in vitro affects expression of MMP-2 and TGF-β1.

**Keywords:** Relaxin, Fibrosis, Bladder, RXFP1, RXFP2

## Background

Relaxin 2, commonly referred to as "relaxin", is known in urology for its ability to facilitate closure of bladder exstrophy without osteotomy in the first 48 h of life. It binds to relaxin family peptide receptor 1 (RXFP1) and RXFP2 [1]. In addition to its ability to increase pelvic ligament and bone laxity in pregnancy, relaxin can inhibit fibrotic pathways [2] and modulate the extracellular matrix [3]. This antifibrotic effect has led to clinical trials looking at relaxin therapy for fibrotic medical

* Correspondence: eddiaz@gmail.com
[1]Department of Urology, Stanford University Medical Center, 300 Pasteur Drive, Grant S-287, Stanford, CA 94305, USA
[2]Present Address: Division of Pediatric Urology, Advocate Children's Hospital, 8901 West Golf Road, Suite 301, Des Plaines, IL 60016, USA
Full list of author information is available at the end of the article

conditions such as heart failure [4], scleroderma [5], and pulmonary fibrosis [6].

The poorly compliant bladder demonstrates a histologic phenotype of fibrosis. There is an evolution of initial hypertrophy and then loss of detrusor muscle [7], muscle replacement with collagen [8], and decreased elastin in the extracellular matrix [9]. Molecular pathways that contribute to this process are multifactorial [10]. Preliminary in-vivo data suggests a relationship between relaxin and bladder fibrosis. Using a radiated murine model, a group demonstrated that relaxin therapy reverses radiation-induced fibrosis and restores bladder function [11]. This evidence supports further investigation as to whether relaxin-related mechanisms also exist in the human bladder which, to our knowledge, has not been documented. The objective of this study is to characterize relaxin receptor expression in the human bladder and assess the in-vitro effect of relaxin on expression of proteins involved in tissue remodeling and fibrosis in human bladder smooth muscle cells.

## Methods

### Procurement of primary bladder specimens

IRB exemption and external approval from Donor Network West's (federally designated organ procurement organization) Internal Research Council and Medical Advisory Board Research Subcommittee was obtained for collection of primary bladder tissue from brain dead cadaveric organ transplant donors. Brain dead donation was selected to eliminate warm ischemia time. Bladder tissue (Dome and trigone) was procured by a board certified urologist after removal of organs allocated for human transplant and immediately cryopreserved, placed in formalin, and processed into cell culture.

### Immunohistochemistry of primary tissue

Primary tissue was processed into paraffin blocks. 5 um sections were made and hematoxylin and eosin stain was performed. Slides were reviewed by a genitourinary pathologist.

### Immunofluorescence for RXFP1 and RXFP2 in primary tissue

5 um cryostat sections were fixed in 4% paraformaldehyde, permeabilized with 0.5% Triton X-100 in phosphate-buffered saline (PBS), and blocked in 1% bovine serum albumin. Primary antibodies: mouse anti-human cytokeratin (AE1/AE3) IgG (5μg/ml, Chemicon International), mouse anti-human desmin IgG (1:50, Sigma-Aldrich), rabbit anti-human RXFP1 IgG (10μg/ml, Abcam), rabbit anti-human RXFP2 IgG (10μg/ml, Lifespan Biosciences). Secondary antibody used: Alexa Fluor 488-conjugated goat anti-mouse IgG (1:300, Invitrogen), Alexa Fluor 594-conjugated donkey anti-rabbit IgG (1:200, Invitrogen).

### Quantitative reverse transcriptase-PCR (qRT-PCR)

RNA was extracted with RNA Stat-60 reagent (Tel-Test Inc.). Primers for target proteins were created using previously described protocols [12–16]. Samples were performed in duplicate. Brilliant SYBR Green qPCR Master Mix (Stratagene) was used. A 10 min hot start at 95 °C with forty cycles of 30 s of denaturation (94 °C), 1 min of annealing (60 °C), and extension at 72 °C for 30 s was used. Glyceraldehyde 3-phosphate dehydrogenase (GAPDH) was used as the endogenous reference. Human vaginal cuff tissue was used as a positive control for RXFP1 and RXFP2 expression.

### Bladder smooth muscle cell culture and Relaxin treatment

Primary human bladder smooth muscle cell (bSMC) line was obtained commercially from Lonza. Cells were grown in Dulbecco's Modified Eagle Medium (DMEM) with 10% charcoal-stripped Fetal Bovine Serum (FBS) at 37 °C and 5% CO2 incubator. Cells (passage 4) were plated in triplicate. At 80–90% confluency, cells were then starved in serum-free DMEM with 0.2% lactalbumin enzymatic hydrolysate for 24 h, and then treated with various concentrations of human relaxin-2 (0–100 ng/mL, PeproTech) for 24 or 48 h as described previously by our group [17].

Supernatant was concentrated 100-fold using Vivaspin filtration tubes (Sartorius AG). To acquire proteins, cell layers were washed with (PBS) and lysed by 3 successive 10- min treatments with Complete-Mini Protease Inhibitor Cocktail (1 tab/10 mL, Sigma- Aldrich) in radioimmunoprecipitation assay (RIPA) buffer at 4 °C. Cell debris was removed by centrifugation.

Extracellular matrix (ECM) was prepared according to Pedrozo et al. [18] Cells were removed with RIPA buffer, the remaining cell-free, non-solubilized ECM was washed 3 times with PBS and plates dried overnight at room temperature. Isolated ECM samples were digested with plasmin (MP Biomedicals) in DMEM for 3 h at 37° to release TGFβ-118 [19]., Reaction was stopped by the addition of aprotinin (5 μg/mL, Sigma- Aldrich). Plasmin-digested ECM samples were collected and concentrated 200-fold with Vivaspin filtration tubes.

### ELISA measurement of active and latent TGF-β1

An ELISA kit (Promega Corp) was used. Nunc MaxiSorp 96-well plates were coated with TGF-β1 monoclonal antibody. Plates were washed and blocked and 100 μL of acid-treated and non-acid treated samples were then added to the wells in duplicate. After washing, anti-TGF-β1 polyclonal antibody was applied. Horseradish peroxidase HRP–conjugated antibody was used for detection. Absorbance at 450 nm was measured on a plate reader (Molecular Devices). Levels of both active and total TGF-β1 in the samples were normalized by protein concentration. Total protein concentration was determined using the Bradford method (Bio-Rad).

### Zymography of proteinases

Equal amounts of protein underwent sodium dodecyl sulfate polyacrylamide gel electrophoresis (SDS-PAGE) in 10% polyacrylamide containing 0.1% gelatin. Gels were soaked in 2.5% Triton X-100, incubated overnight at 37 °C in 0.05 mol/L Tris (pH 8.5), 5.0 mmol/L calcium chloride, and 0.02% sodium azide, then stained with 1% coomassie-blue R-250, 25% ethanol, and 15% formaldehyde. After staining, the enzyme activity appeared as clear bands against the blue-stained background. Activities of MMPs were identified by molecular weight. The area of lysis for each band detected was analyzed using Bio-Rad Quality One Software.

### Western blot

Protein from 24 h and 48 h supernatant and cell lysate were subjected to SDS-PAGE on 8% or 10% polyacrylamide gels. Gels were blotted onto nitrocellulose membranes. Blots were blocked and probed with mouse anti-TIMP-1 (1.0 μg/ml, EMD Bioscience) orTIMP-3 (3.0 μg/ml, EMD Bioscience). Secondary antibody was rabbit anti-mouse IgG (1:10,000, Amersham Pharmacia Biotech) conjugated to HRP. GAPDH was used as an endogenous reference. Membranes were re-blocked and reprobed with goat anti-GAPDH polyclonal IgG (1:500, Abcam) and HRP-conjugated mouse antigoat/ sheep monoclonal IgG (1:10,000, Abcam), for the primary and secondary antibodies respectively. Blots were developed by chemiluminescence.

### Statistical analysis

Statistical analysis for the dose–response studies was performed by using unpaired one-way ANOVA in IBM SPSS Statistics 21.0 software (IBM, Armonk, NY, USA). *P* value < 0.05 was considered statistically significant.

## Results

### Primary bladder procurement

Over a 6 month period, there were 26 offers for bladder tissue. Age range: 2–59, Gender: 17 male donors and 9 female. Patients with a history of a urologic condition, urologic surgery, malignancy, diabetes mellitus, elevated HGB A1c, were excluded. Eleven offers were accepted, but two were withdrawn due to hospital scheduling. A total of 9 bladders were procured. There were 5 male and 4 female donors with an age range of 2 to 55 years and mean age of 30.9 years and median age of 30 years. There was no warm ischemia time for donor tissue as organs were immediately flushed with ice cold UW solution and packed with ice after cross clamp. Cold ischemia time (Cross clamp to bladder tissue preservation) for the nine primary bladders was a mean of 68.6 min, with a median of 64 min. Pathology review for all donors confirmed benign urothelium, lamina propria and muscularis propria at the dome and trigone. Most bladders obtained were normal (Fig. 1a). Benign pathology was seen in donor 4 (Fig. 1b, cystitis cystica et glandularis), donor 7 (Fig. 1c, Squamous metaplasia), and donor 8 (mild chronic inflammation). A description of cadaveric donors is provided in Table 1.

### Relaxin receptor expression

*PCR:* qRT-PCR performed on dome and trigone for all 9 primary bladders ($n = 18$). All 18 samples demonstrated RXFP1 expression, and 17/18 samples demonstrated RXFP2 expression. The dome specimen for the 50 yo female donor did not have detectable RXFP2 transcript. The number of primary bladder specimens ($n = 9$) was too small to detect any significant differences between groups such as: male v. female, prepubertal v. postpubertal. The PCR data, however, confirms expression of both relaxin receptors at both trigone and dome. See Fig. 2.

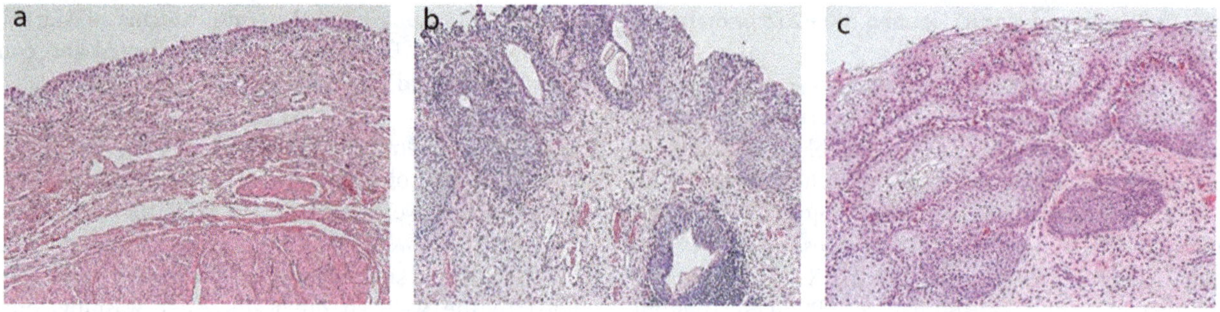


**Fig. 1** Hematoxylin and Eosin staining of donor bladders: **a** normal from donor 5 (10x), (**b**) cystitis cystica et glandularisfrom donor 4 (40x), and (**c**) non-keratinzing squamous metaplasia from donor 7 (40x)

**Table 1** Cadaveric donor summary for primary bladder tissue

| Donor | Gender | Age (Yrs) | Cold Ischemia Time (min) | Cause of Brain Death | Comorbidities | Pathology Assessment |
|---|---|---|---|---|---|---|
| 1 | Male | 19 | 75 | Traumatic Brain Injury | None | Dome: Normal Trigone: Normal |
| 2 | Male | 26 | 83 | Traumatic Brain Injury | None | Dome: Normal Trigone: Normal |
| 3 | Male | 2 | 60 | Traumatic Brain Injury | None | Dome: Normal Trigone: Normal |
| 4 | Male | 43 | 58 | Hemorrhagic stroke from Arteriovenous malformation | None | Dome: Normal Trigone: Benign with chronic inflammation and cystitis cystica et glandularis |
| 5 | Male | 20 | 71 | Anoxic brain injury from asthma exacerbation | Asthma | Dome: Normal Trigone: Normal |
| 6 | Female | 55 | 64 | Anoxic brain injury from cardiovascular event | None | Dome: Normal Trigone: Normal |
| 7 | Female | 33 | 49 | Hemorrhagic stroke from ruptured aneurysm | Non-recurrent urinary tract infection | Dome: Benign with chronic inflammation Trigone: Benign with non-keratinizing squamous metaplasia |
| 8 | Female | 50 | 64 | Anoxic Brain Injury from suicide | Gastroesophageal Reflux Disease, Irritable Bowel Syndrome, Fibroids | Dome: Benign, chronic inflammation Trigone: Benign with chronic inflammation |
| 9 | Female | 30 | 93 | Anoxic Brain Injury from asthma exacerbation | Asthma, atopic dermatitis, gastroesophageal reflux disease, hypertension | Dome: Normal Trigone: Normal |

### *Immunofluorescence*

Immune fluorescence demonstrated RXFP1 and RXFP2 expression within the urothelium, lamina propria and muscularis propria. This pattern of receptor distribution was consistent between male and female donors and RXFP1 and RXFP2 receptor distribution was similar between trigone and dome specimens. Figure 3a, and b demonstrates localization of relaxin receptors (RXFP1 and RXFP2, respectively) to urothelium and Fig. 3c, and d demonstrates localization of relaxin receptors (RXFP1 and RXFP2, respectively) to smooth muscle cell layers.

## Effect of relaxin on tissue remodeling and fibrosis pathways

### *Extracellular matrix proteins*

qPCR of cell lysate after 24 h of relaxin stimulation demonstrated no statistically significant change or discernible trend in expression for Collagen 1, Collagen 3, TGF-β1, TIMP-1, and TIMP-3. However, there did appear to be a dose dependent trend for MMP-2 and elastin that did not reach statistical significance. There was a dose dependent trend of upward expression for MMP-2 and a dose dependent downward trend in elastin expression. Refer to Fig. 4.

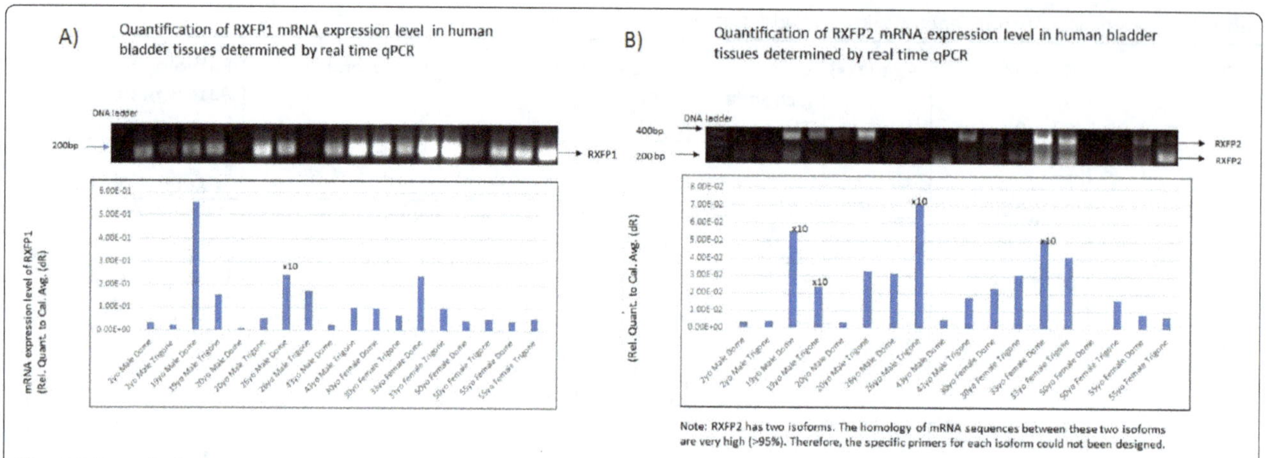


**Fig. 2** PCR results for Primary Human Bladders. **a** Primers amplified for RXFP1 demonstrate robust expression at the trigone, and dome. Quantification of expression was compared to PCR positive control of human vaginal epithelium. **b** Primers amplified for RXFP2 demonstrate amplification for all donors. Quantification of expression was compared to PCR positive control of human vaginal epithelium

***TGF-β1***

In cell lysate, there was increase in active TGF-β1 and total TGF-β1 at all concentrations used for relaxin stimulation. Relaxin stimulation at a concentration of 10 ng/mL resulted in a 19 fold change ($p < 0.005$) in active TGF-β1 and an 82 fold change ($p = 0.03$) for total TGF-β1. See Fig. 5a. These results contrast with supernatant and extracellular matrix where there was a decrease in active and total TGF-β1. In supernatant, active TGF-β1 had a 0.12 fold change at 1 ng/mL and 0.27 fold change at 100 ng/mL ($p < 0.005$, $< 0.005$, respectively) and for total TGF-β1 there was a 0.10 fold change at 1 ng/mL, and 0.08 fold change at 100 ng/mL ($p < 0.005$, $< 0.005$, respectively). In extracellular matrix, active TGF-β1 had a 0.08 change at 1 ng/mL, 0.54 fold change at 10 ng/mL, 0.09 fold change at 100 ng/mL ($p < 0.005$, $=0.01$, $< 0.005$, respectively) and for total TGF-β1 there was a 0.9 fold change at 10 ng/mL ($p = 0.01$).

***MMPs***

At 24 h of stimulation there was no discernable trend and no statistically significant change in protein expression or activity for active MMP2 ($p$ value range = 0.665 to 0.999). At 48 h there was no statistical change in active or latent MMP9 expression in cell lysate ($p$ value range: 0.06 to 0.294 for active MMP9, $p$ value range: 0.912 to 0938 for latent MMP9). In contrast, active and latent MMP2 expression increased in cell lysate and active MMP2 was increased in cell supernatant. See Fig. 5b. In supernatant active MMP2 had a 1.6 fold change at 10 ng/mL, and 1.7 fold change at 100 ng/mL ($p = 0.08$, $=0.04$, respectively). In cell lysate active MMP2 had a 1.4 fold change at 10 ng/mL, and 1.7 fold change at 100 ng/mL ($p = 0.02$, $< 0.005$, respectively). In cell lysate latent MMP2 had a 1.6 fold change at 100 ng/mL ($p = 0.03$, respectively). For cell lysate there was a dose dependent response with increased relaxin concentration resulting in increased MMP2 expression.

***TIMPs***

TIMP1 and TIMP3 expression was assessed in cell lysate at 48 h. There was no discernible trend for TIMP 3. In cell lysate there was an upward trend in TIMP1 expression. For TIMP-1 in cell lysate there was a 2.4 fold change at 1 ng/mL, 3.4 fold change at 10 ng/mL, and 2.1 fold change at 100 ng/mL ($p = 0.56$, $=0.16$, $=0.73$, respectively). Expression for TIMP-1 was also assessed in the supernatant at 48 h and did not demonstrate any trend or statistically significant change.

## Discussion

### Relaxin receptor expression in benign human bladder

Our results demonstrate RXFP1 and RXFP2 expression at the urothelium and muscularis propria within benign human bladder. Our in vitro data also provides preliminary evidence that relaxin signaling in bladder smooth muscle cells affects protein pathways involved in tissue remodeling and fibrosis. Further work is necessary to understand the role of relaxin signaling within urothelial cells. Urothelial signaling is an important component to overall bladder physiology and homeostasis. Urothelial pathways are regulated through mechanical stretch, and/or by molecules within the cellular and extracellular milieu, urine or blood. Molecular pathways that have been characterized for urothelial signaling include purinergic, muscarinic, nitric oxide, prostaglandin and nerve growth factor. These pathways affect cellular and neurovascular signaling within the lamina propria which in turn provides communication with the muscularis propria [20]. Given relaxin receptors ubiquity (dome and trigone and being present in all benign donor tissue), we suspect it plays a role in homeostatic bladder function. In addition

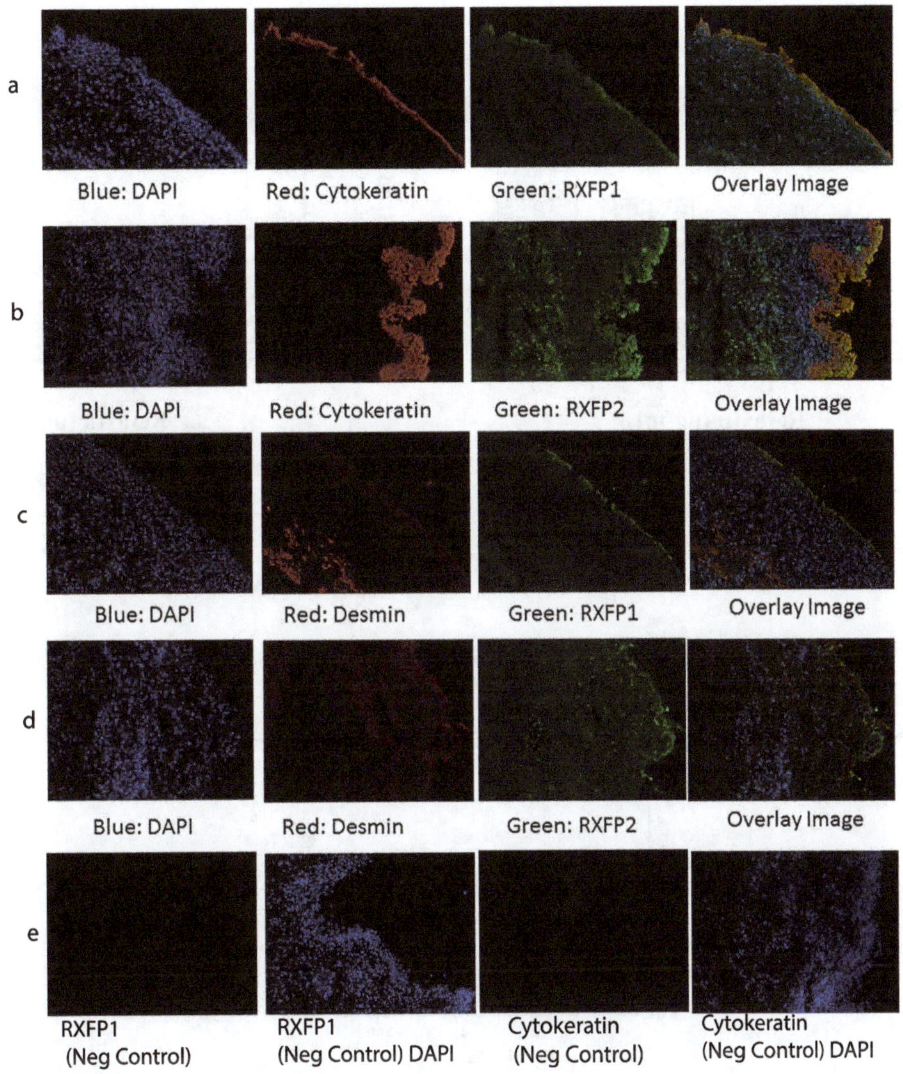


**Fig. 3 a** Immunofluorescence for RXFP1 and Cytokeratin demonstrating urothelial localization (**b**) Immunofluorescence for RXFP2 and Cytokeratin demonstrating urothelial localization (**c**) Immunofluorescence for RXFP1 and Desmin demonstrating localization to lamina propria and muscularis propria (**d**) Immunofluorescence for RXFP2 and Desmin demonstrating localization to lamina propria and muscularis propria (**e**) RXFP1 negative control (primary antibody omitted) with DAPI and Cytokeratin negative control (primary antibody omitted)

to directly influencing fibrotic pathways, changes in urothelial relaxin signaling may impact urothelial homeostatic pathways and ultimately contribute to a pathologic phenotype, such as fibrosis. Researchers have suggested that changes in urothelial cell proliferation, permeability of the urothelium, and recruitment of immune cells mediate pathologic change [21]. Neurovascular signaling can also be impacted and can result in pathologic muscle activity.

The significance of two relaxin receptors in the bladder remains to be elucidated. RXFP1 and RXFP2 have similar protein structure and regulate adenylate cyclase and cAMP [1]. There is evidence in an animal model looking at knee laxity that RXFP receptor expression can be influenced by hormones such as testosterone and estrogen [22]. Hormonal regulation may be one explanation for two relaxin receptors being present in the bladder. INSL3 (primary protein substrate for RXFP2 [23]) signaling may also explain the presence of two relaxin receptors in the bladder. INSL3 is found in both men and women and it is consistently detectable in men and varies by pubertal and menopausal status in women. Its role has been mostly characterized in testicular descent and germ cell maturation. However, it is now being studied in various organ systems and has been found to affect bone metabolism and is elevated in conditions such as polycystic ovarian syndrome [24]. Characterization of relaxin receptor function is ongoing, and within the human bladder it will be essential to identify overlap, synergy or antagonism of RXFP1 and RXFP2 signaling. Researchers

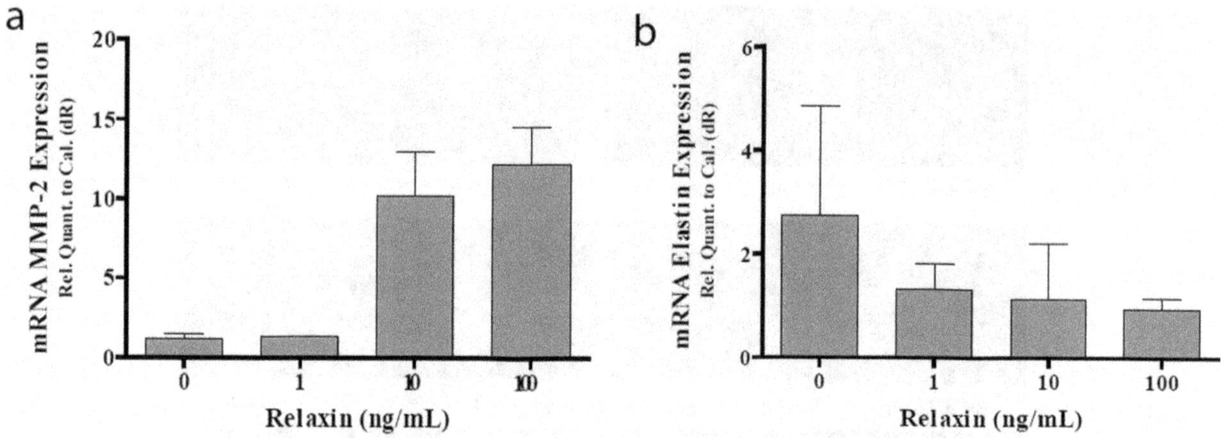


**Fig. 4** **a** mRNA MMP-2 Expression in 24 h Relaxin-2 treated human bladder smooth muscle cell lysate. **b** mRNA Elastin Expression in 24 h Relaxin-2 treated human bladder smooth muscle cell lysate

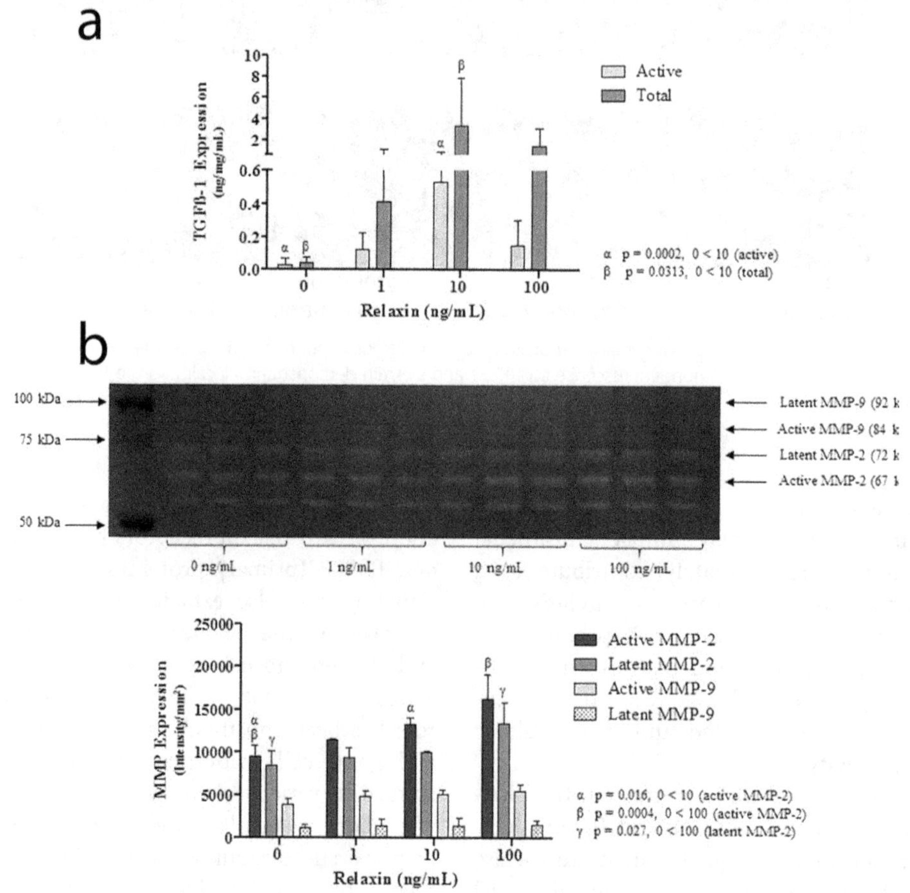


**Fig. 5** **a** TGF-beta 1 expression in cell lysate after 48 h of relaxin stimulation (**b**) MMP2 and MMP9 expression in cell lysate after 48 h of relaxin stimulation

have developed fluorochrome and radioisotope tagged relaxin 2 and INSL3 and small molecules to selectively target individual receptors [25]. These molecules will be useful tools for the future.

Characterization of relaxin receptor expression in normal human bladder also provides important information on the appropriate animal model for future studies. Ideally the chosen animal model would have similar relaxin/relaxin receptor interaction and receptor distribution as the human bladder. In the mouse model of radiation cystitis previously mentioned [11], the histologic evaluation of relaxin receptor distribution in the mouse did not conform to our findings of urothelial expression in the human bladder. The mouse model, however, does illustrate both RFXP1 and RXFP2 in bladder smooth muscle cells similar to humans. Given differences in receptor distribution between human and mouse bladders, further exploration into the role of these receptors within the urothelium and smooth muscle layers can help determine whether a murine model best reflects human physiology. Various researchers have been assessing an appropriate animal model to study relaxin receptor signaling. One group found that macaque and pig models to have the most promise [26], but there are groups that have recently developed a transgenic mouse model to further preclinical study of relaxin [27].

Localization of the relaxin receptors to the urothelium, lamina propria, and muscularis propria also has significant translational implications. This suggests that intravesical instillation may be a potential route of administration for relaxin. In theory this would have less side effects compared to systemic administration. Systemic side effects were problematic in the phase 3 clinical trial looking at relaxin treatment of scleroderma. In that trial, patients were treated systemically with relaxin through a subcutaneous infusion pump for 24 weeks. Abrupt withdrawal of the relaxin treatment resulted in hypertension and decreased creatinine clearance and also resulted in menorrhagia [5].

### In vitro relaxin stimulation on primary human bladder smooth muscle cells

There are many molecular pathways involved in fibrosis. Frequently studied extracellular proteins, and signaling cascades were evaluated in our study. Our goal was to assess whether relaxin can affect tissue remodeling pathways in bladder smooth muscle cells derived from a person without bladder pathology.

After 24 h of stimulation there was no effect on transcriptional levels of studied proteins. This may have been due to lack of time to affect molecular change. Twenty four hours of stimulation with relaxin also did not result in changes to protein expression or activity. However, 48 h of stimulation did result in statistically significant findings. Both active and latent forms of MMP-2 were noted to be upregulated with relaxin stimulation. This upregulation was not demonstrated for MMP-9. In the literature, active MMPs digest surrounding matrix and create binding sites and molecules that can further promote or inhibit various biologic effects. Activation of mitogen activated protein kinase (MAPK)1 and MAPK3 by denatured extracellular matrix results in proliferation of bladder smooth muscle cells in vitro [28]. This proliferative effect on smooth cells as well as the ability of MMP2 to contribute to the breakdown of collagen can be viewed as an antifibrotic effect if one considers a fibrotic bladder to have decreased detrusor muscle and increased collagen deposition. The combination of increased MMP2 and decreased TGF-β1 has previously been described as anti-fibrotic in studies looking at heart failure [2, 3].

Results of relaxin stimulation at 48 h demonstrated increased levels of active and total TGF-β1 in cell lysate but decreased levels in supernatant and ECM. TGF-β1 is found within the cell, supernatant, and ECM. In the cell it is synthesized as an inactive/latent form that require endoproteolytic modification and ultimately binding of a latency TGF-β1 binding protein (LTBP) before it is secreted and deposited in the ECM. Within the ECM, latent TGF-β1 is stored for later activation. In order for TGFβ-1 to become active and bind to its receptor on the cell it needs to be released from its LTBP [29]. Understanding the complex processing and activation of TGF-β1 can help one conjecture the seen effects with relaxin stimulation. Increasing levels of TGF-β1 cell lysate can be related to decrease secretion and intracellular retention of the protein. In addition the decrease in supernatant and ECM can be explained by the presence of increased protein inhibitors of TGF-β1. Overall our findings of inhibition of the TGF-β1 pathway is similar to findings seen in heart failure. Within cardiac fibroblasts relaxin's antifibrotic effect is believed to be due to inhibition of TGF-β1 Smad phosphorylation2 and inhibition of TGF-β1 Stat3 phosphorylation dependent autophagy [30].

## Conclusion

This data demonstrates the expression of relaxin receptors in the human bladder and that it localizes to both the urothelium, lamina propria, and muscularis propria and is expressed at both the trigone and dome of male and females of various age groups. Relaxin stimulation on normal human bladder smooth muscle cells affects expression of proteins involved in tissue remodeling and fibrosis. Further work is necessary to assess the role of relaxin and its receptors in pathologic bladder states.

**Authors' contributions**

ED developed the idea of investigating relaxin in the human bladder, developed protocol for bladder tissue procurement and procured primary bladder tissue, and drafted the manuscript. BC helped design the study, served as a faculty mentor to ED, and provided lab space and personnel. CK provided pathology review of primary bladder specimens and provided Fig. 1 of the manuscript. MB, and YW designed and performed assays described in the methods section with the assistance of GZ, AD and SW. MB and YW also compiled the data, analyzed the data, and created figures and drafted the Methods section for the manuscript. All authors reviewed the manuscript and provided critical review and editing.

**Acknowledgements**

Stanford University and our research team express our thanks for the cooperation of Donor Network West and all of the organ and tissue donors and their families, for giving the gift of life and the gift of knowledge, by their generous donation.

**Author details**

[1]Department of Urology, Stanford University Medical Center, 300 Pasteur Drive, Grant S-287, Stanford, CA 94305, USA. [2]Present Address: Division of Pediatric Urology, Advocate Children's Hospital, 8901 West Golf Road, Suite 301, Des Plaines, IL 60016, USA. [3]Department of Obstetrics and Gynecology, Stanford University Medical Center, 300 Pasteur Drive, Rm A370, MC 5317, Stanford, CA 94305, USA. [4]Department of Pathology, Stanford University Medical Center, 300 Pasteur Drive, Rm L235, Stanford, CA 94305, USA.

**References**

1. Bathgate RA, Halls ML, van der Westhuizen ET, et al. Relaxin family peptides and their receptors. Physiol Rev. 2013;93(1):405–80.
2. Sassoli C, Chellini F, Pini A, et al. Relaxin prevents cardiac fibroblast-myofibroblast transition via notch-1-mediated inhibition of TGF-β/Smad3 signaling. PLoS One. 2013;8(5). Article ID: e63896.
3. Samuel CS, Zhao C, Bathgate RA, et al. The relaxin gene-knockout mouse: a model of progressive fibrosis. Ann N Y Acad Sci. 2005;1041:173–81.
4. Teerlink JR, Cotter G, Davison BA, et al. RELAXin in acute heart failure (RELAXAHF) investigators. Serelaxin, recombinant human relaxin-2, for treatment of acute heart failure (RELAX-AHF): a randomised, placebo-controlled trial. Lancet. 2013;381(9860):29–39.
5. Khanna D, Clements PJ, Furst DE, et al. Relaxin Investigators and the Scleroderma Clinical Trials Consortium.. Recombinant human relaxin in the treatment of systemic sclerosis with diffuse cutaneous involvement: a randomized, double-blind, placebo controlled trial. Arthritis Rheum. 2009; 60(4):1102–11.
6. Tan J, Tedrow JR, Dutta JA, et al. Expression of RXFP1 Is Decreased in Idiopathic Pulmonary Fibrosis. Implications for Relaxin-based Therapies. Am J Respir Crit Care Med. 2016;194(11):1392–402.
7. Aitken KJ, Bägli DJ. The bladder extracellular matrix. Part I: architecture, development and disease. Nat Rev Urol. 2009;6(11):596–611.
8. Deveaud CM, Macarak EJ, Kucich U, et al. Molecular analysis of collagens in bladder fibrosis. J Urol. 1998;160(4):1518–27.
9. Djavan B, Lin V, Kaplan EP, et al. Decreased elastin gene expression in noncompliant human bladder tissue: a competitive reverse transcriptase-polymerase chain reaction analysis. J Urol. 1998;160(5):1658–62.
10. Fusco F, Creta M, De Nunzio C, et al. Progressive bladder remodeling due to bladder outlet obstruction: a systematic review of morphological and molecular evidences in humans. BMC Urol. 2018;18(1):15.
11. Ikeda Y, Zabbarova IV, Birder LA, et al. Relaxin-2 therapy reverses radiation induced fibrosis and restores bladder function in mice. Neurourol Urodyn. 2018;37(8):2441–51.
12. Lee JH, et al. The effect of raloxifene, a SERM, on extracellular matrix protein expression of pelvic fibroblasts. Int Urogynecol J. 2012;23(3):349–55.
13. Li Y, et al. Cell sex affects extracellular matrix protein expression and proliferation of smooth muscle progenitor cells derived from human pluripotent stem cells. Stem Cell Res Ther. 2017;8(1):156.
14. Mazella J, Tang M, Tseng L. Disparate effects of relaxin and TGFbeta1: relaxin increases, but TGFbeta1 inhibits, the relaxin receptor and the production of IGFBP-1 in human endometrial stromal/decidual cells. Hum Reprod. 2004;19(7):1513–8.
15. Wen Y, Polan ML, Chen BC. Do extracellular matrix protein expressions change with cyclic reproductive hormones in pelvic connective tissue from women with stress urinary incontinence? Hum Reprod. 2006;21(5):1266–73.
16. Wen Y, et al. Reprogramming of fibroblasts from older women with pelvic floor disorders alters cellular behavior associated with donor age. Stem Cells Transl Med. 2013;2(2):118–28.
17. Wen Y, et al. Effect of relaxin on TGF-beta1 expression in cultured vaginal fibroblasts from women with stress urinary incontinence. Reprod Sci. 2008;15(3):312–20.
18. Pedrozo HA, et al. Potential mechanisms for the plasmin-mediated release and activation of latent transforming growth factor-beta1 from the extracellular matrix of growth plate chondrocytes. Endocrinology. 1999; 140(12):5806–16.
19. Taipale J, et al. Latent transforming growth factor-beta 1 associates to fibroblast extracellular matrix via latent TGF-beta binding protein. J Cell Biol. 1994;124(1–2):171–81.
20. Birder LA, Ruggieri M, Takeda M, et al. How does the urothelium affect bladder function in health and disease? Neurourol Urodyn. 2012;31(3):293–9.
21. Keay SK, Birder LA, Chai TC. Evidence for bladder urothelial pathophysiology in functional bladder disorders. Biomed Res Int. 2014. Article ID: 865463.
22. Dehghan F, Muniandy S, Yusof A, Salleh N. Testosterone reduces knee passive range of motion and expression of relaxin receptor isoforms via 5α-dihydrotestosterone and androgen receptor binding. Int J Mol Sci. 2014; 15(3):4619–34.
23. Hsu SY, Nakabayashi K, Nishi S, et al. Activation of orphan receptors by the hormone relaxin. Science. 2002 Jan 25;295(5555):671–4.
24. Ivell R, Anand-Ivell R. Insulin-like peptide 3 (INSL3) is a major regulator of female reproductive physiology. Hum Reprod Update. 2018;6:639–51.
25. Xiao J, Huang Z, Chen CZ, et al. Identification and optimization of small-molecule agonists of the human relaxin hormone receptor RXFP1. Nat Commun. 2013;4:1953.
26. Huang Z, Myhr C, Bathgate RA, et al. Activation of Relaxin family receptor 1 from different mammalian species by Relaxin peptide and small-molecule agonist ML290. Front Endocrinol (Lausanne). 2015;6. Article ID: 128.
27. Kaftanovskaya EM, Soula M, Myhr C, et al. Human Relaxin receptor is fully functional in humanized mice and is activated by small molecule agonist ML290. J Endocr Soc. 2017;1(6):712–25.
28. Herz DB, Aitken K, Bagli DJ. Collagen directly stimulates bladder smooth muscle cell growth in vitro: regulation by extracellular regulated mitogen activated protein kinase. J Urol. 2003;170:2072–6.
29. Hyytiäinen M, Penttinen C, Keski-Oja J. Latent TGF-beta binding proteins: extracellular matrix association and roles in TGF-beta activation. Crit Rev Clin Lab Sci. 2004;41(3):233–64.
30. Yuan Y, Zhang Y, Han X, et al. Relaxin alleviates TGFβ1-induced cardiac fibrosis via inhibition of Stat3-dependent autophagy. Biochem Biophys Res Commun. 2017;493(4):1601–7.

# 20

# Intravesical gemcitabine versus mitomycin for non-muscle invasive bladder cancer

Rongxin Li[1†], Ye Li[1†], Jun Song[1,2†], Ke Gao[1], Kangning Chen[1], Xiaogang Yang[1], Yongqiang Ding[1], Xinlong Ma[1], Yang Wang[1], Weipeng Li[1], Yanan Wang[1], Zhiping Wang[1] and Zhilong Dong[1*]

## Abstract

**Background:** Mitomycin (MMC) has been frequently used as the compound for intravesical treatment. The relatively new pyrimidine analog gemcitabine (GEM) has exhibited anticancer effect on various solid cancers, such as the advanced bladder cancer. In this study, the GEM and MMC in treating non-muscle invasive bladder cancer (NMIBC) cases was compared through systemic review.

**Methods:** In accordance with the Preferred Reporting Items for Systematic Reviews and Meta-Analyses (PRISMA) statement, the electronic databases, including Embase, PubMed, Chinese biomedicine literature database, the Cochrane Library, the National Institute for Health and Clinical Excellence, NHS Evidence, Chinese technological periodical full-text database, and Chinese periodical full-text database, were systemically reviewed from inception to October 2018. Then, the RevMan 5.0 software was applied for data analysis. Five randomized controlled trials (RCTs) involving a total of 335 patients were included.

**Results:** For MMC group, the recurrence rate in the mitomycin arm increased compared with that in GEM group (OR = 0.44 95% CI [0.24, 0.78]), and the difference was statistically significant between the two groups. GEM was associated with reduced incidence of chemical cystitis compared with that of MMC (OR = 0.23 95% CI [0.12, 0.44]). Differences in hematuria (OR = 0.46 95% CI [0.16, 1.31]), skin reaction (OR = 0.49 95% CI [0.14, 1.70]) and liver and kidney function damage (OR = 0.51 95% CI [0.09, 2.85]) displayed no statistical significance between the two groups.

**Conclusion:** Findings in our study demonstrate the superior efficacy of GEM over MMC in reducing the relapse rate among NMIBC patients following transurethral resection (TUR). In addition, GEM is associated with reduced local toxic effects on the bladder compared with those of MMC. However, more future studies are needed to examine GEM safety when used as the monotherapy or polytherapy for bladder patients. More RCTs with high quality are also required to validate our findings due to the limitations of the current meta-analysis.

**Keywords:** Bladder cancer, Gemcitabine, Mitomycin, Systematic evaluation, Meta-analysis

* Correspondence: 562691313@qq.com
†Rongxin Li, Ye Li and Jun Song made equal contribution to this manuscript and should be regarded as co-first authors.
[1]Lanzhou University Second Hospital, Lanzhou City, Gansu Province, China
Full list of author information is available at the end of the article

## Background

Bladder cancer has become a common cancer worldwide, and 430,000 new cases and over 165,000 deaths are reported in 2012 [1]. Transitional cell carcinoma is dominant in bladder cancer, in addition, adenocarcinoma (cancer originating from the mucus-making and releasing cells) and squamous cell carcinoma (cancer originating from the thin and flat cells) are also observed [2]. Generally, bladder cancer is associated with the following symptoms, frequent urination, bloody urine (rendering the slight rusty to deep red color of urine), urination pain, or urination sensation with no urine indeed [3].

The incidences of bladder cancer in male and female are reported to be 3.4 and 1.2%, respectively, however, that in patients aged over 70 years is twice to thrice higher than that among patients aged 55–65 years, and 15 to 20 times greater than for patients aged 30–54 years [4]. As estimated by the World Health Organization, there were 132,432 bladder cancer-related deaths in the world in 2000 [5].

About 80% bladder cancers are non-muscle invasive bladder cancers (NMIBC) restricted to the urothelium (clinical stage Ta) or lamina propria (stage T1) at first, which is featured by the in-situ flat carcinoma (stage Tis) [6]. Tumor relapse following transurethral resection (TUR) has been identified as a main issue in treating non-muscle invasive bladder cancer. Specifically, the mechanisms regarding NMIBC relapse following TUR are shown as follows, (1) residual tumor originated from the incomplete resection; (2) floating cancer cell implantation in traumatized bladder sites; (3) incidence of new neoplasm due to high cancer aggressiveness; (4) relapses at the urothelial instability sites (atypia, hyperplasia and dysplasia) [7]; (5) over 50–70% tumor relapse since no adjuvant treatment is given, and approximately 15% cases develop muscle-invasive cancers eventually [8].

The intravesical chemotherapy has been considered as the standard treatment for patients receiving following TUR to eradicate underlying disorders, inhibit cancer relapse, prevent tumor development and extend patient survival [9]. Mitomycin (MMC) is a frequently used compound in intravesical treatment. In addition, gemcitabine (GEM), the relatively new pyrimidine analog, displays anticancer effect on various solid cancers, such as the advanced bladder cancer [10]. MMC and GEM have been classically used as the cytotoxic agents for affecting the DNA integrity, but these two display distinctly different mechanisms of action. Among them, GEM, the difluoro-2, 2-deoxy-cytidine, can be activated upon the stimulation of deoxycytidine kinase, meanwhile, its phosphorylated metabolites may impact the synthesis of deoxy-nucleotide through resulting in DNA injuries and interfering with DNA repair [11]. On the other hand, MMC can be triggered within cancer cells through forming the reducing equivalents, thereby affecting cancer cell replication through forming the damage-induced DNA adducts [12]. Nonetheless, it remains unclear about the efficacy and side effects between the two agents. In this regard, the current systematic review was carried out aiming to evaluate the therapeutic effects and safety between GEM versus MMC on treating NMIBC patients.

## Methods

### Search strategy

In accordance with Preferred Reporting Items for Systematic Reviews and Meta-Analyses (PRISMA) statement [13], the electronic databases, including Embase, PubMed, Chinese biomedicine literature database, the Cochrane Library, the National Institute for Health and Clinical Excellence, NHS Evidence, Chinese periodical full-text database, and Chinese technological periodical full-text database, were systemically reviewed from inception to October 2018 to identify the randomized controlled trials (RCTs) that compared the efficacy and safety of GEM and MMC in treating NMIBC cases. Additionally, the critical Chinese magazines in relevant fields were also retrieved manually, corresponding search engines were employed to identify the relevant references, and each reference in the enrolled articles was retrieved as well to discover other possible relevant publications. Related terms were used for study retrieval. Moreover, the reference lists from those enrolled articles and reviews were also manually retrieved, and experts in this field were contacted if necessary, while those non-published articles were not found. The study retrieval was not restricted by language.

In this study, the following search terms were used in retrieval strategy, including intravesical pharmacotherapy, non-muscle invasive bladder cancer, gemcitabine and mitomycin, so as to find out the titles and abstracts of relevant studies. To be specific, the entire retrieval strategy adopted in the current work for the PubMed database included (irrigation of bladder OR intravesical therapy OR bladder instillation OR intravesical instillation OR intravesical infusion OR infusion of bladder) AND (non-muscle-invasive bladder cancer OR NMIBC OR non-muscle invasive bladder cancer OR superficial bladder cancer) AND (GEM OR gemcitabine) AND (MMC OR mitomycin OR mitomycin-c).

### Data collection

Two researchers independently reviewed those retrieved titles and abstracts in accordance with the study inclusion criteria, and the inappropriate articles were excluded. Any disagreement between them was settled down through the opinion from a third author. Afterwards, data were extracted by the same authors independently by the use of the uniform data collection forms. Besides, the evaluated quality items included the concealment of allocation, randomization, blinding (subjects, researchers, outcome measures, data analysis), as well as follow-up completeness [14].

#### Inclusion and exclusion criteria

The study inclusion criteria were shown as follows: (1) randomized controlled trials (RCTs) as well as quasi-RCTs (namely, RCTs adopting the quasi-random method for participating allocation into various intervention groups); (2) studies that comprised medium- to high-risk patients (with high-grade papillary stage Ta or T1 tumors and any patient with carcinoma in situ) who occupies 15–44% NMIBC cases in certain series [15]; (3) studies that mentioned clinical outcomes, Ta or T1 tumor and included patients receiving intravesical gemcitabine comparing with mitomycin.

The study exclusion criteria were as follows: (1) non-RCTs; (2) studies in which cases with other neoplasm; (3) studies with incomplete information to analysis; (4) duplicate articles.

#### Outcome measure types

Tumor relapse rate, and local side effects (including chemical cystitis, hematuria, skin reaction, and liver and kidney function damage).

#### Intervention types

Intravesical treatment with GEM or MMC following TUR.

#### Statistical analysis

All dichotomous outcomes (such as recurrence, mortality, progression of tumor staging, distant metastasis, systemic and local adverse reaction, treatment delay or withdrawal) were presented in the manner of relative risk (RR) and the corresponding 95% confidence intervals (CI). The data were extracted and pooled using the random-effects model. For guaranteeing our model robustness and outlier susceptibility, we also adopted the fixed-effect model for analysis. The statistical heterogeneities across different trials were tested using the chi-square heterogeneity test while the inconsistency degree was assessed by $I^2$ statistic, with the threshold of $p =$ 0.10, and $p < 0.1$ indicated the presence of statistical heterogeneity across various studies. Thereafter, subgroup analyses, sensitivity analysis, and the random effects model were carried out in the presence of heterogeneity. The potential heterogeneity sources were explored through subgroup analysis. The putative factor impacts on the effect size were explored through sensitivity analysis. The descriptive approaches were adopted for tabulating and assessing the adverse effects, as they were possibly distinct for our examined agents.

## Results

#### Search results

Figure 1 displays the study retrieval and screening procedure. A total of 213 preliminary studies were retrieved initially, among which, 208 were ruled out from this study later. Finally, 5 RCTs including 335 cases were included [16–20], all of which mentioned outcomes including recurrence rate and toxicity evaluation (chemical cystitis, hematuria, skin reaction, and liver and kidney function damage).

#### Included study features and quality

Table 1 displays the enrolled study features and quality. Table 2 presents the patient features and drug administration schedule.

#### Meta-analysis results

##### *Treatment efficacy*

For MMC group, the recurrence rate increased compared with that of GEM group (OR = 0.44 95% CI [0.24, 0.78]), and the difference was of statistical significance between the two groups, as shown in Figs. 2 and 3.

##### *Adverse effects*

Five trials reported the local adverse effects. The most commonly reported adverse effects in both groups were chemical cystitis (OR = 0.23 95% CI [0.12, 0.44]), hematuria (OR = 0.46 95% CI [0.16, 1.31]), skin reaction (OR = 0.49 95% CI [0.14, 1.70]) and liver and kidney function damage (OR = 0.51 95% CI [0.09, 2.85]). According to our results, GEM was associated with reduced local toxicity relative to mitomycin. Overall, these two doses were well tolerable among a majority of cases with reduced adverse reactions.

## Discussion

Meta-analysis is an approach adopted to statistically pooled and examined the findings from several independent RCTs [21]. NMIBC is generally associated with favorable clinical outcomes, but it is refractory due to the increased tumor relapse rate following TUR. As a matter of fact, 40–85% cases develop tumor relapse in 2–5 years following standardized TUR, while approximately 10% among such relapse patients are at the more advanced grade and stage [22]. In clinical practice, TUR is performed prior to intravesical injection with chemotherapeutic or the agents for modulating immunity, so as to lower the bladder cancer relapse and development.

Various anti-cancer agents are administered intravesically to prevent tumor relapse, which is validated as

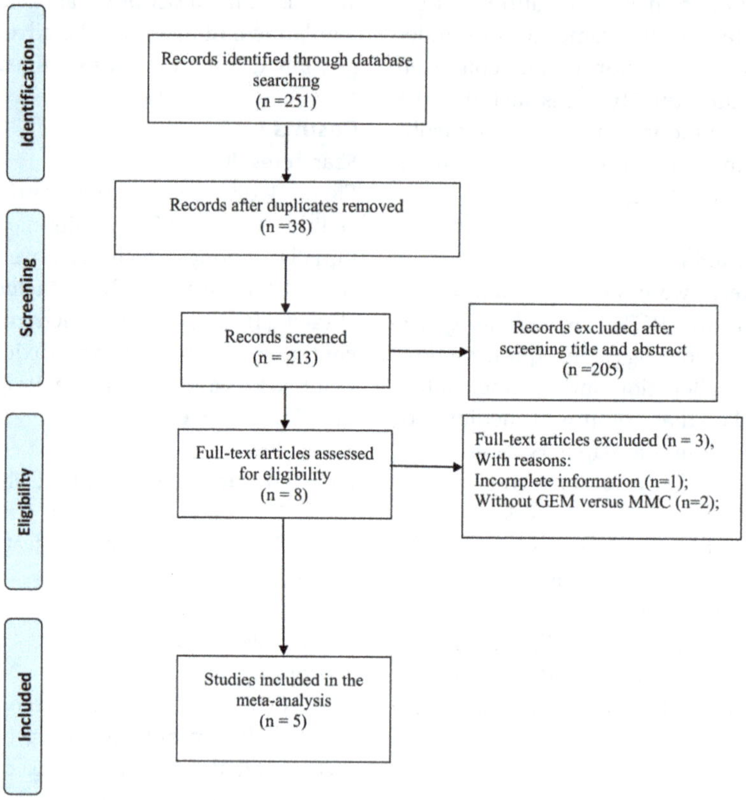


**Fig. 1** PRISMA flow diagram: the study selection process

effective. The classical intravesical agents, Bacille Calmette-Guérin (BCG) as well as MMC are effective on postponing and lowering the postoperative tumor relapse rate; nonetheless, they are also associated with obvious adverse reactions and may be ineffective for some cases. Based on clinical research, GEM is effective on reducing the relapse of non-muscle invasive bladder cancer with lower toxicity, which deserves more investigation [23]. In this study, the meta-analysis was carried out to examine the intravesical GEM and MMC safety and efficacy among the NMIBC patients on the basis of the five enrolled clinical trials including 335 bladder cancer cases. Three of those 5 articles mentioned disease grade and stage [17, 19, 20]. Our results showed that the recurrence rate of MMC group increased compared with that of GEM group (OR = 0.44 95% CI [0.24, 0.78]), and the difference was statistically significant between the two groups; besides, GEM led to a lower incidence of chemical cystitis than MMC (OR = 0.23 95% CI [0.12, 0.44]). But differences in the incidences of hematuria (OR = 0.46 95% CI [0.16, 1.31]), skin reaction (OR = 0.49 95% CI [0.14, 1.70]) and liver and kidney function damage (OR = 0.51 95% CI [0.09, 2.85]) were not statistically significant between the two groups., suggesting that GEM had lower toxicity than MMC. Overall, these two doses were well-tolerable among a majority of cases with lower adverse reactions. Nonetheless, the above conclusions must be interpreted carefully and validated in more articles.

For the low risk disorder, post-operative intravesical MMC treatment is still the vital part of intravesical therapy, meanwhile, there is level-one evidence to prove the

**Table 1** The quality and characteristics of included studies

| Study | Randomization | Allocated Concealment | Blinding | Gemcitabine (sample size) | Mitomycin (sample size) | Grade |
|---|---|---|---|---|---|---|
| Dong 2017 [16] | adequate | not used | clear | 12 | 16 | **C** |
| Lin 2016 [17] | adequate | not used | clear | 42 | 42 | **C** |
| Sun 2016 [18] | adequate | used | clear | 30 | 28 | **B** |
| Xiaohong 2015 [19] | adequate | not used | clear | 27 | 29 | **C** |
| Raffaele 2010 [20] | adequate | used | clear | 54 | 55 | **B** |

**Table 2** Characteristics of studies and the schedule of drug administration among the included studies

| Study | Cases | Sex(M/F) | Age (year) | Type of patients | Stage | Grade | Comparison | Dosage of intervention | Follow-up |
|---|---|---|---|---|---|---|---|---|---|
| Dong 2017 [16] | 28 | NA | NA | NMIBC | NA | NA | GEM | 1000 mg weekly for 8 weeks followed by monthly instillations | 12 months |
| | | | | | | | MMC | 20 mg weekly for 8 weeks followed by monthly instillations | |
| Lin 2016 [17] | 84 | 56/28 | GEM:61 ± 4.2<br>MMC:62 ± 3.5 | NMIBC | Tis: 3<br>Ta: 24<br>T1: 59 | G1: 40 G2: 27<br>G3: 17 | GEM | 1000 mg weekly for 8 weeks followed by monthly instillations (a total of 1 year or 2 years) | 24 months |
| | | | | | | | MMC | 30 mg weekly for 8 weeks followed by monthly instillations (a total of 1 year or 2 years) | |
| Sun 2016 [18] | 58 | 45/13 | GEM: 37 ~ 83<br>MMC: 31 ~ 81 | NMIBC | NA | NA | GEM | 1000 mg weekly for 8 weeks followed by 10 monthly instillations (a total of 1 year) | 2 years |
| | | | | | | | MMC | 20 mg weekly for 8 weeks followed by 10 monthly instillations (a total of 1 year) | |
| Xiaohong 2015 [19] | 56 | 45/11 | GEM:51.26 ± 13.42<br>MMC:51.64 ± 12.39 | NMIBC | Tis: 1<br>Ta: 10<br>T1: 45 | G1: 13 G2: 41<br>G3: 2 | GEM | 1000 mg weekly for 8 weeks followed by 10 monthly instillations (a total of 1 year) | 1 year |
| | | | | | | | MMC | 40 mg weekly for 8 weeks followed by 10 monthly instillations (a total of 1 year) | |
| Raffaele 2010 [20] | 109 | 93/16 | GEM: 64.9 ± 10.5<br>MMC: 67.9 ± 10.2 | NMIBC | Ta: 72<br>T1: 37 | G1: 25<br>G2: 55<br>G3: 29 | GEM | 2000 mg weekly for 6 weeks followed by 10 monthly infusion during the first year | 36 months |
| | | | | | | | MMC | 40 mg weekly for 4 weeks followed by 10 monthly infusion during the first year | |

*M* Male, *F* Female, *NMIBC* Non-muscle invasive bladder cancer, *GEM* Gemcitabine, *MMC* Mitomycin, *NA* Not Available (Insufficient Information Provided)

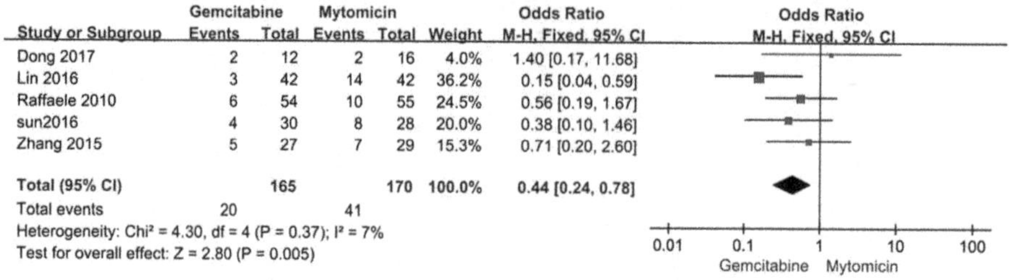


**Fig. 2** Recurrence rates: gemcitabine versus mitomycin

effectiveness of GEM on bladder cancer, yet it has not been recommended in guidelines [24]. Many therapeutic methods are effective on the treatment of NMIBC cases. The intravesical chemotherapy using MMC and GEM has achieved certain favorable results [25]. Gemcitabine is an effective pyrimidine antimetabolite, with only mild toxicity relative to other chemotherapeutic agents [26]. According to Messing EM et al. [27], for the low-grade NMIBC cases ($n = 215$), those receiving intravesical GEM treatment following TUR were associated with the 4-year tumor relapse rate of 34%, while that in the saline-alone control group was 54%. In addition, 5 cases of GEM group and 10 in control group progressed to muscle invasive bladder cancer, and 17 of GEM group as well as 25 of saline group died. Based on Dalbagni et al., for the 30 BCG-refractory NMIBC cases (including uncontrollable Ta, multiple unresected T1, and refractory cancer in situ) who underwent intravesical GEM treatment regularly, 50% achieved a complete response (CR), and adverse effects were reported among 23% cases with a very low toxicity [28]. Moreover, according to Bartoletti et al., no 1-year tumor relapse was reported among 18 out of the 24 medium-risk patients, as well as among 9 out of the 16 high-risk BCG-refractory cases (pTa ~ pT1) treated with weekly intravesical GEM therapy. In that study, no side effect was reported in 94 of the 116 patients in the 1-year treatment process [29]. Jones et al. reviewed 6 GEM treatment-related RCTs in their

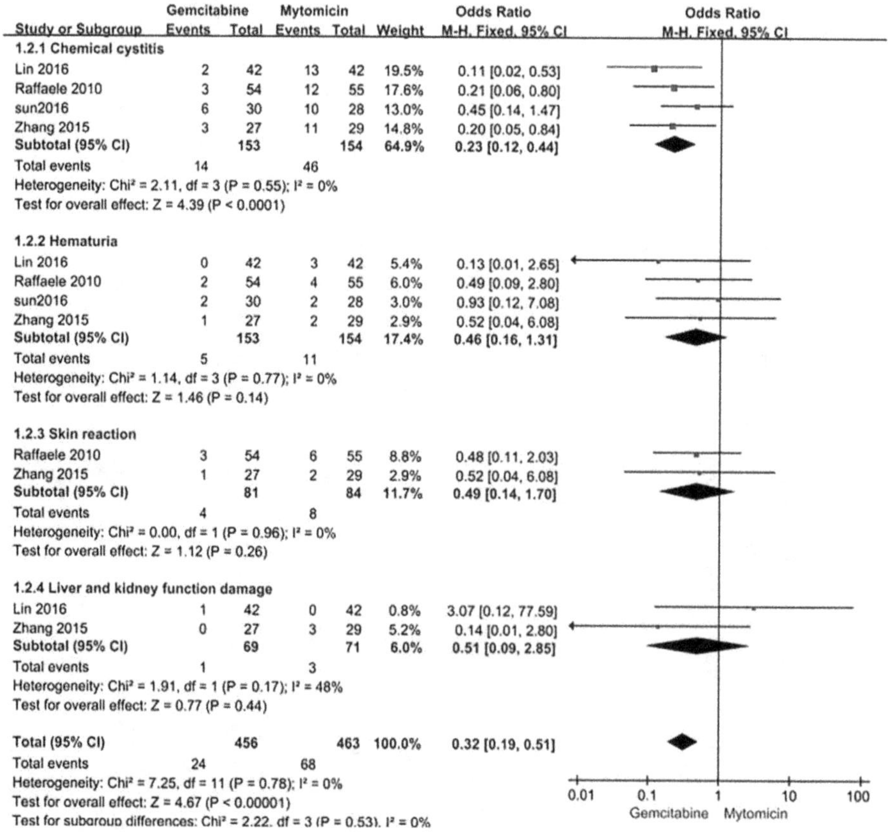


**Fig. 3** Local side effects: gemcitabine versus mitomycin

Cochrane review, and indicated that, intravesical GEM treatment potentially exerted an important part in managing NMIBC cases with moderate and high risk, particularly when it was adopted to be the alternative to MMC for high-risk cases [30].

Auxiliary intravesical treatment can lower the relapse and development rates of NMIBC in the meantime of inducing local and systemic adverse reactions. In terms of the toxic effects, chemical cystitis, hematuria, skin reaction, and liver and kidney function damage were observed in 0–30% cases of each group. The frequency of these side effects of GEM arm markedly decreased compared with that of MMC arm. Such findings validated that, chemical cystitis, the irritable symptom in lower urinary tract, stands for the typical MMC side reaction [31]. GEM led to minimal local toxicity, which was self-resolved rapidly. By contrast, MMC treatment resulted in the more serious local toxicity that required treatment delay. On the other hand, economic influence is also a factor potentially affecting the treatment decision-making. Recently, the mean sales price for 40 mg MMC markedly increases compared with that for 2 g GEM, suggesting that the GEM-based intravesical chemotherapy is advantageous over MMC in price [32].

Some limitations should be noted in the current meta-analysis: 1) the risk of tumor relapse was not compared between GEM and MMC of Ta or T1 group due to the limited total sample size, so more high-quality RCTs should be carried out. 2) The administration does and schedules of these two agents were similar among those five enrolled studies, but the conclusion might be disturbed by the clinical heterogeneity because of the differences in operating methods, like whether the positional changes were allowed, as well as the duration of each infusion. 3) All included RCTs in the current review did not apply the double-blinding method, which might potentially impact our results. 4) The publication bias was not totally ruled out, which possibly led to conclusion distortion.

## Conclusions

In conclusion, our meta-analysis supports that GEM can be a potential agent of intravesical therapy with better efficiency than MMC in preventing recurrence of patients with non-muscle invasive bladder cancer after TUR. At the same time, we observed that GEM produce lower local toxic effects than MMC during intravesical therapy. In addition, more studies are needed to examine the GEM safety, and more high-quality RCTs are warranted to validate our conclusions due to the limitations.

#### Abbreviations

BCG: Bacille Calmette-Guérin; CI: Confidence intervals; GEM: Gemcitabine; MMC: Mitomycin C; NMIBC: Non-muscle-invasive bladder cancers; PRISMA: Preferred Reporting Items for Systematic Reviews and Meta-Analyses; RCTs: Randomized controlled trials; TUR: Transurethral resection

#### Acknowledgments

None.

#### Authors' contributions

WZP, DZL, LRX and SJ were responsible for study conception and design. LRX, LY, and SJ were in charge of manuscript writing and editing. LRX, GK, CKN, DYQ, YXG, MXY, and WY contributed to data collection. LRX, GK, CKN, DYQ, YXG, MXY, WY, LWP, and WYN were responsible for data management/analysis. Each of the author had carefully read and approved the final manuscript for publication.

#### Author details

[1]Lanzhou University Second Hospital, Lanzhou City, Gansu Province, China.
[2]Sanya People's Hospital, Sanya City, Hainan Province, China.

#### References

1. Antoni S, Ferlay J, Soerjomataram I, et al. Bladder Cancer incidence and mortality: a global overview and recent trends. Eur Urol. 2017;71:96–108.
2. Tanaka T, Miyazawa K, Tsukamoto T, Kuno T, Suzuki K. Pathobiology and chemoprevention of bladder Cancer. J Oncol. 2011;2011:528–53.
3. Cabello MJ, Grau L, Franco N, Orenes E, Alvarez M, Blanca A, Heredero O, Palacios A, Urrutia M, Fernández JM, López-Beltrán A, Sánchez-Carbayo M. Multiplexed methylation profiles of tumor suppressor genes in bladder Cancer. J MolDiagn. 2011;13:29–40.
4. Pasbos CL. Bladder cancer, epidemiology, diagnosis, and management. Cancer Pract. 2002;10:311–22.
5. Ferlay J, Bray F, Pisani P, Parkin DM. GLOBOCAN 2000: Cancer incidence, mortality and prevalence worldwide. IARC CancerBase no. 5. Lyon: IARC Press; 2001.
6. Uekado Y, Hirano A, Shinka T, Ohkawa T. The effects of intravesical chemoimmunotherapy with epirubicin and bacillus Calmette-Guerin for prophylaxis of recurrence of superficial bladder cancer: a preliminary report. Cancer Chemother Pharmacol. 1994;35:65–8.
7. Ray ER, O'Brien TS. Approaches to reducing recurrence in superficial bladder cancer. Eur Kidney Urol Dis. 2006;1:1–6.
8. Herr HW, Laudone VP, Whitmore WF Jr. An overview of intravesical therapy for superficial bladder tumors. J Urol. 1987;138:1363–8.
9. Whelan P. The treatment of non-muscle-invasive bladder Cancer with Intravesical chemotherapy and immunotherapy. Eur Urol Suppl. 2007;6:568–71.
10. Stadler WM, Kuzel T, Roth B, et al. Phase II study of single-agent gemcitabine in previously untreated patients with metastatic urothelial cancer. J Clin Oncol. 1997;15:3394–8.
11. Plunkett W, Huang P, Searcy CE, et al. Gemcitabine: preclinical pharmacology and mechanisms of action. Semin Oncol. 1996;23:3–15.
12. Joudi FN, O'Donnel MA. Second-line intravesical therapy versus cystectomy for Bacile Calmette-Gue'rin (BCG) failure. Curr Opin Urol. 2004;14:271–5.
13. Liberati A, Altman DG, Tetzlaff J, et al. The PRISMA statement for reporting systematic reviews and meta-analyses of studies that evaluate health care interventions: explanation and elaboration. J Clin Epidemiol. 2009;62(10):e1–e34.
14. Dong ZL, Yang KH, Liu YL, Mi DH, Wang ZP, Tian JH. Intravesical doxorubicin versus epirubicin for superficial bladder cancer. Cochrane Database Syst Rev. 2010, Issue 1. Art. No.:CD008181. https://doi.org/10.1002/14651858.CD008181.
15. Oosterlinck. Guidelines on bladder cancer. Eur Urol. 2002;41:105–12.
16. Dong X, Song L, Zhang F. Curative effect analysis of different chemotherapeutics at intravesical instillation in the prevention of tumor recurrence after TUR-Bt. Zhejiang J Traumat Surg. 2017;22:109–10.
17. Lin T, Sun L. Comparison of the efficacy of different chemotherapy drugs in the prevention of postoperative recurrence in superficial bladder cancer by intravesical instillation. China Foreign Med Treat. 2016;35:118–9.
18. Sun S, Liu R, Zhao H, et al. Comparison of intravesical perfusion of gemcitabine and mitomycin after non-muscle invasive bladder cancer. J Med Theory Pract. 2016;29:3238–9.

19. Xiaohong Z, Tan J, Wei Y, et al. Clinical effect of antineoplastic drug perfusion in preventing postoperative recurrence of superficial bladder cancer. J Chin Physician. 2015;17:1043–5.
20. Addeo R, Caraglia M, Bellini S, et al. Randomized phase III trial on gemcitabine versus Mitomycin in recurrent superficial bladder Cancer: evaluation of efficacy and tolerance. J Clin Oncol. 2010;28:543–8.
21. Lau J, Ioannidis JP, Schmid CH. Summing up evidence: oneanswer is not always enough. Lancet. 1998;351:123–7.
22. Shariat SF, Chade DC, Karakiewicz PI, Scherr DS, Dalbagni G. Update on intravesical agents for non-muscle-invasive bladder cancer. Immunotherapy, vol. 2; 2010. p. 381–92.
23. Shelley MD, Jones G, Cleves A, et al. Intravesical gemcitabine therapy for non-muscle invasive bladder cancer (NMIBC): a systematic review. BJU Int. 2012;109:496–505.
24. Peyton CC, Chipollini J, Azizi M, et al. Updates on the use of intravesical therapies for non-muscle invasive bladder cancer: how, when and what. World J Urol. 2018. https://doi.org/10.1007/s00345-018-2591-1.
25. Stein JP, Lieskovsky G, Cole R, et al. Radical cystectomy in the treatment of invasive bladder cancer: long term results in 1054 patients. J Clin Oncol. 2001;19:666–75.
26. Schlack K, Boegemann M, Steinestel J, Schrader AJ, Krabbe LM. The safety and efficacy of gemcitabine for the treatment of bladder cancer. Expert Rev Anticancer Ther. 2016;16:255–71.
27. Messing EM, Tangen CM, Lerner SP, et al. Effect of Intravesical instillation of gemcitabine vs saline immediately following resection of suspected low-grade non-muscle-invasive bladder Cancer on tumor recurrence: SWOG S0337 randomized clinical trial. JAMA. 2018;319(18):1880–8.
28. Dalbagni G, Russo P, Bochner B, et al. Phase II trial of intravesical gemcitabine in bacille Calmette Guerin-refractory transitional cell carcinoma of the bladder. J Clin Oncol. 2006;24:2729–34.
29. Bartoletti R, Cai T, Gacci M, et al. Intravesical gemcitabine therapy for superficial transitional cell carcinoma: results of a phase II prospective multicenter study. Urology. 2005;66:726–31.
30. Bolenz C, Cao Y, Arancibia MF, et al. Intravesical mitomycin C for superficial transitional cell carcinoma. Expert Anticancer Ther. 2006;6:1273–82.
31. Jones G, Cleves A, Wilt TJ, Mason M, Kynaston HG, Shelley M. Intravesical gemcitabine for non-muscle invasive bladder cancer. Cochrane Database Syst Rev. 2012;1:CD009294 Published 2012 Jan 18.
32. Centers for Medicare & Medicaid Services. 2020 ASP Drug Pricing Files. https://www.cms.gov/medicare/medicare-part-b-drug-average-sales-price/2020-asp-drug-pricing-files. Accessed 5 Jan 2020.

# 21

# The effects of oral administration of the novel muscarinic receptor antagonist DA-8010 on overactive bladder in rat with bladder outlet obstruction

Jin Bong Choi[1], Seung Hwan Jeon[2], Eun Bi Kwon[3], Woong Jin Bae[4], Hyuk Jin Cho[2], U-Syn Ha[2], Sung-Hoo Hong[2], Ji Youl Lee[2] and Sae Woong Kim[4*]

**Abstract**

**Background:** DA-8010 is a novel compound developed for the treatment of overactive bladder (OAB) and urinary incontinence. The aims of this study were to investigate the effects of DA-8010 on OAB in a rat model.

**Methods:** Study animals were divided into the following five groups of seven animals each: a sham-operated control group, a control group with partial bladder outlet obstruction (BOO) (OAB group), and three DA-8010 (doses of 0.3 mg/kg/day, 1 mg/kg/day, and 3 mg/kg/day, respectively) with partial BOO groups. Oral administration of the drugs was continued for 14 days after 2 weeks of partial BOO. After 4 weeks of partial BOO, cystometrography was performed in all groups. Additionally, pro-inflammatory cytokines, Rho-kinases, and histology of the bladder were analyzed.

**Results:** There was a significant increase in the contraction interval and a decrease in contraction pressure in the 3 mg/kg/day DA-8010 group versus those in the OAB group. Rho kinase was also significantly decreased in the DA-8010 3 mg/kg/day dosage treatment group. The increased ratio of collagen to smooth muscle after partial BOO was significantly attenuated in the DA-8010 3 mg/kg/day dosage group.

**Conclusions:** Oral administration of DA-8010 at 3 mg/kg/day improved findings in an OAB rat model induced by partial BOO. Our results suggest that the novel muscarinic receptor antagonist DA-8010 may be a promising drug for treating patients with OAB.

**Keywords:** Bladder outlet obstruction, Muscarinic antagonists, Overactive bladder

## Background

Overactive bladder (OAB), a syndrome characterized by urgency (with or without urge incontinence), frequency, and nocturia, is common in both men and women and increases in prevalence with age [1]. Because the mean age of the population worldwide is increasing, OAB is causing an increase in socioeconomic costs and has adverse effects on quality of life [2].

Treatment with antimuscarinic and behavioral therapy is one of the first-line management methods for patients with OAB. These drugs inhibit the binding of acetylcholine to the muscarinic receptor in the detrusor muscle and urothelium during detrusor contraction. Examples of these drugs include oxybutynin, tolterodine, trospium, darifenacin, solifenacin, fesoterodine, propiverine, and

* Correspondence: ksw1227@catholic.ac.kr
[4]Department of Urology, Seoul St. Mary's Hospital, College of Medicine, The Catholic University of Korea, Seoul, Republic of Korea and Catholic Integrative Medicine Research Institute, The Catholic University of Korea, Banpo-daero 222, Seocho-gu, Seoul 06591 Seoul, Republic of Korea
Full list of author information is available at the end of the article

flavoxate. While anticholinergics can be effective in OAB, they also carry risk of various complications, such as dry mouth, constipation, acute urinary retention, and visual disturbance. Furthermore, long-term use also increases the risk of psychological problems [3–5]. Therefore, there is a need for new OAB treatments that demonstrate high efficacy and fewer side effects.

DA-8010 ((R)-(1-methylpyrrolidin-3-yl) methyl (3′-chloro-4′-fluoro-[1,1′-biphenyl]-2-yl)carbamate) is a novel compound that has been developed by the Dong-A ST Pharmaceutical Company (Yongin, Korea) for the treatment of OAB and urinary incontinence [6]. DA-8010 is a highly potent $M_3$ antagonist and has appeared more highly selective for the urinary bladder over the salivary glands, large intestine, and heart in preclinical studies compared with other antimuscarinic agents [6]. The aim of this study was to investigate the effects of DA-8010 on OAB in a rat model.

## Methods

### Experimental animals and treatment

Male Sprague-Dawley rats weighing 250 g to 300 g were obtained from Orient Bio Co., Ltd. (Seongnam, Kyeonggi, South Korea) and were randomly divided into five groups of seven animals each. The rats were fed standard rat food and had free access to food and water in an animal room maintained at a constant temperature (18–22 °C) and humidity (40–60%) with a 12-h light/dark cycle. These groups were (1) a sham-operated control group, (2) a partial bladder outlet obstruction (BOO) control group (OAB group), (3) a DA-8010 (0.3 mg/kg/day) with partial BOO group, (4) a DA-8010 (1 mg/kg/day) with partial BOO group, and (5) a DA-8010 (3 mg/kg/day) with partial BOO group. The drugs, which were dissolved in 1 ml of distilled water, were orally administered once a day for 14 days at 2 weeks after BOO in each group.

### Transperitoneal ligation of the urethra

As stated, our OAB rat model was induced by partial BOO. This method has been widely used for the analysis of detrusor overactivity (DO) in rat models. In this study, partial BOO was surgically induced through a transperitoneal approach, as previously described [7, 8]. A 25-gauge polyethylene tube was placed on top of the urethral-vesical junction and ligated using 3–0 silk with similar forces in all rats. The tube was then removed to create a partial BOO.

### Cystometrography

Cystometrography was performed in all groups with the animals in an anesthetized state after 2 weeks of oral drug administration. After exposure of the bladder by a midline lower abdominal incision, a 25-gauge needle connected to a polyethylene tube was inserted through the bladder dome. The polyethylene tube was connected to a pressure transducer and a syringe pump via 3-way stopcock [9]. Saline was infused at a rate of 0.04 mL/min after emptying the bladder, and the nonvoiding contractions during the filling phase of cystometry were measured. The contraction interval and detrusor pressure were recorded on a polygraph through the use of a pressure recording catheter. Uninhibited detrusor contraction was assessed during the 2 min from 4 min before voiding contraction, and contractions were defined by an amplitude higher than 4 cm of $H_2O$ from baseline pressure [10]. At the end of the cystometrography, the rats were sacrificed under sodium pentobarbital anesthesia according to the Guide for the Care and Use of Laboratory Animals [11].

### Western blot analysis

After bladder tissue was ground into powder, the protein was extracted through cell lysis and quantified with the Thermo Scientific Pierce BCA Protein Assay Kit (Thermo Fisher Scientific Waltham, MA, USA). Briefly, 60 μg of quantitative proteins were boiled in loading buffer containing sodium dodecyl sulfate, 100 mM of dithiothreitol, 0.01% bromophenol blue, and 62.6 mM of Tris hydrochloride adjusted to pH 6.8. After sodium dodecyl sulfate polyacrylamide gel electrophoresis, the proteins were moved to Hybond® ECL™ nitrocellulose membranes (Amersham Biosciences, Little Chalfont, UK). The membranes were blocked with 5% nonfat milk in Tris-buffered saline containing 0.1% Tween® 20 (Sigma-Aldrich, St. Louis, MO, USA). Next, the membranes were probed with antibodies against RhoA, Rho-associated protein kinase (ROCK)-I, ROCK-II (BD Pharmingen, San Diego, CA, USA), and β-actin (Santa Cruz Biotechnology, Dallas, TX, USA). After the membranes were washed, they were probed with horseradish peroxidase secondary antibodies (Santa Cruz Biotechnology, Dallas, TX, USA). Expression levels were measured by the density of the bands using a luminescent image analyzer (Fujifilm, Tokyo, Japan) [12].

### Cytokine analyses

To investigate the anti-inflammatory effects of the treatment, we analyzed the levels of interleukin (IL)-6 and IL-8 cytokines. The supernatant was obtained via centrifugation of the blood for 10 min at 3000 rpm. The cytokine concentration was measured using a spectrophotometer with an enzyme-linked immunosorbent assay kit (R&D Systems, Minneapolis, MN, USA) [13].

### Histologic analysis

Bladder tissue samples were fixed with 4% paraformaldehyde for 1 day and then embedded in paraffin. After that, slice sections were made for Masson's trichrome staining for bladder tissue observation. The color distribution was measured using Image-Pro® Plus (Media Cybernetics Inc., Rockville, MD, USA), and the ratio of collagen to smooth muscle was calculated [14].

### Statistical analysis

All data are expressed as the mean ± standard error. Statistical analysis was conducted using SPSS version 22.0 software (IBM Corp., Armonk, NY, USA). Experimental groups were compared using analysis of variance with Tukey's multiple comparison test for post hoc analysis, and $P$ values < 0.05 were considered significant.

## Results

### Cystometrography

The contraction intervals and the contraction pressure in the 3 mg/kg/day DA-8010 group were significantly different from those in the OAB group (Table 1). After 2 weeks of oral medication, the contraction pressure of the OAB group was significantly greater than that of the control group ($P < 0.01$). Additionally, the contraction pressure of the 3 mg/kg/day DA-8010 group was significantly lower than that of the OAB group ($P < 0.05$). Reductions in contraction pressure were also observed in the 0.3 mg/kg/day and 1 mg/kg/day DA-8010 groups, but these changes were not statistically significant. The contraction interval of the OAB group was significantly lower than that of the control group ($P < 0.01$), while the contraction interval of the 3 mg/kg/day DA-8010 group was significantly greater than that of the OAB group ($P < 0.05$). Increases in the contraction interval were also observed in the other DA-8010 (i.e., the 0.3 mg/kg/day and 1 mg/kg/day dosage) groups, but these changes were not statistically significant.

### Western blot analysis

The OAB group showed significantly higher expression of RhoA, ROCK-I, and ROCK-II in the bladder than did the control group ($P < 0.01$). These levels were significantly lower in the 3 mg/kg/day DA-8010 group than in the OAB group ($P < 0.05$). However, there were no statistically significant changes in the other DA-8010 groups receiving 0.3 mg/kg/day or 1 mg/kg/day dosage (Fig. 1).

### Pro-inflammatory cytokine levels

Significantly higher levels of IL-6 and IL-8 were noted in the OAB group than in the control group ($P < 0.01$). After administration of 3 mg/kg/day of DA-8010, a significant decrease in IL-6 and IL-8 levels was observed compared with those in the OAB group ($P < 0.05$). There were no statistically significant changes in the DA-8010 groups receiving 0.3 mg/kg/day or 1 mg/kg/day (Fig. 2).

### Histologic analysis

The ratio of collagen to smooth muscle identified by image analysis was higher in the OAB group than in the control group, indicating increased bladder fibrosis. However, after 3 mg/kg/day DA-8010 treatment, this increased ratio was attenuated significantly ($P < 0.05$). There were no statistically significant changes in either the 0.3 mg/kg/day DA-8010 group or the 1 mg/kg/day DA-8010 group (Fig. 3).

## Discussion

$M_3$ muscarinic receptors are well known to play a predominant role in mediating bladder muscle, although both the $M_2$ and $M_3$ muscarinic receptor subtypes are located on bladder smooth muscle [15, 16]. DA-8010 is a highly potent $M_3$ antagonist with a high binding affinity for the human $M_3$ muscarinic receptor, with a pKi of 8.81 ± 0.05, and is more highly selective for the urinary bladder over the salivary glands compared with other antimuscarinic agents. Intravenous single-dose administration of DA-8010 (0.03 mg/kg and 0.1 mg/kg) demonstrated beneficial effects on the DO induced by partial BOO in conscious rats, with a significant increase in micturition intervals and micturition volume [17]. Therefore, the high potency and selectivity of DA-8010 are expected to provide therapeutic benefit with a lesser frequency/degree of side effects than that observed with other antimuscarinic agents. We observed the functional efficacy of DA-8010 on OAB in a rat model in this study. The main findings were as follows: (1) there was a significant increase in contraction interval and a decrease in contraction pressure in the 3 mg/kg/day DA-8010 group, and (2) the increased ratio of collagen to smooth muscle after partial BOO was significantly attenuated in the 3 mg/kg/day DA-8010 group.

**Table 1** The contraction intervals and the contraction pressure during continuous infusion cystometry

| Parameters | Control | OAB | DA-8010 (0.3 mg) | DA-8010 (1 mg) | DA-8010 (3 mg) |
|---|---|---|---|---|---|
| Contraction interval (seconds) | 60.81 ± 14.84 | 6.97 ± 2.95[a] | 9.22 ± 4.03 | 20.89 ± 8.31 | 22.51 ± 10.89[b] |
| Contraction pressure ($cmH_2O$) | 34.35 ± 11.83 | 51.83 ± 17.95[a] | 46.81 ± 16.38 | 42.09 ± 15.59 | 38.82 ± 17.31[b] |

Data are presented as the mean ± standard error
*Abbreviations*: *OAB* overactive bladder
[a]*P* value < 0.01, OAB group vs. control group
[b]*P* value < 0.05, DA-8010 (3 mg) group vs. OAB group

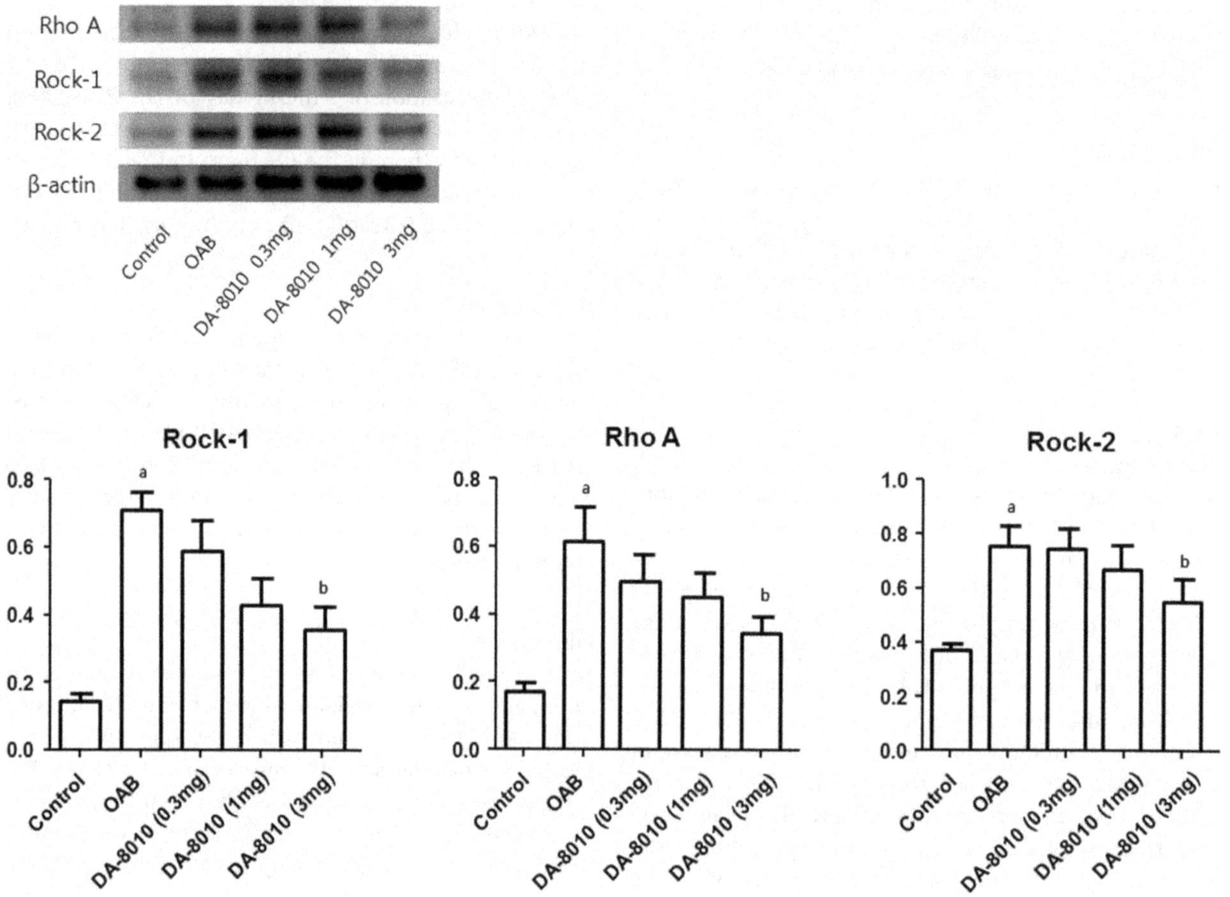


**Fig. 1** Comparison of RhoA, ROCK-I, and ROCK-II. [a]$P < 0.01$ compared with the control group; [b]$P < 0.05$ compared with the OAB group

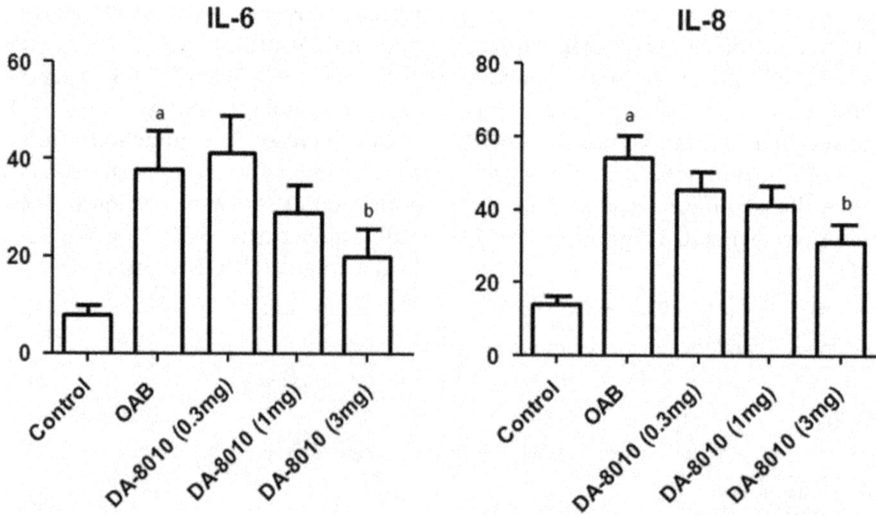


**Fig. 2** Comparison of cytokines. [a]$P < 0.01$ compared with the control group; [b]$P < 0.05$ compared with the OAB group

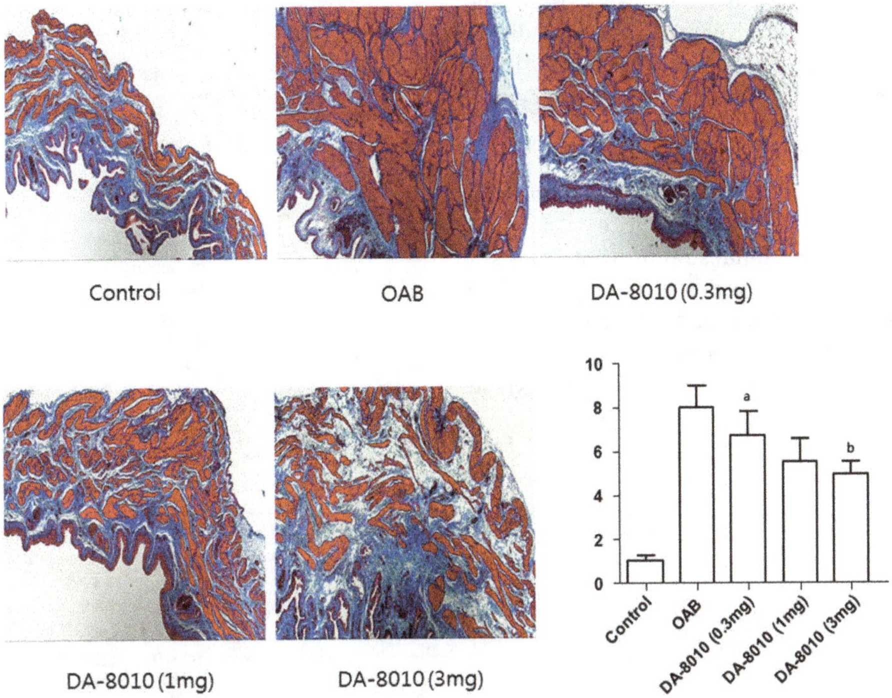


**Fig. 3** Comparison of histologic findings and the ratio of collagen to smooth muscle among the five groups. [a]$P < 0.01$ compared with the control group; [b]$P < 0.05$ compared with the OAB group

Because of the legal and ethical problems associated with using human materials for research, much of our understanding of human voiding function has come from research using animal models [18]. In particular, BOO in humans can be surgically replicated in animal models. Experimental partial BOO in rats is known to increase bladder weight and alter voiding patterns, with changes in central and peripheral nerve control [19]. The most common method to prompt OAB in rats is by inducing partial BOO by silk ligation around the urethra through a transperitoneal approach. In previous reports, bladder pressures, maximal voiding pressure, and frequency of nonvoiding contractions started to increase after 2 weeks of partial BOO using this method [20, 21].

The present study revealed differences in Rho-kinase activity between the OAB group and DA-8010 treatment groups. Rho-kinase was discovered in 1996 by Amano et al. [22]. Kureishi et al. reported that Rho-kinase modulates smooth muscle contraction directly through myosin light-chain phosphorylation without increasing the intracellular $Ca^{2+}$ concentration [23]. Rho-kinase is activated by RhoA GTPase, and RhoA is regulated by guanine nucleotide exchange factors (GEFs), GTPase-activating proteins (GAPs), and guanine nucleotide dissociation inhibitors (GDIs). GEFs are activated by cell stimulation, including that of the muscarinic acetylcholine receptor [24], especially the muscarinic acetylcholine $M_3$ receptor, which activates phospholipase C, stimulates RhoA GTPase activity and induces bladder contraction directly [25]. Therefore, the novel muscarinic receptor antagonist DA-8010 could decrease the expression of RhoA, ROCK-I, and ROCK-II in the bladder.

Pro-inflammatory cytokines such as IL-6 and IL-8 have been reported to be increased in bladders with DO induced by BOO [12, 26]. A clinical study reported that solifenacin improves inflammation by decreasing the levels of inflammatory cytokines [27]. Our results showed that these mechanisms are similar to those of DA-8010. In addition, the inflammatory response due to partial BOO can eventually produce decompensation to fibrosis [28]. Our histologic analysis also revealed that DA-8010 decreased bladder fibrosis significantly compared to BOO alone. These results suggest that DA-8010, by decreasing the inflammatory responses, may have an anti-fibrotic effect.

However, our study has some limitations. First, although we ligated the urethra-vesical junction with similar forces in all rats to produce partial BOO, dominant DO might not have been formed in all rats. Second, changes in bladder function after partial BOO vary with time. Maciejewski et al. reported on urodynamic outcomes in a partial BOO rat model. Outcomes were assessed after four, eight, 12, and 16 weeks, with results indicating an initial increase in bladder capacity and compliance at 4 weeks, followed by a steady decline [21]. Our study investigated urodynamic findings after only

4 weeks of partial BOO. For this reason, we were unable to quantify changes in the urodynamic findings at different stages during the experimental period. Thus, long-term and more detailed preclinical studies are needed.

## Conclusions

OAB is a chronic disease that not only lowers quality of life but is also difficult to treat, although it is not life-threatening. In this study, administration of a 3 mg/kg/day dose of DA-8010 improved the findings of DO induced by partial BOO in a rat model. Our results suggest that the novel muscarinic receptor antagonist DA-8010 could be a promising option for treating OAB in patients.

### Abbreviations

OAB: Overactive bladder; BOO: Bladder outlet obstruction;; DO: Detrusor overactivity; ROCK: Rho-associated protein kinase; IL: Interleukin

### Acknowledgements

Not applicable.

### Authors' contributions

Participated in the conception and initial design: JBC and SWK. Participated in the analysis and interpretation: HJC, USH, SHH, JYL, JBC and WJB. Participated in the drafting of the manuscript: JBC and SWK. Participated in data analysis: SHJ and EBK. All authors reviewed and edited the manuscript and approved the final version of the manuscript.

### Author details

[1]Department of Urology, Bucheon St. Mary's Hospital, College of Medicine, The Catholic University of Korea, Seoul, Republic of Korea. [2]Department of Urology, Seoul St. Mary's Hospital, College of Medicine, The Catholic University of Korea, Seoul, Republic of Korea. [3]Korea Bio Medical Science Institute, Seoul, Republic of Korea. [4]Department of Urology, Seoul St. Mary's Hospital, College of Medicine, The Catholic University of Korea, Seoul, Republic of Korea and Catholic Integrative Medicine Research Institute, The Catholic University of Korea, Banpo-daero 222, Seocho-gu, Seoul 06591 Seoul, Republic of Korea.

### References

1. Abrams P, Cardozo L, Fall M, Griffiths D, Rosier P, Ulmsten U, et al. The standardisation of terminology in lower urinary tract function: report from the standardisation sub-committee of the international continence society. Urology. 2003;61:37–49.
2. Sung W, You H, Yoon TY, Lee SJ. Socioeconomic costs of overactive bladder and stress urinary incontinence in Korea. Int Neurourol J. 2012;16:23–9.
3. Fox C, Smith T, Maidment I, Chan WY, Bua N, Myint PK, et al. Effect of medications with anti-cholinergic properties on cognitive function, delirium, physical function and mortality: a systematic review. Age Ageing. 2014;43: 604–15.
4. Lam S, Hilas O. Pharmacologic management of overactive bladder. Clin Interv Aging. 2007;2:337–45.
5. Ruxton K, Woodman RJ, Mangoni AA. Drugs with anticholinergic effects and cognitive impairment, falls and all-cause mortality in older adults: a systematic review and meta-analysis. Br J Clin Pharmacol. 2015;80:209–20.
6. Lee MJ, Moon JH, Lee HK, Cho CH, Choi SH, Im WB. Pharmacological characterization of DA-8010, a novel muscarinic receptor antagonist selective for urinary bladder over salivary gland. Eur J Pharmacol. 2019;843: 240–50.
7. Jin LH, Andersson KE, Han JU, Kwon YH, Park CS, Shin HY, et al. Persistent detrusor overactivity in rats after relief of partial urethral obstruction. Am J Physiol Regul Integr Comp Physiol. 2011;301:R896–904.
8. Kim WH, Bae WJ, Park JW, Choi JB, Kim SJ, Cho HJ, et al. Development of an improved animal model of overactive bladder: Transperineal ligation versus Transperitoneal ligation in male rats. World J Mens Health. 2016;34:137–44.
9. Kim SJ, Jeon SH, Kwon EB, Jeong HC, Choi SW, Bae WJ, et al. Improvement of persistent detrusor Overactivity through treatment with a Phytotherapeutic agent (WSY-1075) after relief of bladder outlet obstruction. World J Mens Health. 2018;36:153–60.
10. Nishiguchi J, Kwon DD, Kaiho Y, Chancellor MB, Kumon H, Snyder PB, et al. Suppression of detrusor overactivity in rats with bladder outlet obstruction by a type 4 phosphodiesterase inhibitor. BJU Int. 2007;99:680–6.
11. National Research Council Committee for the Update of the Guide for the C, Use of Laboratory A. The National Academies Collection: Reports funded by National Institutes of Health. In: th, editor. Guide for the Care and Use of Laboratory Animals. Washington (DC): National Academies Press (US) National Academy of Sciences.; 2011.
12. Kim SJ, Jeon SH, Kwon EB, Jeong HC, Choi SW, Bae WJ, et al. Improvement of persistent detrusor Overactivity through treatment with a Phytotherapeutic agent (WSY-1075) after relief of bladder outlet obstruction. World J Mens Health. 2018;36(2):153–60.
13. Yoon BI, Bae WJ, Kim SJ, Kim HS, Ha US, Sohn DW, et al. The anti-inflammatory effects of a new herbal formula (WSY-1075) in a nonbacterial prostatitis rat model. World J Mens Health. 2013;31:150–6.
14. Bae WJ, Ha US, Choi JB, Kim KS, Kim SJ, Cho HJ, et al. Protective effects of KH-204 in the bladder of androgen-deprived rats. World J Mens Health. 2015;33:73–80.
15. Eglen RM, Hegde SS, Watson N. Muscarinic receptor subtypes and smooth muscle function. Pharmacol Rev. 1996;48:531–65.
16. Ehlert FJ, Ostrom RS, Sawyer GW. Subtypes of the muscarinic receptor in smooth muscle. Life Sci. 1997;61:1729–40.
17. Choo MS, Moon J-H, Lee HK, Lee MJ, Lee SH, Han JH, et al. MP94-14 urodynamic evaluation of da-8010 in conscious rats with partial bladder outlet obstruction. J Urol. 2017;197:e1251.
18. Gillespie JI. A developing view of the origins of urgency: the importance of animal models. BJU Int. 2005;96(Suppl 1):22–8.
19. Lluel P, Duquenne C, Martin D. Experimental bladder instability following bladder outlet obstruction in the female rat. J Urol. 1998;160:2253–7.
20. Lai H, Tan B, Liang Z, Yan Q, Lian Q, Wu Q, et al. Effect of the Chinese traditional prescription Suo Quan wan on TRPV1 expression in the bladder of rats with bladder outlet obstruction. BMC Complement Altern Med. 2015; 15:424.
21. Maciejewski CC, Tredget EE, Metcalfe PD. Urodynamic improvements following oral medical therapy for partial bladder outlet obstruction in an animal model. Neurourol Urodyn. 2015;34:286–91.
22. Amano M, Ito M, Kimura K, Fukata Y, Chihara K, Nakano T, et al. Phosphorylation and activation of myosin by rho-associated kinase (rho-kinase). J Biol Chem. 1996;271:20246–9.
23. Kureishi Y, Kobayashi S, Amano M, Kimura K, Kanaide H, Nakano T, et al. Rho-associated kinase directly induces smooth muscle contraction through myosin light chain phosphorylation. J Biol Chem. 1997;272:12257–60.
24. Rossman KL, Der CJ, Sondek J. GEF means go: turning on RHO GTPases with guanine nucleotide-exchange factors. Nat Rev Mol Cell Biol. 2005;6:167–80.
25. Schneider T, Fetscher C, Krege S, Michel MC. Signal transduction underlying carbachol-induced contraction of human urinary bladder. J Pharmacol Exp Ther. 2004;309:1148–53.
26. Matsui T, Oka M, Fukui T, Tanaka M, Oyama T, Sagawa K, et al. Suppression of bladder overactivity and oxidative stress by the phytotherapeutic agent, Eviprostat, in a rat model of atherosclerosis-induced chronic bladder ischemia. Int J Urol. 2012;19:669–75.
27. Zhang B, Wei J, Wu X, Wang L, Huo H, Wang J. Clinical optimal dose of solifenacin succinate for nursing patients after transurethral resection of the prostate during the perioperative period. Exp Ther Med. 2018;15:1660–5.
28. Metcalfe PD, Wang J, Jiao H, Huang Y, Hori K, Moore RB, et al. Bladder outlet obstruction: progression from inflammation to fibrosis. BJU Int. 2010; 106:1686–94.

22

# The five primary prostaglandins stimulate contractions and phasic activity of the urinary bladder urothelium, lamina propria and detrusor

Zane Stromberga, Russ Chess-Williams and Christian Moro*

**Abstract**

**Background:** Inflammation is often associated with several bladder dysfunctions, including overactive bladder (OAB) and interstitial cystitis/bladder pain syndrome (IC/PBS). As such, inflammation of the bladder and the actions of inflammatory mediators may contribute to the development of urinary symptoms. This study assessed the actions of $PGE_2$, $PGF_2$, $PGD_2$, $TXA_2$, and $PGI_2$ on urinary bladder urothelium with lamina propria (U&LP), and detrusor smooth muscle.

**Methods:** Studies were carried out using isolated tissue baths, where strips of porcine bladder U&LP or detrusor were exposed to varying concentrations of prostaglandin agonists (1 μM and 10 μM).

**Results:** All assessed prostaglandin agonists contracted both the U&LP and detrusor smooth muscle, with the rank order of contractile response effectiveness as: $PGE_2 > PGF_{2\alpha} > TXA_2 > PGD_2 > PGI_2$. In U&LP, treatment with $PGE_2$ (10 μM) increased tonic contractions by $1.36 \pm 0.09$ g ($n = 42$, $p < 0.001$) and phasic contractions by $40.4 \pm 9.6\%$ ($n = 42$, $p < 0.001$). In response to $PGF_{2\alpha}$ (10 μM), U&LP tonic contractions increased by $0.79 \pm 0.06$ g ($n = 14$, $p < 0.001$) and phasic activity by $13.3\% \pm 5.3\%$ ($n = 15$, $p < 0.05$). In detrusor preparations, $PGE_2$ (10 μM) increased tonic contractions by $1.32 \pm 0.13$ g ($n = 38$, $p < 0.001$) and $PGF_{2\alpha}$ (10 μM) by $0.97 \pm 0.14$ g ($n = 12$, $p < 0.001$). Only 34% ($n = 48$) of all detrusor preparations exhibited spontaneous activity prior to the addition of any agonist at a frequency of $2.03 \pm 0.12$ cpm. In preparations that did not exhibit initial phasic activity, all of the prostaglandin agonists were capable of commencing phasic activity.

**Conclusions:** The urinary bladder U&LP and detrusor respond to a variety of prostaglandin agonists, with their activation resulting in direct contractions, as well as increases to spontaneous contractile activity. This study presents the prostaglandin receptor system as a potential therapeutic target for lower urinary tract dysfunction.

**Keywords:** Inflammation, Prostaglandins, Urinary bladder, Urothelium, Detrusor

* Correspondence: cmoro@bond.edu.au
Centre for Urology Research, Faculty of Health Sciences and Medicine, Bond University, Gold Coast, Queensland 4226, Australia

## Background

The involvement of prostaglandins in bladder physiology was first recognised from their release after urinary bladder distension or injury to the urothelium [1, 2]. An increase of prostaglandins in the urine of patients suffering from OAB has been well-reported previously [3–6], suggesting the prostaglandin system as a potential future therapeutic target in various bladder dysfunctions. The exact role and mechanisms of endogenous prostaglandins in the urinary bladder are not well understood. However, previous studies utilising exogenous prostaglandins have shown that these chemicals can alter contractility and micturition reflex in human bladders [7].

Prostaglandin production is generally low in healthy tissue but can increase immediately following acute inflammation [8]. They are synthesised in the bladder by cyclooxygenase (COX) and then subsequently converted into five primary prostanoids via their respective synthases: $PGE_2$, $PGD_2$, $PGF_{2\alpha}$, prostacyclin ($PGI_2$) and thromboxane ($TXA_2$) [9]. Prostaglandins are synthesised in both the bladder urothelium with lamina propria (U&LP) and in detrusor smooth muscle in response to stretch, nerve stimulation, U&LP damage or other inflammatory mediators [10, 11]. The production of prostaglandins is determined by the cells present at sites of inflammation capable of synthesising prostaglandins and the activity of the two cyclooxygenase isoenzymes, namely COX-1 and COX-2. For example, macrophages predominantly generate $PGE_2$ and $TXA_2$, whereas mast cells produce $PGD_2$ [12]. COX-1 is present in most cells, whereas the expression of COX-2 is generally low in cells, but can increase dramatically upon stimulation by immune cells [13]. Prostaglandin $I_2$ is the main prostaglandin synthesised in the human bladder, followed by $PGE_2$, $PGF_{2\alpha}$ and $TXA_2$ [14, 15].

Although past studies have explored the effects of the different prostaglandins on the urinary bladder with a large focus on the actions of $PGE_2$, a complete understanding of the contractile effects of the other four prostaglandins on the urinary bladder remain unclear. Specifically, of interest is to determine how the actions of the prostaglandins affect urothelium with lamina propria that is separated from the detrusor smooth muscle. Therefore, this study aimed to assess the influence of $PGE_2$, $PGF_{2\alpha}$, $PGD_2$, $TXA_2$ and $PGI_2$ on the urinary bladder urothelium with lamina propria and detrusor smooth muscle contractions and phasic activity.

## Methods

### Tissue preparation

Urinary bladders were obtained from Large White-Landrace pigs (approximately six months old, weighing between 80 and 100 kg) from the local abattoir after slaughter for the routine commercial provision of food. All methods were carried out in accordance with relevant Australian guidelines and regulations, and all experimental protocols were in accordance the Australian Code of Practice for the Care and Use of Animals for Scientific Purpose [16]. As no animals were bred, harmed, culled, interfered, or interacted with as part of this research project, Animal Ethics Approval was not required for offal use [17]. Urothelium with lamina propria was dissected from the underlying detrusor layer, consistent with methods carried out in past studies [18–21], and cut in strips. Adjacent strips of U&LP and detrusor (10 mm × 5 mm) were tied vertically between an isometric force transducer (MCT050/D, ADInstruments, Castle Hill, Australia) and a fixed hook in 10 mL organ baths (Labglass, Brisbane, Australia), and superfused with Krebs-bicarbonate solution (NaCl 118.4 mM, $NaHCO_3$ 24.9 mM, $CaCl_2$ 1.9 mM, $MgSO_4$ 2.41 mM, KCl 4.6 mM, $KH_2PO_4$ 1.18 mM and D-glucose 11.7 mM) and carbogen gas (95% oxygen and 5% carbon dioxide) at 37 °C. After tissue mounting, strips of U&LP and detrusor were washed three times, tension adjusted to 1.5–2.0 g and tissues left to equilibrate for 30 min. After the equilibration period, a single dose of a prostaglandin receptor agonist was added to the tissue strip.

### Pharmaceutical agents

The following compounds were used in this study: prostaglandin $E_2$, prostaglandin $F_{2\alpha}$, prostaglandin $D_2$, prostaglandin $I_2$ and thromboxane $A_2$ (U-46619, Cayman Chemicals, Michigan, USA). Prostaglandin $E_2$, prostaglandin $F_{2\alpha}$, prostaglandin $D_2$, and prostaglandin $I_2$ were dissolved in 100% ethanol and diluted with distilled $H_2O$. U-46619 was supplied as a solution in methyl acetate, which was diluted with distilled $H_2O$. Two concentrations of each prostaglandin receptor agonists were selected, 1 μM and 10 μM.

### Data analysis

Data were graphed and analysed using GraphPad Prism version 8.3 for Windows (GraphPad Software, La Jolla, California, USA). Statistical analysis was conducted using a paired Student's *t*-test, where $p < 0.05$ was considered as significant. All values were reported as mean change ± SEM. *n* equates to the number of individual bladders used in this study.

## Results

### Prostaglandin agonists for increasing U&LP spontaneous phasic activity

Strips of U&LP exhibited spontaneous phasic contractions in the absence of any stimulation at a mean frequency of 3.26 ± 0.07 cycles per minute (cpm, $n = 146$). Treatment with $PGE_2$ caused the most prominent increases to U&LP spontaneous contractile activity. When

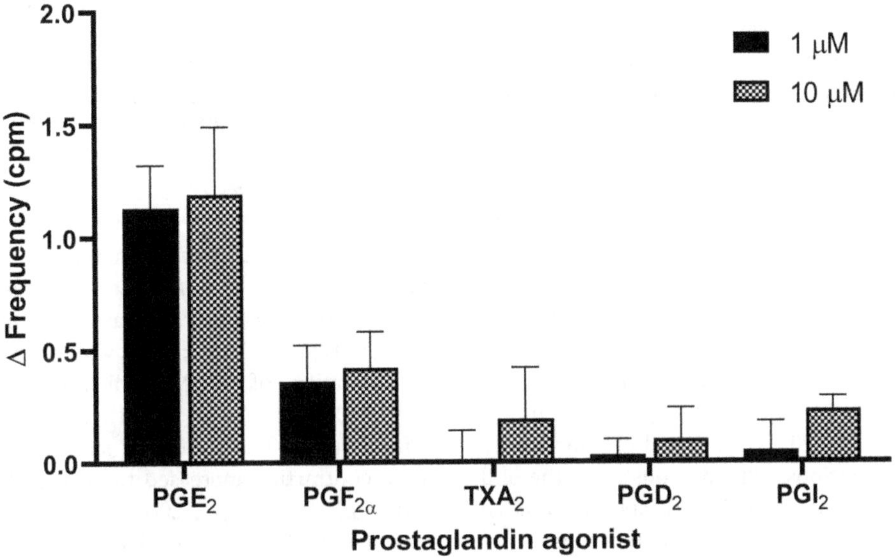


**Fig. 1** U&LP changes in the frequency of spontaneous phasic contractions after the treatment with 1 μM and 10 μM of each specific prostaglandin agonists $E_2$, $F_{2\alpha}$, $TXA_2$, $D_2$, and $I_2$. There were no statistically significant differences in frequency changes between the 1 μM and 10 μM concentrations for any of the agonists (unpaired Student's 2-tailed *t*-test)

$PGE_2$ (1 μM) was added to isolated tissues, spontaneous activity increased by 39.2% ± 6.7% ($n = 38$, $p < 0.001$, Fig. 1). A greater concentration of $PGE_2$ (10 μM) showed similar increases of 40.4% ± 9.6% to the U&LP spontaneous activity ($n = 42$, $p < 0.001$). Treatment with $PGF_{2\alpha}$ showed smaller increases of 10.5% ± 4.6% to spontaneous activity when treated with 1 μM ($n = 10$, $p < 0.05$) and 13.3% ± 5.3% when treated with 10 μM ($n = 14$, $p < 0.05$). The addition of $PGI_2$ (10 μM) increased spontaneous activity by 6.2% ± 1.6% ($n = 8$, $p < 0.01$) but had no effect at a lower concentration (1 μM, $n = 8$). The frequency was not significantly affected by $PGD_2$ (1–10 μM, $n = 12$) or $TXA_2$ (1–10 μM, $n = 16$).

The average amplitude of these spontaneous phasic contractions exhibited in U&LP strips in the absence of any stimulation was 0.57 ± 0.02 g ($n = 146$). In response to treatment with 1 μM $PGE_2$, amplitude decrease of 0.14 ± 0.04 g ($n = 38$, $p < 0.001$, Table 1) were observed. Similar decreases of 0.16 ± 0.03 g were also observed in response to a higher $PGE_2$ concentration (10 μM, $n = 42$, $p < 0.01$). Treatment with $TXA_2$ (1 μM) showed a significant decrease in the amplitude by 0.28 ± 0.06 g ($n = 8$, $p < 0.01$), which was not observed at a higher concentration (10 μM, $n = 6$). The addition of $PGI_2$ (10 μM) decreased amplitude of spontaneous activity by 0.14 ± 0.05 ($n = 8$, $p < 0.05$) but had no effect at a lower concentration (1 μM, $n = 8$). The amplitude of spontaneous contractions was not altered by the addition of either $PGF_{2\alpha}$ (1–10 μM, $n = 24$) or $PGD_2$ (1–10 μM, $n = 12$, Table 1). None of the decreases in the amplitude of spontaneous phasic contractions of the U&LP were significantly affected by the two different prostaglandin receptor agonist concentrations (1 μM and 10 μM).

#### Prostaglandin agonists in stimulating phasic contractions in detrusor

Total of 34% ($n = 48$) of the detrusor preparations that were set up in the organ baths exhibited spontaneous activity prior to the addition of any agonists. These

**Table 1** U&LP changes in the amplitude of phasic contractions in response to the five primary prostaglandin agonists (mean ± SEM)

| | 1 μM of agonist | | | 10 μM of agonist | | |
|---|---|---|---|---|---|---|
| Agonist | Absence (g) | Presence (g) | n | Absence (g) | Presence (g) | n |
| $PGE_2$ | 0.53 ± 0.05 | 0.40 ± 0.03*** | 38 | 0.53 ± 0.04 | 0.37 ± 0.03** | 42 |
| $PGF_{2\alpha}$ | 0.30 ± 0.03 | 0.29 ± 0.01 | 10 | 0.51 ± 0.06 | 0.46 ± 0.08 | 14 |
| $TXA_2$ | 0.90 ± 0.16 | 0.62 ± 0.14** | 8 | 0.75 ± 0.16 | 0.71 ± 0.25 | 6 |
| $PGD_2$ | 0.59 ± 0.10 | 0.46 ± 0.04 | 4 | 0.55 ± 0.08 | 0.43 ± 0.06 | 8 |
| $PGI_2$ | 0.64 ± 0.07 | 0.56 ± 0.07 | 8 | 0.57 ± 0.09 | 0.43 ± 0.06* | 8 |

*$p < 0.05$, **$p < 0.01$, ***$p < 0.001$. Paired Student's *t*-test

contractions occurred at an average frequency of 2.03 ± 0.12 cpm ($n = 48$) with an average amplitude of 0.26 ± 0.02 g ($n = 48$). However, the majority of the detrusor preparations, that were otherwise quiescent developed spontaneous phasic contractions after the addition of the agonist.

Of those detrusor preparations that did not exhibit initial phasic activity during baseline: $PGE_2$ (1 μM) sparked contractions in 68% of preparations ($n = 19$) and $PGE_2$ (10 μM) in 69% ($n = 22$); $PGF_{2\alpha}$ (1 μM) initiated contractions in in 56% ($n = 5$) and $PGF_{2\alpha}$ (10 μM) in 88% ($n = 7$); $TXA_2$ (1 μM) initiated contractions in 63% ($n = 5$) and $TXA_2$ (10 μM) in 80% ($n = 4$); $PGD_2$ (1 μM) initiated phasic activity in 50% ($n = 2$) and $PGD_2$ (10 μM) in 75% ($n = 6$); and lastly $PGI_2$ (10 μM) initiated contractions in 40% ($n = 2$) of preparations. This demonstrates the ability of prostaglandin agonists to induce spontaneous activity in otherwise quiescent detrusor tissue strips.

**Prostaglandin agonists in stimulating tonic contractions in U&LP**

All assessed prostaglandin agonists contracted the U&LP with the rank order of contractile response effectiveness as: $PGE_2 > PGF_{2\alpha} > TXA_2 > PGD_2 > PGI_2$. The addition of $PGE_2$ (1 μM) to isolated U&LP induced tissue contractions, with increases of 1.01 ± 0.08 g ($n = 38$, $p < 0.001$) to the tonic contractions. When a greater concentration of $PGE_2$ (10 μM) was selected, increases of 1.36 ± 0.09 g ($n = 42$, $p < 0.001$, Fig. 2) were observed. Treatment with 1 μM $PGF_{2\alpha}$ showed a small increase to tonic contractions of 0.15 ± 0.04 g ($n = 10$, $p < 0.01$) when compared to a higher concentration of 10 μM, which exhibited increases of 0.79 ± 0.06 g ($n = 14$, $p < 0.001$). The addition of two concentrations of $TXA_2$ induced similar contractions, where tonic contraction increased by 0.70 ± 0.07 g when treated with 1 μM ($n = 8$, $p < 0.001$), and by 0.65 ± 0.12 g after treatment with 10 μM ($n = 6$, $p < 0.001$).

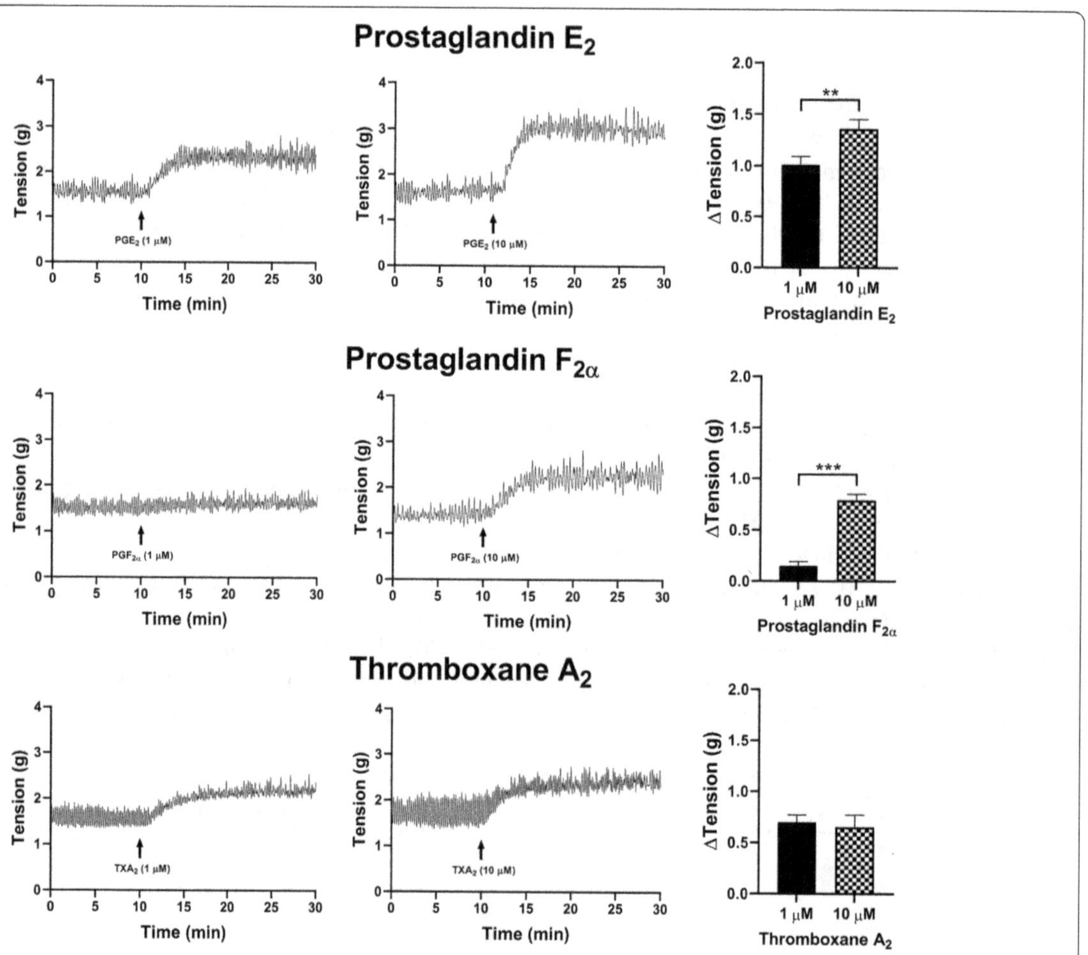


**Fig. 2** U&LP changes in tonic contractions in response to the treatment with 1 μM and 10 μM of prostaglandin $E_2$ (*top row*), $F_{2\alpha}$ (*middle row*) and $TXA_2$ (*bottom row*). Sample traces of the responses observed to two concentrations of prostaglandin agonist (*left & middle columns*). Increases in tonic contractions after treatment with each agonist are represented as mean change ± SEM (*right column*). Significant changes in the tonic contractions between 1 μM and 10 μM were evaluated using an unpaired Student's two-tailed *t*-test, where $^{*}p < 0.05$, $^{**}p < 0.01$, $^{***}p < 0.001$

When $PGD_2$ (1 μM) was added to the U&LP tissue preparations, tonic contractions increased by 0.19 ± 0.04 g ($n = 4$, $p < 0.05$, Fig. 3). Treatment with a higher concentration of $PGD_2$ (10 μM) exhibited increases of 0.63 ± 0.09 g ($n = 8$, $p < 0.001$). The addition of $PGI_2$ showed small increases in tonic contractions of 0.11 ± 0.02 g in response to 1 μM $PGI_2$ ($n = 8$, $p < 0.001$), and 0.22 ± 0.03 g in response to 10 μM $PGI_2$ ($n = 8$, $p < 0.001$, Fig. 3).

### Prostaglandin agonists in stimulating tonic contractions in detrusor

All assessed prostaglandin agonists contracted the detrusor smooth muscle preparations with the rank order of contractile response effectiveness as: $PGE_2 > PGF_{2\alpha} > TXA_2 > PGD_2 > PGI_2$. In detrusor preparations, $PGE_2$ (1 μM) increased the tonic contractions by 0.73 ± 0.09 g ($n = 34$, $p < 0.001$), whereas $PGE_2$ (10 μM) nearly doubled the response, producing an average increase of 1.32 ± 0.13 g ($n = 38$, $p < 0.001$, Fig. 4). Treatment with 1 μM $PGF_{2\alpha}$ showed a small increase of 0.20 ± 0.05 g ($n = 10$, $p < 0.01$), whereas 10 μM of $PGF_{2\alpha}$ increased the tonic contractions by 0.97 ± 0.14 g ($n = 12$, $p < 0.001$). When $TXA_2$ was added, tonic contractions increased by 0.47 ± 0.12 g when treated with 1 μM ($n = 8$, $p < 0.001$), and by 1.03 ± 0.14 g ($n = 6$, p < 0.001, Fig. 4) when treated with 1 μM $TXA_2$.

$PGD_2$ showed a small increase in the tonic contractions of 0.12 ± 0.04 g when 1 μM was added ($n = 4$, $p < 0.05$), and an increase of 0.36 ± 0.06 g when 10 μM $PGD_2$ was added ($n = 6$, p < 0.01, Fig. 5). $PGI_2$ showed small increases in tonic contractions at both concentrations, showing an increase of 0.16 ± 0.02 g when treated with 1 μM ($n = 8$, $p < 0.001$), and 0.13 ± 0.03 g when treated with 10 μM $PGI_2$ ($n = 8$, $p < 0.001$, Fig. 5). The effects of prostaglandin agonists on tonic contractions of the detrusor smooth muscle were significantly different between the two concentrations (1 μM and 10 μM) for $PGE_2$ ($p < 0.001$), $PGF_{2\alpha}$ ($p < 0.001$) and $PGD_2$ ($p < 0.05$).

## Discussion

Previous research has shown that stimulation of the M3 muscarinic receptor in U&LP causes immediate contractions, as well as increases in the frequency of spontaneous phasic contractions, and reduction in their amplitude [22, 23]. In our study, the prostaglandin agonists have shown similar contractile responses to both tonic contractions and spontaneous activity, thereby associating the actions of prostaglandins with many of the bladder contractile dysfunctions, such as OAB and IC/BPS.

The ability to contract the tissue was varied between the different prostaglandin agonists. The rank order of agonist response in stimulating contractions in U&LP and detrusor was: $PGE_2 > PGF_{2\alpha} > TXA_2 > PGD_2 > PGI_2$. This furthers previous research which reported the involvement of $PGE_2$ in the initiation of micturition in both humans and animals [24], suggesting a contribution

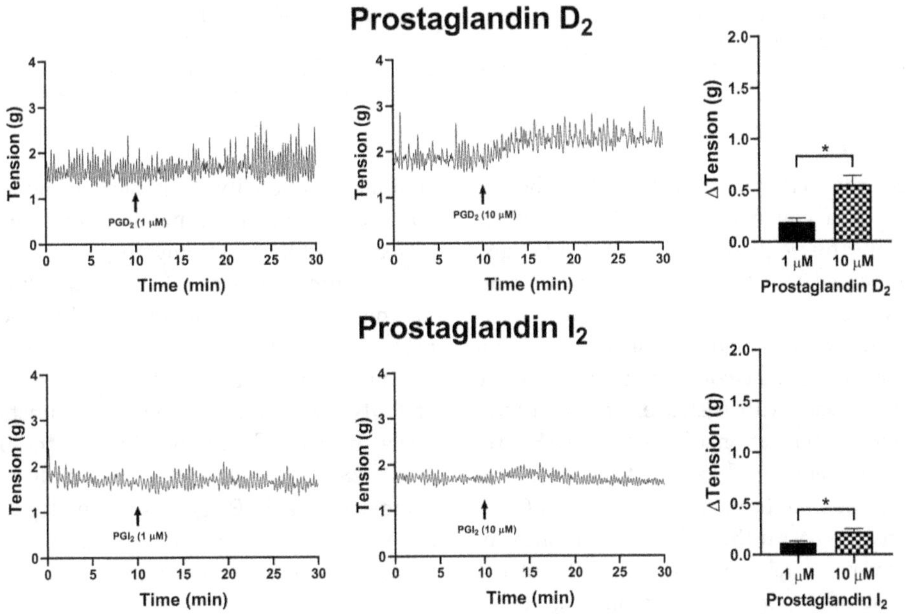


**Fig. 3** U&LP changes in tonic contractions in response to the treatment with 1 μM and 10 μM of prostaglandin agonists $D_2$ (*top row*) and $I_2$ (*bottom row*). Sample traces of the responses observed to two concentrations of prostaglandin agonist (*left & middle columns*). Increases in tonic contractions after treatment with each agonist are represented as mean change ± SEM (*right column*). Significant changes in the tonic contractions between 1 μM and 10 μM were evaluated using an unpaired Student's two-tailed *t*-test, where *$p < 0.05$, **$p < 0.01$, ***$p < 0.001$

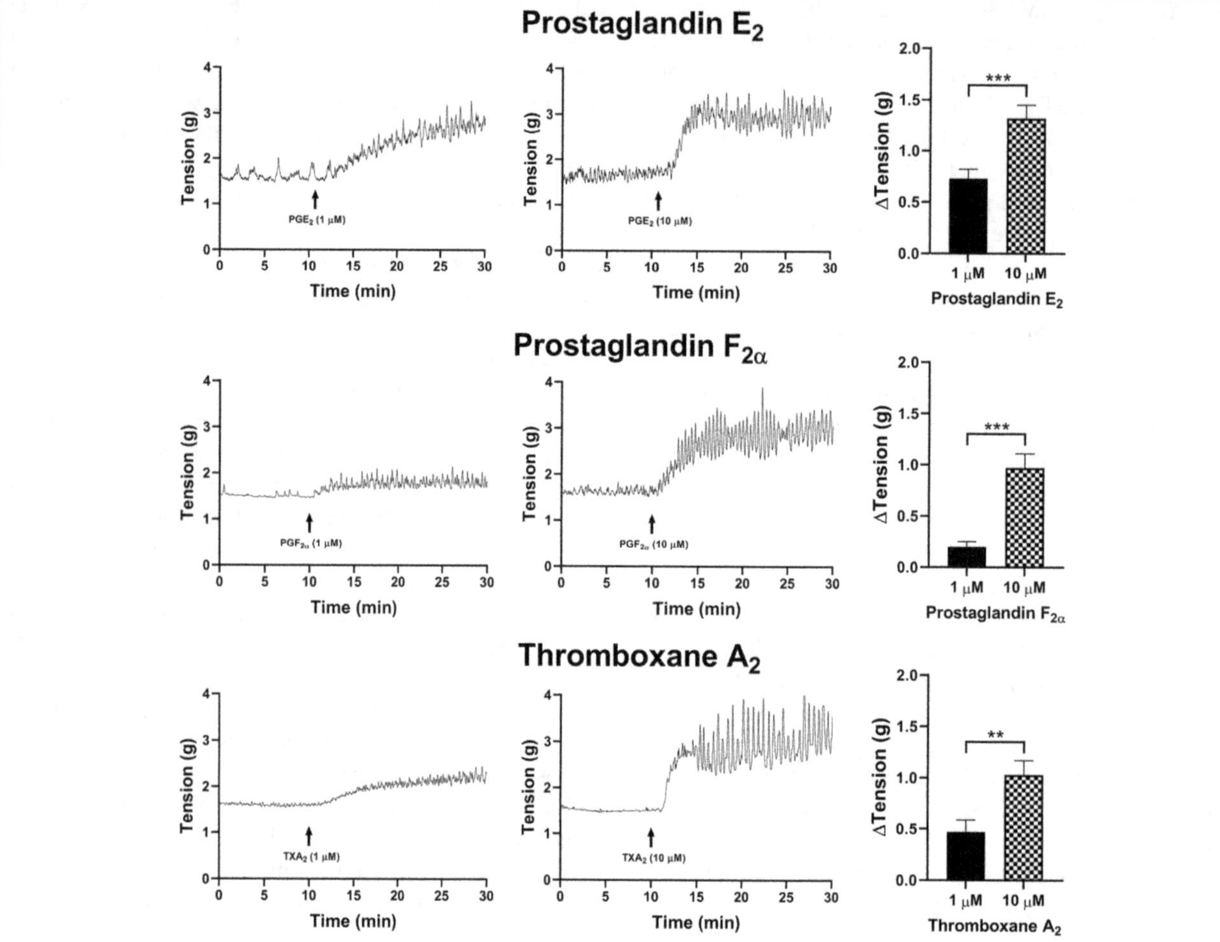


**Fig. 4** Detrusor changes in tonic contractions in response to the treatment with 1 μM and 10 μM of prostaglandin $E_2$ (*top row*), $F_{2\alpha}$ (*middle row*) and $TXA_2$ (*bottom row*). Sample traces of the responses observed to two concentrations of prostaglandin agonist (*left & middle columns*). Increases in tonic contractions after treatment with each agonist are represented as mean change ± SEM (*right column*). Significant changes in the tonic contractions between 1 μM and 10 μM were evaluated using an unpaired Student's two-tailed *t*-test, where $*p < 0.05$, $**p < 0.01$, $***p < 0.001$

to bladder overactivity. Treatment with $PGF_{2\alpha}$ showed minimal increases at a concentration of 1 μM, yet responses were significantly enhanced in both U&LP and detrusor when increased to 10 μM. At the smaller concentration of 1 μM, treatment with $TXA_2$ reached maximal contractile responses, and as such, was not enhanced at the higher agonist concentration of 10 μM. This was not the case with detrusor preparations, wherein the higher concentration of $TXA_2$ (10 μM) resulted in significantly enhanced contractions. The responses observed in porcine tissue in response to $PGF_{2\alpha}$, and $TXA_2$ are consistent with the Palea [25] findings. In addition, our study has established that U&LP isolated tissue is also capable of responding and producing definite increases in tonic contractions in response to these prostaglandin agonists.

Of the five prostaglandins, $PGD_2$ and $PGI_2$ had the smallest effect on both tonic contractions and spontaneous activity. This lack of increases to the tonic contractions or spontaneous contractile frequency may be explained by $PGD_2$ having potential inhibitory actions via the stimulation of DP receptor [26]. An explanation for the small contractile effects observed in our study in response to $PGI_2$, the main prostaglandin synthesised in the human bladder [14, 27], is that the aqueous solutions of $PGI_2$ are extremely chemically unstable with a relatively short half-life, depending on the buffer concentration [28]. As such, future studies utilising more chemically stable $PGI_2$ agonist analogous might provide further insights into the actions of this inflammatory mediator on the urinary bladder.

## Conclusions

The urinary bladder is capable of responding to all five major prostaglandins produced in the urinary bladder. Out of these prostaglandins, $PGE_2$ and $PGF_{2\alpha}$ had the

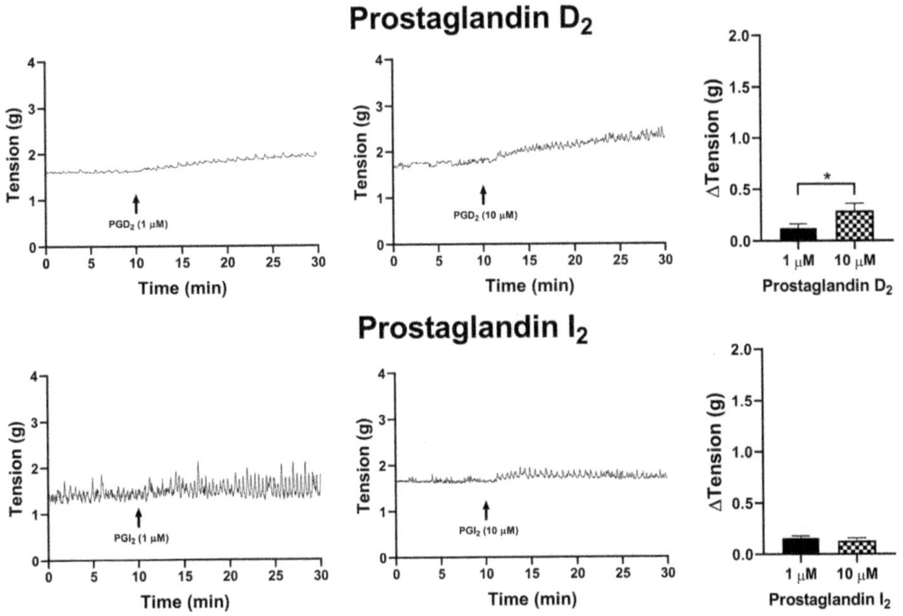


**Fig. 5** Detrusor changes in tonic contractions in response to the treatment with 1 μM and 10 μM of prostaglandin agonists $D_2$ (*top row*) and $I_2$ (*bottom row*). Sample traces of responses observed to two concentrations of a prostaglandin agonist (*left & middle columns*). Increases in the tonic contractions after treatment with an agonist are represented as mean change ± SEM (*right column*). Significant changes in the tonic contractions between 1 μM and 10 μM were evaluated using an unpaired Student's *t*-test, where $^*p < 0.05$, $^{***}p < 0.001$

most significant impact on both contraction and increases to the spontaneous contractile frequency in the U&LP. All five prostaglandin receptor agonists were also capable of inducing spontaneous phasic contractions in otherwise quiescent detrusor tissue strips.

### Abbreviations

PG: Prostaglandin; IC/BPS: Interstitial cystitis/bladder pain syndrome; OAB: Overactive bladder; U&LP: Urothelium and lamina propria; TX: Thromboxane


### Acknowledgements

This research was supported by the Australian Bladder Foundation managed by the Continence Foundation of Australia. ZS was supported by an Australian Government Research Training Program Scholarship.


### Authors' contributions

Data was collected by ZS. CM, RCW and ZS were all equally responsible for the study design, data analysis, and preparation of manuscript. All authors read and approved the manuscript.

### References


1. Gilmore NJ, Vane JR. Hormones released into the circulation when the urinary bladder of the anaesthetized dog is distended. Clin Sci. 1971;41:69–83.
2. Rahnama'i MS, van Kerrebroeck PE, de Wachter SG, van Koeveringe GA. The role of prostanoids in urinary bladder physiology. Nat Rev Urol. 2012;9(5):283–90.
3. Tanaka I, Nagase K, Tanase K, Aoki Y, Akino H, Yokoyama O. Improvement in neurogenic detrusor overactivity by peripheral C fiber's suppression with cyclooxygenase inhibitors. J Urol. 2010;183(2):786–92.
4. Reyes AA, Klahr S. Bladder contributes to eicosanoids excreted in urine. Am J Phys. 1990;259(5 Pt 2):F859–F61.
5. Kim JC. Changes of urinary nerve growth factor and prostaglandins in male patients with overactive bladder symptom. Int J Urol. 2005;12:875–80.
6. Kim JC, Park EY, Seo SI, Park YH, Hwang TK. Nerve growth factor and prostaglandins in the urine of female patients with overactive bladder. J Urol. 2006;175:1773–6.
7. Andersson KE, Ek A, Persson CG. Effects of prostaglandins on the isolated human bladder and urethra. Acta Physiol Scand. 1977;100(2):165–71.
8. Ricciotti E, FitzGerald GA. Prostaglandins and inflammation. Arterioscler Thromb Vasc Biol. 2011;31(5):986–1000.
9. Khan MA, Thompson CS, Mumtaz FH, Jeremy JY, Morgan RJ, Mikhailidis DP. Role of prostaglandins in the urinary bladder: an update. Prostaglandins Leukot Essent Fat Acids. 1998;59(6):415–22.
10. Rahnama'i MS, Van Koeveringe GA, Van Kerrebroeck PE. Overactive bladder syndrome and the potential role of prostaglandins and phosphodiesterases: an introduction. Nephrourol Mon. 2013;5(4):934–45.
11. Andersson KE. Overactive bladder - pharmacological aspects. Scand J Urol Nephrol Suppl. 2002;210:72–81.
12. Tilley SL, Coffman TM, Koller BH. Mixed messages: modulation of inflammation and immune responses by prostaglandins and thromboxanes. J Clin Invest. 2001;108(1):15–23.
13. Smith WL, Dewitt DL. Prostaglandin endoperoxide H synthases-1 and -2. Adv Immunol. 1996;62:167–215.
14. Masunaga K. Prostaglandin E2 release from isolated bladder strips in rats with spinal cord injury. Int J Urol. 2006;13:271–6.
15. Jeremy JY. Eicosanoid synthesis by human urinary bladder mucosa: pathological implications. Br J Urol. 1987;59:36–9.
16. Australia Government. Australian code for the care and use of animals for scientific purposes 2013 [Available from: https://www.nhmrc.gov.au/about-us/publications/australian-code-care-and-use-animals-scientific-purposes.
17. Queensland Government. Using Animals in Science 2016 [Available from: https://www.business.qld.gov.au/industries/farms-fishing-forestry/agriculture/livestock/animal-welfare/animals-science/activities/dead-animals.
18. Strombergа Z, Chess-Williams R, Moro C. Histamine modulation of urinary bladder urothelium, lamina propria and detrusor contractile activity via H1 and H2 receptors. Sci Rep. 2019;9(1):3899.
19. Stromberga Z, Chess-Williams R, Moro C. Alterations in histamine responses between juvenile and adult urinary bladder urothelium, lamina propria and detrusor tissues. Sci Rep. 2020;10(1):4116.
20. Moro C, Edwards L, Chess-Williams R. 5-HT2A receptor enhancement of contractile activity of the porcine urothelium and lamina propria. Int J Urol. 2016;23(11):946–51.

21. Moro C, Chess-Williams R. Non-adrenergic, non-cholinergic, non-purinergic contractions of the urothelium/lamina propria of the pig bladder. Auton Autacoid Pharmacol. 2012;32(3 Pt 4):53–9.
22. Moro C, Uchiyama J, Chess-Williams R. Urothelial/lamina propria spontaneous activity and the role of M3 muscarinic receptors in mediating rate responses to stretch and carbachol. Urology. 2011;78(6):1442.e9–15.
23. Moro C, Leeds C, Chess-Williams R. Contractile activity of the bladder urothelium/lamina propria and its regulation by nitric oxide. Eur J Pharmacol. 2012;674(2–3):445–9.
24. Lee T, Hedlund P, Newgreen D, Andersson KE. Urodynamic effects of a novel EP (1) receptor antagonist in normal rats and rats with bladder outlet obstruction. J Urol. 2007;177(4):1562–7.
25. Palea S. Pharmacological characterization of thromboxane and prostanoid receptors in human isolated urinary bladder. Br J Pharmacol. 1998;124:865–72.
26. Guan NN, Svennersten K, de Verdier PJ, Wiklund NP, Gustafsson LE. Receptors involved in the modulation of Guinea pig urinary bladder motility by prostaglandin D2. Br J Pharmacol. 2015;172(16):4024–37.
27. Jeremy JY, Tsang V, Mikhailidis DP, Rogers H, Morgan RJ, Dandona P. Eicosanoid synthesis by human urinary bladder mucosa: pathological implications. Br J Urol. 1987;59(1):36–9.
28. Moncada S. Biology and therapeutic potential of prostacyclin. Stroke. 1983; 14(2):157–68.

# 23

# Expression of epithelial-Mesenchymal transition related markers in Plasmacytoid Urothelial carcinoma of the urinary bladder

Shunichiro Nomura[1*], Yasutomo Suzuki[1], Jun Akatsuka[1], Yuki Endo[1], Akira Shimizu[2], Tsutomu Hamasaki[1], Go Kimura[1] and Yukihiro Kondo[1]

**Abstract**

**Background:** Plasmacytoid urothelial carcinoma (PUC) of the urinary bladder is a variant of urothelial carcinoma that carries a poor prognosis. The epithelial-mesenchymal transition (EMT) has been demonstrated to contribute to tumor progression. As the cause of the increased aggressiveness of PUC is unknown, we investigated PUC and EMT-related marker expression.

**Methods:** A total of 633 bladder carcinoma cases diagnosed from 2006 to 2015 at the Nippon Medical School Hospital were analyzed. Twelve patients were found to have plasmacytoid histology and diagnosed with PUC. Slides were evaluated for percentage of plasmacytoid variant, and stained for E-cadherin, N-cadherin, Vimentin, Fibronectin and Snail expression.

**Results:** The incidence of PUC was 1.9% (12/633). The median patient age at diagnosis was 71 years (range, 60–80 years) and the male-female ratio was 11:1. All but three patients had stage T2b or higher. The median overall survival was 10 months. In 10/12 cases, Snail and N-cadherin were positive. Vimentin was positive in 9/12 cases. Fibronectin was positive in 8/12 cases. While E-cadherin was negative in 10/12 cases. Nine cases showed > 10% plasmacytoid component. Eight of the nine patients (88.9%) with > 10% plasmacytoid component died.

**Conclusions:** The results indicate that PUC may induce EMT and may be associated with high invasion.

**Keywords:** Bladder, Urinary bladder, Plasmacytoid, Urothelial carcinoma, E-cadherin, Snail, Epithelial-mesenchymal transition

## Background

Plasmacytoid urothelial carcinoma (PUC) of the urinary bladder was first reported in 1991 as a similar histological type to plasma cell [1]. The World Health Organization (WHO) working group classified PUC as a variant of urothelial carcinoma (UC). These tumor cells have eosinophilic cytoplasm and eccentrically placed, enlarged hyperchromatic nuclei with small nucleoli [2]. The prognosis of PUC of the bladder is worse than that of conventional UC [3]. However, why PUC is more aggressive is unknown.

Later inquire about proposes that the epithelial-mesenchymal transition (EMT) is a vital figure related to tumor progression and metastasis [4, 5]. EMT could be a handle at first watched in embryonic improvement in which cells lose epithelial characteristics and pick up mesenchymal properties to extend motility and invasion [4]. Besides, a later ponder detailed that Snail could be a key controller of EMT [6]. Snail is a superfamily of zinc-finger transcription factors that was, to begin with

* Correspondence: s-nomura@nms.ac.jp
[1]Department of Urology, Nippon Medical School, 1-1-5 Sendagi, Bunkyo-ku, Tokyo 113-8603, Japan
Full list of author information is available at the end of the article

distinguished in *Drosophila melanogaster* [7]. Snail actuates EMT, in portion, by straighforwardly repressing epithelial markers such as E-cadherin and by upregulating mesenchymal markers such as N-cadherin, Vimentin, and Fibronectin. Immunohistochemistry has appeared downregulated or negative E-cadherin expression in the majority of PUC [3, 8]. Hence, PUC may actuate EMT. Therefore, EMT may be associated with PUC progression. The present study examined the expression status of EMT-related markers (E-cadherin, N-cadherin, Vimentin, Fibronectin and Snail) in PUC.

Whether survival is related to the proportion of plasmacytoid variant histology is unknown. Thus, we assessed the association between the proportion of plasmacytoid variant histology and survival in PUC patients. Furthermore, we also report clinical outcome information.

## Methods

### Patients and samples

The cohort under investigation comprised 12 patients who had bladder carcinoma with plasmacytoid histology at our institution between March 2006 and August 2015. All hematoxylin and eosin stained glass slides were retrieved and reviewed to confirm the diagnosis using the WHO definition of "plasmacytoid variants" [2]. Having been compiled for research purposes, this group represents patients for whom pretreatment archival paraffin-embedded tissue blocks and data from complete clinical follow-up were available. Tumors were graded histologically in accordance with WHO classifications and were staged as per the TNM staging system of the Union for International Cancer Control (2009). The amount of PUC as a percentage was evaluated in the transurethral resection of bladder tumor (TURBT) and compared with that in the cystectomy when available.

### Immunohistochemistry

Immunostaining was performed on at least one representative paraffin section using routine laboratory standard protocols. The antibodies used on paraffin-embedded tissues included EMA (Dako, Glostrup, Denmark), CK7 (Dako), CK20 (Dako), E-cadherin (Nichirei, Tokyo, Japan), N-cadherin (TaKaRa, Otsu, Japan), Vimentin (Dako), Fibronectin (Abcam, Cambridge, UK), Snail (Abcam) and CD138 (Dako). The stained tumor tissues were evaluated blindly with respect to clinical patient data. Staining was assessed using a semiquantitative scoring system (0, 1+, 2+, and 3+). Immunohistochemical staining was evaluated as follows: 0, no staining of tumor cells; 1+, faint staining in less than 10% of tumor cells; 2+, weak or moderate staining in more than 10% of tumor cells; and 3+, strong staining in more than 10% of tumor cells. Staining intensity of 0 or 1+ was considered negative, while 2+ or 3+ staining was considered positive. Negative controls were incubated without the primary antibody.

### Statistical analysis

Associations between E-cadherin and IHC characteristics of PUC were analyzed using the Fisher's exact test. $P$-values $< 0.05$ were considered significant. All statistical analyses were performed with SPSS Version 21.0 statistical software package (IBM Corp, Armonk, NY, USA).

## Results

### Clinical data

Among the 633 patients with bladder carcinoma that were initially identified, 12 were classified as PUC. Tumors diagnosed as PUC comprised 1.9% (12/633) of all bladder carcinomas. The clinicopathologic features of the 12 patients are shown in Table 1. The median patient age at diagnosis was 71 years (range, 60–80 years) and there was only one female patient.

TNM stage was cT1N0 in three patients, cT2bN0 in three, cT3b-4aN0 in four, cT2bN1 in one, and cT3bN2 in one. The initial diagnosis of plasmacytoid carcinoma of the bladder was made on TURBT in 11 cases and cystoprostatectomy in one case. The pathologic T stage was pT1 in three patients, pT2b in seven, pT3b in one, and pT4a in one. None of the 12 cases had a prior history of bladder cancer.

The treatment outcomes of the 12 patients are shown in Table 2. One patient underwent radical cystectomy preceded by neoadjuvant chemotherapy. However, this surgical specimen was not pathologically free of cancer (pT2<). One patient underwent radical cystectomy alone, and two patients underwent palliative cystectomy. In all available specimens from patients who underwent

**Table 1** Clinical and pathologic features of 12 cases of plasmacytoid urothelial carcinoma

| Case No. | Presenting Symptoms | TNM Clinical Stage | Pathologic T stage | Plasmacytoid Component (%) |
|---|---|---|---|---|
| 1 | Hematuria | T3aN0M0 | 2b | > 10 |
| 2 | Hematuria | T1N0M0 | 1 | > 10 |
| 3 | Hematuria | T2bN0M0 | 2b | > 10 |
| 4 | Hematuria | T3bN0M0 | 3b | > 10 |
| 5 | Frequent urination | T4aN0M0 | 4a | > 10 |
| 6 | incidental | T1N0M0 | 1 | > 10 |
| 7 | Residual urine | T3bN0M0 | 2b | < 10 |
| 8 | Hematuria | T3bN2M0 | 2b | > 10 |
| 9 | Hematuria | T2bN1M0 | 2b | > 10 |
| 10 | Hematuria | T1N0M0 | 1 | < 10 |
| 11 | Hematuria | T2bN0M0 | 2b | > 10 |
| 12 | Hematuria | T2bN0M0 | 2b | < 10 |

**Table 2** Treatment outcomes in 12 patients with plasmacytoid histology

| Case | | Post-treatment | Follow-Up | |
|---|---|---|---|---|
| No. | Treatment | Progression site | Months | Status |
| 1 | Radical cystectomy | Pelvic | 7 | Died of disease |
| 2 | Chemotherapy | Retroperitoneal lymph nodes | 10 | Died of disease |
| 3 | TURBT | Bladder | 9 | Died of disease |
| 4 | Radical cystectomy | Lung | 5 | Died of disease |
| 5 | Chemoradiation | Retroperitoneal lymph nodes | 9 | Died of disease |
| 6 | Chemotherapy alone | No progression | 35 | Alive with disease |
| 7 | TURBT | No progression | 36 | Alive with disease |
| 8 | Radical cystectomy and Chemotherapy | No progression | 11 | Died of chemotherapy |
| 9 | Chemotherapy | Retroperitoneal lymph nodes | 3 | Died of disease |
| 10 | BCG | No progression | 30 | Alive with disease |
| 11 | TURBT | Retroperitoneal lymph nodes | 3 | Died of disease |
| 12 | Radical cystectomy | Retroperitoneal lymph nodes | 15 | Died of disease |

surgery, the negative margin and negative lymph node status rate at surgery were 75% (3 of 4) and 0% (0 of 2). Three patients received chemotherapy alone, and one of the three patients remained alive with disease and the other patient died of disease. All chemotherapy regimen was GC (gemcitabine and cisplatin). One patient received chemoradiotherapy alone and one patient received intravesical bacillus Calmette-Guerin immunotherapy alone. Two patients rejected any further treatment after TURBT. One patient did not receive any further treatment after TURBT due to a rapid worsening cancer.

At the time of analysis in August 2015, disease progression was objectively documented in 8 of the 12 patients. Disease recurrence was observed in the retroperitoneal lymph nodes in 5 of these 12 patients (42%), while 1 (8%) had recurrence in lung, and 1 patient each showed recurrence in bladder or pelvis.

Eleven patients had follow-up information available, while one was lost to follow-up. Eight of the patients died of their disease from 3 to 15 months (median 9 months), while three patients were alive from 29 to 36 months (median 36 months). One patient death was attributed to chemotherapy. With a median follow-up of 9.5 months, the overall median survival was 10 months. The 1-year survival rate was 33.3% for all patients.

Cases were stratified based on the percentage of plasmacytoid variant histology. Nine cases (75%) showed > 10% plasmacytoid component, while three cases (25%) showed < 10% plasmacytoid component. Eight of the nine (88.9%) patients with > 10% plasmacytoid component died. The 1-year survival of patients was 11.1% (8/9 cases) for > 10% plasmacytoid patients. Conversely, the 1-year survival of patients was 100% (3/3 cases) for < 10% plasmacytoid patients.

### Immunohistochemistry

The immunohistochemical findings in the 12 cases are summarized in Table 3. EMA was positive in 5/12 cases (41.7%), CK7 was positive in 7/12 cases (58.3%), CK20 was positive in only 2/12 cases (16.7%). E-cadherin was negative in 10/12 cases (83.3%). N-cadherin and Snail were positive in 10/12 cases (83.3%). Vimentin was positive in 9/12 cases (75%). Fibronectin was positive in 8/12 cases (66.7%). There was no difference in these EMT-related markers expression between E-cadherin positive and negative PUC cells (Table 4). CD138 was negative in all cases. Snail was localized in the nucleus of PUC cells. E-cadherin and N-cadherin were localized in the cytoplasm of PUC cells. Typical UC was positive for E-cadherin. Representative cases of immunohistochemical staining are presented in Fig. 1.

## Discussion

PUC is recognized as a rare and aggressive variant of UC, which often presents at a high stage and carries a poor prognosis [3]. Sahin et al. first described this tumor in 1991 [1]. Mai et al. reported an incidence of 2.7% of PUC in a series of muscle invasive UC [9]. In this study, 9 of 12 tumors were invasive. 9 of 12 PUC patients died during follow-up. The median age at diagnosis was 71 years, a finding similar to other recent reports. We recognized that the poor prognoses of these cases are due to the high invasion and the high clinical stage at presentation [3]. However, it is unclear how often PUC shows high invasion.

**Table 3** Summary of the immunostaining results

| Case No. | EMA | CK7 | CK20 | E-cadherin | N-cadherin | Vimentin | Fibronectin | Snail | CD138 |
|---|---|---|---|---|---|---|---|---|---|
| 1 | – | – | – | – | + | + | + | + | – |
| 2 | + | – | – | – | + | + | + | + | – |
| 3 | – | – | – | – | + | + | + | + | – |
| 4 | – | + | – | – | + | + | + | + | – |
| 5 | + | + | – | + | + | + | + | + | – |
| 6 | – | + | + | + | + | – | – | + | – |
| 7 | + | + | – | – | + | + | – | + | – |
| 8 | – | – | – | – | – | + | – | + | – |
| 9 | + | + | – | – | + | + | + | + | – |
| 10 | – | – | – | – | – | – | – | – | – |
| 11 | – | + | – | – | + | + | + | + | – |
| 12 | + | + | + | – | + | – | + | – | – |

EMT is an essential step amid epithelial tumor metastasis [10]. EMT causes changes in cell-cell and cell-extracellular matrix interactions coming about in transmigration of cancer cells, in this way driving to metastasis [11, 12]. E-cadherin may be a cell-cell intersection protein that is regularly downregulated or misplaced amid EMT, while expression of N-cadherin, Vimentin, Fibronectin, and Snail are obtained amid this process. In this study, E-cadherin expression was largely negative, while N-cadherin, Vimentin, Fibronectin and Snail were mostly positive. The present study reported a possibility of EMT in PUC.

E-cadherin is a key structure protein in maintaining both the stability of adhesion between epithelial cells and the stability of tissues [13]. Recent studies have demonstrated that loss of E-cadherin expression may correlate with high grade and advanced stage of UC [14, 15]. Other studies reported that the majority of PUC cases show low E-cadherin expression [3, 8]. Keck et al. reported that most PUC with loss of membranous E-cadherin show a nuclear accumulation of E-cadherin. E-cadherin also serves as an independent prognostic factor for reduced overall survival of patients with muscle-invasive bladder cancer who were treated with radical cystectomy and adjuvant chemotherapy [16]. In this study, 10 of 12 cases (83.3%) showed largely negative membranous E-cadherin.

Snail is considered a fundamental controller of EMT and, thus, of tumor movement. Bruyere et al. detailed that Snail expression predicts tumor recurrence in superficial bladder cancer [17]. Kosaka et al. reported that Snail expression might be a prognostic indicator of disease-free survival and disease-specific survival in upper urinary tract UC [18]. We moreover already detailed that Snail expression may anticipate poor results in bladder cancer patients treated with neoadjuvant chemotherapy [19]. In this study, Snail was mostly positive in 83.3%. PUC also may predict the poor outcome by Snail. Further studies with a large cohort of PUC patients are needed to confirm this result.

Fibronectin is an essential component of extracellular matrix. It has been found highly expressed in a few kinds of cancer, indicating a potential role in progression [20, 21]. Malmstrom et al. reported the level of urine fibronectin in bladder cancer patients were significantly higher than that in patients with benign urothelial diseases and the health groups [22]. Furthermore, muscle invasive bladder cancer patients have a significantly higher level of urine fibronectin [23]. In this study, fibronectin was all negative in the patient had no progression. Although our study is the small number of cases, fibronectin may predict the recurrence of PUC patients.

**Table 4** IHC characteristics of PUC stratified according to the presence of E-cadherin

| | EMA neg. | CK7 neg. | CK20 neg. | N-cadherin pos. | Vimentin pos. | Fibronectin pos. | Snail pos. |
|---|---|---|---|---|---|---|---|
| E-cad. Neg. | 6/10 | 5/10 | 9/10 | 8/10 | 8/10 | 7/10 | 8/10 |
| | 60% | 50% | 90% | 80% | 80% | 70% | 80% |
| E-cad. Pos. | 1/2 | 0/2 | 1/2 | 2/2 | 1/2 | 1/2 | 2/2 |
| | 50% | 0% | 50% | 100% | 50% | 50% | 100% |
| *P* Value | 1 | 0.47 | 0.318 | 1 | 0.455 | 1 | 1 |

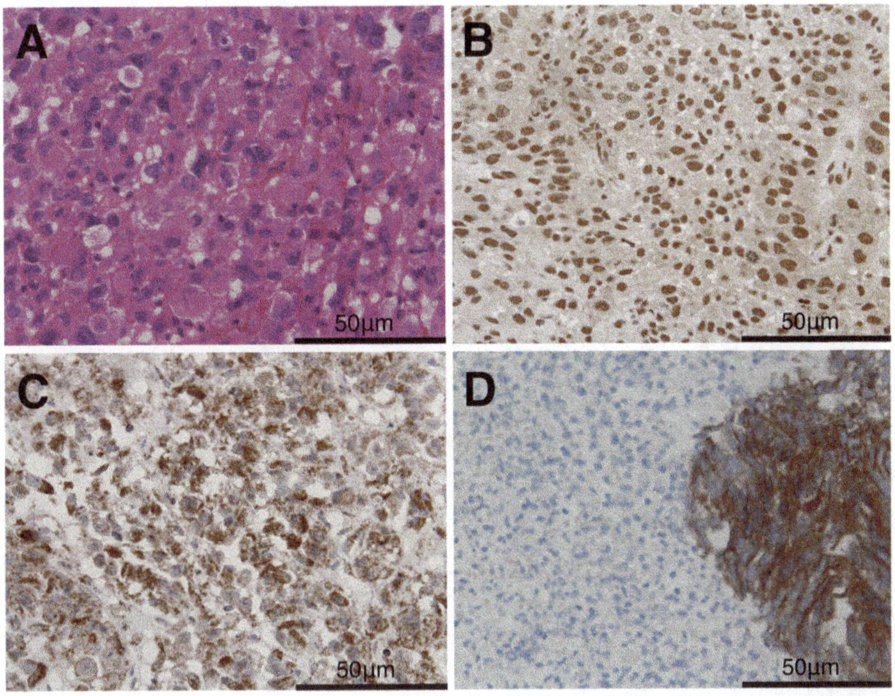


**Fig. 1 a.** Hematoxylin and eosin staining: the tumor cells have eosinophilic cytoplasm and eccentrically placed, enlarged hyperchromatic nuclei with small nucleoli. **b.** Snail-positive tumor cells. **c.** N-cadherin-positive tumor cells. **d.** E-cadherin-negative tumor cells of PUC with an E-cadherin-positive typical urothelial carcinoma

CD138 expression has been reported as a specific marker for PUC. However, Goto et al. reported the frequency of CD138 positivity in PUC was relatively low, compared with that observed in the conventional types and other variants [24]. In this study, CD138 was negative in all cases. Therefore, PUC should be correctly diagnosed using their characteristic cytomorphology.

Whether survival is related to the proportion of plasmacytoid variant histology has been unknown. Here we assessed the association between the proportion of plasmacytoid variant histology and survival in PUC patients. Analysis of the correlation between the amount of PUC and outcome revealed that the three patients with < 10% plasmacytoid component did not die from cancer, while eight of the nine patients (88.9%) with > 10% plasmacytoid component died from disease. This result may demonstrate the importance in identifying the amount of PUC.

It remains unknown how PUC patients should be treated. Qiang et al. reported PUC was not associated with worse overall mortality compared with pure UC on multivariable analysis in a large cohort of patients treated with radical cystectomy [25]. Radical cystectomy may improve survival for patients with PUC. In this study, only four PUC patients underwent radical cystectomy and three patients underwent only TURBT. Radical cystectomy should be considered as the first line choice for PUC.

## Conclusions

Our study is the first to elucidate immunohistochemical evidence of EMT in PUC. PUC may induce EMT and may be associated with high invasion. More detailed studies are needed to address this question.

### Abbreviations

PUC: Plasmacytoid urothelial carcinoma; WHO: World Health Organization; UC: Urothelial carcinoma; EMT: Epithelial-mesenchymal transition; TURBT: Transurethral resection of bladder tumor

### Acknowledgments

Kyoko Wakamatsu provided technical support.

### Authors' contributions

SN evaluated immunohistochemical staining, performed the statistical analyses, and drafted the manuscript. YS assisted with the statistical analysis and helped draft the manuscript. JA and YE supervised the research and helped write the manuscript. AS evaluated the immunohistochemistry and helped draft the manuscript. TH revised the manuscript. GK did the histological review of the samples and reviewed the manuscript. YK participated in the study conception and design, data analysis, interpretation, drafting, and final approval of the manuscript. All authors have read and approved the final manuscript.

### Author details

[1]Department of Urology, Nippon Medical School, 1-1-5 Sendagi, Bunkyo-ku, Tokyo 113-8603, Japan. [2]Analytic Human Pathology, Nippon Medical School, 1-1-5 Sendagi, Bunkyo-ku, Tokyo 113-8603, Japan.

**References**


1. Sahin AA, Myhre M, Ro JY, Sneige N, Dekmezian RH, Ayala AG. Plasmacytoid transitional cell carcinoma. Report of a case with initial presentation mimicking multiple myeloma. Acta Cytol. 1991;35(3):277–80.
2. Eble J, Sauter G, Epstein J. Pathology and genetics: tumours of the urinary system and male genital organs. . WHO Classification of Tumours. Lyon: IARC press; 2004.
3. Keck B, Stoehr R, Wach S, Rogler A, Hofstaedter F, Lehmann J, Montironi R, Sibonye M, Fritsche HM, Lopez-Beltran A, et al. The plasmacytoid carcinoma of the bladder--rare variant of aggressive urothelial carcinoma. Int J Cancer. 2011;129(2):346–54.
4. Thiery JP. Epithelial-mesenchymal transitions in tumour progression. Nat Rev Cancer. 2002;2(6):442–54.
5. Thiery JP, Chopin D. Epithelial cell plasticity in development and tumor progression. Cancer Metastasis Rev. 1999;18(1):31–42.
6. Guaita S, Puig I, Franci C, Garrido M, Dominguez D, Batlle E, Sancho E, Dedhar S, De Herreros AG, Baulida J. Snail induction of epithelial to mesenchymal transition in tumor cells is accompanied by MUC1 repression and ZEB1 expression. J Biol Chem. 2002;277(42):39209–16.
7. Boulay JL, Dennefeld C, Alberga A. The Drosophila developmental gene snail encodes a protein with nucleic acid binding fingers. Nature. 1987; 330(6146):395–8.
8. Lim MG, Adsay NV, Grignon DJ, Osunkoya AO. E-cadherin expression in plasmacytoid, signet ring cell and micropapillary variants of urothelial carcinoma: comparison with usual-type high-grade urothelial carcinoma. Mod Pathol. 2011;24(2):241–7.
9. Mai KT, Park PC, Yazdi HM, Saltel E, Erdogan S, Stinson WA, Cagiannos I, Morash C. Plasmacytoid urothelial carcinoma of the urinary bladder report of seven new cases. Eur Urol. 2006;50(5):1111–4.
10. Thiery JP, Acloque H, Huang RY, Nieto MA. Epithelial-mesenchymal transitions in development and disease. Cell. 2009;139(5):871–90.
11. Ghoul A, Serova M, Astorgues-Xerri L, Bieche I, Bousquet G, Varna M, Vidaud M, Phillips E, Weill S, Benhadji KA, et al. Epithelial-to-mesenchymal transition and resistance to ingenol 3-angelate, a novel protein kinase C modulator, in colon cancer cells. Cancer Res. 2009;69(10):4260–9.
12. Nijkamp MM, Span PN, Hoogsteen IJ, van der Kogel AJ, Kaanders JH, Bussink J. Expression of E-cadherin and vimentin correlates with metastasis formation in head and neck squamous cell carcinoma patients. Radiother Oncol. 2011;99(3):344–8.
13. Baranwal S, Alahari SK. Molecular mechanisms controlling E-cadherin expression in breast cancer. Biochem Biophys Res Commun. 2009;384(1):6–11.
14. Bringuier PP, Umbas R, Schaafsma HE, Karthaus HF, Debruyne FM, Schalken JA. Decreased E-cadherin immunoreactivity correlates with poor survival in patients with bladder tumors. Cancer Res. 1993;53(14):3241–5.
15. Syrigos KN, Krausz T, Waxman J, Pandha H, Rowlinson-Busza G, Verne J, Epenetos AA, Pignatelli M. E-cadherin expression in bladder cancer using formalin-fixed, paraffin-embedded tissues: correlation with histopathological grade, tumour stage and survival. Int J Cancer. 1995;64(6):367–70.
16. Keck B, Wach S, Kunath F, Bertz S, Taubert H, Lehmann J, Stockle M, Wullich B, Hartmann A. Nuclear E-cadherin expression is associated with the loss of membranous E-cadherin, plasmacytoid differentiation and reduced overall survival in urothelial carcinoma of the bladder. Ann Surg Oncol. 2013;20(7): 2440–5.
17. Bruyere F, Namdarian B, Corcoran NM, Pedersen J, Ockrim J, Voelzke BB, Mete U, Costello AJ, Hovens CM. Snail expression is an independent predictor of tumor recurrence in superficial bladder cancers. Urol Oncol. 2010;28(6):591–6.
18. Kosaka T, Kikuchi E, Mikami S, Miyajima A, Shirotake S, Ishida M, Okada Y, Oya M. Expression of snail in upper urinary tract urothelial carcinoma: prognostic significance and implications for tumor invasion. Clin Cancer Res. 2010;16(23):5814–23.
19. Nomura S, Suzuki Y, Takahashi R, Terasaki M, Kimata R, Hamasaki T, Kimura G, Shimizu A, Kondo Y. Snail expression and outcome in T1 high-grade and T2 bladder cancer: a retrospective immunohistochemical analysis. BMC Urol. 2013;13:73.
20. Ioachim E, Charchanti A, Briasoulis E, Karavasilis V, Tsanou H, Arvanitis DL, Agnantis NJ, Pavlidis N. Immunohistochemical expression of extracellular matrix components tenascin, fibronectin, collagen type IV and laminin in breast cancer: their prognostic value and role in tumour invasion and progression. Eur J Cancer. 2002;38(18):2362–70.
21. Rybak JN, Roesli C, Kaspar M, Villa A, Neri D. The extra-domain a of fibronectin is a vascular marker of solid tumors and metastases. Cancer Res. 2007;67(22):10948–57.
22. Malmstrom PU, Larsson A, Johansson S. Urinary fibronectin in diagnosis and follow-up of patients with urinary bladder cancer. Br J Urol. 1993;72(3):307–10.
23. Menendez V, Fernandez-Suarez A, Galan JA, Perez M, Garcia-Lopez F. Diagnosis of bladder cancer by analysis of urinary fibronectin. Urology. 2005;65(2):284–9.
24. Goto K. CD138 expression is observed in the Urothelial epithelium and in various Urothelial carcinomas, and cannot be evidence for Plasmacytoid Urothelial carcinoma. Int J Surg Pathol. 2016;24(7):614–9.
25. Li Q, Assel M, Benfante NE, Pietzak EJ, Herr HW, Donat M, Cha EK, Donahue TF, Bochner BH, Dalbagni G. The impact of Plasmacytoid variant histology on the survival of patients with Urothelial carcinoma of bladder after radical cystectomy. Eur Urol Focus. 2019;5(1):104–8.

24

# Current status of genetic urinary biomarkers for surveillance of non-muscle invasive bladder cancer

F. Lozano[1,2*], C. X. Raventos[1], A. Carrion[1], E. Trilla[1] and J. Morote[1,2]

**Abstract**

**Background:** Genetic biomarkers are a promising and growing field in the management of bladder cancer in all stages. The aim of this paper is to understand the role of genetic urinary biomarkers in the follow up of patients with non muscle invasive bladder cancer where there is increasing evidence that they can play a role in avoiding invasive techniques.

**Methods:** Following PRISMA criteria, we have performed a systematic review. The search yielded 164 unique articles, of which 21 articles were included involving a total of 7261 patients. Sixteen of the articles were DNA based biomarkers, analyzing different methylations, microsatellite aberrations and gene mutations. Five articles studied the role of RNA based biomarkers, based on measuring levels of different combinations of mRNA. QUADAS2 critical evaluation of each paper has been reported.

**Results:** There are not randomized control trials comparing any biomarker with the gold standard follow-up, and the level of evidence is 2B in almost all the studies. Negative predictive value varies between 55 and 98.5%, being superior in RNA based biomarkers.

**Conclusions:** Although cystoscopy and cytology are the gold standard for non muscle invasive bladder cancer surveillance, genetic urinary biomarkers are a promising tool to avoid invasive explorations to the patients with a safe profile of similar sensitivity and negative predictive value. The accuracy that genetic biomarkers can offer should be taken into account to modify the paradigm of surveillance in non muscle invasive bladder cancer patients, especially in high-risk ones where many invasive explorations are recommended and biomarkers experiment better results.

**Keywords:** Biomarkers, Surveillance, Bladder, Genetic

* Correspondence: flozano@vhebron.net
[1]Urology Department, Vall d'Hebron University Hospital, Pg. Vall d'Hebron 119-129, 08035 Barcelona, Spain
[2]Universitat Autònoma de Barcelona, Barcelona, Spain

## Background

Bladder cancer (BC) is the fifth most common neoplasm worldwide, with more than 54,000 new cases estimated per year in the United States alone [1] . BC is a heterogeneous tumour that is associated with very high economic costs and a substantial impact on patients' quality of life owing to its characteristically high risk of recurrence and the complexity of follow up [2]. Guidelines from the European Association of Urology (EAU) and the American Urological Association (AUA) suggest a combination of cystoscopy, cytology and imaging for the surveillance of patients with non-muscle invasive bladder cancer (NMIBC) [3, 4]. Cystoscopy is an invasive procedure that carries the risks of painful micturition, urinary frequency and macroscopic haematuria of 50, 37 and 19%, respectively [5], while cytology has a very low sensitivity, especially for low-grade tumours [6, 7] .

For this reason there has been an increase in research over the past years into urinary biomarkers for the three scenarios of haematuria, diagnosis and surveillance. The role of these new tests is to increase the sensitivity and the specificity of the available gold-standard techniques, while sparing the patient the discomfort of an invasive test and its potential complications. Although many types of urinary biomarkers have been investigated, biomarkers that use genetic materials such as DNA and RNA seem to be the most promising due to their potential to identify a genetic signature. Such a signature would not only prove useful in disease detection and follow-up but also in the facilitation of more precise treatment by avoiding unhelpful therapies that may delay the best oncological pathway.

The field of urinary biomarker research in BC is focused on balancing a non-invasive, safe method with a cost-effective strategy that can be used to improve the sensitivity of bladder tumour detection in the initial phase of the disease and during patient follow-up, compared with the current gold standard.

Selecting a biomarker must be based on the given scenario and follow the principles of the international guidelines [8, 9] . The current literature clearly differentiates between different biomarker tests and characteristics depending on whether the BC is low or high risk. For low-risk tumours, marker-guided testing of lesions is suggested to detect possible progression to high-risk tumours. For high-risk tumours, however, where early detection is the main objective, selection of high-sensitivity biomarkers is recommended [9].

The aim of this study is to analyse the current literature for the use of genetic urinary biomarkers in the surveillance of NMIBC.

## Methods

FLP performed a bibliographic search of Medline (http://www.ncbi.nlm.nih.gov), Embase (http://www.embase.com) and the Cochrane library (http://www.cochrane.org) up to March 2020. MeSH terms used were Bladder cancer AND surveillance AND biomarkers AND DNA OR RNA OR methylation, yielding 2241 articles. After that, two authors (FLP and CXR) screened all published original articles appearing in the above search for eligibility. Studies using genetic urinary biomarkers for surveillance in non muscle invasive bladder cancer in humans were selected. Studies were excluded if they were not original research papers, used a language other than English, had less than 20 patients or did not report biomarker performance in terms of sensitivity, specificity, or area under the curve (AUC); or reported the performance of genetic markers only in combination with other factors (clinical data or non genetic biomarkers), yielding 164 articles.

After applying the PRISMA (Preferred Reporting Items for Systematic Reviews and Meta-analyses) criteria narrowed this down to 21 original articles (Fig. 1).

After reviewing each of the selected articles using the REMARK checklist [10], we designed a QUADAS-2 table to evaluate each study's risk of bias and quality (Fig. 2). The main bias observed was reference to the index test. Although we identified a 50% risk of bias, most of the articles reviewed met most of the QUADAS-2 criteria [11], using the four considerations (patient selection, index, reference and flux and timming) which suggested that the studies were of moderately high quality.

We have also used the SWIM (Synthesis without meta-analysis) reporting guideline [12] to clarify the reporting methodology of the article (Fig. 3). The evidence was reported in terms of sensitivity and specificity for each biomarker (for low grade and high grade tumors in case of studies that indicated that subestratification). Area under de curve has been informed in eleven of the seventeen studies. We have also reported negative and positive predictive value of the markers. Recurrence rate has been calculated using the positive cases (positive pathology) and the total number of samples. We have prioritized articles identified as low risk of bias based on QUADAS-2 table to draw the conclusions of this review. We have also performed exploratory analyses to determine whether different study characteristics varied the effects of the interventions. Almost all the studies accepted as confirmed positive case if there is a pathology report. Some studies generate artificial cohort. We examined whether this different type of targeted behaviour modified, on average, the effect of the interventions.

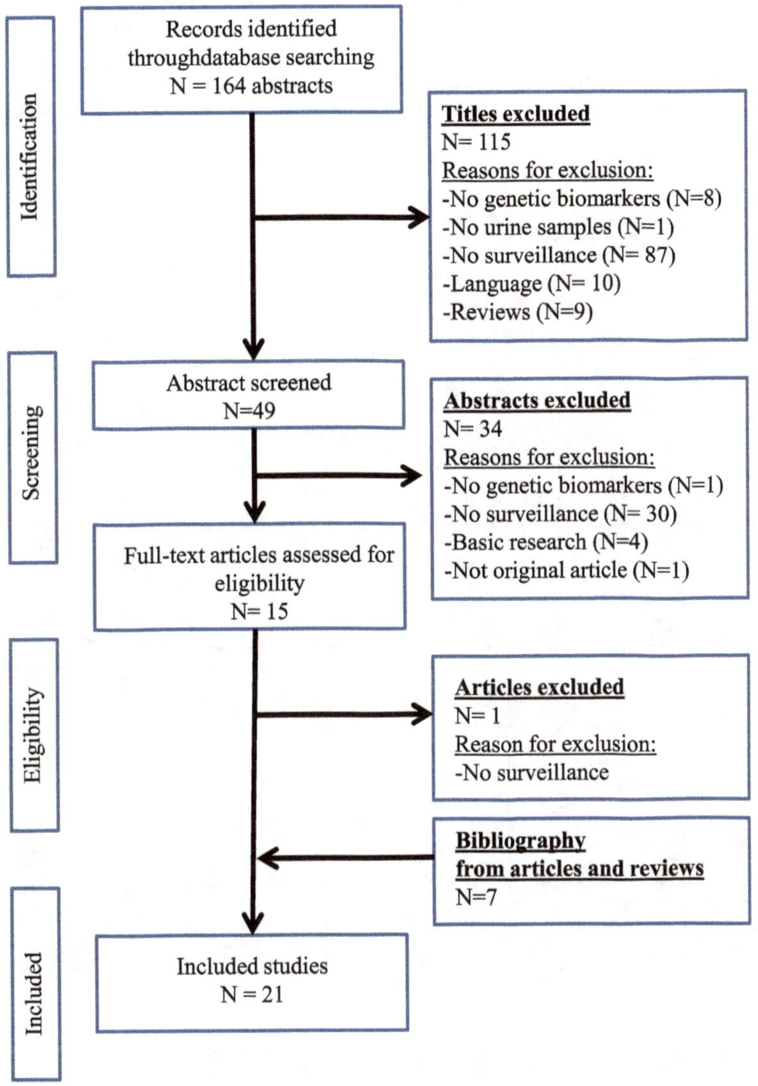


**Fig. 1** Flow chart following PRISMA criteria

## Results

In order to obtain a practical and visual description of the different studies, we divided the biomarkers by method into DNA-based (Table 1) and RNA-based (Table 2) tests.

### DNA tests (Table 1)

DNA tests used for surveillance are based on microsatellite analysis (MA). They are employed to detect loss of heterozygosity, gene methylation levels and gene mutations in cells collected from urine.

Microsatellite markers are highly polymorphic tandem repeat DNA sequences distributed throughout the genome and easily amplifiable by standard polymerase chain reaction [34] . Rouprêt et al. [13] compared this biomarker with methylation biomarkers in a comparative cohort study of 40 patients. In this study, MA appeared to yield better results for detecting recurrences (AUC 0.81 vs 0.44). When a Bayesian network analysis was performed that combined variables and biomarkers, the panel of markers generated a sensitivity of 85% and a specificity of 86%. Van der Aa et al. [14] designed a multicentre study to evaluate the clinical utility of MA in low-grade tumours in combination with *FGFR3* mutations described previously [35]. The sensitivity in this study was 58% and the specificity 73%, with a negative predictive value of 94%.

DNA methylation has been recognized to be important in the developmental biology and cancer aetiology of many neoplasms [36–38]. DNA methylation is an epigenetic marker that mainly affects CpG dinucleotides. These dinucleotides are distributed throughout the genome and usually have a normal methylation status. Hypermethylation of CpG dinucleotides in the promoter

| | Risk of bias | | | | Concerns regarding applicability | | |
|---|---|---|---|---|---|---|---|
| | Patient selection | Index test(s) | Reference standard | Flow and timing | Patient selection | Index test(s) | Reference standard |
| Roupret 2008 | (-) | (-) | (+) | (+) | (+) | (+) | (+) |
| Van der Aa 2009 | (+) | (+) | (-) | (+) | (+) | (+) | (+) |
| Zuuiverloon 2010 | (-) | (+) | (+) | (+) | (+) | (+) | (+) |
| Reinert 2012 | (+) | (-) | (+) | (-) | (+) | (+) | (+) |
| Zuiverloon 2011 | (-) | (-) | (+) | (+) | (+) | (-) | (+) |
| Allory 2013 | (+) | (-) | (+) | (+) | (+) | (+) | (+) |
| Abern 2014 | (-) | (+) | (-) | (+) | (-) | (+) | (+) |
| Su 2014 | (+) | (-) | (+) | (-) | (+) | (+) | (+) |
| Sapre 2015 | (-) | (-) | (+) | (+) | (+) | (+) | (-) |
| Fantony 2015 | (+) | (-) | (-) | (+) | (+) | (-) | (-) |
| Baukers 2016 | (+) | (+) | (+) | (+) | (+) | (+) | (+) |
| Kavalieris 2016 | (+) | (-) | (+) | (+) | (+) | (+) | (+) |
| Roperch 2016 | (-) | (+) | (+) | (-) | (+) | (+) | (+) |
| Lotan 2017 | (+) | (+) | (+) | (+) | (+) | (+) | (+) |
| Pilcher 2017 | (+) | (-) | (+) | (+) | (+) | (+) | (+) |
| Van der Heijden 2018 | (+) | (-) | (+) | (+) | (+) | (+) | (+) |
| Wallace 2018 | (+) | (-) | (+) | (-) | (+) | (+) | (+) |
| Witjes 2018 | (-) | (+) | (+) | (+) | (+) | (-) | (+) |
| Springer 2018 | (-) | (+) | (+) | (+) | (-) | (+) | (+) |
| D'Andrea 2019 | (-) | (+) | (-) | (+) | (-) | (+) | (+) |
| Batista 2019 | (+) | (-) | (+) | (+) | (+) | (-) | (+) |

Risk of bias (-) High (+) Low

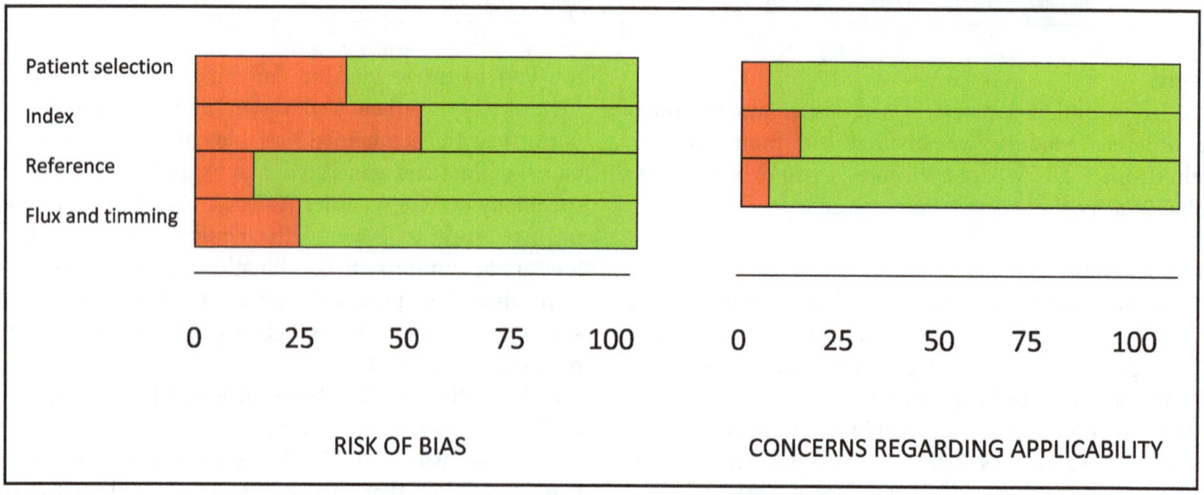


**Fig. 2** QUADAS 2 table evaluating quality of the studies

## Synthesis Without Meta-analysis (SWiM) reporting items

The citation for the Synthesis Without Meta-analysis explanation and elaboration article is: Campbell M, McKenzie JE, Sowden A, Katikireddi SV, Brennan SE, Ellis S, Hartmann-Boyce J, Ryan R, Shepperd S, Thomas J, Welch V, Thomson H. Synthesis without meta-analysis (SWiM) in systematic reviews: reporting guideline BMJ 2020;368:l6890 http://dx.doi.org/10.1136/bmj.l6890

| SWiM is intended to complement and be used as an extension to PRISMA | | | |
|---|---|---|---|
| **SWiM reporting item** | **Item description** | **Page in manuscript where item is reported** | **Other*** |
| *Methods* | | | |
| **1** Grouping studies for synthesis | 1a) Provide a description of, and rationale for, the groups used in the synthesis (e.g., groupings of populations, interventions, outcomes, study design) | 3 | |
| | 1b) Detail and provide rationale for any changes made subsequent to the protocol in the groups used in the synthesis | - | |
| **2** Describe the standardised metric and transformation methods used | Describe the standardised metric for each outcome. Explain why the metric(s) was chosen, and describe any methods used to transform the intervention effects, as reported in the study, to the standardised metric, citing any methodological guidance consulted | 3 | |
| **3** Describe the synthesis methods | Describe and justify the methods used to synthesise the effects for each outcome when it was not possible to undertake a meta-analysis of effect estimates | - | |
| **4** Criteria used to prioritise results for summary and synthesis | Where applicable, provide the criteria used, with supporting justification, to select the particular studies, or a particular study, for the main synthesis or to draw conclusions from the synthesis (e.g., based on study design, risk of bias assessments, directness in relation to the review question) | 3 | |
| **SWiM reporting item** | **Item description** | **Page in manuscript where item is reported** | **Other*** |
| **5** Investigation of heterogeneity in reported effects | State the method(s) used to examine heterogeneity in reported effects when it was not possible to undertake a meta-analysis of effect estimates and its extensions to investigate heterogeneity | 3 | |
| **6** Certainty of evidence | Describe the methods used to assess certainty of the synthesis findings | 3 | |
| **7** Data presentation methods | Describe the graphical and tabular methods used to present the effects (e.g., tables, forest plots, harvest plots).<br>Specify key study characteristics (e.g., study design, risk of bias) used to order the studies, in the text and any tables or graphs, clearly referencing the studies included | 4 | |
| *Results* | | | |
| **8** Reporting results | For each comparison and outcome, provide a description of the synthesised findings, and the certainty of the findings. Describe the result in language that is consistent with the question the synthesis addresses, and indicate which studies contribute to the synthesis | 4-6 | |
| *Discussion* | | | |
| **9** Limitations of the synthesis | Report the limitations of the synthesis methods used and/or the groupings used in the synthesis, and how these affect the conclusions that can be drawn in relation to the original review question | 6-7 | |

PRISMA=Preferred Reporting Items for Systematic Reviews and Meta-Analyses.
*If the information is not provided in the systematic review, give details of where this information is available (e.g., protocol, other published papers (provide citation details), or website (provide the URL)).

**Fig. 3** Synthesis Without Meta-analysis (SWiM) reporting items

**Table 1** DNA based biomarkers used in follow-up for non muscle invasive bladder cancer patients

| Reference | Patients/ samples | Recurrence rate | Sensitivity(%) | Specificity(%) | NPV (%) | PPV (%) | AUC | Method | Markers |
|---|---|---|---|---|---|---|---|---|---|
| Roupret *et al* 2008 [13] | 40/40 | 38% | 80 (microsatellite)<br>86 (methylation)<br>85 (combination) | 68 (microsat)<br>8 (methyl)<br>86 (combination) | | | 0.81 (microsat)<br>0.44 (methyl) | DNA PCR | Microsatellite[a] vs methylation[b] |
| Van der Aa *et al* 2009 [14] | 228/815 | 10.3% | 58 | 73 | 94 | 61-77 | NA | DNA PCR | Microsatellite + FGFR3 mutation |
| Zuiverloon *et al* 2010 [15] | 134/463 | 9.7% | 58 | NA | 89 | 25 | NA | DNA PCR | FGFR3 mutations[c] |
| Reinert *et al* 2012 [16] | 158/206 | 67.4% | 87-94 | 28-47 | 55-78 | 72-78 | 0.68-0.78 | DNA PCR | Methylation [d] |
| Zuiverloon *et al* 2012 [17] | NA/94 | 69.1% | 72.3 | 55.2 | NA | NA | NA | DNA PCR | Methylation genes APC_a , TERT_a , TER _b ,EDNRB |
| Allory *et al* 2013 [18] | 194/395 | 44.8% | 19(FGFR3)<br>42(TERT)<br>50(FGFR3+TERT) | 73 (TERT)<br>90(FGFR3)<br>71(FGFR3+TERT) | NA | NA | NA | DNA PCR | Gene mutations (TERT and FGFR3) |
| Abern *et al* 2014 [19] | 111/111 | 21.6% | 75-79 | 63-71 | 92 | 37-42 | 0.74 (TWIST1)<br>0.68 (NID2) | DNA PCR | Methylation genes TWIST1, NID2 |
| Su *et al* 2014 [20] | 90/368 | 37.7% | 80 | 97 | NA | NA | 0.95 | DNA PCR | Hyper and hypomethylated genes (SOX1, IRAK3, L1-MET) |
| Fantony *et al* 2015 [21] | 126/126 | 25% | 58-67 | 61-69 | 83-85 | 36-38 | 0.66 (TWIST1)<br>0.63 (NID2) | DNA PCR | Methylation genes TWIST1, NID2 |
| Beukers *et al* 2016 [22] | NA/2191 | 64% | 57 (LG)<br>72 (HG) | 59% LG | NA | NA | NA | DNA PCR | FGFR3 mutation, TERT mutation and OTX1 methylation |
| Roperch *et al* 2016 [23] | 158/613 | 45.5% | 94.5<br>96 (HG) | 75.9 | 98.5 | NA | 0.82 | DNA PCR | FGFR3 mutation +DNA methylation HS3ST2, SLIT2 and SEPTIN9 |
| Van der Heijden *et al* 2018 [24] | NA/458 | 37.7% | 90 | 31 | 82 | 50 | 0.74 | DNA PCR | DNA gene Methylation (CFTR, SALL3, TWIST1) |
| Witjes *et al* 2018 [25] | 353/353 | 13% | 68.2<br>92.6 (HG) | 88 | 95.1<br>99.3( HG) | 44.8 | 0.82 | DNA PCR | 15 DNA methylation genes (Epicheck®) |
| Springer *et al* 2018 [26] | 322/322 | 58% | 68<br>71 (HG) | 80 | NA | NA | NA | DNA PCR | 10 gen mutations[e] plus detection of aneuploidy (UroSEEK®) |
| D'Andrea *et al* 2019 [27] | 357/357 | 13.7% | 67.3<br>88.9 (HG) | 88<br>88(HG) | 94<br>99 (HG) | 47<br>30 (HG) | 85.9 | DNA PCR | 15 DNA methylation genes (Epicheck®) |
| Batista *et al* 2019 [28] | 122/122 | 28% | 73.5 | 73.2 | NA | NA | NA | DNA PCR | TERT promoter and FGFR3 mutations (Uromonitor®) |

*LG* low grade, *HG* high grade, *NA* not allowed

[a]FGA (4q28), D4S171(4q35)), 5 (ACTBP2(5q14)), 9 (D9S162 (9p), IFNA (9p21)), 14 (MJD52(14q32)), 16 (D16S310 (16q21)) and 18 (D18S51 (18q21), MBP (18qter).

[b](RASSF1a (3p21.3),E-cadherin (16q22.1), APC (5q21), DAPK (9q22.1), MGMT (10q26), BCL2 (18q21.33), h-TERT (5p15.33), EDNRB (13q22), WIF-1 (12q14.3), TNFRSF25 (1p36.31), IGFBP3 (7p13))

[c]R248C and S249C (exon 7); G372C,S373C, Y375C, G382R, and A393E (exon 10); and K652M, K652T, K652E, and K652Q (exon 15)

[d]EOMES, HOXA9, POU4F2, TWIST1, VIM, ZNF154

[e]FGFR3, TP53, CDKN2A, ERBB2, HRAS, KRAS, PIK3CA, MET, VHL, MLL and TERT promoter.

**Table 2** RNA based biomarkers used in follow-up for non muscle invasive bladder cancer patients

| Reference | Patients/samples | Recurrence rate | Sensitivity | Specificity | NPV | PPV | AUC | Method | Markers |
|---|---|---|---|---|---|---|---|---|---|
| Sapre *et al* 2016 [29] | 131/131 | NA | 88 | 48 | 75 | 63 | 0.74 | miRNA PCR | 6 miRNA signature[a] |
| Kavalieris *et al* 2017 [30] | 736/1036 | 15.1% | 92 | NA | 96 | NA | 0.73 | mRNA PCR | 5 genes mRNA expression (Cx Bladder Monitor® )[b] |
| Lotan *et al* 2017 [31] | 748/1016 | 14.8% | 91<br>95 (HG) | NA | 96 | NA | NA | mRNA PCR | 5 genes mRNA expression (Cx Bladder Monitor® )[b] vs NMP22 ELISA vs NMP22 BladderChek |
| Pilcher *et al* 2018 [32] | 140/155 | 30.7% | 84<br>100 (HG) | 91 | 93 | 72 | 0.87 | mRNA RT-PCR | ABL1, CRH, IGF2, UPK1B, ANXA10 (Xpert Bladder Cancer Monitor®) |
| Wallace *et al* 2018 [33] | 370/370 | 13.2% | 73<br>83 (HG) | 77 | 92 | 44 | 0.87 | mRNA RT-qPCR | ABL1, CRH, IGF2, ANXA10, UPK1B (Xpert Bladder Cancer Monitor®) |

*HG* high grade, *NA* not allowed
[a]miR16, miR200c, miR205, miR21, miR221 and miR34a
[b]IGFBP5, HOXA13, MDK, CDK1, CXCR2

regions of tumour suppressor genes can repress their transcription in human cells [39, 40]. Methylation status is one of the most studied biomarkers in the follow-up scenario because it is both chemically stable and quantifiable [41]. Zuiverloon et al. [17] developed a retrospective four-step test, selecting methylation of the *APC_a*, *TERT_a*, *TER_b* and *EDNRB* genes as the combination providing a higher sensitivity and specificity (63.3 and 58.3%, respectively) than other combinations investigated in this study. Based on their previous study [42], Reinert et al. evaluated the methylation of *EOMES*, *HOXA9*, *POU4F2*, *TWIST1*, *VIM* and *ZNF154*. Their study consisted of a first step, validating the markers and establishing the cut-off levels, and a second step in the surveillance scenario excluding those patients who showed no aberrant methylation of their tumour marker genes. The authors reported a sensitivity of between 87 and 94% and a specificity ranging from 43 to 67%. Combining the different biomarkers did not improve the accuracy of the test [16]. Su et al. [20] tested six DNA methylation markers before building a model with *SOX1*, *IRAK3* and *L1-MET* as the best combination to detect recurrences. Using this model they obtaining a sensitivity of 80% and a very high specificity of 97%. Roperch et al. [23] combined four different *FGFR3* mutations and eighteen methylation markers based on the literature [43, 44]. Finally, they selected three of these markers (the genes *HS3ST2*, *SLIT2* and *SEPTIN9*) for combination with the *FGFR3* mutations in a logistic regression model, obtaining a sensitivity of 94.5% (96% in high-grade tumours) and a specificity of 75.9%. Van der Heijden et al. [24] evaluated seven selected genes that are found at significantly increased levels in the urine sediment from patients with BC. After testing a training set, they selected the *CFTR*, *SALL3* and *TWIST1* genes for validation in a large series (458 samples) and obtained a sensitivity of 90% (96% in combination with cytology). Witjes et al. [25] evaluated a combination of 15 methylated genes (Epicheck®), obtaining a sensitivity of 68.2% (92.6% for high-grade tumours) and a specificity of 88%. D'Andrea et al. [27] published another multicentric and independent study using the same test, supporting the sensitivity (67.3, 88.9% for high grade) and specificity (88%) described in the previous publication by Witjes. Abern [19] studied the role of two methylated genes, TWIST1 and NID2 based on Renard work [45] due to their high sensitivity and specificity for urothelial carcinoma. They observed that TWIST1 methylation had better AUA than NID2 or the combination of both genes. They also showed that adjusting the thresholds, the test had a sensitivity and specificity of 75 and 71%, respectively. Fantony et al. [21] published a more recent multi-institutional study using the same methylated genes, obtaining similar conclusions and results of sensitivity (58–67%) and specificity (61–69%). In this paper, prior BCG treatment for NMIBC reduced the accuracy of the test.

Many of the gene mutations investigated are related to the carcinogenesis of urothelial carcinomas, which are among the most heterogeneous tumours [46]. One of the most studied among these genes is fibroblast growth factor receptor 3 (*FGFR3*), mutations of which are found in almost 80% of the low-grade tumours and associated with a good prognosis [35, 47].

Zuiverloon et al. [15] evaluated this marker in non-high grade tumours, achieving a sensitivity of 58%. Beukers et al. [22] combined *FGFR3* mutation with *TERT* mutation and *OTX1* gene methylation in a large prospective European cohort study, obtaining a sensitivity of 57% for low-grade and 72% for high-grade BC. Allory investigated the role of telomerase reverse transcriptase (TERT) promoter mutations, frequently founded in many other non urothelial tumors [48] in combination with FGFR3 mutation [18]. This study showed that combination of TERT and FGFR3 has higher sensitivity (50%) than TERT or FGFR3 individually. Moreover, FGFR3 had higher specificity than TERT mutation.

In a more recent multicentric study, Batista et al. [48] have developed a biomarker based on two TERT mutations (c. 1-124C > T and c.1-146C > T) plus FGFR3 (p.R248C and p.S249C) hotspot mutations. After a technical validation of the test, they achieved a73.5% of sensitivity and 93.2% of specificity. Springer et al. [26] have also analyzed mutations in TERT promoter, mutations in FGFR3 in combination with other nine gen mutations (TP53, CDKN2A, ERBB2, HRAS, KRAS, PIK3CA, MET, VHL, MLL) plus detection of aneuploidy,an abnormal chromosome number, that has been estimated to be present in > 90% of the cancer of most histopathologic types [49]. They found that this combination could detect recurrences with a sensitivity of 68% and a specificity of 80%.

#### RNA tests (Table 2)

RNA biomarkers are less well studied in the field of BC surveillance.

MicroRNAs (miRNAs) are B22-nucleotide long, single-stranded, non-coding RNAs that bind to complementary 'seed' regions found in the 30-untranslated region of particular messenger RNA (mRNA) species. MiRNAs can modulate the expression of their mRNA targets and are involved in many physiological processes, but also in carcinogenesis [50]. Sapre et al. [29] evaluated a 12-miRNA-panel test, with the aim of selecting the minimum number of miRNAs necessary to achieve an accurate prediction. They found that a selection of six miRNAs (miR16, miR200c, miR205, miR21, miR221 and miR34a) provided a sensitivity of 88% and a specificity of 48%.

Kavalieris et al. [30] and Lotan et al. [31] tested a combination of five mRNAs (*IGFBP5, HOXA13, MDK, CDK1, CXCR2*), commercially available under the brand name Cx Bladder Monitor®, and reported highly consistent results for the evaluation of the mRNA expression from the five genes. The studies included a scoring system, based on variables such as previous tumour status (primary or recurrent) and time since previous tumour in years, to classify the test as positive or negative. The authors reported sensitivities between 91 and 92% (95% in high-grade tumours) and a negative predictive value of 96%.

Wallace et al. [33] and Pichler et al. [32] tested the Xpert BC Monitor®, a commercial kit that measures five target mRNAs (*ABL1, CRH, IGF2, UPK1B, ANXA10*), in a population of 510 patients and obtained sensitivities between 73 and 84% (100% in high-grade tumours) and a negative predictive value of 92–93%. They also confirmed that cytology did not enhance diagnostic accuracy.

### Discussion

Biomarker investigation is a growing field in the management of NMIBC. Many of the investigations are used in different scenarios: diagnosis, surveillance, and risk stratification of patients with NMIBC. Although many molecular marker tests have been developed to improve diagnostic and surveillance accuracy, with some having been approved by the US Food and Drug Administration, none of the currently available tests have been accepted or incorporated into the follow-up algorithms described in the guidelines [51].

Biomarkers can be divided into cellular, protein and genetic markers. The latter are the most recent and, in contrast to cytology, have the advantages of being reliable, easy to perform, and objective.

In fact, they perform significantly better in BC because thousands of genetic changes can be detected accurately and simultaneously compared with the lower-throughput protein-based biomarkers. As aberrant DNA methylation also occurs in non-malignant tissue it is not pathognomonic of malignancy and genetic methylation cannot be used to distinguish between cancer cells and other pre- or non-neoplastic cells [52]. However, this genetic biomarker has the benefits of always occurring in the same DNA location and chemical stability which make it easier to detect than gene mutations.

Protein-based and cell-based biomarkers are also more likely to be affected by benign conditions such as infection, inflammation and bladder treatments.

To date the gold standard for these cases, as outlined in the guidelines, is to use cystoscopy and cytology. Cystoscopy is an invasive procedure that may be associated with pain and discomfort [5]. Moreover, cystoscopy does not detect all lesions and is subject to the experience of the urologist or nurse [53]. Voided urine cytology needs trained cytopathologists and has the potential for inter-observer variability.

Researchers who are developing urinary biomarkers are looking for high sensitivity and a high negative predictive value. This profile is of special interest in the follow-up scenario because the aim of these tests is to reduce the number of cystoscopies by alternating the procedures, rather than avoiding cystoscopy altogether. Thus, cystoscopy will only be performed when the urine test is positive (urine-first strategy).

One of the major limitations of the use of DNA- or mRNA-based techniques is the difficulty in obtaining sufficiently large quantities of high-quality RNA from voided urine. In terms of monitoring, another limitation of non-invasive urine biomarkers is their low sensitivity, particularly for early-stage and low-grade tumours that account for a significant proportion of recurrences.

Almost all the studies had a high percentage of 'false'-positive urine tests for the detection of concomitant recurrences, resulting in low specificity. In many articles, the authors justified these percentages with the well-known phenomenon of the anticipatory effect, i.e. the urine test detects recurrent tumours earlier than cystoscopy. It is accepted in the literature that anticipatory detection would include recurrences that occur within the next 18 months after a positive biomarker test [54]. In any case, performing a cystoscopy because of a false positive is more acceptable than missing a tumour because of a false negative.

Other limitations of the studies included in this review are the retrospective nature of some of the cohorts used for the outcome analysis, artificial oversampling of the recurrence rate by recruiting patients scheduled for transurethral resection of a proven bladder tumour, and using the same population for the training and the validation sets, which increases the possibility that the performance of the biomarker may be artificially inflated due to over-fitting.

In this review, most of the biomarker tests are dichotomous, providing either positive (tumour detected) or negative (no tumour) test results. However, giving a numerical prediction of the probability of a recurrent tumour may be more helpful to urologists in terms of their decision-making.

Moreover, there is a lack of uniformity in the design of the studies. Some of the works describe surveillance programs but they create the cohorts. Many of the biomarkers tested need clinical information to complete an algorithm and yield a positive or negative result, which increases subjectivity and decreases the homogeneity of results.

The main limitations were the lack of randomized control trials and the diverse study outcomes, which made meta-analysis impossible to perform. Comparison between sensitivity and specificity of different biomarkers may generate a bias due to the different incidence and different cohort.

Literature lacks of direct comparison between urinary biomarkers and gold standard maybe due to commercial interests.

## Conclusion

BC is one of the most expensive tumours due to its high recurrence rate and the costs of the follow-up protocols.

This is the reason why there is an increased interest in biomarkers, in order to reduce the number of exploratory investigations and improve the quality of life of patients with BC. In this review, there are some genetic biomarkers with higher negative predictive value and sensitivity, especially for high-grade tumours, compared to the gold standard. European and US guidelines still recommend cystoscopy and cytology for follow-up. Genetic urinary biomarkers are a very heterogeneous group of test that nowadays cannot replace the standard pathway of surveillance with cystoscopy and cytology. Although there are some ongoing clinical trials comparing both options, there is no level 1 evidence to support their recommendation instead of the gold standard.

### Abbreviations

PRISMA: Preferred reporting items for systematic reviews and meta-analyses; QUADAS: Quality Assessment of Diagnostic Accuracy Studies; BC: Bladder cancer; EAU: European Association of Urology; AUA: American Urological Association; NMIBC: Non-muscle invasive bladder cancer; MA: Microsatellite analysis; TERT: Telomerase reverse transcriptase; MiRNA: MicroRNAs; mRNA: Messenger RNA

### Acknowledgements

Not applicable.

### Authors' contributions

F. L and C.X.R. did the evidence acquisition and the tables. All authors (F.L., C.X.R., A.C., E.T., J.M.) contributed writing the manuscript, read and approved the final manuscript.

### References

1. Siegel RL, Miller KD, Jemal A. Cancer statistics, 2019. CA Cancer J Clin. 2019; 69(1):7–34. https://doi.org/10.3322/caac.21551.
2. Leal J, Luengo-Fernandez R, Sullivan R, Witjes JA. Economic burden of bladder Cancer across the European Union. Eur Urol. 2016;69(3):438–47. https://doi.org/10.1016/j.eururo.2015.10.024.
3. Compérat E, Gontero P, Mostafid AH, Palou J, Van Rhijn BWG, Rouprêt M, et al. Non-muscle-invasive Bladder Cancer (TaT1 and CIS) EAU Guidelines; 2018. p. 1–48. Retrieved from http://uroweb.org/wp-content/uploads/EAU-Guidelines-Non-muscle-invasive-Bladder-Cancer-TaT1-CIS-2018.pdf.
4. Daneshmand S, Konety BR. American urological association (AUA) guideline American urological association non-muscle invasive bladder Cancer. AUA Clinical Guidelines, (April); 2016. p. 1–45.
5. Burke DM, Shackley DC, O'Reilly PH. The community-based morbidity of flexible cystoscopy. BJU Int. 2002;89(4):347–9. https://doi.org/10.1046/j.1464-4096.2001.01899.x.
6. Karakiewicz PI, Benayoun S, Zippe C, Lüdecke G, Boman H, Sanchez-Carbayo M, et al. Institutional variability in the accuracy of urinary cytology for predicting recurrence of transitional cell carcinoma of the bladder. BJU Int. 2006;97(5):997–1001. https://doi.org/10.1111/j.1464-410X.2006.06036.x.
7. Lotan Y, Roehrborn CG. Sensitivity and specificity of commonly available bladder tumor markers versus cytology: results of a comprehensive literature review and meta-analyses. Urology. 2003;61(1):109–18. https://doi.org/10.1016/S0090-4295(02)02136-2.
8. Bensalah K, Montorsi F, Shariat SF. Challenges of Cancer biomarker profiling {a figure is presented}. Eur Urol. 2007;52(6):1601–9. https://doi.org/10.1016/j.eururo.2007.09.036.
9. Kamat AM, Karakiewicz PI, Xylinas E, Hegarty PK, Hegarty N, Jenkins LC, et al. ICUD-EAU international consultation on bladder Cancer 2012: screening, diagnosis, and molecular markers. Eur Urol. 2012;63(2013):4–15.
10. Altman DG, McShane LM, Sauerbrei W, Taube SE, Cavenagh MM. REMARK (REporting recommendations for tumor MARKer prognostic studies). Guidelines for Reporting Health Research: A User's Manual. 2014:241–9. https://doi.org/10.1002/9781118715598.ch23.
11. Whiting, Penny F. ; Rutjes, Anne W.S.; Westwood, Marie E. ; Mallett, Susan ; Deeks, Jonathan J. ; Reitsma, Johannes B., ; Leeflang, Mariska M.G. ; Sterne, Jonathan A.C. ; Bossuyt, P. M. M. ; (2011). QUADAS-2: a revised tool for the quality assessment of diagnostic accuracy studies. Ann Internal Med Res RepMethods, 155(4), 529–536.

12. Campbell M, McKenzie JE, Sowden A, Katikireddi SV, Brennan SE, Ellis S, et al. Synthesis without meta-analysis (SWiM) in systematic reviews: reporting guideline. The BMJ. 2020;368:1–6. https://doi.org/10.1136/bmj.l6890.
13. Rouprêt M, Hupertan V, Yates DR, Comperat E, Catto JWF, Meuth M, et al. A comparison of the performance of microsatellite and methylation urine analysis for predicting the recurrence of urothelial cell carcinoma, and definition of a set of markers by Bayesian network analysis. BJU Int. 2008; 101(11):1448–53. https://doi.org/10.1111/j.1464-410X.2008.07591.x.
14. van der Aa MNM, Zwarthoff EC, Steyerberg EW, Boogaard MW, Nijsen Y, van der Keur KA, et al. Microsatellite analysis of voided-urine samples for surveillance of low-grade non-muscle-invasive Urothelial carcinoma: feasibility and clinical utility in a prospective multicenter study (cost-effectiveness of follow-up of urinary bladder Cancer trial C). Eur Urol. 2009; 55(3):659–68. https://doi.org/10.1016/j.eururo.2008.05.001.
15. Zuiverloon TCM, Van Der Aa MNM, Van Der Kwast TH, Steyerberg EW, Lingsma HF, Bangma CH, Zwarthoff EC. Fibroblast growth factor receptor 3 mutation analysis on voided urine for surveillance of patients with low-grade non-muscle - invasive bladder cancer. Clin Cancer Res. 2010;16(11): 3011–8. https://doi.org/10.1158/1078-0432.CCR-09-3013.
16. Reinert T, Borre M, Christiansen A, Hermann GG, Ørntoft TF, Dyrskjøt L. Diagnosis of bladder Cancer recurrence based on urinary levels of EOMES, HOXA9, POU4F2, TWIST1, VIM, and ZNF154 Hypermethylation. PLoS One. 2012;7(10):1–9. https://doi.org/10.1371/journal.pone.0046297.
17. Zuiverloon TCM, Beukers W, Van Der Keur KA, Munoz JR, Bangma CH, Lingsma HF, et al. A methylation assay for the detection of non-muscle-invasive bladder cancer (NMIBC) recurrences in voided urine. BJU Int. 2012; 109(6):941–8. https://doi.org/10.1111/j.1464-410X.2011.10428.x.
18. Allory Y, Beukers W, Sagrera A, Flández M, Marqués M, Márquez M, et al. Telomerase reverse transcriptase promoter mutations in bladder cancer: high frequency across stages, detection in urine, and lack of association with outcome. Eur Urol. 2014;65(2):360–6. https://doi.org/10.1016/j.eururo.2013.08.052.
19. Abern MR, Owusu R, Inman BA. Clinical performance and utility of a DNA methylation urine test for bladder cancer. Urologic Oncol. 2014;32(1):51.e21–6. https://doi.org/10.1016/j.urolonc.2013.08.003.
20. Su S-F, de Castro Abreu AL, Chihara Y, Tsai Y, Andreu-Vieyra C, Daneshmand S, et al. A panel of three markers hyper- and Hypomethylated in urine sediments accurately predicts bladder Cancer recurrence. Clin Cancer Res. 2014;20(7):1978–89. https://doi.org/10.1158/1078-0432.CCR-13-2637.
21. Fantony JJ, Abern MR, Gopalakrishna A, Owusu R, Jack Tay K, Lance RS, Inman BA. Multi-institutional external validation of urinary TWIST1 and NID2 methylation as a diagnostic test for bladder cancer. Urologic Oncol. 2015; 33(9):387.e1–6. https://doi.org/10.1016/j.urolonc.2015.04.014.
22. Beukers W, van der Keur KA, Kandimalla R, Vergouwe Y, Steyerberg EW, Boormans JL, et al. FGFR3, TERT and OTX1 as a urinary biomarker combination for surveillance of patients with bladder Cancer in a large prospective multicenter study. J Urol. 2017;197(6):1410–8. https://doi.org/10.1016/j.juro.2016.12.096.
23. Roperch JP, Grandchamp B, Desgrandchamps F, Mongiat-Artus P, Ravery V, Ouzaid I, et al. Promoter hypermethylation of HS3ST2, SEPTIN9 and SLIT2 combined with FGFR3 mutations as a sensitive/specific urinary assay for diagnosis and surveillance in patients with low or high-risk non-muscle-invasive bladder cancer. BMC Cancer. 2016;16(1):1–9. https://doi.org/10.1186/s12885-016-2748-5.
24. van der Heijden AG, Mengual L, Ingelmo-Torres M, Lozano JJ, van Rijt-van de Westerlo CCM, Baixauli M, et al. Urine cell-based DNA methylation classifier for monitoring bladder cancer. Clin Epigenetics. 2018;10(1):1–10. https://doi.org/10.1186/s13148-018-0496-x.
25. Witjes JA, Morote J, Cornel EB, Gakis G, van Valenberg FJP, Lozano F, et al. Performance of the bladder EpiCheck™ methylation test for patients under surveillance for non–muscle-invasive bladder Cancer: results of a multicenter, prospective, blinded clinical trial. Eur Urol Oncol. 2018;1(4):307–13. https://doi.org/10.1016/j.euo.2018.06.011.
26. Springer SU, Chen CH, Del Carmen Rodriguez Pena M, Li L, Douville C, Wang Y, et al. Non-invasive detection of urothelial cancer through the analysis of driver gene mutations and aneuploidy. ELife. 2018;7:1–27. https://doi.org/10.7554/eLife.32143.
27. D'Andrea D, Soria F, Zehetmayer S, Gust KM, Korn S, Witjes JA, Shariat SF. Diagnostic accuracy, clinical utility and influence on decision-making of a methylation urine biomarker test in the surveillance of non-muscle-invasive bladder cancer. BJU Int. 2019;123(6):959–67. https://doi.org/10.1111/bju.14673.
28. Batista R, Vinagre J, Prazeres H, Sampaio C, Peralta P, Conceição P, et al. Validation of a novel, sensitive, and specific urine-based test for recurrence surveillance of patients with non-muscle-invasive bladder Cancer in a comprehensive multicenter study. Front Genet. 2019;10(December):1–15. https://doi.org/10.3389/fgene.2019.01237.
29. Sapre N, Macintyre G, Clarkson M, Naeem H, Cmero M, Kowalczyk A, et al. A urinary microRNA signature can predict the presence of bladder urothelial carcinoma in patients undergoing surveillance. Br J Cancer. 2016;114(4):454–62. https://doi.org/10.1038/bjc.2015.472.
30. Kavalieris L, O'Sullivan P, Frampton C, Guilford P, Darling D, Jacobson E, et al. Performance characteristics of a multigene urine biomarker test for monitoring for recurrent Urothelial carcinoma in a multicenter study. J Urol. 2017;197(6):1419–26. https://doi.org/10.1016/j.juro.2016.12.010.
31. Lotan Y, O'Sullivan P, Raman JD, Shariat SF, Kavalieris L, Frampton C, et al. Clinical comparison of noninvasive urine tests for ruling out recurrent urothelial carcinoma. Urologic Oncol. 2017;35(8):531.e15–22. https://doi.org/10.1016/j.urolonc.2017.03.008.
32. Pichler R, Fritz J, Tulchiner G, Klinglmair G, Soleiman A, Horninger W, et al. Increased accuracy of a novel mRNA-based urine test for bladder cancer surveillance. BJU Int. 2018;121(1):29–37. https://doi.org/10.1111/bju.14019.
33. Wallace E, Higuchi R, Satya M, McCann L, Sin MLY, Bridge JA, et al. Development of a 90-minute integrated noninvasive urinary assay for bladder Cancer detection. J Urol. 2018;199(3):655–62. https://doi.org/10.1016/j.juro.2017.09.141.
34. Mourah S, Cussenot O, Vimont V, Desgrandchamps F, Teillac P, Cochant-Priollet B, et al. Assessment of microsatellite instability in urine in the detection of transitional-cell carcinoma of the bladder. Int J Cancer. 1998; 79(6):629–33. https://doi.org/10.1002/(SICI)1097-0215(19981218)79:6<629::AID-IJC13>3.0.CO;2-1.
35. Van Oers JMM, Lurkin I, Van Exsel AJA, Nijsen Y, Van Rhijn BWG, Van Der Aa MNM, Zwarthoff EC. A simple and fast method for the simultaneous detection of nine fibroblast growth factor receptor 3 mutations in bladder cancer and voided urine. Clin Cancer Res. 2005;11(21):7743–8. https://doi.org/10.1158/1078-0432.CCR-05-1045.
36. Heller G, Babinsky VN, Ziegler B, Weinzierl M, Noll C, Altenberger C, et al. Genome-wide CpG island methylation analyses in non-small cell lung cancer patients. Carcinogenesis. 2013;34(3):513–21. https://doi.org/10.1093/carcin/bgs363.
37. Kim JG, Takeshima H, Niwa T, Rehnberg E, Shigematsu Y, Yoda Y, et al. Comprehensive DNA methylation and extensive mutation analyses reveal an association between the CpG island methylator phenotype and oncogenic mutations in gastric cancers. Cancer Lett. 2013;330(1):33–40. https://doi.org/10.1016/j.canlet.2012.11.022.
38. Ying J, Li H, Seng TJ, Langford C, Srivastava G, Tsao SW, et al. Functional epigenetics identifies a protocadherin PCDH10 as a candidate tumor suppressor for nasopharyngeal, esophageal and multiple other carcinomas with frequent methylation. Oncogene. 2006;25(7):1070–80. https://doi.org/10.1038/sj.onc.1209154.
39. Kelly TK, Jones PA, Sharma S. Epigenetics in cancer. Carcinogenesis. 2009; 31(1):27–36. https://doi.org/10.1093/carcin/bgp220.
40. Saxonov S, Berg P, D. L. B. A genome-wide analysis of CpG dinucleotides in the human genome distinguishes two distinct classes of promoters. Proc Natl Acad Sci. 2006;18(2):193–204. https://doi.org/10.1080/03071375.1994.9747015.
41. Laird PW. The power and the promise of DNA methylation markers. Nat Rev Cancer. 2003;3(4):253–66. https://doi.org/10.1038/nrc1045.
42. Reinert T, Modin C, Castano FM, Lamy P, Wojdacz TK, Hansen LL, et al. Comprehensive genome methylation analysis in bladder cancer: identification and validation of novel methylated genes and application of these as urinary tumor markers. Clin Cancer Res. 2011;17(17):5582–92. https://doi.org/10.1158/1078-0432.CCR-10-2659.
43. Serizawa RR, Ralfkiær U, Steven K, Lam GW, Schmiedel S, Schüz J, et al. Integrated genetic and epigenetic analysis of bladder cancer reveals an additive diagnostic value of FGFR3 mutations and hypermethylation events. Int J Cancer. 2011;129(1):78–87. https://doi.org/10.1002/ijc.25651.
44. Kandimalla R, Van Tilborg AAG, Kompier LC, Stumpel DJPM, Stam RW, Bangma CH, Zwarthoff EC. Genome-wide analysis of CpG Island methylation in bladder cancer identified TBX2, TBX3, GATA2, and ZIC4 as pTa-specific prognostic markers. Eur Urol. 2012;61(6):1245–56. https://doi.org/10.1016/j.eururo.2012.01.011.

45. Renard I, Joniau S, van Cleynenbreugel B, Collette C, Naômé C, Vlassenbroeck I, et al. Identification and validation of the methylated TWIST1 and NID2 genes through Real-time methylation-specific polymerase chain reaction assays for the noninvasive detection of primary bladder Cancer in urine samples. Eur Urol. 2010;58(1):96–104. https://doi.org/10.1016/j.eururo.2009.07.041.
46. Cancer T, Atlas G. Comprehensive molecular characterization of Urothelial bladder carcinoma:the Cancer genome Atlas research network. Nature. 2013;507(7492):315–22. https://doi.org/10.1038/nature12965.Comprehensive.
47. Billerey C, Chopin D, Bralet M, Lahaye J, Abbou CC, Bonaventure J, et al. Short Communication. 2001;158(6):1955–9.
48. Killela PJ, Reitman ZJ, Jiao Y, Bettegowda C, Agrawal N, Diaz LA, et al. TERT promoter mutations occur frequently in gliomas and a subset of tumors derived from cells with low rates of self-renewal. Proc Natl Acad Sci U S A. 2013;110(15):6021–6. https://doi.org/10.1073/pnas.1303607110.
49. Douville C, Springer S, Kinde I, Cohen JD, Hruban RH, Lennon AM, et al. Detection of aneuploidy in patients with cancer through amplification of long interspersed nucleotide elements (LINEs). Proc Natl Acad Sci U S A. 2018;115(8):1871–6. https://doi.org/10.1073/pnas.1717846115.
50. Kiselev FL. MicroRNA and cancer. Mol Biol. 2014;48(2):232–42.
51. Lotan Y, Shariat SF, Schmitz-Dräger BJ, Sanchez-Carbayo M, Jankevicius F, Racioppi M, et al. Considerations on implementing diagnostic markers into clinical decision making in bladder cancer. Urologic Oncol. 2010;28(4):441–8. https://doi.org/10.1016/j.urolonc.2009.11.004.
52. Esteller M. CpG island hypermethylation and tumor suppressor genes: a booming present, a brighter future. Oncogene. 2002;21(35 REV. ISS. 3):5427–40. https://doi.org/10.1038/sj.onc.1205600.
53. van der Aa MNM, Steyerberg EW, Bangma C, van Rhijn BWG, Zwarthoff EC, van der Kwast TH. Cystoscopy revisited as the gold standard for detecting bladder Cancer recurrence: diagnostic review Bias in the randomized, prospective CEFUB trial. J Urol. 2010;183(1):76–80. https://doi.org/10.1016/j.juro.2009.08.150.
54. Wolff EM, Chihara Y, Pan F, Weisenberger DJ, Siegmund KD, Sugano K, et al. Unique DNA methylation patterns distinguish noninvasive and invasive urothelial cancers and establish an epigenetic field defect in premalignant tissue. Cancer Res. 2010;70(20):8169–78. https://doi.org/10.1158/0008-5472.CAN-10-1335.

# 25

# Cognitive behavioral therapy for overactive bladder in women: Study protocol for a randomized controlled trial

Satoshi Funada[1,2,3*], Norio Watanabe[2], Takayuki Goto[1], Hiromitsu Negoro[4], Shusuke Akamatsu[1], Kentaro Ueno[5], Ryuji Uozumi[5], Kentaro Ichioka[6], Takehiko Segawa[7], Tatsuo Akechi[3], Toshiaki A. Furukawa[2] and Osamu Ogawa[1]

**Abstract**

**Background:** Overactive bladder (OAB) symptoms affect daily life by decreasing health-related quality of life (HRQol). However, there remain no very effective treatment for OAB. Pharmacotherapy is one of the best treatments, but it is not always efficient and may incur adverse events. Although behavioral therapy is another effective treatment, there are very few structured treatment manuals on how to prescribe behavioral therapy to treat OAB for whom.

Cognitive behavioral therapy (CBT) is a psychotherapy consisting of structured sessions to solve problems with the collaborative empiricism between therapists and patients. OAB symptoms are supposed to worsen with cognitive distortion, and CBT is expected to be effective in treating OAB by modifying such cognitive processes. In this trial, we will evaluate the efficacy of CBT for OAB.

**Methods:** A randomized, controlled, open-label, multicenter parallel-group superiority trial will be conducted. Participants with moderate to severe OAB symptoms with or without pharmacotherapy will be recruited and will be randomly allocated 1:1 to two different groups by minimization (age, baseline OAB severity, treatment status, types of intervention, and treating institutions). The intervention group will be prescribed an individual CBT program covering six techniques in 4 sessions (30 min each), with or without pharmacotherapy. The primary outcome is the change scores in an OAB-questionnaire (OAB-q) from baseline to the end of the trial (week 13). Secondary outcomes will include other patient reported outcome measures and the frequency volume chart. All analyses will be conducted on an intention-to-treat principle.

**Discussion:** This trial will determine the efficacy of CBT to treat OAB using a rigorous methodology. The effectiveness of CBT with a structured manual may not only lead to a new treatment option for patients suffering from OAB symptoms, but may also reduce the social burden by OAB.

**Keywords:** Cognitive behavioral therapy, Overactive bladder, Randomized control trial

* Correspondence: sfunada@kuhp.kyoto-u.ac.jp
[1]Department of Urology, Kyoto University Graduate School of Medicine, 54 Shogoinkawahara-cho, Sakyo-ku, Kyoto 606-8507, Japan
[2]Department of Health Promotion and Human Behavior, Kyoto University School of Public Health, Kyoto, Japan
Full list of author information is available at the end of the article

## Background

Overactive bladder (OAB) is defined as "urgency, with or without urgency incontinence, usually with frequency and nocturia." [1] The prevalence of OAB is estimated to range between 10 and 20%, and increases with age [2–4]. OAB has a negative impact on lives. Firstly, it decreases health-related quality of life (HRQoL), and the more severe the OAB symptoms, the higher the decrease [5]. Secondly, it incurs an economic burden as the estimated total cost on OAB in six Western countries was €9.7 billion [6]. To make matters worse, 43 to 83% of OAB patients discontinued pharmacotherapy within 1 month either because these were not effective or adverse events were incurred [7].

Behavioral therapy consists of lifestyle modifications, bladder training and pelvic floor muscle training (PFMT), and clinical guidelines recommend this as a first-line therapy to treat OAB because it is safe [8, 9]. A systematic review showed that behavioral therapy was more effective in treating urgent urinary incontinence (UUI) than were anticholinergics [10]. However, behavioral therapy is superseded by drug therapy. One of the reasons may be a lack of structured treatment manuals with regard to whom and how to prescribe behavioral therapy to treat OAB.

Cognitive behavioral therapy (CBT) is a psychotherapy originally developed to treat depression in 1960s [11]. CBT consists of structured sessions to address challenges through the collaborative empiricism between therapists and patients. The techniques were generalized and applied to other psychological disorders, such as panic disorder and posttraumatic stress disorder. The effectiveness CBT was demonstrated not only in the context of psychological disorders, but also in the context of functional diseases, such as irritable bowel disease [12] and chronic pain [13]. Accordingly, CBT has been increasingly applied to many diseases in addition to psychological disorders. A previous report has shown that urinary voiding is not only induced by sensation, but also by cognitive processes, and OAB is suspected to worsen as a result of cognitive distortions [14]. Therefore, we deemed that CBT may be effective in treating OAB by modifying certain cognitive processes. Previously, we had developed CBT for drug-resistant OAB and evaluated its clinical feasibility and acceptability as treatment [15].

To establish a new program to treat OAB, we will use CBT techniques and develop a structured treatment manual based on conventional behavioral therapy. In this randomized controlled trial (RCT), we will evaluate the efficacy of our new program to treat OAB.

## Methods/design

### Trial design

This study is designed as a randomized, controlled, open-label, multicenter parallel-group superiority trial. Patients will be randomly allocated 1:1 into two groups in order to evaluate the efficacy of CBT to treat OAB. The study protocol follows the Standard Protocol Items: Recommendations for Interventional Trials (SPIRIT) [16] and Template for Intervention Description and Replication (TIDieR) checklist and guide [17]. This study was approved by the Institutional Review Boards at Kyoto University Graduate School of Medicine (No. C1423) and was registered in the clinical trial registry (UMIN000035734). Written informed consent will be obtained from all participants.

### Participants

The participants will be recruited at one university hospital, two general hospitals, and one private clinic. The following inclusion criteria will be used for this trial:

(1) Women between 20 to 80 years;
(2) Participants not having undergone any OAB treatment or taking pharmacotherapy for OAB lasting more than 6 weeks;
(3) Participants diagnosed with OAB based on their OAB symptom score (OABSS) (a total OABSS score ≥ 3, with an urgency score ≥ 2), with the total score being higher than 6 (OABSS; 6 to 11 points indicate moderate severity, 12 to 15 points indicate severity of severe nature) [18];
(4) An Eastern Cooperative Oncology Group (ECOG) Performance Status of Grade 0; and
(5) Participants who are able to understand explanations and sign a written informed consent.

The following exclusion criteria will be used for this trial:

(1) Abnormalities around the bladder (e.g., bladder cancer, bladder calculus, interstitial cystitis, endometriosis);
(2) Urinary tract infection;
(3) Surgery for urinary incontinence;
(4) Pregnancy;
(5) Disability to understand Japanese;
(6) Depression;
(7) Dementia; and
(8) Participants judged otherwise unsuitable for participation by the researchers. For example, participants with serious comorbidities or living far from the recruiting institution will be excluded because they are assumed to drop out from the intervention or assessment.

### Interventions

Participants will be prescribed a face-to-face, individual CBT program added onto their baseline therapy. After the start of the study, the study protocol was revised to add a treatment option via a remote teleconferencing service such as Zoom (©Zoom Video Communications, Inc) because of the spread of the coronavirus disease 2019 (COVID-19). When possible and/or necessary, sessions will be conducted via Zoom. If participants have not started or have quit drug therapy for more than 6 weeks, they will only receive CBT.

### *Development of the cognitive behavioral therapy program for overactive bladder*

The research team consists of urologists, gynecologist, psychiatrists, psychologists, and physiotherapists. We have developed a CBT program based on conventional behavioral therapy [8, 19] to treat drug-resistant OAB and CBT techniques for panic disorder, [20, 21] and evaluated the clinical feasibility and acceptability as a pilot study [15]. We simplified the CBT program to treat OAB since most participants were expected to be elderly or aging. As a result, we developed a training program based on 4 sessions (30 min each) and 6 techniques carried out over the course of 4 to 12 weeks (Fig. 1). Each session is divided into three parts, reviewing homework, providing new techniques, and reviewing the current day's session. All sessions will be provided face-to-face, individually, at each institution or via Zoom. Brief descriptions of each of the 4 sessions are shown in Fig. 2. (1) Participants collect frequency volume charts (FVC) for self-monitoring during the intervention period. (2) Participant education consists of teaching them about the normal urinary tract system, abnormal voiding function, and epidemiology and physiology of OAB. We develop a CBT model applied to OAB and explain the targets of each CBT technique (Fig. 3). (3) Lifestyle modifications are carried out based on participants' habits, such as by restricting water and coffee intake, as appropriate. (4) PFMT is conducted with abdominal breathing and taught by using photos and a yoga ball to enable easy imagination. (5) Exposure is modified to treat OAB based on bladder training techniques. For example, if a participant and a therapist set a goal, such as going on a bus tour for 3 h without urinary voiding, they set up several steps to achieve this goal, such as step 1: Be patient with urinary urgency and void every 2 h at home, step 2: Be patient with urinary urgency and void every 3 h at home, step 3: Be patient with urinary urgency and void every 3 h outside (Fig. 4). (6) Relapse prevention consists of planning for the future and encouraging the continuation of the taught techniques. Weekly homework is assigned in order for participants to learn the techniques and to assess participant adherence to subsequent sessions.

### *Therapist and treatment integrity*

Our therapist is a urologist with 10 years of experience in urological treatment and a Japanese Board-Certified Instructor. He has attended a 2-day CBT workshop held by the Ministry of Health, Labour and Welfare of Japan. We developed a treatment manual for this study and the therapist followed the manual to ensure the reproducibility of the delivered intervention. We also attached worksheets to assist with the acquisition of each technique and homework practice. The therapist used a procedure checklist at each session to ensure adherence.

### *Waiting list control group*

The control group is a waiting list. Participants will keep receiving their baseline therapy during the study period. If they are naïve or quit drug therapy for more than 6 weeks, they will not receive any therapy. After completing the trial, they will receive CBT treatment.

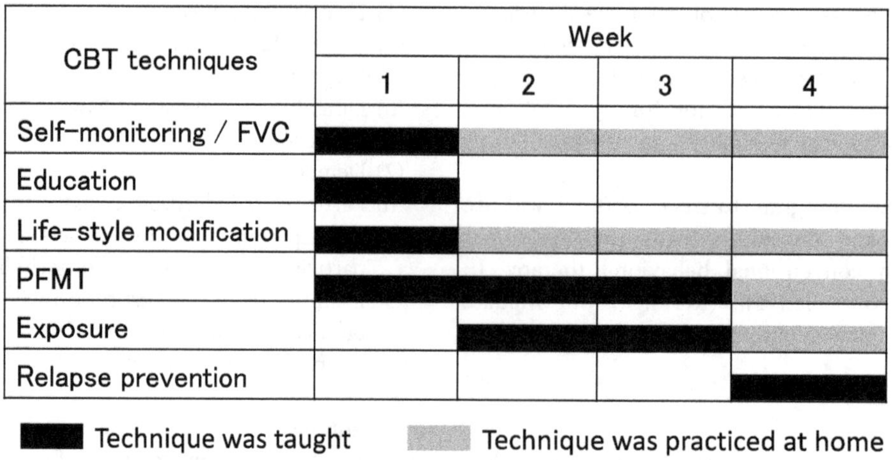


**Fig. 1** Overview of CBT for drug-resistant OAB

| Sessions | Description |
|---|---|
| 1 | **Education**<br>Education about voiding function, OAB and CBT<br>**Life-style modification**<br>Check drinking water and coffee, taking exercise<br>Modify bad life-styles<br>**PFMT**<br>Teach by using photos and a yoga-ball<br>Ten minutes/session and more then 3 sessions each day<br>**Review and homework** |
| 2 | **Review session 1 and homework**<br>**PFMT**<br>**Exposure**<br>Set a goal and several steps to achieve the goal<br>**Review and homework** |
| 3 | **Review session 2 and homework**<br>**PFMT**<br>**Exposure**<br>Set the next steps and goal<br>**Review and Give homework** |
| 4 | **Review session 3 and homework**<br>**Relapse prevention**<br>Plan the future's goal and encourage to continue the techniques<br>**Total review** |

**Fig. 2** Brief summary of CBT manual for drug-resistant OAB

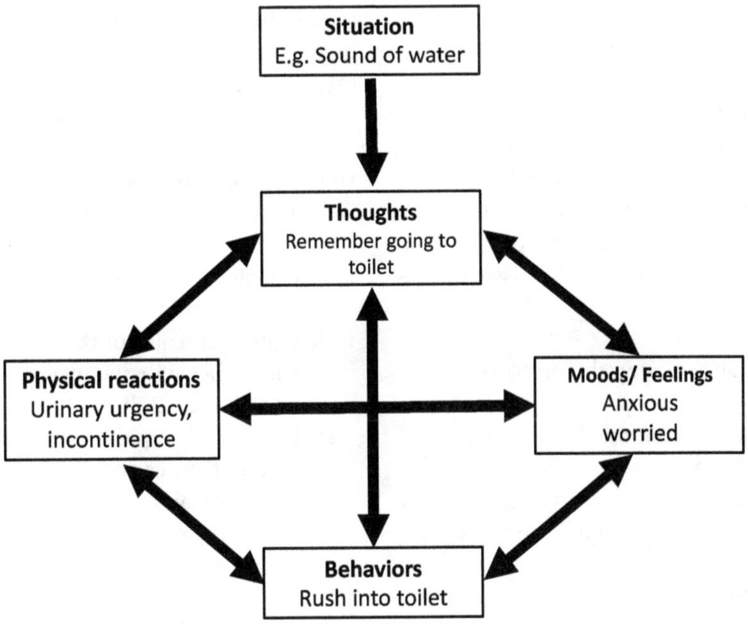


**Fig. 3** CBT model for OAB and target of each techniques

## Exposure

Rushing to the toilet can avoid urinary urgency, but it makes a vicious circle.
Exposure to urinary urgency, which increases tolerance.

ex.)

| Goal : Trip to somewhere by bus without toilet for 3 hours | | |
|---|---|---|
| Step | | Anxiety |
| 1 | Make urinary interval for 2 hours at home | 50% |
| 2 | Make urinary interval for 3 hours at home | 70% |
| 3 | Spend 3 hours outside without voiding | 90% |

**Fig. 4** The example of the technique of exposure

**Rules with regard to participant cessation**

***Deviation from protocol treatment***

The following cases will be determined as deviations from the treatment protocol. However, the participants will not be determined to have dropped out of the trial at this stage and will be able to receive protocol assessments unless they withdraw consent for assessments (as below):

1) When a participant does not receive any intervention;
2) When interventions are separated by more than 3 weeks;
3) When a participant receives another treatment for OAB during the trial;
4) When there is no outcome-related data.

***Discontinuation of the protocol treatment***

The following cases will be considered as discontinuations from the treatment protocol. However, the participants will not be determined to have dropped out of the trial at this stage and will be able to receive protocol assessments unless they withdraw consent for assessments (as below):

1) If the participant wishes to stop the protocol treatment;
2) If the participant cannot continue the protocol treatment due to adverse events;
3) When the trial physician considers that the risk will be more than the benefit to continue the protocol treatment for any reason;
4) When the trial physician considers that it is not appropriate to continue the protocol treatment for any other reason.

***Cessation of assessments***

If the participant withdraws consent for assessments, he/she will not be followed up.

**Outcomes**

***Primary outcome measure***

We will use the changes in HRQoL total scores of the OAB questionnaire (OAB-q) [22] from baseline to week 13 as a primary outcome in this study. The OAB-q reflects OAB-related QoL outcomes, consisting of 33 questionnaires and six subscales, assessing symptom bother, coping behaviors, concerns/worries, sleep patterns, social interaction, and total HRQoL score. Each subscale score ranges from 0 to 100, and lower symptom scores but higher scores on the other subscales reflect improvement. The minimum clinical important difference (MCID) of the OAB-q was reported to be 10 points [23].

***Secondary outcome measures***

Secondary outcomes include the following:

1) Changes in HRQoL total scores of the OAB-q at weeks 5 and 9 [22];
2) Other subscales of the OAB-q (symptom bother, coping behaviors, concern/worry, sleep and social interaction) [22];
3) King's health questionnaire (KHQ: OAB-related QoL outcomes consist of 21 questionnaires and nine subscales [24]. Each score of the subscales ranges from 0 to 100, and lower scores indicate improvement);
4) OABSS (questionnaires to diagnose OAB and also to classify the severity [25]. The total score ranges from 0 to 15, and the severity is classified as mild (0

to 5), moderate (6 to 11), and severe (11 to 15). The MCID of the OABSS was 3 points);

5) Patient Global Impression-Improvement (PGI-I: measures patient-perceived impression of changes in symptoms with a 7-point Likert-type scale ranging from (1) "very much improved" to (7) "very much worse" [26]), which scales will be classified into 2 categories for analysis as responses (1) or (2) ("very much improved" or "much improved") compared with all other categories;
6) Patient Global Impression-Severity (PGI-S: measures patient-perceived severity of symptoms with a 4-point Likert-type scale ranging from (1) "normal", (2)" mild", (3)" moderate", or (4) "severe" [26]), which will be dichotomized into 2 categories for analysis as responses (1) or (2) ("normal" or "mild") compared with all other categories;
7) Frequency volume chart (FVC: voiding frequency, urgency, and incontinence are documented in 3-day bladder diaries [27]);
8) Hospital Anxiety and Depression Scale (HADS: measures to assess anxiety and depression, and both scores range between 0 to 21 [28]. The status is classified as "mild" (0 to 7), "borderline" (8 to 10), and "severe" (11 to 21));
9) Five-level EuroQol five-dimensional questionnaire (EQ-5D-5L: health status is assessed with 5 items, 5 subscales [29]);
10) Treatment satisfaction (5 points Likert scale questions, "How is your satisfaction with your treatment?"; (1) "very satisfied," (2) "satisfied," (3) "neutral," (4) "dissatisfied," and (5) "very dissatisfied"), which will be dichotomized into 2 categories for analysis as responses (1) or (2) ("very satisfied" or "satisfied") compared with all other categories;
11) Drop-out rate;
12) Change in pharmacotherapy ("Did you change your medication during the treatment period?"; (1) "no change," (2) "add medication," (3) "decrease medication," or (4) "quit medication");
13) Adherence (evaluated as the week rate of homework completion).

#### *Baseline characteristics measures*

Participants will complete a form on demographics including age, height, weight, comorbidity, medicine, delivery, menopause, education, marital and job status, and history of OAB treatment.

#### *Participant timeline*

Fig. 5 shows the participant timeline reflecting enrollment, intervention, and assessment. Enrollment will be carried out at each institution. Following screening, the trial will be explained to eligible participants. After completing informed consent, participants will fill out the questionnaires about baseline characteristics. Participants will complete a self-report questionnaire in a written paper format or via electronic data capture at baseline (week 0), immediately after intervention (week 5), and at follow-up (week 9 and week 13)).

#### *Sample size*

The primary outcome is change from baseline to week 13 in HRQoL total scores of the OAB-q between groups. A total of 128 participants are required to detect a moderate effect size of 0.5 between the groups based on a two-sided significance level of 0.05 and 80% power [30]. Assuming a 15% drop out rate based on a previous RCT to evaluate behavioral therapy in women with mixed urinary incontinence [31], we set the target sample size at 150 participants.

| | STUDY PERIOD | | | | | | | |
|---|---|---|---|---|---|---|---|---|
| | Enrolment | Allocation | Post-allocation | | | Post intervention | Follow-up | Close-out |
| TIMEPOINT: | 0 | 1 | 2 | 3 | 4 | 5 | 9 | 13 |
| ENROLMENT | | | | | | | | |
| Eligible screen | X | | | | | | | |
| Informed consent | X | | | | | | | |
| Baseline characteristics | X | | | | | | | |
| Allocation | | X | | | | | | |
| INTERVENTION: | | | | | | | | |
| Intervention group | X | | | | | X | X | X |
| Control group | X | X | | | | X | X | X |
| ASSESMENTS: | | | | | | | | |
| Primary outcome | X | | | | | X | X | X |
| Secondary outcome | X | | | | | X | X | X |
| Adverse Events | | X | X | X | X | X | X | X |
| Drop out | | X | X | X | X | X | X | X |
| Adherence | | X | X | X | X | | | |

**Fig. 5** The schedule of this study

*Recruitment*

General hospitals and private clinic providers will identify potential participants during clinic visits. Screening interviews will be carried out to assess participant eligibility. When possible and/or necessary, the recruitment and screening interview will be conducted via Zoom. We are planning to recruit participants within two and a half years from trial start.

**Assignment of interventions**

*Sequence generation*

The random allocation will be carried out by UMIN INDICE (UMIN Internet Data and Information Center of Clinical Research, https://www.umin.ac.jp/indice/cloud.html) cloud, an internet-based central randomization cloud system. A minimization algorithm will be used to ensure balance across age (20- to 64-year-olds vs 65- to 80-year-olds), baseline OAB severity (moderate (OABSS: 6 to 11) vs severe (OABSS: 11 to 15)), treatment status (no treatment vs past treatment vs under treatment), types of intervention (face-to-face vs online remote session), and treating institutions.

*Allocation concealment and implementation*

In week 1, the therapist will access the UMIN INDICE cloud in front of participants. The random allocation to either group at a 1:1 ratio will be centrally generated via the UMIN INDICE cloud after the necessary baseline information is entered, and opened at the same time to the therapist. Allocation concealment will therefore be ensured. Immediately after this, the intervention group will be prescribed CBT, and the waiting list control group will be informed of the schedule.

*Blinding*

In this open label study, participants and a therapist will be aware of the intervention assigned. Not all outcome assessments will be blinded due to the nature of the patient reported outcome measures (PROM). The statistician will be blinded to the allocation during the analyses.

**Data collection**

*Data collection methods*

Outcome data will be collected at baseline (week 0), immediately after intervention (week 5), and at follow-up (week 9 and week 13) using self-reported questionnaires in paper form or via electronic data capture.

*Data management*

Outcome data will be transferred into a Research Electronic Data Capture (REDcap) system (https://www.project-redcap.org/). The therapist will enter the data on baseline characteristics, allocation, drop out, changes of pharmacotherapy, homework adherence, and adverse events into REDcap. If any missing data is detected via the REDcap system, the researcher will contact the participants by telephone.

*Statistical methods*

All analyses will be carried out based on an intention-to-treat principal, considering all participants as randomized, regardless of whether they received the randomized treatment. We do not plan to conduct any interim analyses.

*Analysis of primary outcome*

We will use a linear mixed-effects model with repeated-measures analysis to estimate the least-squares mean difference in score changes from baseline at weeks 5, 9, and 13 in the HRQoL of the OAB-q between group comparisons. This model assumes that primary outcome data are missing at random and includes study group (intervention and control), assessment points (week 5, week 9, and week 13), OAB severity (moderate and severe), baseline score, and the interaction of study group with assessment points. Week 13 is the assessment point for the primary analysis. A multiple-testing procedure will be used to control for the familywise type I error rate at a two-sided significance level of 0.05. If the primary analysis at week 13 shows statistical significance, testing of other assessment points of the primary outcome is to be performed in a hierarchical manner: week 9 and week 5.

*Analysis of secondary outcomes*

Secondary outcomes are important in order to measure the wider effects for participants, and will be similarly analyzed (as appropriate for continuous or dichotomous outcomes). No adjustments for multiplicity are made for the secondary outcomes except the HRQoL total scores of the OAB-q, as shown above. Thus, point estimates and 95% confidence intervals will be reported, without *P* values. The 95% confidence intervals are not adjusted for multiple comparisons, and inference drawn from these may not be reproducible. These analyses will be exploratory in nature in order to complement the primary analyses.

*Adverse events*

We will convey the numbers and frequencies (%) of adverse events.

*Subgroup analyses*

We will perform the following subgroup analyses:

1) Participants: aged 20 to 64 years vs 65 to 80 years;
2) OAB severity: moderate (OABSS: 6 to 11 points) vs severe (OABSS: 12 to 15 points);

3) Pharmacotherapy: naïve vs past vs under treatment;
4) Incontinence: no (OABSS Q4 = 0 point) vs yes (OABSS Q4 = 1 to 5 point);
5) HADS Anxiety score: normal (0 to 7 points) vs borderline or abnormal (8 to 21 points)
6) HADS Depression score: normal (0 to 7 points) vs borderline or abnormal (8 to 21 points).

When possible and/or necessary,

7) Intervention type: face-to-face vs online remote session

### *Sensitivity analyses*

Participants who (1) receive all intervention treatment; (2) have had intervention intervals lasting less than 3 weeks; (3) have not received any other treatment for OAB; and (4) have generated full outcome data will be analyzed as per protocol set (PPS). Furthermore, sensitivity analyses including multiple imputation approach for imputing missing data will be performed, with missing-at-random assumptions.

## Monitoring

### *Data monitoring*

There was no composition of data monitoring committee no interim analysis in this study.

## Reporting of adverse events and protection of participants

### *Definition of adverse events*

An adverse event is defined as any unintended or unwanted symptom, sign, or disease seen in participants. The Japanese Ministry of Health, Labor and Welfare publish, "Ethical Guidelines for Clinical Studies: Questions and Answers, " and it defines severe adverse events as following: a) death; b) threatened death; c) admission or prolongation of admission for treatment; d) enduring and severe impairment and dysfunction; or e) congenital anomaly.

When such a serious adverse event will happened, the trial physician must inform the principal investigator within 48 h, with or without the causal relationship to the protocol treatment. The principal investigator will report to the Institutional Review Boards in Kyoto University Graduate School of Medicine within 72 h, also inform all collaborators at all participating institutions. If it occurs an unexpected serious adverse event, the principal investigator will report it to the Ministry of Health, Labor and Welfare.

### *Auditing*

Any formal audits will not be performed, because this study's intervention can be classified as a "minimally invasive intervention".

## Ethics and dissemination

### *Research ethics approval*

This study protocol was approved by the Institutional Review Boards of Kyoto University Graduate School of Medicine (No. C1457) on January 15, 2020. The protocol was revised to add a treatment option via Zoom because of the spread of the coronavirus disease 2019 (COVID-19) and re-approved on June 30, 2020.

### *Protocol amendments*

The steering committee will determine any revisions of the protocol. Any amendments of the protocol will be submitted to the Institutional Review Boards of Kyoto University Graduate School of Medicine for approval. The amended protocol will also be submitted to the Institutional Review Boards of the other participating institutions and reported to the participants as necessary.

### *Consent or assent*

Informed consent will be obtained at each institution. Following the screening, the trial will be explained to eligible participants. Next, researchers will obtain full informed written consent from participants.

### *Confidentiality*

An identification number will be assigned to each participant on enrollment. This number will be used for data registration. The correspondence list is kept securely in the computer on which the password has been set. After completion of the trial, the raw data will be kept in a locked drawer at the Kyoto University Graduate School of Medicine for 10 years following the publication of the first survey results.

### *Access to date*

The final trial dataset will be able to access to all members of the steering committee and the statistician. After the dataset will be de-identified and anonymized, it will be uploaded to the UMIN-ICDR website (http://www.umin.ac.jp/icdr/index-j.html), and researchers who will be approved by the steering committee will be able to access to the dataset.

### *Ancillary and post-trial care*

Because all protocol interventions are administered within the scope of the approved regulations in Japan, any health hazards will be covered by Japan's National Health Insurance.

### *Dissemination policy*

The study results will be disseminated to the public in academic conferences and journals. The steering committee will determine authorship of the planned primary and secondary publications. The order of the authors will be decided by the contributions of each member. The authors of the paper and the conference presenters will be based on the Uniform Requirements for Manuscripts Submitted to Biomedical Journals of the International Committee of Medical Journal Editors.

## Discussion

We have reported the protocol for a randomized, controlled, open-label, multicenter superiority trial seeking to evaluate the efficacy of CBT for OAB. To our knowledge, this is the first trial investigating the efficacy of CBT for OAB in a clinical setting. We have previously developed a CBT program for drug-resistant OAB and evaluated the clinical feasibility and acceptability of the treatment in a pilot study [15]. We will rigorously evaluate the efficacy of CBT for OAB in this RCT.

There are several limitations to this study. First, this will be an open-label designed RCT, with unblinded participants, therapist, and outcome assessors. The primary outcome, OAB-q, is a PRO questionnaire, and the unblinding will result in a certain degree of assessment bias, which may favor the intervention group. Although we have considered relatively hard outcomes, such as voiding frequency, the purpose of treatment is to improve patients' QOL, to which end we have selected OAB-q as the primary outcome. Secondly, although this treatment will be administered using a manual, it will be conducted by a urologist, meaning that its general applicability cannot be fully ascertained. To improve generalizability, more therapists will be needed to participate in further evaluations of this approach.

This study has some critical implications for clinicians and patients. This new approach is expected to treat OAB with few adverse events compared with drug therapy. Moreover, this CBT treatment consists of a structured manual that enables therapists of various backgrounds to administer the therapy in an efficient, consistent way. As it may be applied to group therapy, or smartphone therapy, more and more patients may eventually benefit from this CBT approach. It may solve the issue of the shortage of CBT therapists and increasing the medical cost.

### Abbreviations

CBT: Cognitive behavioral therapy; FVC: Frequency volume chart; HRQoL: Health-related quality of life; MCID: Minimum clinical important difference; OAB: Overactive bladder; OABSS: OAB symptom score; PFMT: Pelvic floor muscle training; PPS: Per protocol set; RCT: Randomized controlled trial; UUI: Urgent urinary incontinence

### Authors' contributions

All authors contributed to the conception and conduct of this clinical trial. OO is the principal investigator of this trial. SF, NW, TG, SA, TAF, and OO designed the overall framework of the trial and HN, KI, TS and TA helped with implementation. KU and RU are responsible for the statistical design to test efficacy. SF, NW, TG, SA, TAF, and OO in particular, conceived the treatment implementation and coordinated the research. SF will monitor adverse events and take necessary medical action if they occur. SF, NW, TG, SA, TAF, and OO arranged the infrastructure essential to execute the trial. SK, NW, and TAF drafted the manuscript, and all co-authors read it and provided critical comments. All authors approved the final manuscript.

### Competing interests

SF has a research grant from JSPS KAKENHI Grant Number JP 20K18964. NW has received a research grant from the Fujiwara Memorial Foundation for this work. He has also received royalties from Sogensha and Advantage Risk Management, for other than this work. RU has received personal fees from Eisai, Sawai Pharmaceutical, and CAC Croit, for other than this work. TA has received lectures fees from Astellas, AstraZeneca, Daiichi-Sankyo, Dainippon-Sumitomo, Hisamitsu, Janssen, Kyowa-hakko Kirin, Kyowa, Lilly, MSD, Meiji-seika Pharma, Mochida, Mundipharma, Nipro, Otsuka, Pfizer, Shionogi, Takeda, and Tsumura. He has received royalties from Igaku-shoin, and also has received research funds from Daiichi-Sankyo, Eisai, FUJIFILM RI Pharma, MSD, Otsuka, and Shionogi. TAF reports personal fees from Mitsubishi-Tanabe, MSD and Shionogi, and a grant from Mitsubishi-Tanabe, for other than the submitted work; TAF has a patent 2018–177688 pending. All of the other authors declare that they have no competing interests.

### Author details

[1]Department of Urology, Kyoto University Graduate School of Medicine, 54 Shogoinkawahara-cho, Sakyo-ku, Kyoto 606-8507, Japan. [2]Department of Health Promotion and Human Behavior, Kyoto University School of Public Health, Kyoto, Japan. [3]Department of Psychiatry, Nagoya City University Graduate School of Medical Sciences, Nagoya, Japan. [4]Department of Urology, University of Tsukuba Hospital, Tsukuba, Japan. [5]Department of Biomedical Statistics and Bioinformatics, Kyoto University Graduate School of Medicine, Kyoto, Japan. [6]Ichioka Urological Clinic, Kyoto, Japan. [7]Department of Urology, Kyoto City Hospital, Kyoto, Japan.

### References

1. Abrams P, Cardozo L, Fall M, Griffiths D, Rosier P, Ulmsten U, et al. The standardisation of terminology of lower urinary tract function: report from the standardisation sub-committee of the international continence society. Neurourol Urodyn. 2002;21:167–78. https://doi.org/10.1016/S0090-4295(02)02243-4.
2. Stewart WF, Van Rooyen JB, Cundiff GW, Abrams P, Herzog AR, Corey R, et al. Prevalence and burden of overactive bladder in the United States. World J Urol. 2003;20:327–36.
3. Irwin DE, Milsom I, Hunskaar S, Reilly K, Kopp Z, Herschorn S, et al. Population-based survey of urinary incontinence, overactive bladder, and other lower urinary tract symptoms in five countries: results of the EPIC study. Eur Urol. 2006;50:1306–15.
4. Funada S, Kawaguchi T, Terada N, Negoro H, Tabara Y, Kosugi S, et al. Cross-sectional epidemiological analysis of the Nagahama study for correlates of overactive bladder: genetic and environmental considerations. J Urol. 2018; 199:774–8.
5. Vaughan CP, Johnson TM, Ala-Lipasti MA, Cartwright R, TLJ T, Taari K, et al. The prevalence of clinically meaningful overactive bladder: bother and quality of life results from the population-based FINNO study. Eur Urol. 2011;59:629–36. https://doi.org/10.1016/j.eururo.2011.01.031.
6. Irwin DE, Mungapen L, Milsom I, Kopp Z, Reeves P, Kelleher C. The economic impact of overactive bladder syndrome in six Western countries. BJU Int. 2009;103:202–9.
7. Sexton CC, Notte SM, Maroulis C, Dmochowski RR, Cardozo L, Subramanian D, et al. Persistence and adherence in the treatment of overactive bladder syndrome with anticholinergic therapy: a systematic review of the literature. Int J Clin Pract. 2011;65:567–85.
8. Nambiar AK, Bosch R, Cruz F, Lemack GE, Thiruchelvam N, Tubaro A, et al. EAU guidelines on assessment and nonsurgical Management of Urinary Incontinence. Eur Urol. 2018;73:596–609. https://doi.org/10.1016/j.eururo.2017.12.031..

9. Lightner DJ, Gomelsky A, Souter L, Vasavada SP. Diagnosis and Treatment of Overactive Bladder (Non-Neurogenic) in Adults: AUA/SUFU Guideline Amendment 2019. J Urol. 2019;:101097JU0000000000000309. https://doi.org/10.1097/JU.0000000000000309.
10. Balk EM, Rofeberg VN, Adam GP, Kimmel HJ, Trikalinos TA, Jeppson PC. Pharmacologic and nonpharmacologic treatments for urinary incontinence in women. Ann Intern Med. 2019;170:465. https://doi.org/10.7326/M18-3227.
11. BECK AT. Thinking and depression. I. idiosyncratic content and cognitive distortions. Arch Gen Psychiatry. 1963;9:324–33 http://www.ncbi.nlm.nih.gov/pubmed/14045261.
12. Laird KT, Tanner-Smith EE, Russell AC, Hollon SD, Walker LS. Comparative efficacy of psychological therapies for improving mental health and daily functioning in irritable bowel syndrome: a systematic review and meta-analysis. Clin Psychol Rev. 2017;51:142–52. https://doi.org/10.1016/j.cpr.2016.11.001.
13. Williams AC de C, Eccleston C, Morley S. Psychological therapies for the management of chronic pain (excluding headache) in adults. Cochrane Database Syst Rev. 2012;11:CD007407. https://doi.org/10.1002/14651858.CD007407.pub3.
14. Harvey J, Finney S, Stewart L, Gillespie J. The relationship between cognition and sensation in determining when and where to void: the concept of cognitive voiding. BJU Int. 2012;110:1756–61.
15. Funada S, Watanabe N, Goto T, Negoro H, Akamatsu S, Uozumi R, et al. Clinical feasibility and acceptability of adding cognitive behavioral therapy to pharmacotherapy for drug-resistant overactive bladder in women: a single-arm pilot study. Low Urin Tract Symptoms. 2020. https://doi.org/10.1111/luts.12333.
16. Chan AW, Tetzlaff JM, Gøtzsche PC, Altman DG, Mann H, Berlin JA, et al. SPIRIT 2013 explanation and elaboration: guidance for protocols of clinical trials. BMJ. 2013;346:1–42.
17. Hoffmann TC, Glasziou PP, Boutron I, Milne R, Perera R, Moher D, et al. Better reporting of interventions: Template for intervention description and replication (TIDieR) checklist and guide. BMJ. 2014;348:1–12. https://doi.org/10.1136/bmj.g1687.
18. Yamaguchi O, Nishizawa O, Takeda M, Yokoyama O, Homma Y, Kakizaki H, et al. Clinical guidelines for overactive bladder. Int J Urol. 2009;16:126–42. https://doi.org/10.1111/j.1442-2042.2008.02177.x.
19. Gormley EA, Lightner DJ, Faraday M, Vasavada SP. American urological association, Society of Urodynamics FPM. Diagnosis and treatment of overactive bladder (non-neurogenic) in adults: AUA/SUFU guideline amendment. J Urol. 2015;193:1572–80. https://doi.org/10.1016/j.juro.2015.01.087.
20. Barlow D, Craske M, Mercier M. Mastery of your anxiety and panic II: client workbook. 1999. https://scholar.google.com/scholar_lookup?title=Mastery+of+your+anxiety+and+panic:+Client+workbook&author=DH+Barlow&author=MG+Craske&publication_year=2006&. Accessed 17 Aug 2019.
21. Wells A, White J, Carter K. Attention training: effects on anxiety and beliefs in panic and social phobia. Clin Psychol Psychother. 1997;4:226–32. https://doi.org/10.1002/(SICI)1099-0879(199712)4:4<226::AID-CPP129>3.0.CO;2-M.
22. Coyne K, Revicki D, Hunt T, Corey R, Stewart W, Bentkover J, et al. Psychometric validation of an overactive bladder symptom and health-related quality of life questionnaire: the OAB-q. Qual Life Res. 2002;11:563–74 http://www.ncbi.nlm.nih.gov/pubmed/12206577.
23. Dyer KY, Xu Y, Brubaker L, Nygaard I, Markland A, Rahn D, et al. Minimum important difference for validated instruments in women with urge incontinence. Neurourol Urodyn. 2011;30:1319–24. https://doi.org/10.1002/nau.21028.
24. Kelleher CJ, Cardozo LD, Khullar V, Salvatore S. A new questionnaire to assess the quality of life of urinary incontinent women. Br J Obstet Gynaecol. 1997;104:1374–9 http://www.ncbi.nlm.nih.gov/pubmed/9422015.
25. Gotoh M, Homma Y, Yokoyama O, Nishizawa O. Responsiveness and minimal clinically important change in overactive bladder symptom score. Urology. 2011;78:768–73. https://doi.org/10.1016/j.urology.2011.06.020.
26. Busner J, Targum SD. The clinical global impressions scale: applying a research tool in clinical practice. Psychiatry (Edgmont). 2007;4:28–37 http://www.ncbi.nlm.nih.gov/pubmed/20526405.
27. Wyman JF, Choi SC, Harkins SW, Wilson MS, Fantl JA. The urinary diary in evaluation of incontinent women: a test-retest analysis. Obstet Gynecol. 1988;71(6 Pt 1):812–7 http://www.ncbi.nlm.nih.gov/pubmed/3368165.
28. Zigmond AS, Snaith RP. The hospital anxiety and depression scale. Acta Psychiatr Scand. 1983;67:361–70. https://doi.org/10.1111/j.1600-0447.1983.tb09716.x.
29. Herdman M, Gudex C, Lloyd A, Janssen M, Kind P, Parkin D, et al. Development and preliminary testing of the new five-level version of EQ-5D (EQ-5D-5L). Qual Life Res. 2011;20:1727–36. https://doi.org/10.1007/s11136-011-9903-x.
30. Cohen J. A power primer. Psychol Bull. 1992;112:155–9. https://doi.org/10.1037//0033-2909.112.1.155.
31. Sung VW, Borello-France D, Newman DK, Richter HE, Lukacz ES, Moalli P, et al. Effect of behavioral and pelvic floor muscle therapy combined with surgery vs surgery alone on incontinence symptoms among women with mixed urinary incontinence: the esteem randomized clinical trial. JAMA. 2019;322:1066–76.

# 26

# Hyperpolarization-activated cation currents in medium-size dorsal root ganglion cells are involved in overactive bladder syndrome in rats

Chao Tan[1†], Fei Yan[1†], Li-Ping Yao[2†], Jun-Ling Xing[3†], Wei-Jun Qin[1], Kun Zhang[1], Guo-Jun Wu[1], Jian-Lin Yuan[1*] and Fei Liu[1*]

**Abstract**

**Background:** To investigate the functions of the hyperpolarization-activated cation currents in medium-size dorsal root ganglion cells in a rat model of overactive bladder syndrome.

**Methods:** Rats with OAB were screened using a urodynamic testing device. The whole-cell patch clamp technique was used to investigate changes in excitability and hyperpolarization-activated cation current ($I_h$) of medium-size cells in the L6 dorsal root ganglia (DRG) of the OAB rats. Intrathecal injection of the specific $I_h$ inhibitor ZD7288 was used to investigate changes of voiding function and $I_h$ of medium-size cells in the L6 DRG.

**Results:** The urinary bladder weight of the OAB rats was significantly increased ($p < 0.01$); However, 7 days after intrathecally administration of ZD7288 (2 μM), the weight of rat bladder was significantly reduced ($p < 0.01$). The excitability of the medium-size cells in the L6 DRG of the OAB rats was significantly increased, and the number of action potentials elicited by a 500 pA stimulus was also markedly increased. Furthermore, ZD7288 significantly reduced the excitability of the medium-size DRG cells. The medium-size cells in the DRG of the OAB rats had a significantly increased $I_h$ current density, which was blocked by ZD7288.

**Conclusions:** The $I_h$ current density significantly increased in medium-size cells of the L6 DRG in the OAB model. A decrease of the $I_h$ current was able to significantly improve the voiding function of the OAB rats, in addition to lowering their urinary bladder weight. Our finding suggested that the observed increase of $I_h$ current in the medium-size DRG neurons might play an important role in the pathological processes of OAB.

**Keywords:** Overactive bladder, $I_h$, Dorsal root ganglion, Hyperpolarization, ZD7288

* Correspondence: jianliny@fmmu.edu.cn; liufeiyh@163.com
†Chao Tan, Fei Yan, Li-Ping Yao and Jun-Ling Xing contributed equally to this work.
[1]Department of Urology, Xijing Hospital, Air Force Medical University, 15 Changle West Road, Xi'an 710032, Shaanxi, China
Full list of author information is available at the end of the article

## Background

Overactive bladder syndrome (OAB) is characterized by urinary urgency accompanied by frequent urination and nocturia, with or without urinary urge incontinence [1]. OAB severely affects the patients' quality of life, since frequent urination can cause severe inconvenience, whereas long-term incontinence can lead to urinary tract infections, possibly leading to severe clinical complications affecting the patient's physical and mental well-being [2]. Therefore, the micturition reflex which is subject to complex control from both the central and the peripheral nervous system, is attracting more attention. Anatomic studies have uncovered that the relevant afferent nerves mainly pass through the pelvic posterior, mainly from the L6 and S1 dorsal root ganglia (DRG) to the spinal cord, to trigger the micturition reflex [3]. According to the diameter of the neurons, the afferent DRG nerve fibers are classified as large, medium and small, which are further categorized into $A_{\alpha/\beta}$, $A_{\delta}$ and C-type fibers [4, 5]. The afferent nerves controlling of the urinary bladder include the myelinated $A_{\delta}$ and the unmyelinated C-type fibers [6]. The hyperpolarization-activated cyclic nucleotide-gated cation (HCN) currents ($I_h$) have been reported to be expressed by many cell types, such as cardiac pacemaker cells and retinal photoreceptor cells, as well as central and peripheral nerve cells, including DRG cells.

It has been discovered that small- and medium-size nerve cells of the DRG which can control urinary bladder all possess $I_h$ currents, and the $I_h$ current of the medium-sized neurons is significantly higher than that of the small neurons [7]. This indicates that the $I_h$ current is predominantly present in the medium-size DRG neurons. Even though the afferent neurons that control the bladder include C and $A_{\delta}$ type fibers, in normal physiological conditions, the $A_{\delta}$ fibers are solely responsible for the mechanical nociceptive reflex when the bladder expands to threshold pressure. This indicates that the medium-size neurons of the DRG play an important role in the micturition reflex. The $I_h$ current activated by hyperpolarization of the HCN-gated channels has been shown to be involved in many important physiological functions, including the pacemaker function of the heart and brain as well as maintaining the resting membrane potential and cell excitability [8, 9].

Masuda and coworkers have discovered that ZD7288, a specific inhibitor of HCN-gated channels, can inhibit the $I_h$ current in the medium-size cells that control the bladder, markedly increasing the duration of the afterhyperpolarization potential of an action potential [7]. This in turn implies that the $I_h$ current influences the excitability of the medium-size DRG neurons that innervate the bladder. In order to find out the relationship between OAB and the $I_h$ current in medium-size DRG neurons, this study was performed to characterize the electrophysiological properties of the $I_h$ current in the medium-size cells of the L6 dorsal root ganglion in a rat model of overactive bladder, and to investigate its influence on the model animals' urodynamics.

## Methods

### Experimental animals

Experiments were performed using adult female SD rats, aged 7–8 weeks, weighing 200–220 g, provided by the Air Force Medical University animal facility. Under standard experimental conditions, the animals were kept on a 12 h day and night cycle, at 25 °C, and were provided with rat chow (Allentown, USA) and water ad libitum. The rats were allowed to acclimatize to the laboratory environment for 1 week prior to starting the experiments. The experiments were approved by the Air Force University animal experiment ethics committee.

### Animal grouping and establishment of the rat model of overactive bladder syndrome

The investigators were blinded to group allocation during the experiments and analysis. The animals were fasted for 12 h before beginning the experiments. By random number table grouping method, the animals were randomly assigned to the sham intervention group, sham+saline group, sham+ZD7288 group, OAB group, OAB + saline group, and OAB + ZD7288 group. The sample size calculation of each group was based upon our pilot study. In our pilot study, we used 3 animals in each of the six groups and totally 18 rats. And we got the preliminary data from the urodynamic studies from the six experimental groups. And mean ± SD of Micturition Interval (Sec) in the six groups were 65.83 ± 11.27, 65.42 ± 10.42, 67.22 ± 14.16, 45.89 ± 9.76, 42.35 ± 9.54, 54.28 ± 6.60 respectively. Method of one-way analysis of variance was used to estimate sample size. According to pilot study results, the means of six groups were set to 66, 65, 67, 46, 42, 54. And the standard deviation was preset to 14, because the largest SD was 14.16. Significance level was set to 0.05 for two-sided tests ($\alpha = 0.05$), and the power was set to 0.9 ($\beta = 0.1$). Estimation results showed that the sample size of each group should be no less than 7. In the present study, the real sample size of each group was from our actual experiments, and more than 7 animals were used in each group. We have not ruled out any raw data. Consequently, 8 to 11 animals from each group were used for this study, and the number of animals or DRG cells used were indicated in the tables and figure legends, respectively. Similar researches regarding sample size were reported previously [10, 11]. An intraperitoneal injection comprising 1% sodium pentobarbital (50 mg/kg body weight, sigma, USA) was administered to anaesthetize the animals, A 1.1 mm diameter indwelling catheter (PE20, Smith Medical, England), lubricated with paraffin oil was gently inserted into the lightly pinched external urethral orifice, and passed through the urethra into the bladder. A 1.5 cm median incision was made in the lower abdomen. The neck of the bladder and the proximal urethra were bluntly separated using a sterilized cotton swab, and the rear of the bladder neck was bluntly separated exposing the bilateral ureters using an ophthalmic forceps in order to avoid ligation. The bladder was lifted, and the potential lacuna between the back of the urethra and the uterus was opened via blunt and sharp dissection, a 3–0 thread was inserted through it, and the proximal urethra ligated. The degree of tightness of the thread knot can be adjusted and it can be moved along with the surrounding tissue when pulling the indwelling catheter, so that the catheter can be easily removed. Four weeks after the initial surgery, the rats were anaesthetized using an intraperitoneal injection of 25% urethane (1.0 mg/kg). The lower abdomen was cut open and the pelvic cavity entered to expose the bladder. The upper part of the bladder was incised, and a plastic bushing inserted and fastened using purse string suture, after which a micro perfusion pump (Promed-Tech., Bellingham, MA, USA) and a three-way connection pressure sensing device (Nidoc970 urodynamic instrument, Yong xin, China) were connected to the other end of the bushing. The pressure measurement parameters were set to pressure mode, scanning speed of 10 s/div, direct current time-constant, acquisition frequency of 400 Hz, and filtering frequency of 30 Hz. In order to calibrate the zero value, physiological saline at 37 °C was administered into the bladder at 0.3 mL/min, with concomitant digital data collection. If during the low-pressure filling period the bladder contraction interval was shortened and the internal bladder pressure surpassed 15 mm $H_2O$, the OAB animal model was considered successfully developed, and further experiments were conducted.

### Determination of urodynamic parameters

In accordance with a published method [12], after having been prevented from drinking but not from eating the night before, the rats were anaesthetized by intraperitoneally administered 25% urethane (1.0 g/kg), and a 24-gauge catheter (Surflo, Terumo Corp., Tokyo, Japan) was buried within the dome of the bladder. A three-channel connector was used to connect the catheter and the pressure sensor (TP-200 T, Nihon Kohden, Tokyo, Japan). The catheter was also connected via a threefold to a pump for continuous administration of physiological saline at 0.1 mL/min. Bladder pressure and urinary volume were recorded by the software on the connected computer during the saline administration process. The measured parameters also included micturition interval (MI), micturition volume (MV), micturition time (MT), pressure difference between the maximal micturition pressure and the basal pressure (MP-BP), and the pressure difference between the threshold pressure and basal pressure [13]. For each animal, 6–8 micturition cycles were recorded, and the average value was taken as the final result [14].

### Electrophysiological characterization of dorsal root ganglia (DRG)

#### *Preparation of DRG samples*

After anesthesia via intraperitoneal injection of sodium pentobarbital (40 mg/kg), the L6 DRG was exposed and completely separated from surrounding muscle tissue using a glass needle. The extracted DRG was placed into artificial cerebrospinal fluid (ACSF, comprising (mM): NaCl 124, $MgCl_2$ 1, KCl 2.5, $NaH_2PO_4$ 1.2, $CaCl_2$ 2, $NaHCO_3$ 25, Glucose 10, pH 7.4 set using 1 N HCl or NaOH, osmotic pressure set to 290–310 mOsm), which had been air-saturated for 30 min. The upper surface of the specimen was cleaned from connective tissue and covering membranes under a dissecting microscope, after which it was placed into a centrifuge tube containing 0.5 mL of a protease solution comprising 1.0 mg/mL collagenase (Sigma, USA) and 0.4 mg/mL trypsin (Sigma, USA) in PBS pH 7.4, and incubated in a water bath at 37 °C for 40 min. After digestion was completed, the DRG specimen was removed and washed three times with 25 mL ACSF, after which it was incubated in air-saturated ACSF for 1 h [15].

### Whole-cell patch-clamp measurements

The DRG sample was carefully transferred to a perfusion chamber (SHD-27LPKIT, DL Nature gene Life Science, China), fastened using a u-shaped platinum sample holder, and irrigated using a perfusion pump (BT100-2 J/DG-2, Longer, China) at a controlled rate of 1–2 mL/min. An upright microscope was used to investigate the intactness and distribution of cells in the DRG sample, and a cell with a clear 35–40 μm outline and clean surface was selected as the patch-clamp target. A glass electrode (TW150F-4, WPI, USA, electrode resistance 3–6 MΩ) filled with the appropriate amount of electrode solution (mM: Glucose 120, $MgCl_2$ 2, KCl 18, $CaCl_2$ 1, EGTA 5, HEPES 10, $Na_2$-ATP 5, $Na_3$-GTP 0.4, pH set to 7.4 using 1 N HCl, osmotic pressure set to 280–300 mOsm) was placed into the electrode holder, after which a 1 mL syringe was used to apply positive pressure to prevent contamination of the electrode tip. As the electrode was slowly moved toward the target cell, an "umbilical" indentation formed. When the electrical resistance in this seal test rose to 0.1–0.3 MΩ, the positive pressure was removed, providing a small amount of negative pressure, forming a high-resistance seal between the cell and the electrode tip. This ensured a GΩ resistance level, which induced the cells to rupture the membrane, thus forming the whole-cell patch clamp. After the clamp was formed, Cm, Vm and Ra were measured. Under the current clamp, the cell's resting potential was measured, and cells exhibiting a Ra value < 20 MΩ and a resting potential below − 50 mV were selected for further experiments [15].

Under the electrical-current clamp, the DRG neuron was stimulated with a 600 ms depolarizing square wave based on the resting potential, at 100-pA intervals. The induced action potentials (AP) were recorded, and their characteristics analyzed. The first action potential was chosen to determine changes of the AP amplitude, AHP amplitude, threshold value and half width, as well as the membrane potential, Cm and Rm. The amplitude of the AP (mV) was defined as the difference in electric potential between its beginning and highest point, the threshold value (mV) was defined as the membrane potential level at 30% of the rising slope after AP differentiation, the half width (ms) refers to the time difference between two corresponding points on the ascending and descending branches starting at the beginning of the AP, and AHP amplitude denotes the difference in electric potential between the membrane potential and the lowest point of the hyperpolarization. The threshold strength of the medium-size DRG cells (expressed in pA), defined as the smallest current that can elicit an AP from the cells, was recorded under the current clamp. During the experiment, the cells were stimulated with a square-wave stimulus, starting from − 100 pA and rising in steps of 10 pA, with a duration of 60 ms. In order to prevent cell damage, the upper limit of the square-wave stimulus was set to 1000 pA. The 1.5-fold current strength of the rheobase was used to record the number of APs in the medium-size DRG cells, yielding the statistical current strength, with a square-wave stimulus duration of 600 ms. The cells were clamped at − 60 mV, in order to stimulate an $I_h$, and a hyperpolarization potential was applied starting from − 110 mV and increasing in 10 mV steps to − 60 mV. The slow depolarization constant τ was fitted from $I_h$ using the formula $It = I_{ss} + I_h \cdot \exp. - t/\tau$, to obtain the size of the current for time t, whereby $I_{ss}$ is the steady-state current value [7].

#### Intrathecal injection of ZD7288

Intrathecal cathetererization was conducted according to a published report [16]. Briefly, an incision encompassing 1.5–2.0 cm was made along the spinous processes of the spine, and the muscle tissue separated via blunt dissection. A PE-10 catheter (Smith Medical, England), was slowly inserted with its port plugged into the intervertebral foramen, and fixed with dental cement once it came in contact with the DRG. The control group animals also had PE-10 catheters inserted into the intervertebral foramen and fixed with dental cement. A 1 cm segment of the fixed catheter was exposed. After burying the tube, the animals' locomotor function was investigated, and individuals with normal mobility were used for further experiments. Three days after surgery, ZD7288 (Sigma, USA) was injected into the exposed catheter (2 μM, in 10 μL of physiological saline, once per day) and continued for 7 days. The control group was injected with the corresponding amount of pure physiological saline. After pharmaceutical administration for 7 days, the urodynamic parameters of the administered group were measured again. Animals were sacrificed via an overdose of sodium pentobarbital at the end of the experiment.

#### Statistical analysis

The experimental data are represented as mean ± SD. The patch clamp data were analyzed using the Clampfit software (Version 9.2, Axon, USA), charts were drawn using Origin 8.0, and statistical analysis was conducted using SPSS 16.0 (SPSS, USA). Statistical analyses were performed by with Student's *t* test when two groups were compared. Results for more than two groups were evaluated by one-way ANOVA followed by Tukey post hoc test. Results were considered statistically significant at $p < 0.05$.

## Results

#### ZD7288 significantly reduces urinary bladder weight in OAB rats

The average whole-body and bladder weights of the rats in each group are listed in Table 1. The OAB rats did not show any statistically significant differences in body weight ($p > 0.05$). One week after the OAB rats were intrathecally administered either ZD7288 or saline at the L6 DRG, the body weight also did not change in a statistically significant way ($p > 0.05$). Furthermore, following the experimental endpoint, the urinary bladders of the SD rats were removed, and their weights were found to be significantly increased in the treatment group compared to the sham- group ($p < 0.01$,). Furthermore, this increase was significantly lowered upon ZD7288 administration ($p < 0.01$ compared to the sham- group). Intrathecal administration of saline did not have a significant effect on the bladder weight of the OAB rats ($p > 0.05$, OAB vs OAB + saline).

#### Decrease of urinary bladder function in the OAB rats

Table 2 lists the micturition time, micturition interval, micturition volume, the difference between maximal micturition pressure and the basal pressure, as well as the difference between the threshold pressure and basal pressure. Statistical analysis revealed that in the OAB

**Table 1** Average whole-body and bladder weights of the rats in different groups after intrathecal pharmaceutical administration for 7 days

| Parameter | Sham intervention | OAB | OAB + saline | OAB + ZD7288 |
|---|---|---|---|---|
| Body weight (g) | 233.21 ± 11.12 | 229.34 ± 12.13 | 235 ± 10.67 | 231.41 ± 13.51 |
| Bladder weight(mg) | 121.32 ± 7.56 | 214.53 ± 11.42** | 211.34 ± 12.28 | 187.38 ± 12.63## |
| n | 8 | 11 | 11 | 11 |

*OAB* Overactive bladder syndrome group; OAB + saline: OAB group treated with saline; OAB + ZD7288: OAB group treated with ZD7288; ** $p < 0.01$, comparison between the OAB and sham-intervention groups; ## $p < 0.01$, comparison between the OAB and OAB + ZD7288 groups (one-way ANOVA)

group, the micturition interval was significantly shortened ($p < 0.01$), micturition volume was significantly decreased ($p < 0.01$), and the duration of micturition was significantly longer ($p < 0.05$), compared to the sham group. The difference between the basal and maximal urination pressure, as well as the difference between the threshold pressure and the basic pressure did not change significantly ($p > 0.05$, OAB vs sham). One week after intrathecal administration of ZD7288, the micturition interval and volume of OAB + ZD7288 rats were significantly increased, compared with OAB rats ($p < 0.01$). The micturition time was also significantly reduced ($p < 0.05$, OAB + ZD7288 vs OAB). However, 2 μM ZD7288 did not significantly affect either the difference between the basal and maximal urine pressure, or the difference between the basal and the threshold pressure ($p > 0.05$, OAB + ZD7288 vs OAB). We also investigated the effects of intrathecal administration of saline on voiding function, without discovering significant differences in any of the experimentally determined parameters ($p > 0.05$, OAB vs OAB + saline).

### Increase of excitability of the medium-size DRG neurons in the OAB rats

In the whole-call patch clam experiment, we recorded the resting membrane potential (RMP), cell capacitance (Cm), and input resistance ($R_{in}$) of the medium-size DRG neurons. As is shown in Table 3, the RMP and $R_{in}$ of the OAB rats were significantly decreased ($p < 0.05$), while the cells' radius and Cm did not exhibit significant changes compared with the sham group ($p > 0.05$).

Thus, the passive membrane characteristics of the medium-size DRG cells did not change significantly under OAB conditions. However, did the active characteristics change? Compared with the sham group, the AP amplitude of the medium-size DRG neurons in the OAB group was significantly increased (from 95.64 ± 5.70 mV to 110.21 ± 12.34 mV), and the half-width decreased from 1.67 ± 0.45 ms to 1.24 ± 0.32 ms (Fig. 1c), the afterhyperpolarization amplitude decreased from 12.45 ± 1.45 mV to 10.37 ± 1.37 mV (Fig. 1c), and the threshold value was significantly less negative (− 31.03 ± 3.24 mV compared to − 38.10 ± 2.31 mV in the control, Fig. 1d) with $p$ values < 0.05 in all cases (OAB vs sham).Taken together, these results indicate that the excitability of the medium-size DRG neurons of the OAB rats was significantly increased. Furthermore, we investigated the lowest stimulus strength of the current (equal to the rheobase) capable of eliciting an AP from the medium-size DRG neurons. The results show that the rheobase was significantly decreased in the OAB group (365.36 ± 10.54 pA in sham vs 234.67 ± 17.45 pA in OAB, $p < 0.05$, Fig. 2a).

In order to quantify the cells' excitability, we measured the number of action potentials (APs) induced by a current corresponding to the 1.5-fold of the rheobase. The results thus represent the number of APs induced by a current of 500 pA, and the number of APs induced in cells from the OAB group was significantly higher than in the sham group (14.63 ± 4.35 in OAB vs 2.42 ± 0.51 in sham, $p < 0.01$, Fig. 2c and d).

**Table 2** Urinary bladder and voiding parameters, determined for each group of animals after intrathecal pharmaceutical administration for 7 days

| Parameter | Sham intervention | OAB | OAB + saline | OAB + ZD7288 |
|---|---|---|---|---|
| Micturition Interval (Sec) | 75.23 ± 5.71 | 32.85 ± 4.32** | 33.45 ± 3.78 | 48.18 ± 6.58## |
| Micturition Volume (ml) | 0.63 ± 0.42 | 0.21 ± 0.05** | 0.34 ± 0.24 | 0.58 ± 0.32## |
| Micturition Time (s) | 10.38 ± 0.74 | 12.65 ± 1.31* | 13.02 ± 1.54 | 10.54 ± 1.53# |
| Difference between the Maximal and Basal Micturition Pressures ($cmH_2O$) | 54.35 ± 4.67 | 52.28 ± 7.49 | 51.76 ± 6.98 | 49.53 ± 4.87 |
| Difference between the Threshold Pressure and Basal Pressure ($cmH_2O$) | 12.86 ± 1.08 | 9.59 ± 6.75 | 9.78 ± 7.31 | 8.87 ± 7.21 |
| n | 8 | 11 | 11 | 11 |

*OAB* Overactive bladder syndrome group; OAB + saline: OAB group treated with saline; OAB + ZD7288: OAB group treated with ZD7288; * $p < 0.05$, ** $p < 0.01$, OAB group compared to the sham-intervention group; # $p < 0.05$, ## $p < 0.01$, OAB group compared to the OAB + ZD7288 group (one-way ANOVA)

**Table 3** Passive electrophysiological characteristics of the middle-size DRG neurons in the OAB and sham-intervention groups

| Parameter | Sham intervention | OAB |
|---|---|---|
| Cell size (μm) | 41.36 ± 1.34 | 42.21 ± 1.25 |
| RMP(mV) | −58.49 ± 1.72 | −51.03 ± 2.45* |
| $R_{in}$ (MΩ) | 54.87 ± 5.36 | 49.38 ± .54* |
| $C_m$ (pF) | 63.41 ± 6.37 | 65.39 ± 7.82 |
| n | 24 | 19 |

*OAB* denotes the overactive bladder syndrome group, n represents the number of individual investigated cells, *RMP* is the resting membrane potential, $R_{in}$ is input resistance, and $C_m$ is cell capacitance. Comparison of DRG in the OAB and sham-intervention groups revealed no significant difference in $C_m$ ($p > 0.05$, Student's *t* test), while the RMP was significantly less negative and $R_{in}$ was significantly decreased in the OAB group (*$p < 0.05$ for both, Student's *t* test)

**ZD7288 significantly decreased the excitability of the medium-size DRG cells in the OAB rats**

Taken together, the above-stated results indicate that the excitability of the medium-size DRG cells increased in the OAB rats. Our research further revealed that an intrathecal injection of ZD7288 was able to significantly decrease the OAB rats' bladder weight as well as to significantly improve their voiding function (Table 2). This in turn means that ZD7288 can influence the excitability of the DRG neurons, reducing the DRG-mediated activation of the bladder, and thus lowering bladder motility. The $I_h$ current induces the slow depolarization of the cell membrane at the beginning of the AP, so that, after the AP burst and until the hyperpolarization potential, there is an inactivation of the $I_h$ load-bearing channel. Therefore, the $I_h$ current can influence the AP threshold

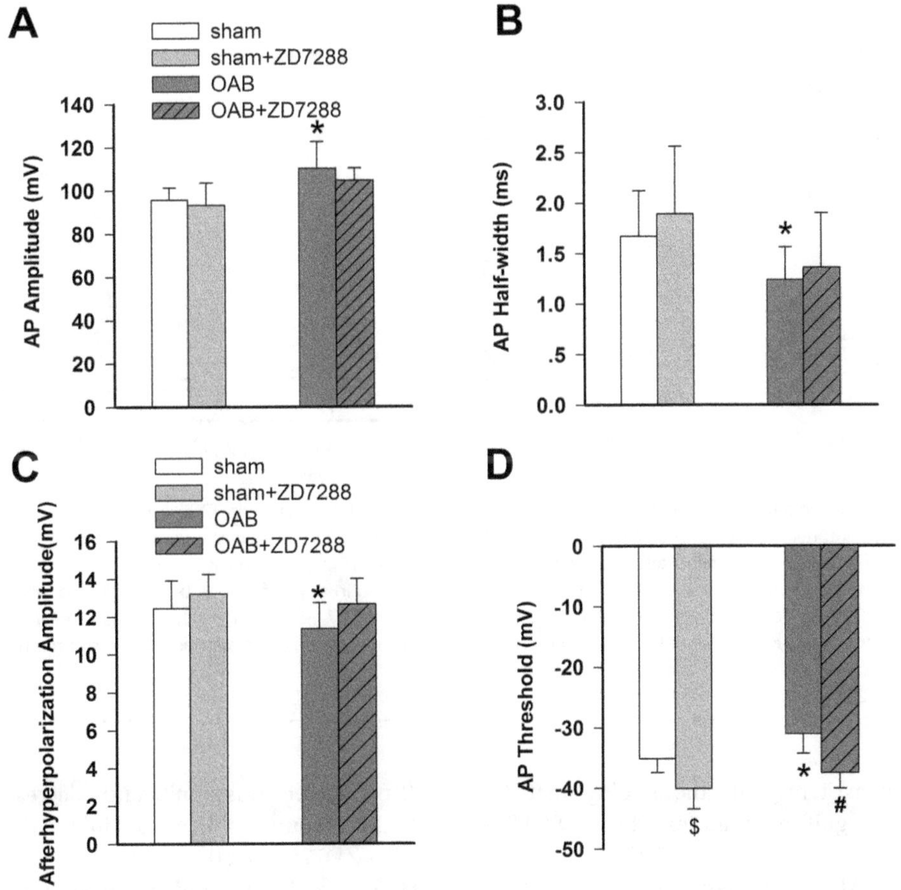


**Fig. 1** Effects of ZD288 on the AP amplitude, half-width, threshold value, and after hyperpolarization amplitude of the medium-size DRG neurons in OAB and sham-intervention rats. The amplitude, half-width, afterhyperpolarization potential (AHP) amplitude and threshold value of the first induced action potential (AP) of the medium-size DRG cells in the OAB rat model were investigated, together with the effect of ZD7288 (2 μM) administration on said parameters. **a**: the amplitude of the action potential was significantly increased in OAB rats, **b**: the action potential half-width was significantly reduced in OAB rats, **c**: the amplitude of the afterhyperpolarization potential was significantly reduced in OAB rats, **d**: the action potential threshold value of OAB rats was significantly lowered; ZD7288 significantly reduced the threshold value of both OAB and sham-intervention rats, but did not affect the AP amplitude, half-width, and AHP amplitude. (*$p < 0.05$, sham vs OAB group, #$p < 0.05$, OAB vs OAB + ZD7288 group,; $p < 0.05, sham vs sham+ZD7288 group,; sham $n = 24$, sham+ZD7288 $n = 24$, OAB $n = 19$, OAB + ZD7288 $n = 19$

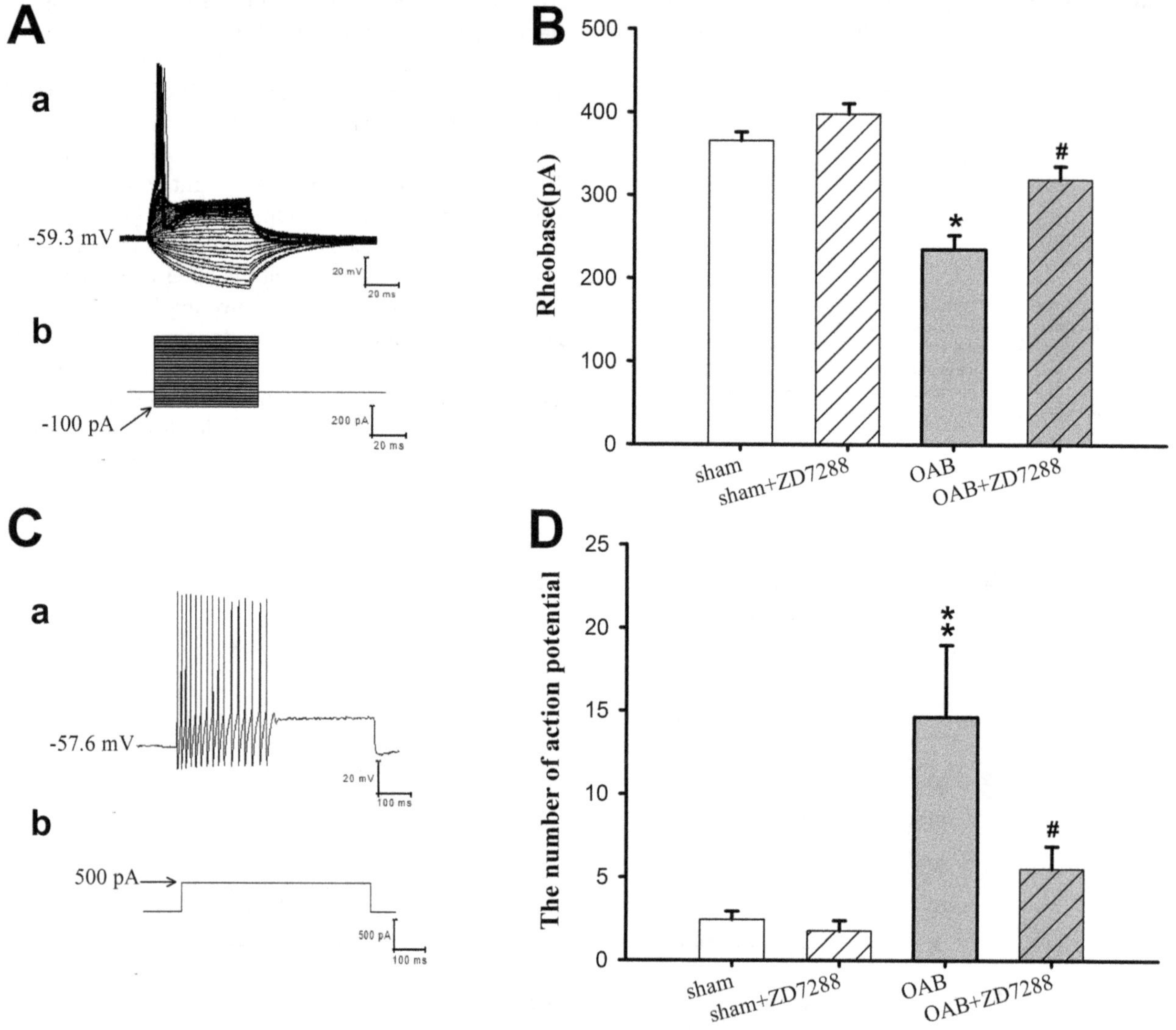


**Fig. 2** Effects of ZD7288 on the threshold value and number of action potentials of the medium-size DRG cells in OAB and sham-intervention rats. The threshold value and number of induced action potentials (AP) of medium-size DRG cells in the rat model of OAB and the effect of ZD7288 on both parameters were investigated. **a**:a shows the diagram of the original action potentials produced by the medium-size DRG cells, b shows the square wave used to induce the APs (starting from − 100 pA, increasing in steps of 10 pA); **b**: the threshold intensity of the cells in the OAB group was significantly decreased, and was significantly increased by 2 μM ZD7288; **c**: a shows the original diagram of the medium-size DRG cells' action potential, b shows the 500 pA square wave used to elicit the action potentials; **d**: statistical analysis of the number of APs revealed a significant increase in the OAB group, which was significantly decreased by ZD7288 (*$p < 0.05$, ** $p < 0.01$, sham vs OAB group; #$p < 0.05$, OAB vs OAB + ZD7288 group; sham $n = 24$, sham+ZD7288 $n = 24$, OAB $n = 19$, OAB + ZD7288 $n = 19$)

value, which is consistent with the finding that the threshold value was significantly increased by ZD7288 in both the OAB and sham groups (− 35.03 ± 2.31 Mv in sham vs − 40.10 ± 3.41 mV in sham+ZD7288; − 31.03 ± 3.24 Mv in OAB vs − 37.46 ± 2.66 mV in OAB + ZD7288, $p < 0.05$ in both cases; Fig. 1d). The rheobase of the medium-size cells in the L6 DRG ganglia of the OAB animals was also significantly increased by ZD7288 (234.67 ± 17.45 pA in OAB vs 318.82 ± 16.39 pA in OAB + ZD7288, $p < 0.05$; Fig. 2b). Additionally, the experiments revealed that the number of APs induced by a 500-pA current was significantly decreased in the OAB + ZD7288 group (14.63 ± 4.35 in OAB vs 5.50 ± 1.37 in OAB + ZD7288, $p < 0.05$; Fig. 2d).

However, ZD7288 did not have any significant effect on the amplitude of the afterhyperpolarization potential or half-width ($p > 0.05$, OAB + ZD7288 vs OAB and sham+ZD7288 vs sham; Figs. 1a, b and c).

During the AP hyperpolarization process, the $I_h$ current is activated and involves in the recovery of the membrane following the AHP [17, 18]. This means that the $I_h$ current may possibly influence the time-course of

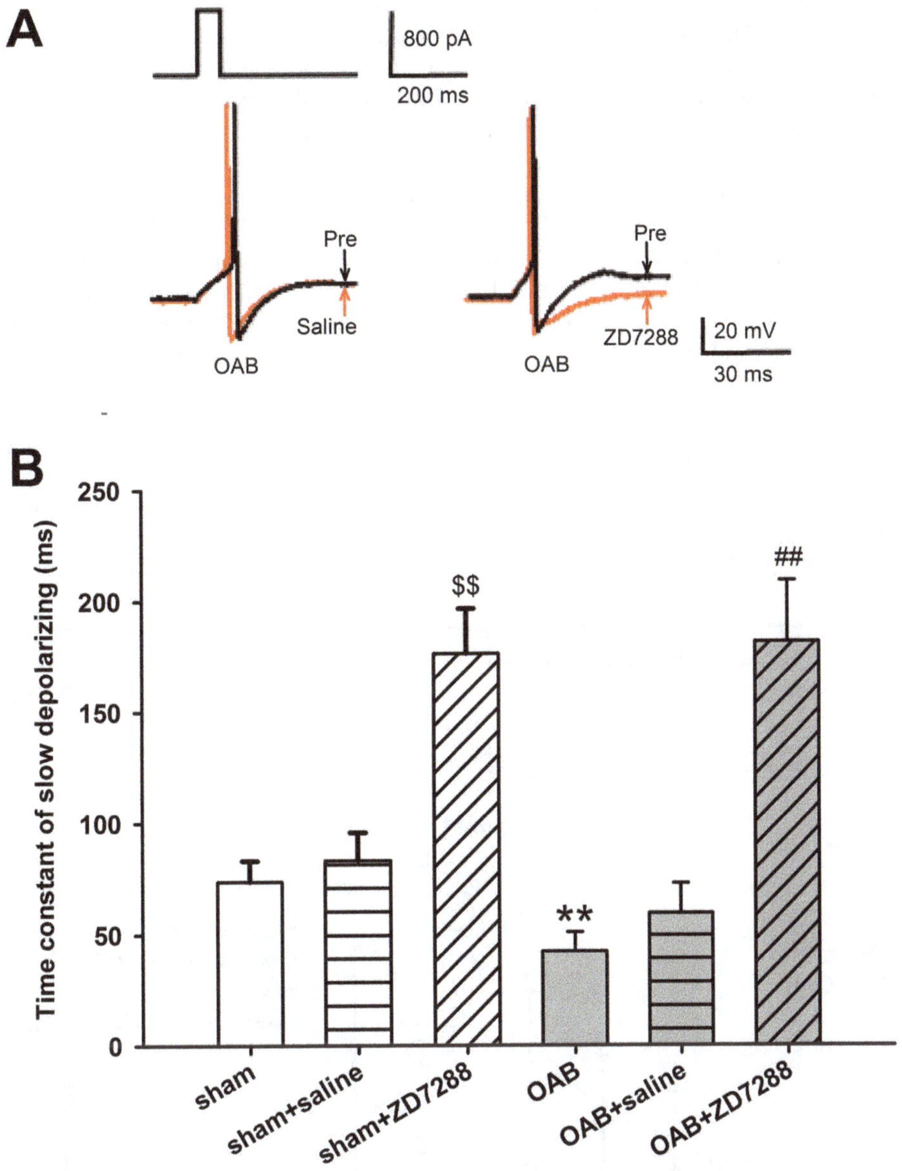


**Fig. 3** Effects of ZD7288 on the τ value of the medium-size cells in the L6 DRG of the OAB and sham-intervention rats. The τ value (time constant of slow depolarizing) of the DRG medium-size cells in the DRG of the OAB model rats was investigated, along with the effect of ZD7288 on this parameter. **a**: Square-wave stimulation of DRG medium-size cells under current-clamp conditions (800 pA, 60 ms, first row). ZD7288 significantly increased the τ value in the OAB model, whereas saline did not have an effect. **b**: Change of the τ value. The τ value was significantly decreased in the OAB rats, and ZD7288 was able to significantly increase it in both OAB and sham groups ($^{\$\$}p < 0.01$, sham vs sham+ZD7288 group; $^{**}p < 0.01$, sham vs OAB group; $^{\#\#}p < 0.01$, OAB vs OAB + ZD7288 group; sham $n = 12$, sham+ZD7288 $n = 12$, OAB $n = 13$, OAB + ZD7288 $n = 13$)

the recovery of the hyperpolarization potential towards the level of the membrane potential. The experiments have uncovered that the τ value in the OAB model was significantly reduced (73.7 ± 9.4 ms in sham vs 42.35 ± 8.67 ms in OAB; $p < 0.01$; Fig. 3b), indicating that the excitability of the OAB rats' medium-size DRG cells increased, which was in agreement with the increase of the number of preceding discharges. ZD7288 (2 μM) was able to significantly increase the τ values of both the OAB and sham animals (73.7 ± 9.4 ms in sham vs 176.34 ± 20.30 ms in sham+ZD7288; 42.35 ± 8.67 ms in OAB vs 181.56 ± 27.45 ms in OAB + ZD7288; $p < 0.01$, in both cases; Fig. 3b).

At the same time, saline administration did not have a significant effect on the τ value of either the OAB or the sham group (73.7 ± 9.4 ms in sham vs 83.26 ± 12.56 ms in sham+saline; 42.35 ± 8.67 ms in OAB vs 59.44 ± 13.43 ms in OAB+ saline; $p > 0.05$ in both cases; Fig. 3b).

**Measurement of $I_h$ current density in the medium-size DRG cells of the OAB rats with ZD7288 treatment**

The above-described experiments revealed that ZD7288 is able to significantly reduce the threshold value, threshold intensity, and number of APs, in addition to significantly increasing the τ value of the L6 DRG neurons in the OAB rats. These results thus indicate that the formation of the $I_h$ current in the OAB model might play an inordinately important role. In the voltage clamp experiments, the cells were clamped at – 60 mV, and the hyperpolarization potential was increased in 10 mV steps from – 110 mV to – 60 mV, inducing a slow inward cation current (Fig. 4a). Furthermore, this type of hyperpolarization-activating inward current could be completely blocked by 2 μM ZD7288, confirming that the recorded current is indeed the $I_h$ current. When the potential was clamped at – 90, – 100 and – 110 mV, the $I_h$ current density was significantly higher in OAB group compared with control (at – 90 mV: 2.68 ± 1.67 pA/pF in sham vs 8.43 ± 2.10 pA/pF in OAB; at – 100 mV: 4.56 ± 1.79 pA/pF in sham vs 9.73 ± 2.67 pA/pF in OAB; at – 110 mV: 6.12 ± 2.13 pA/pF in sham vs 14.39 ± 2.87 pA/pF in OAB; $p < 0.05$, Fig. 4b). In contrast, 15 min after 2 μM ZD7288 was added to the measurement buffer in

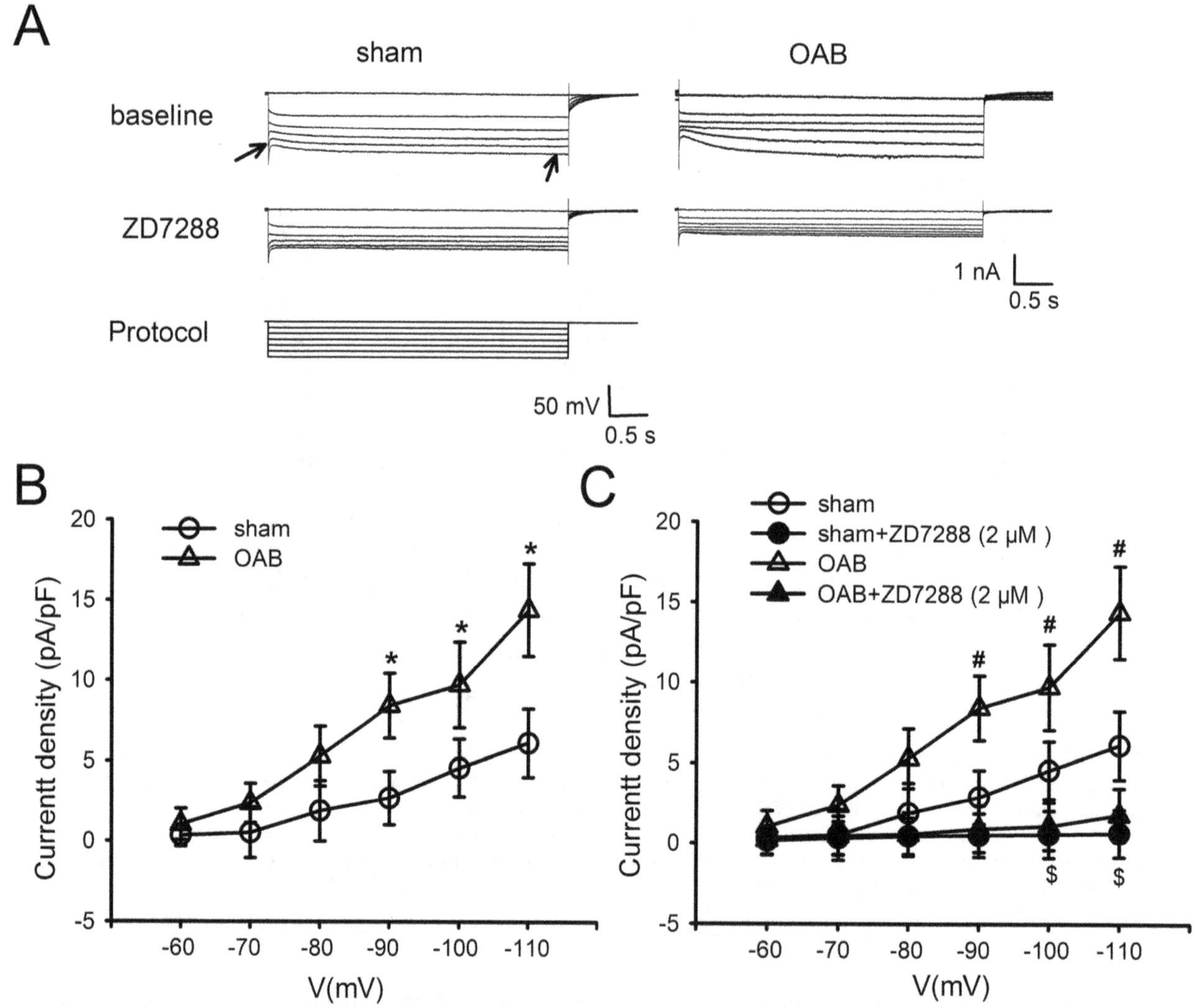


**Fig. 4** Measurement of $I_h$ current density in the medium-size DRG cells of the OAB and sham-intervention rats. **a**: The $I_h$ current eliciting a hyperpolarization potential in the medium-size DRG cells of the sham group (left side) and OAB group (right side). The magnitude of the $I_h$ current is the current difference corresponding to the vertical distance from the instantaneous starting point to the steady state (the two arrows in the diagram indicate the endpoints of the magnitude). The ratio of the $I_h$ amplitude and the capacitance of the neural cells is the $I_h$ current density. After the addition of 2 μM ZD7288 to the perfusion fluid, the $I_h$ current of both the OAB and sham groups was significantly inhibited (middle row). The final row shows the $I_h$ current induced by the square-wave stimulus (starting from – 110 mV, increasing in 10 mV steps). **b**: When said cells were clamped at – 110, – 100 and – 90 mV, the $I_h$ current density was significantly increased. C: The $I_h$ current density of the both the OAB and sham groups was significantly reduced by ZD7288 (*$p < 0.05$, sham vs OAB group; #$p < 0.05$, OAB vs OAB + ZD7288 group; \$$p < 0.05$, sham vs sham+ZD7288 group; sham $n = 11$, sham+ZD7288 $n = 11$, OAB $n = 13$, OAB + ZD7288 $n = 13$)

which the cells were immersed, the $I_h$ current density of the DRG neurons in the OAB group was significantly lower (at − 90 mV, 8.43 ± 2.10 pA/pF in OAB vs 0.91 ± 1.45 pA/pF in OAB + ZD7288; at − 100 mV, 9.73 ± 2.67 pA/pF in OAB vs 1.08 ± 1.48 pA/pF in OAB + ZD7288; at − 110 mV, 14.39 ± 2.87 pA/pF in OAB vs 1.78 ± 1.67 pA/pF in OAB + ZD7288; $p < 0.05$, Fig. 4c).

During the same experiment, it was discovered that ZD7288 was able to significantly reduce the $I_h$ current density of the DRG neurons in the sham rats (at − 100 mV: 4.56 ± 1.79 pA/pF in sham vs 0.57 ± 1.46 pA/pF in sham+ZD7288; at − 110 mV: 6.12 ± 2.13 pA/pF in sham vs 0.64 ± 1.47 pA/pF in sham+ZD7288; $p < 0.05$; Fig. 4c). However, the reduction range of current density of DRG neurons after ZD7288 administration were obviously wider in OAB rats than sham rats (Fig. 4c). These results suggested that ZD7288 could inhibit cell excitability of DRG cells relatively more strongly in OAB group than in sham group.

## Discussion

The urinary bladder weight of the overactive bladder syndrome (OAB) model rats, as well as the excitability and $I_h$ current density of the animals' medium-size DRG neurons were significantly increased. Intrathecal injection of the specific $I_h$ current inhibitor ZD7288 was able to alleviate the observed changes in the OAB rats, including a prolonged micturition time and shortened micturition interval. At the same time, ZD7288 completely blocked the $I_h$ current density, and lowered the excitability of the medium-size DRG cells. Taken together, these results strongly suggest that the $I_h$ current may be a factor in the development of OAB.

The partial bladder outlet obstruction rat model is a good approximation of the condition seen in clinical patients with urinary bladder overactivity and urethral blockage syndromes, including a high degree of agreement in the observed pathological changes [19]. Therefore, the partial bladder outlet obstruction rat model was used in this study, and the urinary bladder weight of the successfully induced OAB rats was significantly increased, in agreement with the literature [13]. Recordings of the micturition process have uncovered that the micturition interval of the OAB rats was significantly shortened, their micturition time was significantly increased, and micturition volume was significantly decreased, indicating that the rats with the partially-blocked urethra indeed had an abnormally enhanced micturition reflex.

According to anatomical studies, the neural fibers that innervate the bladder include the myelinated $A_\delta$ and the myelin-free C-type fibers [6, 19, 20]. One part of these afferent fibers transverses the pelvis, arriving at the L6 and S1 DRG of the spine, and takes part in the initial stage of the micturition signal, while another part transverses the lower abdomen, arriving at the L1 and L2 level of the spine [3, 21, 22]. The DRG neurons are classified into small, medium and large types according to their cross-sectional diameter, and further separated according to the $A_{\alpha/\beta}$, $A_\delta$ and C typology [4, 5]. A subset of the nerve fibers that control the micturition process terminate at the L6 DRG, making the question pertinent whether the excitability of the OAB rats' L6 DRG has exhibited any changes. The results of present study indicated that the AP amplitude and number of APs elicited by a 500-pA stimulus were significantly increased, whereas the half-width, threshold strength, threshold value and the afterhyperpolarization potential, as well as the input resistance were significantly decreased. The membrane potential also had an obvious depolarization tendency. All these results suggested that the medium-size L6 DRG cells of the OAB rats had a significantly increased excitability. The membrane potential of the L6 DRG neurons of the OAB rats also displayed obvious depolarization, with an increase in the number of APs elicited by a 500-pA stimulus, as well as a decrease of the input resistance and τ value. Thus, the hyperpolarization-induced cation current ($I_h$) might play an important role in the observed increased excitability of the medium-size neurons in the L6 DRG of the OAB rats. The $I_h$ current is present in excitable cells in both the center and the periphery of the body, including the photoreceptor cells of the retina and the cardiac pacemaker cells, as well as cells of the central and peripheral nervous system [23, 24]. The $I_h$ current channel is activated when the AHP is rapidly increasing, and the influx of $Na^+$ causes a slow depolarization of the cell membrane. In peripheral nerves, $I_h$ is found in the sensory DRG neurons [25]. Within these sensory neurons, it participates in the AHP process, and induces the cell membrane to recover to the resting potential after depolarization, shortening the AHP amplitude and duration [26, 17, 27]. Studies have also reported that the $I_h$ current plays a role in the maintenance of membrane potential, influencing the cells' spontaneous and repeated discharge, as well as related phenomena [28, 29]. In our experiments, it was shown that the specific $I_h$ current inhibitor ZD7288 is able to clearly inhibit the excitability of the medium-size DRG cells in the OAB rats, including a reduction of the number of APs elicited by a 500-pA stimulus and an increase of the τ value, indicating that the $I_h$ current within the L6 DRG neurons plays an important role in the etiology of OAB. After administration of ZD7288, DRG in sham+ZD7288 group also showed elevated τ value and reduction in current density, suggested that $I_h$ current inhibitor could reduce the cell membrane excitability in sham rats. However, the reduction range of current density of DRG neurons after ZD7288 administration were obviously wider in OAB + ZD7288 group than sham+ZD7288 group. These results suggested that ZD7288 could inhibit cell excitability of DRG cells relatively more strongly in OAB rats than in sham rats.

A study by Masuda and coworkers has found that the $I_h$ current is primarily present in the medium-size DRG neurons that control the urinary bladder, and that inhibition of the current significantly increases the time from the highest AHP point until the return to the resting potential, and reduces the excitability of the medium-size DRG neurons [7]. These results imply that the excitability of the medium-size mechanical nociceptor cells in the DRG that control the urinary bladder may be influenced by the $I_h$ current. This raises the question whether the $I_h$ current in the medium-size DRG cells of the OAB mice experienced changes. Our results show that the $I_h$ current density was significantly increased, and functional experiments have shown that intrathecal injection of ZD7288 significantly improved the micturition parameters of the OAB rats. The experimental results indicate that an increase in the strength of the $I_h$ current in the medium-size cells of the L6 DRG might be an important component of the OAB development process. Furthermore, the hyperpolarization-activated cyclic nucleotide-gated cation channel (HCN) mediates the $I_h$ current, and an investigation of HCN expression in the neurons that control the bladder, which are found in the L6-S1 DRG, has uncovered rich expression of HCN2 in the average medium-size DRG cells.

It is thus theoretically possible that the significant increase of the $I_h$ current in the medium-size neurons of the L6 DRG of OAB rats is related to the HCN2 channel, and this notion merits further research. Furthermore, these experimental results demonstrate that the half-width, amplitude, and afterhyperpolarization potential of the action potential are not influenced by ZD7288, which is in agreement with other studies, which have also found that ZD2788 cannot influence the shape of the AP or the AHP amplitude [28, 29]. This indicates that the observed changes of the $I_h$ current may be part of the electrophysiological mechanism responsible for the increase of excitability in the medium-size DRG cells of the OAB rats. The limitations of current study is that the precise functional activity of the $I_h$ current in the medium-size DRG neurons of OAB rats has not been fully unveiled, and we do not observe the small-size DRG neurons. Further studies using structurally dissimilar HCN channel blockers such as ivabradine will be needed to strengthen our present behavioral and electrophysiological findings. Further electrophysiological mechanisms influencing the cells' excitability still remain to be resolved. Since the etiology of OAB is complicated and multifactorial, additional studies are needed in different animal models and different OAB related cells to clarify the real role of $I_h$ current in bladder dysfunction.

## Conclusions

This study reveals that the excitability of medium-size cells in the L6 DRG of OAB model rats was significantly increased, and that the $I_h$ current correlates with a part of the parameters of this heightened nerve-cell excitability. The medium-size cells in the L6 DRG of the OAB rats had a significantly increased $I_h$ current density, and their micturition reflex was significantly improved under the influence of ZD7288, which indicates that the $I_h$ current in these cells may be an important part of the electrophysiological mechanism leading to the development of OAB.

### Abbreviations

OAB: OVERACTIVE bladder syndrome; DRG: Dorsal root ganglia; MI: Micturition interval;; MV: Micturition volume; MT: Micturition time; MP-BP: Maximal micturition pressure and the basal pressure; HCN: Hyperpolarization-activated cyclic nucleotide-gated cation; RMP: Resting membrane potential; AP: Action potentials; RMP: Resting membrane potential; Cm: Cell capacitance

### Acknowledgements

Not applicable.

### Authors' contributions

C.T., F.Y., L.Y., and J.X. conceived and designed the experiments; W.Q., K.Z., and G.W. performed the experiments; C.T., F.Y., L.Y., and J.X. analyzed the data; F.L. provided all the funding, direction of the detail of experiments and design of the research. F.L. and J.Y. contributed reagents/materials/analysis tools. J.Y. has also designed the work and contributed to the data interpretation. C.T., F.Y., L.Y., and J.X. wrote the manuscript. All authors read and approved the final manuscript.

### Author details

[1]Department of Urology, Xijing Hospital, Air Force Medical University, 15 Changle West Road, Xi'an 710032, Shaanxi, China. [2]Xijing Hospital of Digestive Diseases, Xijing Hospital, Air Force Medical University, Xi'an, Shaanxi, China. [3]Institute of neuroscience, Air Force Medical University, Xi'an, Shaanxi, China.

### References

1. Lee U, Scott V, Rashid R, Behniwal A, Wein A, Maliski S, Anger J. Defining and managing overactive bladder: disagreement among the experts. Urology. 2013;81(2):257–62.
2. Leong R, De Wachter S, van Kerrebroeck P. Current information on sacral neuromodulation and botulinum toxin treatment for refractory idiopathic overactive bladder syndrome: a review. Urol Int. 2010;84(3):245–53.
3. de Groat W, Yoshimura N. Anatomy and physiology of the lower urinary tract. Handb Clin Neurol. 2015;130:61–108.
4. Light A, Perl E. Spinal termination of functionally identified primary afferent neurons with slowly conducting myelinated fibers. J Comp Neurol. 1979; 186(2):133–50.
5. Réthelyi M. Preterminal and terminal axon arborizations in the substantia gelatinosa of cat's spinal cord. J Comp Neurol. 1977;172(3):511–21.
6. de Groat W, Nadelhaft I, Milne R, Booth A, Morgan C, Thor K. Organization of the sacral parasympathetic reflex pathways to the urinary bladder and large intestine. J Auton Nerv Syst. 1981;3(2–4):135–60.
7. Masuda N, Hayashi Y, Matsuyoshi H, Chancellor M, de Groat W, Yoshimura N. Characterization of hyperpolarization-activated current (Ih) in dorsal root ganglion neurons innervating rat urinary bladder. Brain Res. 2006;1096(1): 40–52.

8. Beaumont V, Zucker R. Enhancement of synaptic transmission by cyclic AMP modulation of presynaptic Ih channels. Nat Neurosci. 2000;3(2):133–41.
9. Chevaleyre V, Castillo P. Assessing the role of Ih channels in synaptic transmission and mossy fiber LTP. Proc Natl Acad Sci U S A. 2002;99(14): 9538–43.
10. Yoshimura N, Bennett NE, Hayashi Y, Ogawa T, Nishizawa O, Chancellor MB, de Groat WC, et al. Bladder overactivity and hyperexcitability of bladder afferent neurons after intrathecal delivery of nerve growth factor in rats. J Neurosci. 2006;26(42):10847–55.
11. Zotova EG, Christ GJ, Zhao W, Tar M, Kuppam SD, Arezzo JC. Effects of fidarestat, an aldose reductase inhibitor, on nerve conduction velocity and bladder function in streptozotocin-treated female rats. J Diabetes Complicat. 2007;21(3):187–95.
12. Liu HP, Chen GL, Liu P, Xu XP. Amlodipine alone or combined with terazosin improves lower urinary tract disorder in rat models of benign prostatic hyperplasia or detrusor instability: focus on detrusor overactivity. BJU Int. 2009;104(11):1752–7.
13. Jang H, Dong SH, Yuk SM. Changes of neuregulin-1(NRG-1) expression in a rat model of overactive bladder induced by partial urethral obstruction: is NRG-1 a new biomarker of overactive bladder? BMC Urol. 2013;13(1):54.
14. Liu F, Yao L, Yuan J, Liu H, Yang X, Qin W, Wu G, et al. Protective effects of inosine on urinary bladder function in rats with partial bladder outlet obstruction. Urology. 2009;73(6):1417.
15. Zhang M, Han W, Zheng J, Meng F, Jiao X, Hu S, Xu H. Inhibition of hyperpolarization-activated Cation current in medium-sized DRG neurons contributed to the Antiallodynic effect of Methylcobalamin in the rat of a chronic compression of the DRG. Neural Plast. 2015;2015:197392.
16. Yaksh TL, Rudy TA. Chronic catheterization of the spinal subarachnoid space. Physiol Behav. 1976;17(6):1031–6.
17. Linden DR, Sharkey KA, Mawe GM. Enhanced excitability of myenteric AH neurones in the inflamed guinea-pig distal colon 2003. 589–601.
18. Mallory B, Steers WD, Groat WCD. Electrophysiological study of micturition reflex in rats. Am J Physiol. 1989;257(2 Pt 2):R410.
19. Parsons BA, Drake MJ. Animal models in overactive bladder research. Handb Exp Pharmacol. 2011;202(202):15.
20. Vera PL, Nadelhaft I. Conduction velocity distribution of afferent fibers innervating the rat urinary bladder. Brain Res. 1990;520(1–2):83.
21. Su TH, Wang KG, Hsu CY, Wei HJ, Hong BK. Prospective comparison of laparoscopic and traditional colposuspensions in the treatment of genuine stress incontinence. Acta Obstet Gynecol Scand. 1997;76(6):576.
22. Vera PL, Nadelhaft I. Afferent and sympathetic innervation of the dome and the base of the urinary bladder of the female rat. Brain Res Bull. 1992;29(5): 651–8.
23. Bader C, Macleish P, Schwartz E. A voltage-clamp study of the light response in solitary rods of the tiger salamander. J Physiol Lond. 1979;296: 1–26.
24. Difrancesco D, Tortora P. Direct activation of cardiac pacemaker channels by intracellular cyclic AMP. Nature. 1991;351(6322):145.
25. Doan TN, Kunze DL. Contribution of the hyperpolarization-activated current to the resting membrane potential of rat nodose sensory neurons. J Physiol. 1999;514(( Pt 1)(1)):125.
26. Mayer M, Westbrook G. A voltage-clamp analysis of inward (anomalous) rectification in mouse spinal sensory ganglion neurones. J Physiol Lond. 1983;340:19–45.
27. Pape HC. Queer current and pacemaker: the hyperpolarization-activated cation current in neurons. Annu Rev Physiol. 1996;58(1):299.
28. Funahashi M, Mitoh Y, Kohjitani A, Matsuo R. Role of the hyperpolarization-activated Cation current ( I h ) in pacemaker activity in area Postrema neurons of rat brain slices. J Physiol. 2003;552(1):135–48.
29. Rusznák Z, Pál B, Kőszeghy Á, Fu Y, Szücs G, Paxinos G. The hyperpolarization-activated non-specific cation current (I h ) adjusts the membrane properties, excitability, and activity pattern of the giant cells in the rat dorsal cochlear nucleus. Eur J Neurosci. 2013;37(6):876–90.

27

# Small cell carcinoma of the bladder with coexisting prostate adenocarcinoma: Two cases report and literature review

Yanxia Liu[1], Hongming Xu[1], Bin Wu[2], Shuguang Liu[3] and Qiang Luo[2*]

**Abstract**

**Background:** Primary small cell carcinoma of the bladder (SCCB) is a rare disease of the genitourinary tract and reported limitedly. SCCB is very aggressive and always mixed with other histologic components, but coexistence of SCCB and prostate adenocarcinoma is extremely rare.

**Cases presentation:** Two aged males (72 and 58 years) were included in this study. Both of them presented with gross hematuria as initial symptom. Magnetic resonance imaging (MRI) demonstrated protruding lesions in the urinary bladder. Pathological examination after radical cystectomy and prostatectomy showed the concurrence of SCCB and prostate adenocarcinoma. One patient died of liver and lung metastasis 8 months after surgery, and the other patient was still alive after 19 months of follow-up.

**Conclusion:** In this paper, we reported two unusual cases of coexistence of SCCB and prostate adenocarcinoma, and reviewed relative literatures with respect to the epidemiology, clinical features, pathologic features, diagnosis, treatment and prognosis of SCCB.

**Keywords:** Small cell carcinoma, Urinary bladder, Prostate, Adenocarcinoma

## Background

Small cell carcinoma occurs mainly in the lung, which occupies about 15–20% pulmonary malignant tumors. Besides, this disease could also exist in extra pulmonary sites, such as skin, gastrointestinal and urinary tract [1, 2]. Small cell carcinoma of the bladder (SCCB) accounts for 0.35–0.7% of bladder tumors and indicates aggressive biological behavior and poor prognosis [3]. SCCB is usually admixed with other pathological subtypes, like urothelial carcinoma and squamous cell carcinoma [4]. Prostate cancer is the most commonly diagnosed cancer and the second leading cause of cancer related death in men around the world. Nevertheless, coexistence of SCCB and prostate adenocarcinoma in one patient was extremely scarce, which brought certain challenges to the treatment and prognosis of patients [5, 6]. Here, we described two cases of such rare malignancy who underwent surgery in our institution.

## Cases presentation

### Case 1 #

A 72-years-old hypertensive man visited our hospital with gross hematuria and odynuria for 2 months (Table 1). Urinary Doppler ultrasound revealed a neoplasm located in the left posterior bladder wall, no enlarged prostate or obvious hydronephrosis. The serum total prostate specific antigen (PSA) was 16.40 ng/ml. The patient stated a smoking history of 40 years and quitted smoking for 8 years. Magnetic resonance imaging (MRI) indicated an oval-shaped tumor mass involving the entire layer of bladder (Fig. 1). Small cell

* Correspondence: drluoqiang@163.com
[2]Department of Urology, Jiangyin People's Hospital, Affiliated Jiangyin Hospital of the Southeast University Medical College, Jiangyin 214400, Jiangsu Province, China
Full list of author information is available at the end of the article

**Table 1** The clinical characteristics of two patients

| | Case 1 | Case 2 |
|---|---|---|
| Age (years) | 72 | 58 |
| Bladder size (cm) | 11.0 × 8.0 × 6.0 | 10.0 × 6.5 × 5.0 |
| Prostate size (cm) | 4.0 × 3.5 × 2.5 | 5.5 × 4.0 × 3.5 |
| SCCB size (cm) | 4.0 × 3.0 × 2.5 | 3.0 × 2.5 × 1.5<br>1.5 × 1.0 × 1.0 |
| SCCB location | left posterior wall | posterior wall top wall |
| Initial symptoms | gross hematuria odynuria | gross hematuria dysuria |
| Serum PSA (ng/ml) | 16.40 | 8.56 |

carcinoma and urothelial carcinoma cells were detected through cytological examination.

The patient underwent radical cystectomy and prostatectomy. Post-operative pathological examination revealed small round cells containing scant cytoplasm full of the microscope views (Fig. 2a). Mitotis images could be observed as well. Immunohistochemical (IHC) staining displayed intense positivity of neuroendocrine markers, including chromogranin A (CgA), synaptophysin (Syn) and neuron specific enolase (NSE) (Fig. 2c- e). The representative feature of prostate adenocarcinoma was also be discovered, and PSA and P504s were positive (Fig. 2b and f). The IHC results of two cases were shown in Table 2.

The patient accepted regular CE-based chemotherapeutic regimen (Carboplatin, 200 mg, 1d/21d; VP-16, 100 mg, 1-4d/21d) for six sessions and died of liver and lung metastasis 8 months after surgery. The postoperative serum PSA after one and 2 months were 0.34 ng/ml and 0.55 ng/ml, which reminded the biochemical recurrence (BCR) of prostate cancer. During the follow up, the patient accepted endocrine therapy (Bicalutamide, 250 mg/d) as well.

### Case 2 #

A 58-year-old male was hospitalized in our center due to painlessness gross hematuria lasted for 2 weeks and dysuria for half a year. Urinary Doppler ultrasound showed two neoplasms attached to bladder wall, and the prostate volume slightly increased. The serum total PSA was 8.56 ng/ml. MRI subsequently revealed two masses located at the posterior and top wall of the bladder, respectively (Fig. 3). Cystoscopy detection indicated the tumors invaded into the muscle layer. Therefore, we performed radical cystectomy and prostatectomy.

As shown in Fig. 4, pathological examination revealed coexistence of SCCB and prostate adenocarcinoma. CgA, Syn, NSE and P504s were all positive by IHC staining (Fig. 4c-f), while CK7, LCA, CD3, P63 and CK34βE12 were negative (Table 2). The patient received serum PSA examination monthly within 3 months after operation, and the levels were consistently < 0.2 ng/ml. Regular CE regimen was performed for eight sessions. Six months after operation, the patient accepted chest and abdomen CT scan, whichreminded no apparent metastatic lesions in distant

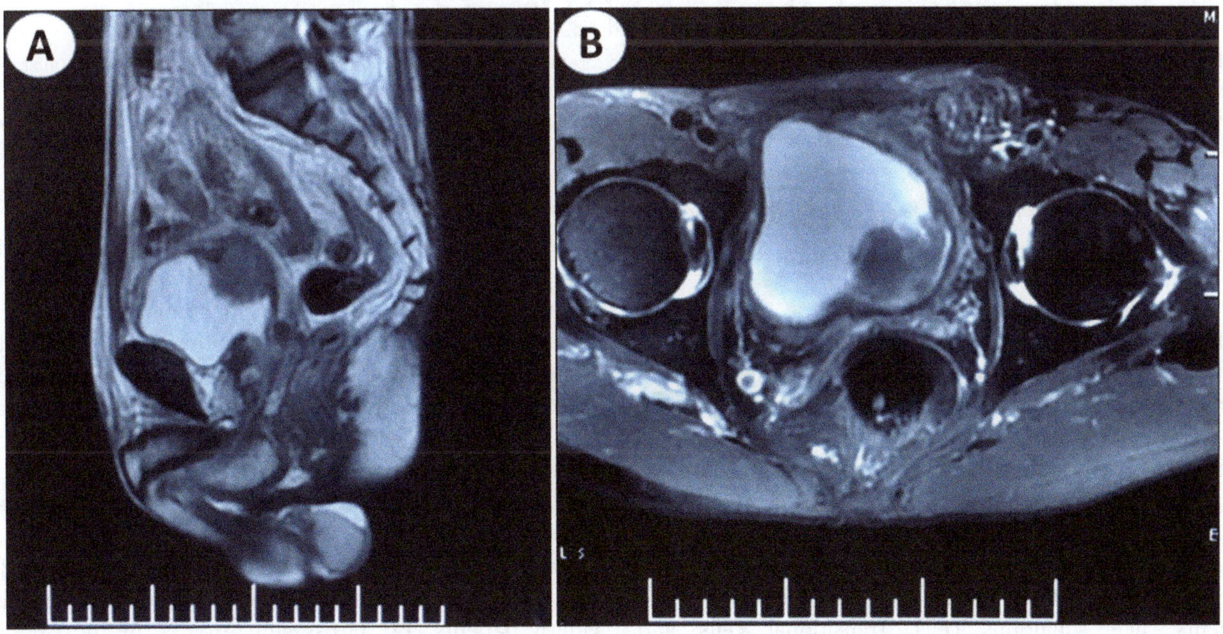


**Fig. 1** Sagittal (**a**) and horizontal plane (**b**) MRI demonstrated an oval-shaped tumor mass invading the entire layer of bladder in the left posterior bladder wall

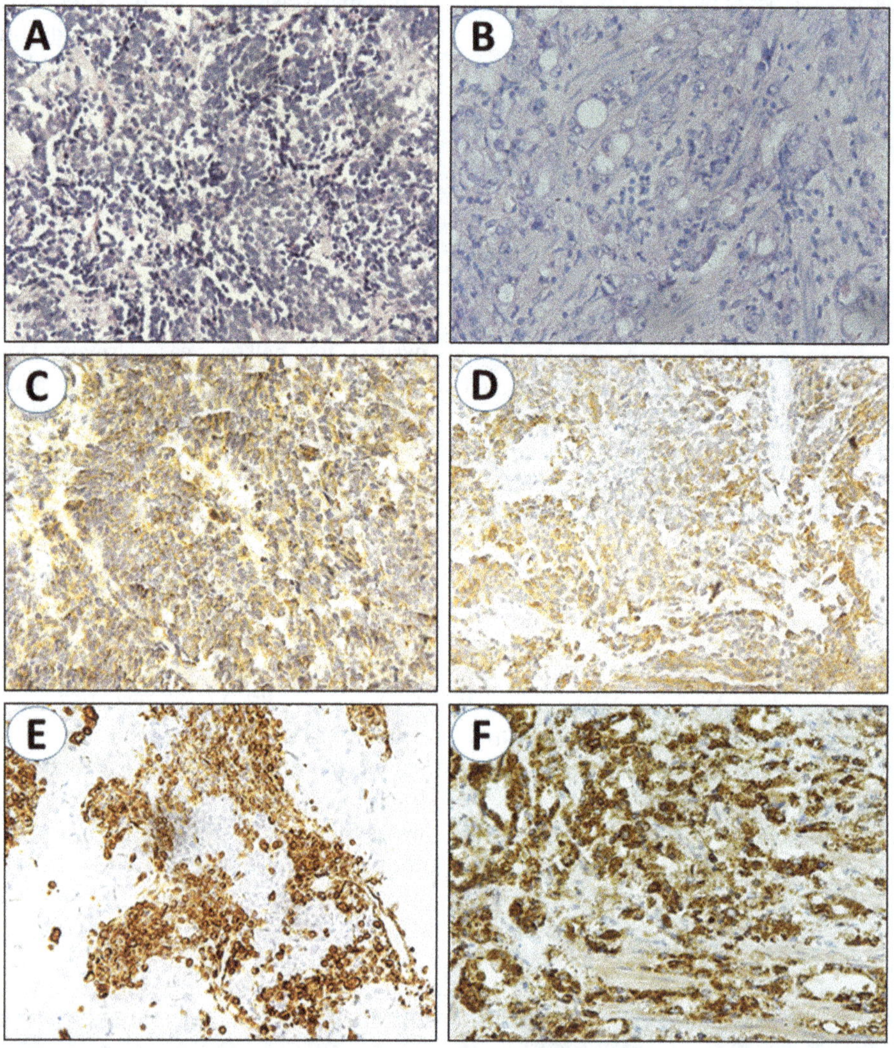


**Fig. 2** 100X magnification of the resected tissues. HE staining showed typical small cells with scant cytoplasm arranged in sheets of SCCB (**a**) and disorder of glands structure, glandular hyperplasia and cell atypia of prostate adenocarcinoma (**b**). Positive staining for CgA (**c**), Syn (**d**), NSE (**e**) and P504s (**f**)

organs. The patient has been followed up for 19 months and is still alive up to now.

## Discussion and conclusion

In present study, we described two unusual SCCB cases with combination of prostate adenocarcinoma. HE and IHC staining of tissue sections with demonstration of NSE, CgA, Syn, P504s and PSA supported the diagnosis. Prostate cancer is the most common malignancy in men and a major cause of cancer deaths in western countries [7]. SCCB is extremely infrequent with a proportion about 0.35–0.7% of all bladder tumors, and has a tendency to present with mixed histological accompaniments, like squamous cells, transitional cells and urothelial carcinoma [3, 8]. SCCB has an evident male predominance (male: female = 7: 1) with an average age of 60–80 years [9]. The mechanism of SCCB is still controversial at present. The most widely accepted theory is that it derives from multi-potential stem cells. Such conjecture could also explain the phenomenon that more than half of SCCB coexisted with other histological patterns [10]. The second theory considers that SCCB originates from neuroendocrine cells among the urothelial cells, just like the enterochromaffi cells in the intestinal tract. Another theory suggests it arises from the neuroendocrine cells within the normal or metaplastic urothelium [3, 11].

Bladder tumors often cause hematuria, so unusually subtype of tumors should be kept in mind, especially in elderly patients [12]. Gross hematuria is the most common symptom in SCCB because of the ulcerative growth of invasive lesion into bladder wall. Both the two

**Table 2** The immunohistochemical (IHC) characteristics of two patients

| | Patient 1 | Patient 2 |
|---|---|---|
| IHC staining | | |
| CgA | + | + |
| Syn | + | + |
| NSE | + | + |
| CK7 | + | − |
| LCA | − | − |
| CD20 | − | no |
| CD3 | no | − |
| P504s | + | + |
| PSA | + | + |
| P63 | − | − |
| CK34βE12 | − | − |
| GATA3 | + | − |
| ERG | − | − |
| TTF-1 | − | + |
| Gleason score | 3 + 4 = 7 | 3 + 3 = 6 |

patients presented with gross hematuria, and odynuria/ dysuria. Paraneoplastic syndromes (hypercalcaemia, Cushing syndrome, sensory neuropathy and so on) were commonly in patients of small cell carcinoma of prostate or lung, extremely rare in SCCB [4]. Prostate tumor often cause the elevation of PSA level. According to pre-operative serum chemistries, both patients had higher PSA level than normal (4 ng/ml). Macroscopically, SCCB is usually round or oval without pedicles, and infiltrates into the bladder wall [13]. It is difficult to diagnose SCCB by clinical manifestation or imaging examination. The diagnosis of SCCB mainly depend on histopathological examination. Small and round-shaped cancer cells are representative features of SCCB. Meanwhile, the nest-like structures, overlapping nucleoli, scarce cytoplasm, tumor necrosis and substantial mitotic images are also commonly seen. Neuroendocrine markers are typical for small cell carcinoma, including Syn, NSE and CgA. The appearance of disorder of glands structure, glandular hyperplasia, cell atypia, invasive growth pattern and positive expression of P504S and PSA are essential for the diagnosis of prostate adenocarcinoma [14, 15]. As shown in Figs. 2 and 4, all these pathological characteristics were observed in the resected tissues.

SCCB tends to metastasize to lymph nodes and distant organs early. Koay et al. [16] analyzed 642 SCCB patients and found muscular layer infiltrated in > 90% cases and lymphatic or distant organic metastasis in > 80% cases. But in this study, no obvious metastatic lesions were detected via pre-operative examinations. Proven treatments for SCCB have been explored over the years, while no significant progress has been verified. The curative strategy of SCCB is similar to that of small cell lung cancer (SCLC), with comprehensive treatment including surgery, chemotherapy and radiation therapy. Howbeit, no standard therapeutic regimens have been established currently, and the treatment depends on the stage and

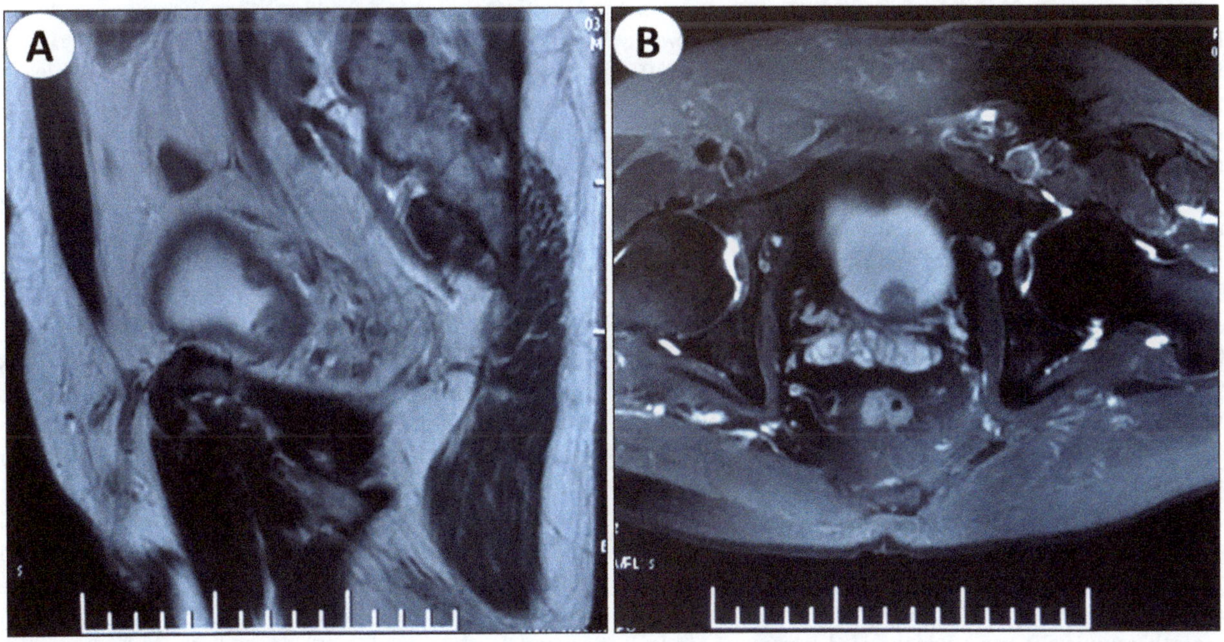


**Fig. 3** Sagittal (**a**) and horizontal plane (**b**) MRI demonstrated two tumor masses located at the posterior and top wall of the bladder, respectively

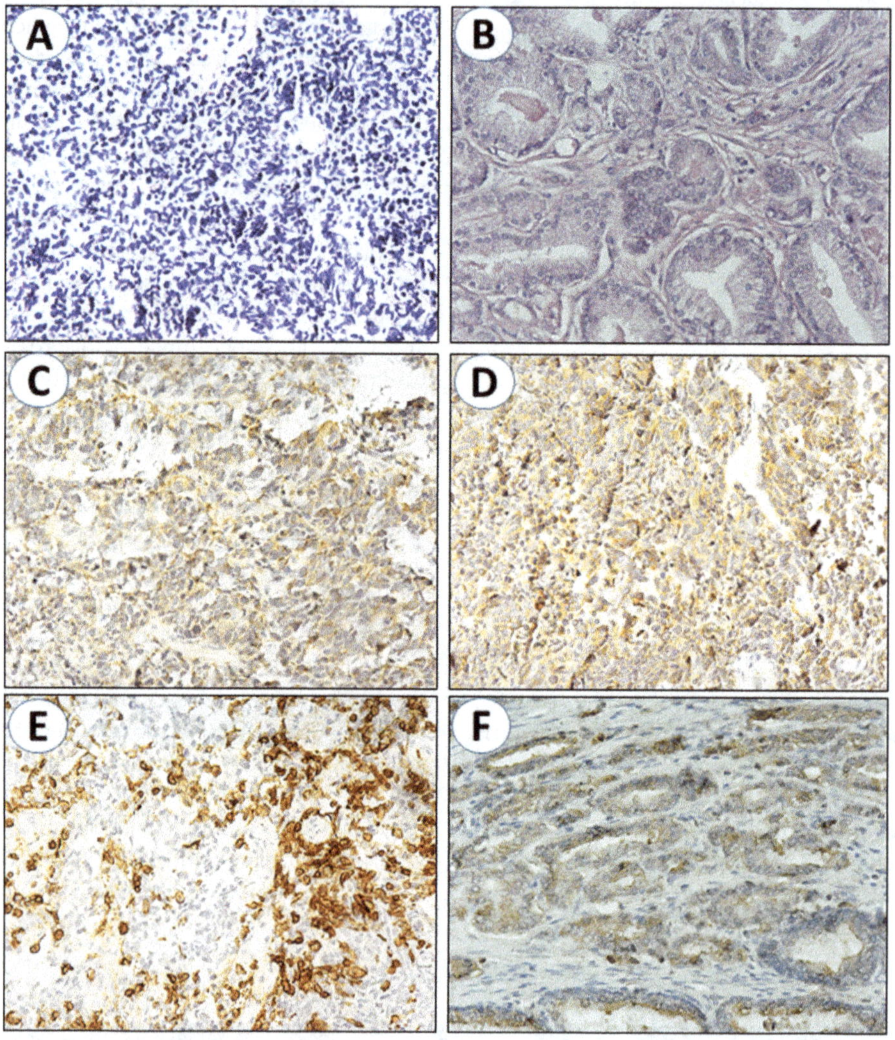


**Fig. 4** 100X magnification of the resected tissues. HE staining showed typical small cells with scant cytoplasm arranged in sheets of SCCB (**a**) and disorder of glands structure, glandular hyperplasia and cell atypia of prostate adenocarcinoma (**b**). Positive staining for CgA (**c**), Syn (**d**), NSE (**e**) and P504s (**f**)

progress of SCCB basically [4, 17]. Transurethral resection of bladder tumors (TUR-BT) is not effective enough in controlling SCCB progression, even for localized lesions. Siefker et al. [18] compared the effects of different cooperative therapy (neoadjuvant chemotherapy + surgery vs. surgery + post-operative chemotherapy) for SCCB and found the 5-year survival rates of two groups were 78 and 36%, respectively. Pre-neoadjuvant chemotherapy was able to prolong the survival time of SCCB patients significantly ($p < 0.05$). Carranza et al. [19] also agreed with the benefit of neoadjuvant chemotherapy according to their clinical experience. Pre-neoadjuvant chemotherapy was not used in our study because we could not know the accurate pathological subtype of tumor lesions before operation. Radical cystectomy plus chemotherapy is the most widely used treatment for localized SCCB. At present, cisplatin, cyclophosphamide, VP16 and Adriamycin are frequently used and combined regimen is proven better than monotherapy [20]. Mixed SCCB had a good response to the MVAC protocol (methotrexate + vincristine + adriamycin + cisplatin), while pure SCCB responded to cisplatin-etoposide or ifosfamide/adriamycin regimen better. Since cisplatin has strong side effects of nephrotoxicity and neurotoxicity, it is feasible to choose carboplatin instead of cisplatin in patients with poor conditions [3, 21]. In our study, both patients accepted CE-based chemotherapy regimens after surgery.

Radical prostatectomy (RP) is the optimal strategy for limited prostate cancer. Biochemical recurrence (BCR) is defined as consecutive serum PSA > 0.2 ng/ml twice after RP [22]. Proper treatment for BCR after RP is still controversial, the usual options include radiotherapy of prostate region, anti-androgen drugs in combination with 5α-reductase inhibitors, chemotherapy and observational waiting [22]. In our study, one patient progressed to BCR with successive post-operative serum PSA of 0.34 and 0.55 ng/ml. This patient only took Bicalutamide orally for remedy because of physical and financial reasons, and died of liver and lung metastasis 8 months after operation eventually. Owing to the lack of post-mortem pathological examination, we are not clear whether the metastatic foci derived from prostate adenocarcinoma or SCCB. The other patient just underwent CE chemotherapy regimen after surgery and no BCR of prostate cancer or distant metastasis was detected after a follow up of 19 months.

In conclusion, We reported two extremely unusual cases of coexistence of SCCB and prostate adenocarcinoma and reviewed relative articles in this paper. SCCB is an infrequent pattern of neuroendocrine tumor with low differentiation and high malignancy. There are still many "blind areas" for its pathogenesis, diagnosis and treatment. Although a variety of therapeutic measures are applied currently, the mortality rate of SCCB patients remains high. The discovery of specific diagnostic method and optimal remedial policy should be the keynotes of future research.

## Supplementary information

**Additional file 1.**

#### Abbreviations

SCCB: Small cell carcinoma of the bladder; MRI: Agnetic resonance imaging; PSA: Prostate specific antigen; CgA: Chromogranin A; Syn: Synaptophysin; NSE: Neuron specific enolase; LCA: Leukocyte common antigen; BCR: Biochemical recurrence; IHC: Immunohistochemical

#### Acknowledgements

Not applicable.

#### Authors' contributions

YX L collected and analyzed data, and performed the histological examination. HM X performed the histological examination and drafted the manuscript. B W treated the patients and performed the follow-up. SG L analyzed data and revised the manuscript. Q L designed this study and treated the patients. All authors read and approved the final manuscript.

#### Author details

[1]Department of Pathology, Jiangyin People's Hospital, Affiliated Jiangyin Hospital of the Southeast University Medical College, Jiangyin 214400, Jiangsu Province, China. [2]Department of Urology, Jiangyin People's Hospital, Affiliated Jiangyin Hospital of the Southeast University Medical College, Jiangyin 214400, Jiangsu Province, China. [3]Department of Urology, Tianjin Jinnan Hospital, Tianjin 300350, China.

#### References

1. Berniker AV, Abdulrahman AA, Teytelboym OM, Galindo LM, Mackey JE. Extrapulmonary small cell carcinoma: imaging features with radiologic-pathologic correlation. Radiographics. 2015;35(1):152–63.
2. Salhab M, Migdady Y, Donahue M, Xiong Y, Dresser K, Walsh W, Chen BJ, Liebmann J. Immunohistochemical expression and prognostic value of PD-L1 in Extrapulmonary small cell carcinoma: a single institution experience. J ImmunoTher Cancer. 2018;6(1):42.
3. Ghervan L, Zaharie A, Ene B, Elec FI. Small-cell carcinoma of the urinary bladder: where do we stand? Clujul Med. 2017;90(1):13–7.
4. Erdem GU, Ozdemir NY, Demirci NS, Sahin S, Bozkaya Y, Zengin N. Small cell carcinoma of the urinary bladder: changing trends in the current literature. Curr Med Res Opin. 2016;32(6):1013–21.
5. Hatano K, Kawamura N, Kakuta Y, Fukuhara S, Takada T, Harai T, Yamaguchi S, Adachi S. Three cases of small cell carcinoma of the urinary bladder: a case report. Hinyokika Kiyo. 2008;54(4):297–300.
6. Siegel RL, Miller KD, Jemal A. Cancer statistics, 2017. CA Cancer J Clin. 2017; 67(1):7–30.
7. Attard G, Parker C, Eeles RA, Schroder F, Tomlins SA, Tannock I, Drake CG, de Bono JS. Prostate cancer. Lancet. 2016;387(10013):70–82.
8. Pasquier D, Barney B, Sundar S, Poortmans P, Villa S, Nasrallah H, Boujelbene N, Ghadjar P, Lassen-Ramshad Y, Senkus E. Small cell carcinoma of the urinary bladder: a retrospective, multicenter rare Cancer network study of 107 patients. Int J Radiat Oncol. 2015;92(4):904–10.
9. Cerulli C, Busetto GM, Antonini G, Giovannone R, Di Placido M, Soda G, De Berardinis E, Gentile V. Primary metastatic neuroendocrine small cell bladder cancer: a case report and literature review. Urol Int. 2012;88(3):365–9.
10. Wang Y, Li Q, Wang J, Tong M, Xing H, Xue Y, Pan H, Huang C, Li D. Small cell carcinoma of the bladder. the characteristics of molecular alterations, treatment, and follow-up. Med Oncol. 2019;36(12):98.
11. Trias I, Algaba F, Condom E, Espanol I, Segui J, Orsola I, Villavicencio H, Garcia Del Muro X. Small cell carcinoma of the urinary bladder. Presentation of 23 cases and review of 134 published cases. Eur Urol. 2001;39(1):85–90.
12. Yilmaz S, Ipekci T, Akin Y. An extremely rare cause of hematuria: Adamantionma like Neuroectodermal tumor of bladder. Kuwait Med J. 2016;48(4):343–5.
13. Sharma A, Sharma S, Patnaik N, Pradhan D, Satapathy K, Pradhan MR, Mohanty SK. Cytomorphologic and Immunophenotypic profile of a cohort of small cell carcinoma of the urinary bladder. Acta Cytol. 2016;60(5):475–80.
14. Epstein JI. Diagnosis and reporting of limited adenocarcinoma of the prostate on needle biopsy. Modern Pathol. 2004;17(3):307–15.
15. Epstein JI. An update of the Gleason grading system. J Urol. 2010;183(2): 433–40.
16. Koay EJ, Teh BS, Paulino AC, Butler EB. A surveillance, epidemiology, and end results analysis of small cell carcinoma of the bladder: epidemiology, prognostic variables, and treatment trends. Cancer. 2011;117(23):5325–33.
17. Kouba E, Cheng L. Neuroendocrine tumors of the urinary bladder according to the 2016 World Health Organization classification: molecular and clinical characteristics. Endocr Pathol. 2016;27(3):188–99.
18. Siefker-Radtke AO, Dinney CP, Abrahams NA, Moran C, Shen Y, Pisters LL, Grossman HB, Swanson DA, Millikan RE. Evidence supporting preoperative chemotherapy for small cell carcinoma of the bladder: a retrospective review of the M. D. Anderson cancer experience. J Urol. 2004;172(2):481–4.
19. Carranza OE, Castanon E, Abella LE, Zudaire ME, Castillo A, Arevalo E, Fusco JP, Zudaire JJ, Carias R, Cambeiro M. Clinical management of small-cell carcinoma of the urinary tract: a 10-year single-center's experience. Clin Genitourin Canc. 2013;11(2):168–74.
20. Ou WT, Liang QL, Huang X, Li ZY, Liu QL. Small cell carcinoma of the urinary bladder: a case report and review of the literature. Oncol Lett. 2015;9(1): 488–90.
21. Moretto P, Wood L, Emmenegger U, Blais N, Mukherjee SD, Winquist E, Belanger EC, Macrae R, Balogh A, Cagiannos I. Management of small cell carcinoma of the bladder: consensus guidelines from the Canadian Association of Genitourinary Medical Oncologists (CAGMO). Can Urol Assoc. 2013;7(1-2):E44–56.
22. Heidenreich A, Bastian PJ, Bellmunt J, Bolla M, Joniau S, van der Kwast T, Mason M, Matveev V, Wiegel T, Zattoni F. EAU guidelines on prostate cancer. Part II: treatment of advanced, relapsing, and castration-resistant prostate cancer. Eur Urol. 2014;65(2):467–79.

# Knockdown of TRPM7 prevents tumor growth, migration and invasion through the Src, Akt and JNK pathway in bladder cancer

Eun Hye Lee[1†], So Young Chun[2†], Bomi Kim[2], Bo Hyun Yoon[2], Jun Nyung Lee[1,3,4], Bum Soo Kim[1,3,5], Eun Sang Yoo[3,5], Sangkyu Lee[6], Phil Hyun Song[7], Tae Gyun Kwon[1,3,4*] and Yun-Sok Ha[1,3,4*]

**Abstract**

**Background:** Bladder cancer (BC) is one of the most common malignancies of the urinary tract. The role of transient receptor potential melastatin 7 (TRPM7) in BC remains unclear. The aim of this study was to investigate the function and signal transduction pathway of TRPM7 in BC.

**Methods:** T24 and UMUC3 cells were used to evaluate the molecular mechanism of TRPM7 by immunoblot analysis. Small interfering RNA was used to knockdown TRPM7, and the effect of silencing TRPM7 was studied by wound healing, migration, and invasion assays in T24 and UMUC3 cells. Xenograft model study was obtained to analyze the effect of TRPM7 inhibition in vivo.

**Results:** Silencing of TRPM7 decreased the migration and invasion ability of T24 and UMUC3 cells. The phosphorylation of Src, Akt, and JNK (c-Jun N-terminal kinase) was also suppressed by TRPM7 silencing. Src, Akt, and JNK inhibitors effectively inhibited the migration and invasion of T24 and UMUC3 cells. In addition, the TRPM7 inhibitor, carvacrol, limited the tumor size in a xenograft model.

**Conclusion:** Our data reveal that TRPM7 regulates the migration and invasion of T24 and UMUC3 cells via the Src, Akt, and JNK signaling pathway. Therefore, TRPM7 suppression could be a potential treatment for BC patients.

**Keywords:** Bladder cancer, TRPM7, Src, Akt, JNK

## Background

Bladder cancer (BC) is a critical public health issue, and is known as the most common cancer of the urinary tract and the ninth most common cause of cancer related death worldwide [1]. There are approximately 400,000 cases of BC and 150,000 deaths per year [2]. The incidence of BC rises with age and the incidence is three times greater in in men than women. The most common symptom of BC is hematuria without pain [3], and BC is commonly diagnosed by cystoscopy and cytology [4].

The pathologic type of BC can be divided into two groups: non-muscle invasive BC (NMIBC) and muscle invasive BC (MIBC) [5]. NMIBC includes Ta and T1 stages, which are a low grade non-invasive papillary tumors that penetrate the basement membrane without invading the muscle layer of the bladder wall.

* Correspondence: tgkwon@knu.ac.kr; yunsokha@gmail.com
†Eun Hye Lee and So Young Chun contributed equally to this work.
[1]Joint Institute for Regenerative Medicine, Kyungpook National University Hospital, Daegu, Republic of Korea
Full list of author information is available at the end of the article

MIBC includes T2–T4 stages which invade the muscle layer of bladder wall [6]. Around 70% of BC patients are diagnosed with NMIBC; however, these patients show a high reoccurrence rate with occasionally progressed stages with muscle layer invasion within 5 years [7]. The reason for recurrence with muscle invasion remains unclear [3]. Most deaths from BC result from metastasis to other organs due to chemotherapy resistance [8], and the majority of MIBC cases have metastasis, migration, and invasion [9, 10]. Indeed, approximately 25% of MIBC patients show metastasis, and patients with metastasis show poor prognosis [11]. Recently used pathological markers for prognosis require further study to clarify the most appropriate parameter [12]. Thus, there has been a sustained effort to understand the role of pathogical markers in predicting the therapeutic response and prognosis in BC patients [13]. In the clinic, immune check point inhibitors, such as Atezolizumab, have been approved and used in BC. However, the effectiveness is still under investigation, and has followed cisplatin-based chemotherapy for the past decade [14].

TRPM7 is endogenously expressed in several human organs [15] and presents in a tetrameric form [16]. TRPM7 is a member of the transient receptor potential (TRP) channel family which is a non-selective cation channel family [17, 18]. Specifically, TRPM7 is a bifunctional protein that is well known as an essential regulator of $Ca^{2+}$ and $Mg^{2+}$ homeostasis [17]. TRPM7 is a protein kinase that has crucial roles in regulating diverse cellular processes including cell proliferation, adhesion, migration, and survival by phosphorylating itself [19, 20]. As TRPM7 is highly involved in many types of cancers, research onTRPM7 related mechanisms is actively underway. TRPM7 is highly expressed in both glioblastoma [21] and pancreatic adenocarcinoma [22], and has been reported to be associated with tumor migration and invasion [20, 23, 24]. Indeed, somatic mutation of TRPM7 has been found in breast carcinoma [25], colon carcinoma [26], ovarian cancer, and gastric carcinoma [25]. In previous studies, TRPM7 has been reported to regulate cell migration and invasion through the MAPK pathway, as well as the PI3K/Akt, ERK, and JNK pathways in cancer [27–29].

However, the function and the mechanism of TRPM7 in BC is not clearly understood and further studies are required to fully elucidate its role. In the current study, by exploring the role of TRPM7 and its underlying mechanisms using BC cell lines, we suggest TRPM7 as a beneficial treatment for BC patients. In addition, we evaluated whether the TRPM7 inhibitor, carvacrol, inhibited tumor size in a xenograft model.

## Methods

### Reagents

Anti-phospho-Src, anti-Src, anti-phospho-Akt, anti-Akt, anti-phospho-Erk, anti-Erk, anti-phospho-JNK, anti-JNK, anti-phospho-p38, anti-p38, and anti-TRPM7 antibodies were obtained from Cell Signaling Technology (Beverly, MA, USA). Carvacrol, dimethyl sulfoxide (DMSO), crystal violet, cell migration kit, and cell invasion kit were purchased from Sigma-Aldrich (St. Louis, MO, USA).

### Bladder cancer cell lines

T24, J82, UMUC3, 5637, and HT1376 cell lines were purchased from American Type Culture Collection. Each cell line was cultured in RPMI 1640, DMEM high glucose, and MEM alpha media containing 10% FBS and 100 U/ml penicillin-streptomycin (Gibco, Waltham, MA, USA) and incubated at 37 °C in a humidified 5% $CO_2$ atmosphere.

### siRNA treatment

Cells were plated at $2 \times 10^5$ cells per well. AccuTarget Predesigned siRNAs specific for human TRPM7, and scramble siRNAs purchased from Bioneer (Daejeon, Korea) were used to knockdown TRPM7 expression. The sequences for human TRPM7 siRNA were as follows: Fwd 5′-GUC UUG CCA UGA AAU ACU CUU-3′ and Rev. 5′GAG UAU UUC AUG GCA AGA CUU-3′ (siRNA #1), and Fwd 5′-AGG AGA AGA UGC AAU UAA ATT-3′ and Rev. 5′-UUU AAU UGC AUC UUC UCC UAG-3′ (siRNA #2). The negative control (NC) group was treated with a non-targeted sequence, and the sequences for NC were as follows: Fwd 5′- UUC UCC GAA CGU GUC ACG UTT-3′ and Rev. 5′-ACG UGA CAC GUU CGG AGA ATT-3′. For transient transfection, Lipofectamine® RNAiMAX (13778–150; Invitrogen, Carlsbad, CA, USA) was used with siRNA (2–200 pmol/μL) to treat the cells for 6 h. Following treatment, the media was changed to a transfection reagent free media containing 10% FBS, and incubated for 48 h at 37 °C in a humidified 5% $CO_2$ atmosphere.

### Immunoblot analysis

Treated cells were lysed using RIPA buffer as described previously [30]. Protein samples were loaded into SDS-PAGE gels and transferred to nitrocellulose membrane. The primary antibodies were applied overnight at 4 °C at 1:1000 dilutions after blocking with 5% skim milk solution. The secondary antibodies were applied at 1:5000 for 2 h at room temperature. The bands were developed using ECL reagent (Advensta, Menlo Park, CA, USA), images were captured with a chemi-doc image analyzer (iBright 1500, Thermo

Fisher Scientific), and the values were quantified with Image J software (Wayne Rasband, retired from NIH).

#### Wound healing assay

T24 and UMUC3 cells were plated in 6-well plates, and the cell layer was scratched with a pipette tip. Cells were washed with phosphate buffered saline to remove cell debris. The scratched area was monitored photographically and imaged at 0 and 24 h using an Olympus CKX41 inverted microscope coupled with a digital imaging system.

#### Migration and invasion assay

T24 and UMUC3 cells in serum free media were seeded in 8-μm pore size cell culture inserts (#353097, BD Falcon, Franklin Lakes, NJ, USA) and in Matrigel coated inserts (#354480, Corning, NY, USA) for migration and invasion, respectively. Media containing 10% FBS was added to the lower chamber. The cells were removed from the insert after 24 h incubation, and cells on the chamber were stained with crystal violet solution. The stained cells were dissolved in DMSO, and measured with a microplate spectrophotometer (wavelength 590 nm, BioTek Instruments, Winooski, VT, USA).

#### Cell viability assay (MTT assay)

T24 and UMUC3 cells were seeded in 96-well plates at a density of $1 \times 10^4$ per well and treated with different doses of carvacrol or siRNA. Cells were stained with filtered 1 mg/mL MTT solution for 4 h at 37 °C in a humidified 5% $CO_2$ atmosphere. Stained cells were dissolved in DMSO after removing media and MTT solution. Absorbance was measured with a microplate spectrophotometer at 570 nm wavelength.

#### In vivo analysis

All animal study protocols were approved by the Institutional Animal Ethics Committee of Yeungnam University, College of Medicine (YUMC-2017-024). All animals were kept in a controlled specific pathogen free environment under a 12 h light/dark cycle at a temperature of 25.0 °C ± 0.2 °C and humidity of 45% ± 2%. All mice were freely provided with food and water. UMUC3 cells were injected into Balb/c nude mice ($n = 6$, 6-week-old, 18-20 g, female). According to 3R (reduction, replacement, refinement) of Institutional Animal Care and Use Committee (IACUC), we chose the minimal number of animals used. For animal welfare, in case of movement disorder, eating disorder and weight loss (20% of normal

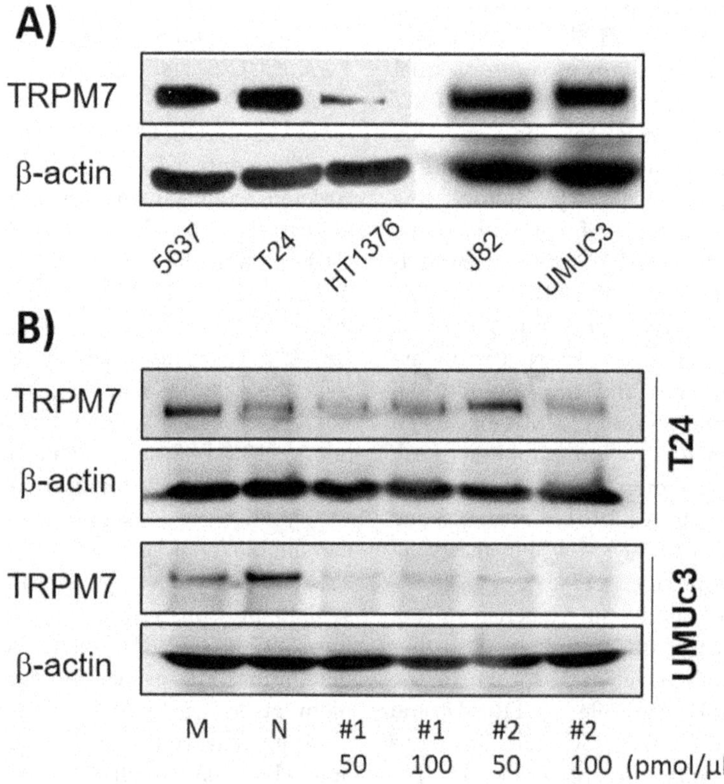


**Fig. 1** Protein expression of TRPM7 in bladder cancer cell lines by immunoblot analysis. **a** Protein expression of TRPM7 in 5637, T24, HT1376, J82, and UMUC3 cells. **b** Downregulation of TRPM7 in T24 and UMUC3 with different doses of siRNA. β-actin served as a loading control. M: Mock, N: Negative

weight) we euthanized the animals in $CO_2$ gas. UMUC3 cells ($5 \times 10^5$) were subcutaneously injected in 200 μL PBS-Matrigel (1:1, Matrigel: PBS). When the tumor reached 4–6 mm in diameter, carvacrol was intraperitoneally injected at a 50 mg/mL concentration once a week for 4 weeks. The tumor size was measured twice a week, for 4 weeks. After 4 weeks from starting day of size measurement, mice were anesthetized with Zoletil 0.006 cc/10 g (30 mg/kg) and Rompun 0.004 cc/10 g (10 mg/kg) and euthanized in $CO_2$ gas.

### Source of animals

Balb/c nude mice were purchased from Orient (Seoul, Korea).

### Immunohistochemistry stain

The tumor tissues were fixed in 10% formalin solution to produce paraffin blocks. The samples were sectioned at a 4 μm thickness and deparaffinized. Slides were heated in citrate buffer and 0.2% triton x solution for 30 mins and 10 mins, respectively, and 5% BSA solution was used as a blocking reagent. The primary antibody was incubated overnight at 4 °C, and the secondary antibody (Alexa Fluor 594 Goat anti-rabbit IgG, 1:1000 dilution, Abcam, Cambridge, MA, USA) was incubated for 1 h at room temperature. The slides were mounted with DAPI containing mounting solution (Vectashield, Vector Laboratories, Burlingame, CA, USA).

### Statistical analysis

One-way analysis of variance was used to assess differences among the treatment groups. The criterion for statistical significance was set at $p < 0.05$ or $p < 0.01$.

## Result

### TRPM7 knockdown suppresses bladder cancer cell viability

In order to select the most suitable cell line, we checked the protein expression of TRPM7 in 5637, T24, HT1376, J82, and UMUC3 BC cell lines by immunoblot (Fig. 1a). Among these five cell lines, T24 and UMUC3 showed higher expression than HT1376. T24 and UMUC3 cell lines belong to transitional cell carcinoma, which is the most common type of bladder cancer, and T24 and UMUC3 showed high siRNA transfection efficacy. Next, we treated T24 and

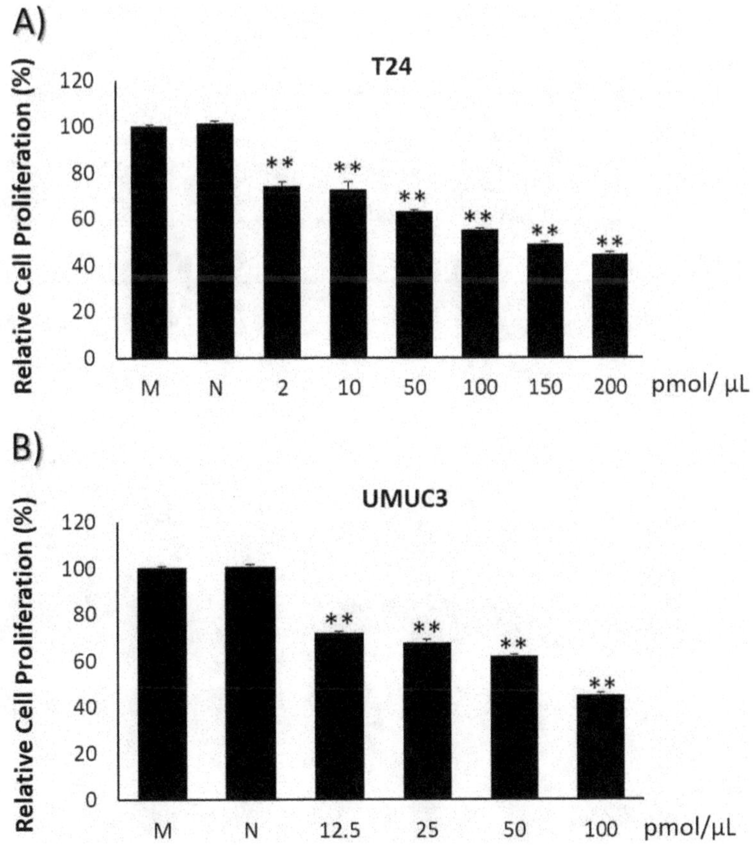


**Fig. 2** Effect of TRPM7 knockdown in bladder cancer cell proliferation. **a** T24 cells and (**b**) UMUC3 cells were treated with different doses of siRNA and incubated for 24 h. All data represent the means ± SD of three independent experiments (*$p < 0.05$ and **$p < 0.01$ between M and siRNA treated groups). M: Mock, N: Negative

UMUC3 cells with two different sequences of siRNA in doses of 50 and 100 pmol/μL. The #2 sequence at dose of 100 pmol/μL siRNA significantly suppressed the expression of TRPM7 in T24 and UMUC3 cell lines, compared to mock and NC groups (Fig. 1b). Furthermore, the proliferation of T24 (Fig. 2a) and UMUC3 (Fig. 2b) cells was significantly inhibited by TRPM7 siRNA treatment, even at 2 pmol/μL, compared to the mock and NC groups. Full-length blots that presented in Fig. 1 are presented in Suppl. Fig. 4.

### TRPM7 knockdown reduces the motility of bladder cancer cells

A wound healing assay, migration assay, and invasion assay performed in order to analyze the effect of TRPM7 knockdown on cell motility. In the wound healing assay, siRNA treated (100 and 50 pmol/μL, non-lethal dose for each cell line) T24 and UMUC3 cells showed relatively wider wound gaps than non-treated groups following 24 h treatment (Fig. 3a and b). In the migration assay, siRNA treated T24 and UMUC3 cells showed significantly inhibited migration ability compared to non-treated groups (Fig. 4a and b). The invasion assay also showed significantly inhibited invasion in siRNA treated T24 and UMUC3 cells (Fig. 5a and b).

### TRPM7 regulates cell proliferation via Src, Akt, and JNK pathways

The protein expression of Src, Akt and JNK (frequently related to cancer cell metastasis and invasion) was examined by immunoblot (Fig. 6). The results demonstrated that siRNA treated cells showed significantly reduced expression of p-Src, p-Akt, and p-JNK protein, while the total forms of Src, Akt, and JNK protein were not significantly changed by siRNA

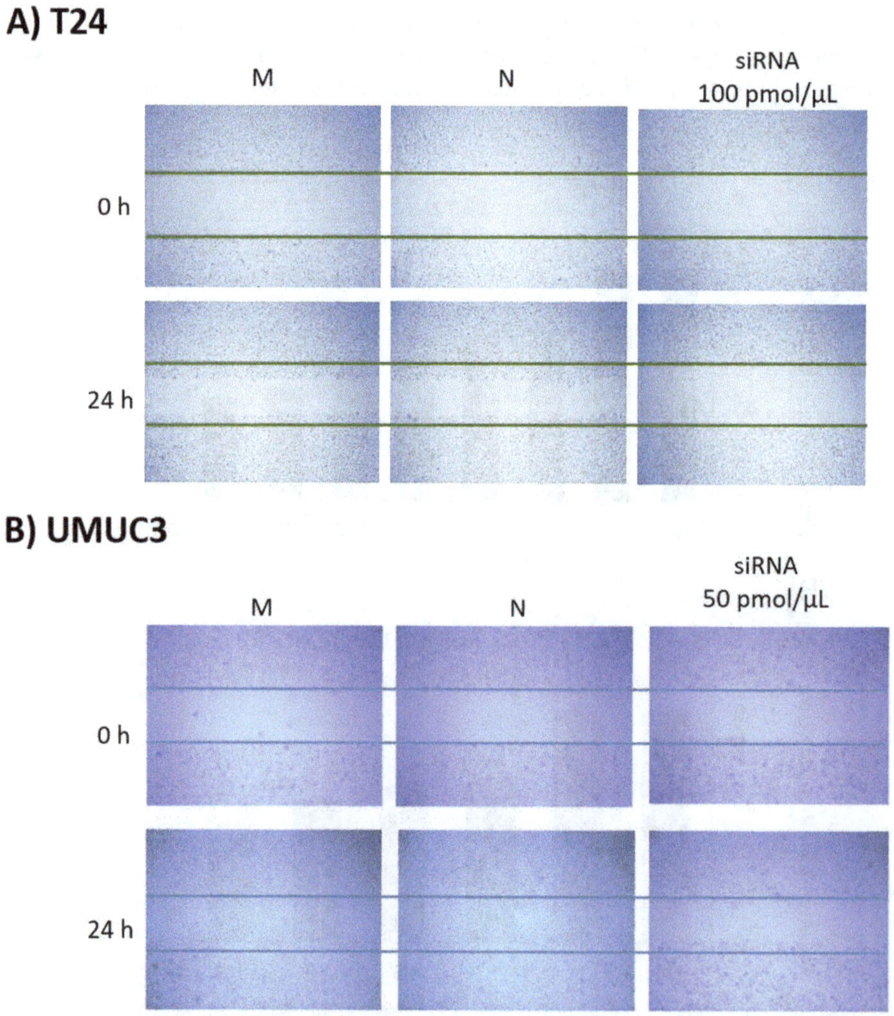


**Fig. 3** Effect of TRPM7 on cell migration in a wound healing assay. **a** T24 and (**b**) UMUC3 cells were treated with 100 pmol/μl and 50 pmol/μl and incubated for 24 h. M: Mock, N: Negative, h: Hour

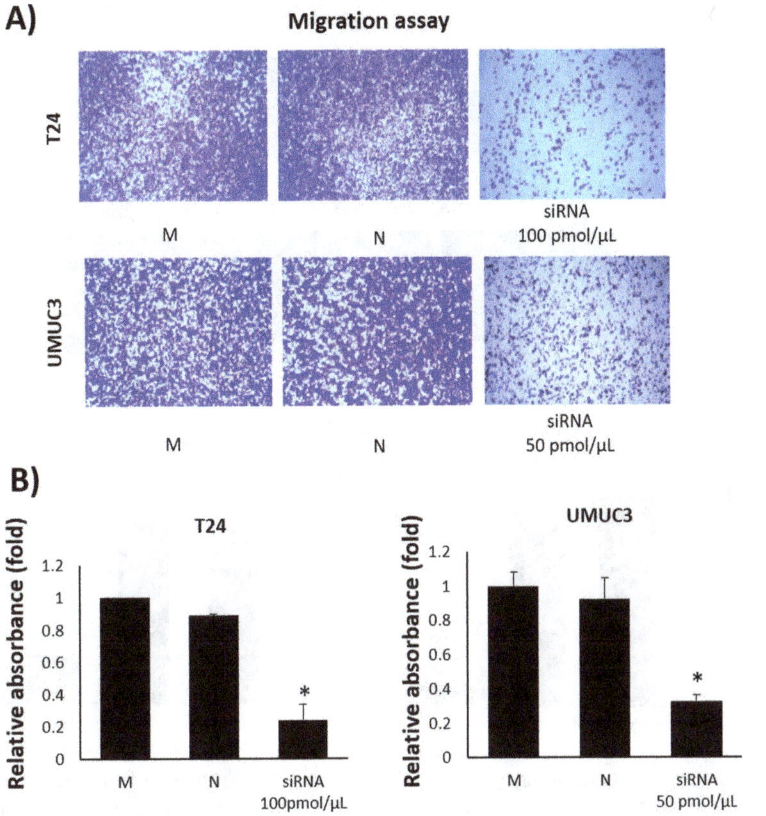


**Fig. 4** Effect of TRPM7 on cell migration in a cell permeable transwell. **a** Migration assay using a transwell with siRNA treatment. **b** Relative absorbance of migrated cells. The cells that passed through the 8 μm pore insert were stained with crystal violet solution. All data represent the means ± SD of three independent experiments (*$p < 0.05$ and **$p < 0.01$ between M and siRNA treated groups). M: Mock, N: Negative

treatment (Fig. 6a). The association of these proteins with TRPM7 regulated cell proliferation was confirmed by treatment with the inhibitor of each protein (Fig. 6b). Both cell lines showed significantly decreased cell proliferation compared to the non-treated groups. Full-length blots that presented in Fig. 6 are presented in Suppl. Fig. 5.

### In vitro responses to TRPM7 inhibitor

To analysis cell responses to the TRPM7 inhibitor, the cell lines were treated with 100–500 μM of carvacrol. In cell proliferation analysis, the proliferation of T24 cells was significantly decreased in a dose dependent manner (from 300 μM) (Suppl. Fig. 1a) compared to UMUC3 (Suppl. Fig. 1b). In the cell migration (Suppl. Fig. 2) and invasion (Suppl. Fig. 3) assays, UMUC3 cells were significantly more sensitive to carvacrol (from 200 μM) compared to T24 cells.

### In vivo responses to TRPM7 inhibitor

Based on in vitro results, the in vivo condition was established using UMUC3 cells treated with 50 mg/mL carvacrol. At Day 24 after cell injection, the tumor volume was significantly reduced in the carvacrol treated group (468.45 ± 291.04 mm3) compared to the ctrl (4361.14 ± 2817.94 mm3) and vehicle (5176.45 ± 1603.25 mm3) groups (Fig. 7a). TRPM7 tumor expression was analyzed by IHC stain, wherein the carvacrol treated group showed significantly down-regulated expression of TRPM7 compared to the other groups (Fig. 7b).

## Discussion

Recently, TRPM7 has been reported to be implicated in carcinogenesis and has been considered as a potential target for diverse cancer treatment [27, 31]. TRPM7, one of the TRP member channels, is permeable to $Ca^{2+}$ and $Mg^{2+}$. Since $Ca^{2+}$ is an important regulator of cell cycle and proliferation, TRPM7 regulation is considered to be critical to the biological function of cancer cells [31]. TRPM7 is reported to be overexpressed in human pulmonary adenocarcinoma, and pancreatic and prostate adenocarcinoma [18, 32]. Furthermore, downregulation of TRPM7 is

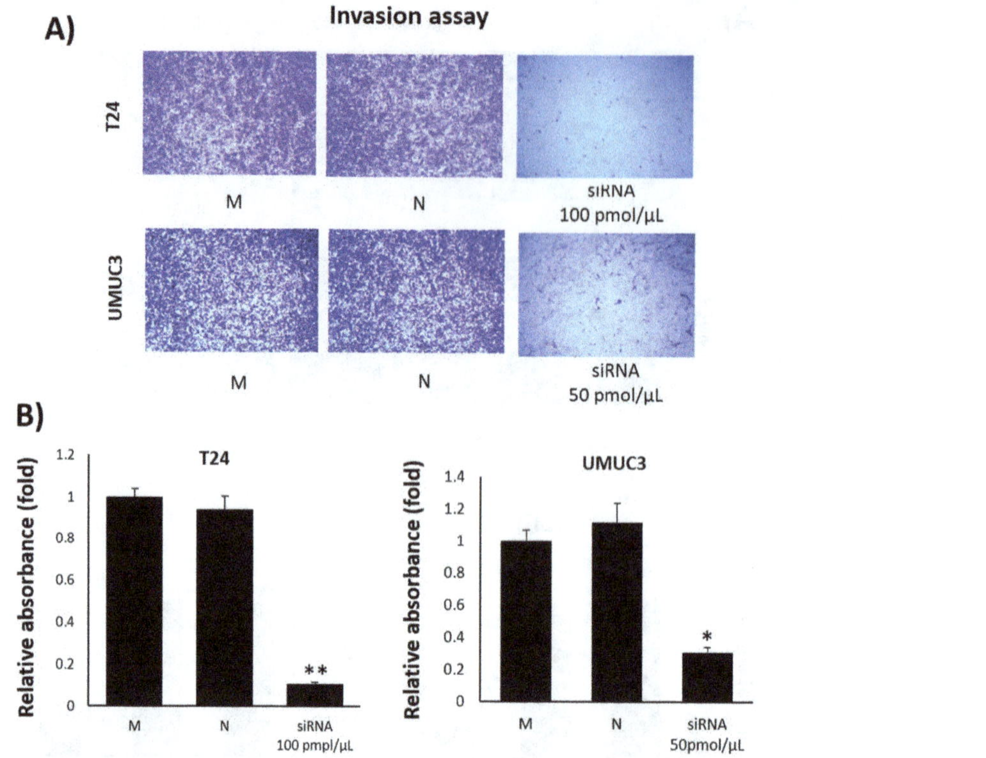


**Fig. 5** Effect of TRPM7 on Invasion. **a** Migration assay using a transwell with siRNA treatment. **b** Relative absorbance of migrated cells. The cells that passed through the 8-μm pore coated insert were stained with crystal violet solution. All data represent the means ± SD of three independent experiments (*$p < 0.05$ and **$p < 0.01$ between M and siRNA treated groups). M: Mock, N: Negative

known to inhibit the migration and invasion of breast cancer cells [27], while up-regulation has been shown to promote migration of lung cancer cells and vascular smooth muscle cells [23, 33].

Although numerous studies support that TRPM7 is involved in cancer cell migration and invasion [34–36], the precise understanding of the TRPM7 signaling pathway that modulates the molecular process of cancer cells remains unclear. According to previous studies, Src, Akt, and JNK are involved in cancer cell metastasis and invasion [37–40]. Indeed, Src was the first discovered oncogene, and it is able to activate caspase 8 by phosphorylation. Phosphorylated caspase-8 switches its function from pro-apoptotic to pro-migratory [41]. It has been reported that Src modulates the invasiveness of prostate cancer cells via regulating the E-cadherin/β-catenin complex [42]. Moreover, phosphorylated Akt serves as a cell proliferation boosting agent [43], while Akt has also been reported to promote invasion in fibrosarcoma and thyroid cancer cells [44, 45]. JNK is well known cancer regulating protein due to its action on oncogenes such as, Ras, c-fos, Met, and Bcr-Abl [46]. Furthermore, activated JNK induces the activation of apoptosis related Bcl-2 family proteins; thus, phosphorylated JNK acts as a pro-apoptotic signal in cancer cells [47]. In this study, we evaluated the TRPM7 mediated signaling pathway involved in BC cell lines, and demonstrated that silenced TRPM7 suppressed the protein expression of phosphorylation of Src, Akt, and JNK by immunoblot analysis. Based on this result, we can deduce TRPM7 regulates the Src, Akt, and JNK signaling pathway as a complex.

Our results also demonstrated that knockdown of TRPM7 by siRNA led to a decrease in proliferation of T24 and UMUC cells compared to the non-treated group, indicating that TRPM7 plays a key role in BC cell growth. In order to determine the effect of silenced TRPM7 on cell motility, we used T24 and UMUC3 cells in wound healing, migration, and invasion assays. Our results demonstrated that the TRPM7 silenced group showed a narrower area gap compared to the non-treated group in the wound healing assay, while the TRPM7 silenced group significantly suppressed the migration and invasion ability of BC cells. Thus, we were able to confirm that

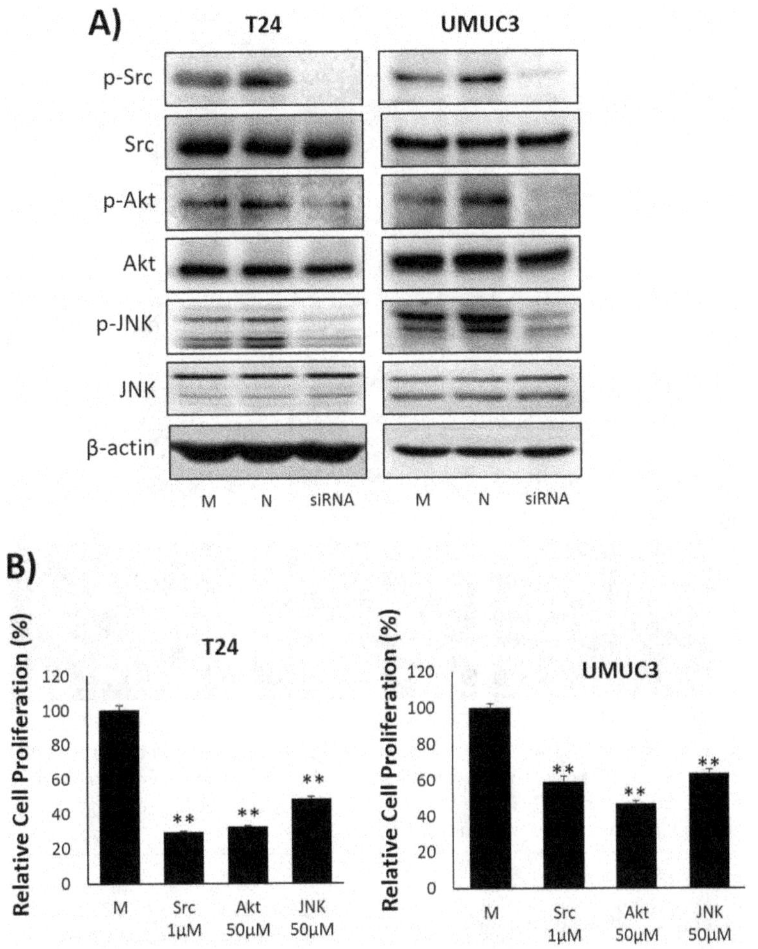


**Fig. 6** Effect of TRPM7 silencing in the Src, Akt, and JNK pathway. **a** Immunoblotting sowed that TRPM7 siRNA down-regulated protein expression of p-Src, p-Akt, and p-JNK. **b** Treatment of T24 and UMUC3 with Src, Akt, and JNK inhibitor induced significantly lowered cell proliferation compared to control. All data represent means ± SD of three independent experiments (*$p < 0.05$ and **$p < 0.01$ between M and inhibitor treated groups). M: Mock, N: Negative

TRPM7 plays a crucial role in cell metastasis and invasion of BC cells.

To verify the effect of each protein (Src, Akt, and JNK) in cancer cell proliferation, we treated T24 and UMUC3 cells with inhibitors of Src, Akt, and JNK. As we expected, inhibition of Src, Akt, and JNK restricted cell proliferation. Based on the suppression of cell viability by Src, Akt, and JNK inhibition, we were able to derive that Src, Akt, and JNK play important roles in BC cell proliferation. In addition, we investigated the importance of TRPM7 in cancer growth by treatment with the TRPM7 inhibitor, carvacrol. In vitro, treatment of carvacrol showed decreased cell proliferation in a dose dependent manner compared to the non-treated group. In migration and invasion assays, as we expected, the migration and invasion capacity was lowest in carvacrol treated cells.

We evaluated the effect of TRPM7 inhibition in vivo by using carvacrol as a TRPM7 inhibitor in a xenograft model. Carvacrol injection reduced tumor size in nude mice, while the vehicle group showed similar tumor sizes to the control group. Furthermore, the carvacrol treated group had low TRPM7 protein expression by IHC. These in vivo results indicate that TRPM7 has a crucial role in tumor growth.

In previous studies regarding the function of TRPM7 in BC, the effect of TRPM7 downregulation induced BC cell apoptosis via the ERK1/2 pathway, while overexpressed TRPM7 promoted proliferation, migration, invasion, and tumor growth of BC [28]. Previous studies have demonstrated that TRPM7 downregulation increases reactive oxygen species, cell proliferation, migration, and invasion via elevated p-ERK1/2 and decreased PI3K/Akt protein expression [28]. According to other reports, overexpressed TRPM7 led to enhanced cell proliferation, migration, and invasion ability of BC cells [48]. In our study, we proved that TRPM7 mediates tumor growth, which is consistent with the findings of previously reports. As

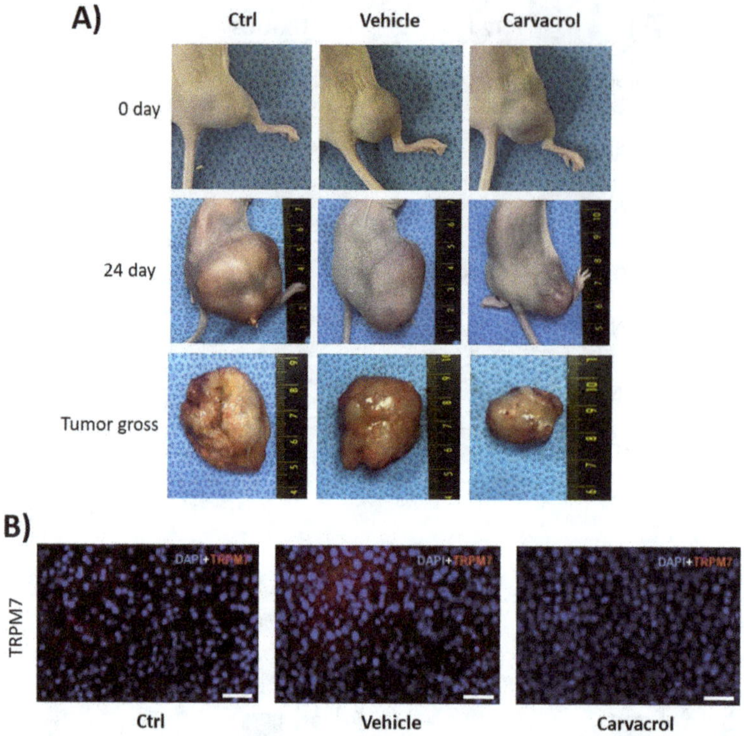


**Fig. 7** Effect of TRPM7 inhibitor on xenograft model. **a** UMUC3 cells were injected subcutaneously into Balb/c nude mice. Day 0 pictures were taken 2 weeks after UMUC3 cell injection, and Day 24 pictures were taken after the third injection of carvacrol. Tumor gross pictures were taken after the fourth injection of carvacrol. **b** Expression of TRPM7 in the control, vehicle, and carvacrol treated groups. Scale bar = 25 μm. Ctrl; no treat group, Vehicle; 1% DMSO injected group, Carvacrol; carvacrol injected group

our limits, we proceeded cell cycle analysis; however, we excluded the results due to complicated understanding of the results. In addition, we were unable to investigate the expression of proteins related to proliferation, although we did examine the effect of TRPM7 knockdown in vivo, in order to extend the findings of our study.

## Conclusion

Taken together, this study provides the function and molecular mechanism of TRPM7 in BC. We demonstrated that knockdown of TRPM7 inhibits the migration and invasion of human BC cells via the Src, Akt, and JNK signaling pathway. Moreover, we demonstrated that suppression of TRPM7 inhibits tumor growth in a xenograft model. These results indicate that TRPM7 plays a crucial role in BC, and regulation of TRPM7 could be a potential treatment of BC.

## Supplementary information

**Additional file 1 Supplementary Fig. 1. Effect of carvacrol on T24 and UMUC3 cell viability.** (a) T24 and (b) UMUC3 cells were seeded in coated 96-well plates and grown until a confluency of 90%. Cells were treated with different doses (100, 200, 300, 400, 500 μM) of carvacrol and incubated for 24 h. All data represent the means ± SD of three independent experiments (*$p < 0.05$ and **$p < 0.01$ between control and carvacrol treated groups). Ctrl: Control.

**Additional file 2 Supplementary Fig. 2. Effect of carvacrol on bladder cancer cell migration.** (a) T24 and UMUC3 cells were seeded in cell transwells and treated with different doses (100, 200, 300, 400, 500 μM) of carvacrol before being incubated for 24 h. (b) The relative absorbance was measured in migrated cells stained with crystal violet at a wavelength of 590 nm. All data represent the means ± SD of three independent experiments (*$p < 0.05$ and **$p < 0.01$ between control and carvacrol treated groups). Ctrl: Control.

**Additional file 3 Supplementary Fig. 3. Effect of carvacrol on bladder cancer cell invasion.** (a) T24 and UMUC3 cells were seeded in the cell transwells and treated with different doses (100, 200, 300, 400, 500 μM) of carvacrol before being incubated for 24 h. (b) The relative absorbance was measured in invaded cells stained with crystal violet at a wavelength of 590 nm. All data represent the means ± SD of three independent experiments (*$p < 0.05$ and **$p < 0.01$ between control and carvacrol treated groups). Ctrl: Control.

**Additional file 4 Supplementary Fig. 4. Original western blot image of** Fig. 1a and b**.** (a) Beta-actin of J82 and UMUC3 in Fig. 1a. (b) TRPM7 of J82 and UMUC3 in Fig. 1a. (c) Beta-actin of siRNA treated T24 in Fig. 1b. (d) TRPM7 of siRNA treated T24 in Fig. 1b. (e) TRPM7 of siRNA treated UMUC3 in Fig. 1b. (f) Beta-actin of siRNA treated UMUC3 in Fig. 1b.

**Additional file 5 Supplementary Fig. 5. Original western blot image of** Fig. 6**a.** (a) Beta-actin of siRNA treated T24 in Fig. 6a. (b) p-Akt of siRNA treated T24 in Fig. 6a. (c) p-JNK of siRNA treated T24 in Fig. 6a.

(d) p-Src of siRNA treated T24 in Fig. 6a. (e) t-Akt of siRNA treated T24 in Fig. 6a. (f) t-JNK of siRNA treated T24 in Fig. 6a. (g) t-Src of siRNA treated T24 in Fig. 6a. (h) Beta-actin of siRNA treated UMUC3 in Fig. 6a. (i) Beta-actin of siRNA treated UMUC3 in Fig. 6a. (j) p-Akt of siRNA treated UMUC3 in Fig. 6a. (k) p-Src of siRNA treated UMUC3 in Fig. 6a. (l) t-Akt of siRNA treated UMUC3 in Fig. 6a. (m) t-JNK of siRNA treated UMUC3 in Fig. 6a. (n) t-Src of siRNA treated UMUC3 in Fig. 6a. Full-length blots are presented in Suppl. Figs. 4 and 5.

**Additional file 6.** Fig. 1a beta-actin. Beta-actin of J82 and UMUC3 in Fig. 1a. Figure 1a TRPM7. TRPM7 of J82 and UMUC3 in Fig. 1a. Figure 1b beta-actin. Beta-actin of siRNA treated T24 in Fig. 1a. Fig. 1b, TRPM7_1. TRPM7 of siRNA treated T24 in Fig. 1b. Fig. 1b, TRPM7_2. TRPM7 of siRNA treated UMUC3 in Fig. 1b. Fig. 1b beta-actin. Beta-actin of siRNA treated UMUC3 in Fig. 1b. Figure 6a beta-actin-1. Beta-actin of siRNA treated T24 in Fig. 6a. Figure 6a p-Akt-1. p-Akt of siRNA treated T24 in Fig. 6a. Figure 6a p-JNK-1. p-JNK of siRNA treated T24 in Fig. 6a. Figure 6a p-Src-1. p-Src of siRNA treated T24 in Fig. 6a. Figure 6a t-Akt-1. t-Akt of siRNA treated T24 in Fig. 6a. Fig. 6a t-JNK-1. t-JNK of siRNA treated T24 in Fig. 6a. Fig. 6a t-Src-1. t-Src of siRNA treated T24 in Fig. 6a. Fig. 6a beta-actin-2. Beta-actin of siRNA treated UMUC3 in Fig. 6a. Fig. 6a p-Akt-2. p-Akt of siRNA treated UMUC3 in Fig. 6a. Fig. 6a p-JNK-2. p-JNK of siRNA treated UMUC3 in Fig. 6a. Fig. 6a p-Src. p-Src of siRNA treated UMUC3 in Fig. 6a. Fig. 6a t-Akt-2/ t-Akt of siRNA treated UMUC3 in Fig. 6a. Fig. 6a t-JNK-2/ t-JNK of siRNA treated UMUC3 in Fig. 6a. Fig. 6a t-Src. t-Src of siRNA treated UMUC3 in Fig. 6a.

### Abbreviations

BC: Bladder cancer; JNK: C-Jun N-terminal kinase; MIBC: Muscle invasive bladder cancer; NMIBC: Non-muscle invasive bladder cancer; TRP: Transient receptor potential; TRPM7: Transient receptor potential melastin 7

### Acknowledgements

Not applicable

### Authors' contributions

EHL: Draft or revision article. SYC: Draft or revision article. BMK: Acquisition of data. BHY: Acquisition of data. JNL: Data analysis. BSK: Data analysis. ESY: Interpretation of data. SKL: Interpretation of data. PHS: Interpretation of data. TG Kwon: Conception and design. YSH: Conception and design. All authors have read and approved the manuscript.

### Author details

[1]Joint Institute for Regenerative Medicine, Kyungpook National University Hospital, Daegu, Republic of Korea. [2]BioMedical Research Institute, Kyungpook National University Hospital, Daegu, Republic of Korea. [3]Department of Urology, School of Medicine, Kyungpook National University, Daegu, Republic of Korea. [4]Department of Urology, School of Medicine, Kyungpook National University, Kyungpook National University Chilgok Hospital, Daegu, Republic of Korea. [5]Department of Urology, School of Medicine, Kyungpook National University, Kyungpook National University Hospital, Daegu, Republic of Korea. [6]BK21 Plus KNU Multi-Omics Based Creative Drug Research Team, College of Pharmacy, Research Institute of Pharmaceutical Sciences, Kyungpook National University, Daegu, Republic of Korea. [7]Department of Urology, Yeungnam University College of Medicine, Daegu, Republic of Korea.

### References

1. Yonemori M, Seki N, Yoshino H, Matsushita R, Miyamoto K, Nakagawa M, Enokida H. Dual tumor-suppressors miR-139-5p and miR-139-3p targeting matrix metalloprotease 11 in bladder cancer. Cancer Sci. 2016; 107(9):1233–42.
2. King MA, Ganley IG, Flemington V. Inhibition of cholesterol metabolism underlies synergy between mTOR pathway inhibition and chloroquine in bladder cancer cells. Oncogene. 2016;35(34):4518–28.
3. Kaufman DS, Shipley WU, Feldman AS. Bladder cancer. Lancet. 2009; 374(9685):239–49.
4. Tilki D, Burger M, Dalbagni G, Grossman HB, Hakenberg OW, Palou J, Reich O, Roupret M, Shariat SF, Zlotta AR. Urine markers for detection and surveillance of non-muscle-invasive bladder cancer. Eur Urol. 2011;60(3): 484–92.
5. Enokida H, Yoshino H, Matsushita R, Nakagawa M. The role of microRNAs in bladder cancer. Investig Clin Urol. 2016;57(Suppl 1):S60–76.
6. Buraschi S, Xu SQ, Stefanello M, Moskalev I, Morcavallo A, Genua M, Tanimoto R, Birbe R, Peiper SC, Gomella LG, et al. Suppression of progranulin expression inhibits bladder cancer growth and sensitizes cancer cells to cisplatin. Oncotarget. 2016;7(26):39980–95.
7. Kawahara T, Inoue S, Ide H, Kashiwagi E, Ohtake S, Mizushima T, Li P, Li Y, Zheng Y, Uemura H, et al. ZKSCAN3 promotes bladder cancer cell proliferation, migration, and invasion. Oncotarget. 2016;7(33):53599–610.
8. Kim EY, Seo JM, Kim C, Lee JE, Lee KM, Kim JH. BLT2 promotes the invasion and metastasis of aggressive bladder cancer cells through a reactive oxygen species-linked pathway. Free Radic Biol Med. 2010;49(6):1072–81.
9. Kong DB, Chen F, Sima N. Focal adhesion kinases crucially regulate TGFbeta-induced migration and invasion of bladder cancer cells via Src kinase and E-cadherin. Onco Targets Ther. 2017;10:1783–92.
10. Park SL, Lee EJ, Kim WJ, Moon SK. p27KIP1 is involved in ERK1/2-mediated MMP-9 expression via the activation of NF-kappaB binding in the IL-7-induced migration and invasion of 5637 cells. Int J Oncol. 2014;44(4):1349–56.
11. Robertson AG, Kim J, Al-Ahmadie H, Bellmunt J, Guo G, Cherniack AD, Hinoue T, Laird PW, Hoadley KA, Akbani R, et al. Comprehensive molecular characterization of muscle-invasive bladder Cancer. Cell. 2018;174(4):1033.
12. van Rhijn BW, Catto JW, Goebell PJ, Knuchel R, Shariat SF, van der Poel HG, Sanchez-Carbayo M, Thalmann GN, Schmitz-Drager BJ, Kiemeney LA. Molecular markers for urothelial bladder cancer prognosis: toward implementation in clinical practice. Urol Oncol. 2014;32(7):1078–87.
13. Friedlander TW, Welty C, Anantharaman A, Schonhoft JD, Jendrisak A, Lee J, Li P, Hough J, Stromlund A, Edwards M, et al. Identification and characterization of circulating tumor cells in men who have undergone prostatectomy for clinically localized. High Risk Prostate Cancer J Urol. 2019; 202(4):732–41.
14. Patel R, Bock M, Polotti CF, Elsamra S. Pharmacokinetic drug evaluation of atezolizumab for the treatment of locally advanced or metastatic urothelial carcinoma. Expert Opin Drug Metab Toxicol. 2017;13(2):225–32.
15. Kim BJ, Park EJ, Lee JH, Jeon JH, Kim SJ, So I. Suppression of transient receptor potential melastatin 7 channel induces cell death in gastric cancer. Cancer Sci. 2008;99(12):2502–9.
16. Zou ZG, Rios FJ, Montezano AC, Touyz RM. TRPM7, Magnesium, and Signaling. Int J Mol Sci. 2019;20(8):1877.
17. Ha YS, Kim YY, Yu NH, Chun SY, Choi SH, Lee JN, Kim BS, Yoo ES, Kwon TG. Down-regulation of transient receptor potential melastatin member 7 prevents migration and invasion of renal cell carcinoma cells via inactivation of the Src and Akt pathway. Investig Clin Urol. 2018; 59(4):263–74.
18. Dhennin-Duthille I, Gautier M, Korichneva I, Ouadid-Ahidouch H. TRPM7 involvement in cancer: a potential prognostic factor. Magnes Res. 2014; 27(3):103–12.
19. Giamarchi A, Padilla F, Crest M, Honore E, Delmas P. TRPP2: Ca2+ –permeable cation channel and more. Cell Mol Biol (Noisy-le-grand). 2006; 52(8):105–14.
20. Wang J, Liao QJ, Zhang Y, Zhou H, Luo CH, Tang J, Wang Y, Tang Y, Zhao M, Zhao XH, et al. TRPM7 is required for ovarian cancer cell growth, migration and invasion. Biochem Biophys Res Commun. 2014;454(4):547–53.
21. Yee NS. Role of TRPM7 in Cancer: Potential as Molecular Biomarker and Therapeutic Target. Pharmaceuticals (Basel). 2017;10(2):39.
22. Yee NS, Chan AS, Yee JD, Yee RK. TRPM7 and TRPM8 ion channels in pancreatic adenocarcinoma: potential roles as Cancer biomarkers and targets. Scientifica (Cairo). 2012;2012:415158.
23. Gao H, Chen X, Du X, Guan B, Liu Y, Zhang H. EGF enhances the migration of cancer cells by up-regulation of TRPM7. Cell Calcium. 2011;50(6):559–68.
24. Chen WL, Barszczyk A, Turlova E, Deurloo M, Liu B, Yang BB, Rutka JT, Feng ZP, Sun HS. Inhibition of TRPM7 by carvacrol suppresses glioblastoma cell proliferation, migration and invasion. Oncotarget. 2015;6(18):16321–40.
25. Greenman C, Stephens P, Smith R, Dalgliesh GL, Hunter C, Bignell G, Davies H, Teague J, Butler A, Stevens C, et al. Patterns of somatic mutation in human cancer genomes. Nature. 2007;446(7132):153–8.
26. Dai Q, Shrubsole MJ, Ness RM, Schlundt D, Cai Q, Smalley WE, Li M, Shyr Y, Zheng W. The relation of magnesium and calcium intakes and a genetic polymorphism in the magnesium transporter to colorectal neoplasia risk. Am J Clin Nutr. 2007;86(3):743–51.

27. Meng X, Cai C, Wu J, Cai S, Ye C, Chen H, Yang Z, Zeng H, Shen Q, Zou F. TRPM7 mediates breast cancer cell migration and invasion through the MAPK pathway. Cancer Lett. 2013;333(1):96–102.
28. Cao R, Meng Z, Liu T, Wang G, Qian G, Cao T, Guan X, Dan H, Xiao Y, Wang X. Decreased TRPM7 inhibits activities and induces apoptosis of bladder cancer cells via ERK1/2 pathway. Oncotarget. 2016;7(45):72941–60.
29. Zeng Z, Leng T, Feng X, Sun H, Inoue K, Zhu L, Xiong ZG. Silencing TRPM7 in mouse cortical astrocytes impairs cell proliferation and migration via ERK and JNK signaling pathways. PLoS One. 2015;10(3):e0119912.
30. Lee EH, Baek SY, Park JY, Kim YW. Rifampicin activates AMPK and alleviates oxidative stress in the liver as mediated with Nrf2 signaling. Chem Biol Interact. 2019;315:108889.
31. Liu H, Dilger JP, Lin J. The Role of Transient Receptor Potential Melastatin 7 (TRPM7) in Cell Viability: A Potential Target to Suppress Breast Cancer Cell Cycle. Cancers (Basel). 2020;12(1):131.
32. Guilbert A, Gautier M, Dhennin-Duthille I, Haren N, Sevestre H, Ouadid-Ahidouch H. Evidence that TRPM7 is required for breast cancer cell proliferation. Am J Phys Cell Phys. 2009;297(3):C493–502.
33. Callera GE, He Y, Yogi A, Montezano AC, Paravicini T, Yao G, Touyz RM. Regulation of the novel Mg2+ transporter transient receptor potential melastatin 7 (TRPM7) cation channel by bradykinin in vascular smooth muscle cells. J Hypertens. 2009;27(1):155–66.
34. Bodding M. TRP proteins and cancer. Cell Signal. 2007;19(3):617–24.
35. Gkika D, Prevarskaya N. Molecular mechanisms of TRP regulation in tumor growth and metastasis. Biochim Biophys Acta. 2009;1793(6):953–8.
36. Su LT, Chen HC, Gonzalez-Pagan O, Overton JD, Xie J, Yue L, Runnels LW. TRPM7 activates m-calpain by stress-dependent stimulation of p38 MAPK and c-Jun N-terminal kinase. J Mol Biol. 2010;396(4):858–69.
37. Yang P, Su C, Luo X, Zeng H, Zhao L, Wei L, Zhang X, Varghese Z, Moorhead JF, Chen Y, et al. Dietary oleic acid-induced CD36 promotes cervical cancer cell growth and metastasis via up-regulation Src/ERK pathway. Cancer Lett. 2018;438:76–85.
38. Huang YL, Chu YL, Ho CT, Chung JG, Lai CI, Su YC, Kuo YH, Sheen LY. Antcin K, an active Triterpenoid from the fruiting bodies of basswood-cultivated Antrodia cinnamomea, inhibits metastasis via suppression of integrin-mediated adhesion, migration, and invasion in human Hepatoma cells. J Agric Food Chem. 2015;63(18):4561–9.
39. Zhang X, Wu J, Luo S, Lechler T, Zhang JY. FRA1 promotes squamous cell carcinoma growth and metastasis through distinct AKT and c-Jun dependent mechanisms. Oncotarget. 2016;7(23):34371–83.
40. Cheng HL, Lin CW, Yang JS, Hsieh MJ, Yang SF, Lu KH. Zoledronate blocks geranylgeranylation not farnesylation to suppress human osteosarcoma U2OS cells metastasis by EMT via rho a activation and FAK-inhibited JNK and p38 pathways. Oncotarget. 2016;7(9):9742–58.
41. Guarino M. Src signaling in cancer invasion. J Cell Physiol. 2010;223(1):14–26.
42. Wei J, Xu G, Wu M, Zhang Y, Li Q, Liu P, Zhu T, Song A, Zhao L, Han Z, et al. Overexpression of vimentin contributes to prostate cancer invasion and metastasis via src regulation. Anticancer Res. 2008;28(1A):327–34.
43. Polivka J Jr, Janku F. Molecular targets for cancer therapy in the PI3K/AKT/mTOR pathway. Pharmacol Ther. 2014;142(2):164–75.
44. Kim D, Kim S, Koh H, Yoon SO, Chung AS, Cho KS, Chung J. Akt/PKB promotes cancer cell invasion via increased motility and metalloproteinase production. FASEB J. 2001;15(11):1953–62.
45. Vasko V, Saji M, Hardy E, Kruhlak M, Larin A, Savchenko V, Miyakawa M, Isozaki O, Murakami H, Tsushima T, et al. Akt activation and localisation correlate with tumour invasion and oncogene expression in thyroid cancer. J Med Genet. 2004;41(3):161–70.
46. Bubici C, Papa S. JNK signalling in cancer: in need of new, smarter therapeutic targets. Br J Pharmacol. 2014;171(1):24–37.
47. Cheng CY, Tang NY, Kao ST, Hsieh CL. Ferulic acid administered at various time points protects against cerebral infarction by activating p38 MAPK/p90RSK/CREB/Bcl-2 anti-apoptotic signaling in the subacute phase of cerebral ischemia-reperfusion injury in rats. PLoS One. 2016;11(5):e0155748.
48. Gao SL, Kong CZ, Zhang Z, Li ZL, Bi JB, Liu XK. TRPM7 is overexpressed in bladder cancer and promotes proliferation, migration, invasion and tumor growth. Oncol Rep. 2017;38(4):1967–76.

# Permissions

All chapters in this book were first published by BioMed Central; hereby published with permission under the Creative Commons Attribution License or equivalent. Every chapter published in this book has been scrutinized by our experts. Their significance has been extensively debated. The topics covered herein carry significant findings which will fuel the growth of the discipline. They may even be implemented as practical applications or may be referred to as a beginning point for another development.

The contributors of this book come from diverse backgrounds, making this book a truly international effort. This book will bring forth new frontiers with its revolutionizing research information and detailed analysis of the nascent developments around the world.

We would like to thank all the contributing authors for lending their expertise to make the book truly unique. They have played a crucial role in the development of this book. Without their invaluable contributions this book wouldn't have been possible. They have made vital efforts to compile up to date information on the varied aspects of this subject to make this book a valuable addition to the collection of many professionals and students.

This book was conceptualized with the vision of imparting up-to-date information and advanced data in this field. To ensure the same, a matchless editorial board was set up. Every individual on the board went through rigorous rounds of assessment to prove their worth. After which they invested a large part of their time researching and compiling the most relevant data for our readers.

The editorial board has been involved in producing this book since its inception. They have spent rigorous hours researching and exploring the diverse topics which have resulted in the successful publishing of this book. They have passed on their knowledge of decades through this book. To expedite this challenging task, the publisher supported the team at every step. A small team of assistant editors was also appointed to further simplify the editing procedure and attain best results for the readers.

Apart from the editorial board, the designing team has also invested a significant amount of their time in understanding the subject and creating the most relevant covers. They scrutinized every image to scout for the most suitable representation of the subject and create an appropriate cover for the book.

The publishing team has been an ardent support to the editorial, designing and production team. Their endless efforts to recruit the best for this project, has resulted in the accomplishment of this book. They are a veteran in the field of academics and their pool of knowledge is as vast as their experience in printing. Their expertise and guidance has proved useful at every step. Their uncompromising quality standards have made this book an exceptional effort. Their encouragement from time to time has been an inspiration for everyone.

The publisher and the editorial board hope that this book will prove to be a valuable piece of knowledge for researchers, students, practitioners and scholars across the globe.

# List of Contributors

**Go Anan, Yasuhiro Kaiho, Hiromichi Iwamura, Jun Ito, Yuki Kohada, Jotaro Mikami and Makoto Sato**
Department of Urology, Tohoku Medical and Pharmaceutical University, Sendai, Japan, 1-15-1 Fukumuro, Miyagino-ku, Sendai, Miyagi 983-8536, Japan

**I Hsu**
Division of plastic surgery, Department of Surgery, Chi-Mei Medical Center, Tainan, Taiwan

**Chia-Chen Lee**
Department of surgery, Kaohsiung Medical University Hospital, Kaohsiung, Taiwan

**Ming-Jenn Chen**
Department of Surgery, Chi-Mei Medical Center, No.901, Zhonghua Rd., Yongkang Dist., Tainan City 710, Taiwan, Republic of China
Department of Sports Management, College of Leisure and Recreation Management, Chia Nan University of Pharmacy and Science, Tainan, Taiwan, Republic of China

**Sofie C. M. Tops, Eva Kolwijck and Heiman F. L. Wertheim**
Department of Medical Microbiology, Radboud Center Infectious Diseases, Radboudumc, huispost 777, Geert Grooteplein Zuid 10, 6525, GA, Nijmegen, the Netherlands

**Evert L. Koldewijn**
Department of Urology, Catharina Hospital, Eindhoven, the Netherlands

**Diederik M. Somford**
Department of Urology, Canisius-Wilhelmina Hospital, Nijmegen, the Netherlands

**Marlies E. J. L. Hulscher and Anita M. P. Huis**
Scientific Center for Quality of Healthcare, Radboud Institute for Health Sciences, Radboudumc, Nijmegen, the Netherlands

**J. P. Michiel Sedelaar**
Department of Urology, Radboudumc, Nijmegen, the Netherlands

**Heikki Seikkula**
Department of Surgery, Central Hospital of Central Finland, Jyväskylä, Finland

**Peter J. Boström**
Department of Urology, Turku University Hospital, Turku, Finland
Department of Urology, University of Turku, Turku, Finland

**Karri Seppä**
Finnish Cancer Registry, Helsinki, Finland

**Janne Pitkäniemi**
Finnish Cancer Registry, Helsinki, Finland
Faculty of Social Sciences (Health Sciences), Tampere, Finland
Department of Public Health, University of Helsinki, Helsinki, Finland

**Nea Malila**
Finnish Cancer Registry, Helsinki, Finland
School of Health Sciences, University of Tampere, Tampere, Finland

**Antti Kaipia**
Department of Urology, Tampere University Hospital, Tampere, Finland

**Marcus Derigs, Rainer Hofmann and Axel Hegele**
Department of Urology and Pediatric Urology, University Hospital, Philipps-University Marburg, Baldingerstr. 1, 35043 Marburg, Germany

**Anika Pehl**
Department of Pathology, University Hospital, Philipps-University Marburg, Baldingerstr 1, 35043 Marburg, Germany

**Jorge Riera-Knorrenschild**
Department of Hematology and Oncology, University Hospital, Philipps-University Marburg, Baldingerstr. 1, 35043 Marburg, Germany

**Youkong Li, Min Zhu, Mengbo Li and Zhenwei Yang**
Department of Urology, Jingzhou Central Hospital and The Second Clinical Medical College, Yangtze University, No.60 Jingzhong Road, Jingzhou District, Jingzhou 434020, Hubei Province, People's Republic of China

**Wen Zhong**
Department of Endocrine, Jingzhou Central Hospital and The Second Clinical Medical College, Yangtze University, Jingzhou 434020, Hubei Province, People's Republic of China

**Haiqing He**
Department of Urology, The Second Xiangya Hospital, Central South University, Changsha 410011, Hunan, China
Vancouver Prostate Centre, Department of Urologic Sciences, Faculty of Medicine, University of British Columbia, Vancouver, BC, Canada

**Shuiqing Wu, Kai Ai, Xuan Zhu, Ran Xu, Xiaokun Zhao, Yinhuai Wang and Zhaohui Zhong**
Department of Urology, The Second Xiangya Hospital, Central South University, Changsha 410011, Hunan, China

**Jun Hao**
Vancouver Prostate Centre, Department of Urologic Sciences, Faculty of Medicine, University of British Columbia, Vancouver, BC, Canada

**Long Wang**
Department of Urology, Xiangya Hospital, Central South University, Changsha 410008, Hunan, China

**Agus Rizal A. H. Hamid, Harun W. Kusuma Putra, Putri Diana, Saras Serani Sesari, Rainy Umbas and Chaidir A. Mochtar**
Department of Urology, CiptoMangunkusumo Hospital - Faculty of Medicine Universitas Indonesia, Jl. Diponegoro No.71, RW.5, Kenari, Senen, RW.5, Kenari, Senen, Kota Jakarta Pusat, Daerah Khusus Ibukota Jakarta 10430, Indonesia

**Ningrum Paramita Sari and Asmarinah**
Department of Biology, CiptoMangunkusumo Hospital - Faculty of Medicine Universitas Indonesia, Jl. Diponegoro No.71, RW.5, Kenari, Senen, RW.5, Kenari, Senen, Kota Jakarta Pusat, Daerah Khusus Ibukota Jakarta, Indonesia

**Eka Novita, Fajar Lamhot Gultom, Meilania Saraswati and Budiana Tanurahardja**
Department of Pathology Anatomy, CiptoMangunkusumo Hospital – Faculty of Medicine Universitas Indonesia, Jl. Diponegoro No.71, RW.5, Kenari, Senen, RW.5, Kenari, Senen, Kota Jakarta Pusat, Daerah Khusus Ibukota Jakarta, Indonesia

**Sandy Srinivas**
Stanford University Medical Center, Palo Alto, California, USA

**Ateesha F. Mohamed, Sreevalsa Appukkuttan, A. Reginald Waldeck and Stacey J Simmons**
Bayer U.S. LLC, Whippany, NJ, USA

**Marc Botteman, Xinyi Ng, Namita Joshi and Erica Horodniceanu**
Pharmerit International, Bethesda, MD, USA

**K. Shyamprasad**
R&D Center for Excellence, Vidya Herbs Pvt. Ltd, #14A, Jigani I phase, Bangalore, Karnataka 560 105, India

**H. V. Sudeep**
R&D Center for Excellence, Vidya Herbs Pvt. Ltd, #14A, Jigani I phase, Bangalore, Karnataka 560 105, India
Leads Clinical Research and Bio services Private Ltd., Bangalore, India

**Jestin V. Thomas**
Leads Clinical Research and Bio services Private Ltd., Bangalore, India

**Hong-wei Zhao**
Department of Urology, Affiliated Yantai Yuhuangding Hospital, Qingdao University, Yantai 264000, Shandong, P. R. China
Department of Urology, First Affiliated Hospital, Sun Yat-Sen University, No.58 ZhongShan 2nd Road, Guangzhou 510080, Guangdong, P. R. China

**Zhen-li Gao and Lei Shi**
Department of Urology, Affiliated Yantai Yuhuangding Hospital, Qingdao University, Yantai 264000, Shandong, P. R. China

**Jin-huan Wei, Zhen-hua Chen, Hao-hua Yao, Yi-hui Pan, Jun-hang Luo, Wei Chen and Yong Fang**
Department of Urology, First Affiliated Hospital, Sun Yat-Sen University, No.58 ZhongShan 2nd Road, Guangzhou 510080, Guangdong, P. R. China

**Jian Li**
State Key Laboratory of Oncology in South China, Department of Ultrasound, Sun Yat-Sen University Cancer Center, Guangzhou 510060, Guangdong, P. R. China

**Jia-Zheng Cao**
Department of Urology, Jiangmen Hospital, Sun Yat-Sen University, Jiangmen 529000, Guangdong, P. R. China

**Juan Lin**
Department of Pediatrics, hird Affiliated Hospital of Sun Yat-sen University, Guangzhou 510630, Guangdong, P. R. China

**Zhu Wang and Jian-yao Lv**
Department of Ultrasound, First Affiliated Hospital, Sun Yat-Sen University, Guangzhou 510080, Guangdong, P. R. China

**Hiroji Uemura**
Department of Urology and Renal Transplantation, Yokohama City University Medical Center, Yokohama, Japan

**Yosuke Koroki**
Medical Affairs, Janssen Pharmaceutical K.K., Tokyo, Japan

**Yuki Iwaki**
Clinical Pharmacology, Janssen Pharmaceutical K.K, Tokyo, Japan

**Keiichiro Imanaka**
Clinical Science, Janssen Pharmaceutical K.K, Tokyo, Japan

**Takeshi Kambara**
Department of Dermatology, Yokohama City University Medical Center, Yokohama, Japan

**Angela Lopez-Gitlitz and Andressa Smith**
Janssen Global Research & Development, Spring House, PA, USA

**Hirotsugu Uemura**
Department of Urology, Kindai University Faculty of Medicine, Osaka, Japan

**Daozhang Yuan and Yiyu Huang**
Department of Urology, GuangDong Second Traditional Chinese Medicine Hospital, No.212, Luogang Road Street, Luogang District, Guangzhou 510700, Guangdong, China

**Jiaxin LI**
Department of Colorectal Surgery, The Sixth Affiliated Hospital, Sun Yat-Sen University, Guangzhou 510655, China

**Shan Yang**
Department of Emergency, Guangdong Provincial Hospital of Chinese Medicine, Guangzhou 510120, China

**Shusheng Wang**
Department of Urology, Guangdong Provincial Hospital of Chinese Medicine, No.261, Datong Road, Yuexiu District, Guangzhou 510030, Guangdong, China

**James McKiernan**
Columbia University Medical Center, New York City, NY, USA

**Mikkel Noerholm, Vasisht Tadigotla, Sonia Kumar, Phillipp Torkler, Grannum Sant, Jason Alter and Johan Skog**
Exosome Diagnostics, a Bio-Techne Brand, Waltham, MA, USA

**Michael J. Donovan**
Exosome Diagnostics, a Bio-Techne Brand, Waltham, MA, USA
Icahn School of Medicine at Mt. Sinai, New York City, NY, USA

**Suchitra K. Hourigan**
Inova Children's Hospital, 3300 Gallows Road, Falls Church, VA 22042, USA
Inova Translational Medicine Institute, 3300 Gallows Road, Falls Church, VA 22042, USA

**Wei Zhu, Wendy S.W.Wong, Nicole C. Clemency, Marina Provenzano and Thierry Vilboux**
Inova Translational Medicine Institute, 3300 Gallows Road, Falls Church, VA 22042, USA

**John E. Niederhuber**
Inova Translational Medicine Institute, 3300 Gallows Road, Falls Church, VA 22042, USA
Public Health Sciences, Center for Genomics in Public Health, School of Medicine, University of Virginia, Charlottesville, VA 22908, USA

**John Deeken**
Inova Translational Medicine Institute, 3300 Gallows Road, Falls Church, VA 22042, USA
Public Health Sciences, Center for Genomics in Public Health, School of Medicine, University of Virginia, Charlottesville, VA 22908, USA
Inova Schar Cancer Institute, 3224 Gallows Road, Fairfax, VA 22031, USA

**Simon Chung**
Inova Schar Cancer Institute, 3224 Gallows Road, Fairfax, VA 22031, USA
Department of Urology, Inova Fairfax Medical Center, 3300 Gallows Road, Falls Church, VA 22042, USA

**Kim McDaniel-Wiley**
Department of Urology, Inova Fairfax Medical Center, 3300 Gallows Road, Falls Church, VA 22042, USA

**Donald Trump**
Inova Schar Cancer Institute, 3224 Gallows Road, Fairfax, VA 22031, USA

**Madhusudan Koya and Sue Osborne**
Waitemata District Health Board, Auckland, New Zealand

**Christophe Chemaslé**
Mid Central District Health Board, Palmerston North, New Zealand

**Sima Porten**
University of California San Francisco, San Francisco, CA, USA

**Anne Schuckman**
USC Institute of Urology, USC/Norris Comprehensive Cancer Center, University of Southern California, Los Angeles, CA, USA

**Andrew Kennedy-Smith**
Capital & Coast District Health Board, Wellington, New Zealand

**Weilin Fang, Lei Xu, Jiabei Sun and Jiayi Li**
Department of Urology, Renji Hospital, School of Medicine, Shanghai Jiaotong University, Shanghai, 200127, People's Republic of China

**Jacques Corcos**
Department of Urology, Jewish General Hospital, 3755 Côte Ste Catherine Road, Suite E-945, Montreal,, QC, Canada

**Tao Jiang, Xiaozhou Zhou, Zhipeng Chen, Tailin Xiong, Jian Fu, Zhengchao Liu, Dishi Yan, Zhansong Zhou and Wenhao Shen**
Department of Urology, Urology Institute of PLA, Southwest Hospital, Third Military Medical University (Army Medical University), Gao Tanyan Street 29#, Sha Pingba, Chongqing 400038, China

**Edward C. Diaz**
Department of Urology, Stanford University Medical Center, 300 Pasteur Drive, Grant S-287, Stanford, CA 94305, USA
Present Address: Division of Pediatric Urology, Advocate Children's Hospital, 8901 West Golf Road, Suite 301, Des Plaines, IL 60016, USA

**Amy D. Dobberfuhl**
Department of Urology, Stanford University Medical Center, 300 Pasteur Drive, Grant S-287, Stanford, CA 94305, USA

**Mason Briggs**
Department of Urology, Stanford University Medical Center, 300 Pasteur Drive, Grant S-287, Stanford, CA 94305, USA
Department of Obstetrics and Gynecology, Stanford University Medical Center, 300 Pasteur Drive, Rm A370, MC 5317, Stanford, CA 94305, USA

**Yan Wen, Guobing Zhuang, Shannon L. Wallace and Bertha C. Chen**
Department of Obstetrics and Gynecology, Stanford University Medical Center, 300 Pasteur Drive, Rm A370, MC 5317, Stanford, CA 94305, USA

**Chia-Sui Kao**
Department of Pathology, Stanford University Medical Center, 300 Pasteur Drive, Rm L235, Stanford, CA 94305, USA

**Rongxin Li, Ye Li, Ke Gao, Kangning Chen, Xiaogang Yang, Yongqiang Ding, Xinlong Ma, Yang Wang, Weipeng Li, Yanan Wang, Zhiping Wang and Zhilong Dong**
Lanzhou University Second Hospital, Lanzhou City, Gansu Province, China

**Jun Song**
Lanzhou University Second Hospital, Lanzhou City, Gansu Province, China
Sanya People's Hospital, Sanya City, Hainan Province, China

**Jin Bong Choi**
Department of Urology, Bucheon St. Mary's Hospital, College of Medicine, The Catholic University of Korea, Seoul, Republic of Korea

**Hyuk Jin Cho, U-Syn Ha, Sung-Hoo Hong, Ji Youl Lee and Seung Hwan Jeon**
Department of Urology, Seoul St. Mary's Hospital, College of Medicine, The Catholic University of Korea, Seoul, Republic of Korea

**Eun Bi Kwon**
Korea Bio Medical Science Institute, Seoul, Republic of Korea

**Woong Jin Bae and Sae Woong Kim**
Department of Urology, Seoul St. Mary's Hospital, College of Medicine, The Catholic University of Korea, Seoul, Republic of Korea and Catholic Integrative Medicine Research Institute, The Catholic University of Korea, Banpo-daero 222, Seocho-gu, Seoul 06591 Seoul, Republic of Korea

**Zane Stromberga, Russ Chess-Williams and Christian Moro**
Centre for Urology Research, Faculty of Health Sciences and Medicine, Bond University, Gold Coast, Queensland 4226, Australia

**Shunichiro Nomura, Yasutomo Suzuki, Jun Akatsuka, Yuki Endo, Tsutomu Hamasaki, Go Kimura and Yukihiro Kondo**
Department of Urology, Nippon Medical School, 1-1-5 Sendagi, Bunkyo-ku, Tokyo 113-8603, Japan

**Akira Shimizu**
Analytic Human Pathology, Nippon Medical School, 1-1-5 Sendagi, Bunkyo-ku, Tokyo 113-8603, Japan

**C. X. Raventos, A. Carrion and E. Trilla**
Urology Department, Vall d'Hebron University Hospital, Pg. Vall d'Hebron 119-129, 08035 Barcelona, Spain

**F. Lozano and J. Morote**
Urology Department, Vall d'Hebron University Hospital, Pg. Vall d'Hebron 119-129, 08035 Barcelona, Spain
Universitat Autònoma de Barcelona, Barcelona, Spain

**Satoshi Funada**
Department of Urology, Kyoto University Graduate School of Medicine, 54 Shogoinkawahara-cho, Sakyo-ku, Kyoto 606-8507, Japan
Department of Health Promotion and Human Behavior, Kyoto University School of Public Health, Kyoto, Japan
Department of Psychiatry, Nagoya City University Graduate School of Medical Sciences, Nagoya, Japan

**Takayuki Goto, Shusuke Akamatsu and Osamu Ogawa**
Department of Urology, Kyoto University Graduate School of Medicine, 54 Shogoinkawahara-cho, Sakyo-ku, Kyoto 606-8507, Japan

**Norio Watanabe and Toshiaki A. Furukawa**
Department of Health Promotion and Human Behavior, Kyoto University School of Public Health, Kyoto, Japan

**Tatsuo Akechi**
Department of Psychiatry, Nagoya City University Graduate School of Medical Sciences, Nagoya, Japan

**Hiromitsu Negoro**
Department of Urology, University of Tsukuba Hospital, Tsukuba, Japan

**Kentaro Ueno and Ryuji Uozumi**
Department of Biomedical Statistics and Bioinformatics, Kyoto University Graduate School of Medicine, Kyoto, Japan

**Kentaro Ichioka**
Ichioka Urological Clinic, Kyoto, Japan

**Takehiko Segawa**
Department of Urology, Kyoto City Hospital, Kyoto, Japan

**Chao Tan, Fei Yan, Wei-Jun Qin, Kun Zhang, Guo-Jun Wu, Jian-Lin Yuan and Fei Liu**
Department of Urology, Xijing Hospital, Air Force Medical University, 15 Changle West Road, Xi'an 710032, Shaanxi, China

**Li-Ping Yao**
Xijing Hospital of Digestive Diseases, Xijing Hospital, Air Force Medical University, Xi'an, Shaanxi, China

**Jun-Ling Xing**
Institute of neuroscience, Air Force Medical University, Xi'an, Shaanxi, China

**Yanxia Liu and Hongming Xu**
Department of Pathology, Jiangyin People's Hospital, Affiliated Jiangyin Hospital of the Southeast University Medical College, Jiangyin 214400, Jiangsu Province, China

**Bin Wu and Qiang Luo**
Department of Urology, Jiangyin People's Hospital, Affiliated Jiangyin Hospital of the Southeast University Medical College, Jiangyin 214400, Jiangsu Province, China

**Shuguang Liu**
Department of Urology, Tianjin Jinnan Hospital, Tianjin 300350, China

**Eun Hye Lee**
Joint Institute for Regenerative Medicine, Kyungpook National University Hospital, Daegu, Republic of Korea

**So Young Chun, Bomi Kim and Bo Hyun Yoon**
BioMedical Research Institute, Kyungpook National University Hospital, Daegu, Republic of Korea

**Jun Nyung Lee, Tae Gyun Kwon and Yun-Sok Ha**
Joint Institute for Regenerative Medicine, Kyungpook National University Hospital, Daegu, Republic of Korea
Department of Urology, School of Medicine, Kyungpook National University, Daegu, Republic of Korea
Department of Urology, School of Medicine, Kyungpook National University, Kyungpook National University Chilgok Hospital, Daegu, Republic of Korea

**Bum Soo Kim**
Joint Institute for Regenerative Medicine, Kyungpook National University Hospital, Daegu, Republic of Korea
Department of Urology, School of Medicine, Kyungpook National University, Daegu, Republic of Korea
Department of Urology, School of Medicine, Kyungpook National University, Kyungpook National University Hospital, Daegu, Republic of Korea

**Eun Sang Yoo**
Department of Urology, School of Medicine, Kyungpook National University, Daegu, Republic of Korea
Department of Urology, School of Medicine, Kyungpook National University, Kyungpook National University Hospital, Daegu, Republic of Korea

**Sangkyu Lee**
BK21 Plus KNU Multi-Omics Based Creative Drug Research Team, College of Pharmacy, Research Institute of Pharmaceutical Sciences, Kyungpook National University, Daegu, Republic of Korea

**Phil Hyun Song**
Department of Urology, Yeungnam University College of Medicine, Daegu, Republic of Korea

# Index

www.ingramcontent.com/pod-product-compliance
Lightning Source LLC
LaVergne TN
LVHW082140200926
848484LV00008B/2082